GRAEME HENDERSON

MECHANISMS OF PAIN AND ANALGESIC COMPOUNDS

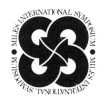

MILES INTERNATIONAL SYMPOSIUM SERIES

Number 11: Mechanisms of Pain and Analgesic Compounds
      Roland F. Beers, Jr., and Edward G. Bassett, editors. 512 pp., 1979.

Number 10: Impact of Recombinant Molecules on Science and Society
      Roland F. Beers, Jr., and Edward G. Bassett, editors. 560 pp., 1977.

Number 9: Cell Membrane Receptors for Viruses, Antigens and Antibodies, Polypeptide Hormones, and Small Molecules
      Roland F. Beers, Jr., and Edward G. Bassett, editors. 540 pp., 1976.

Number 8: The Role of Immunological Factors in Infectious, Allergic, and Autoimmune Processes
      Roland F. Beers, Jr., and Edward G. Bassett, editors. 540 pp., 1976.

Mechanisms of Pain and Analgesic Compounds

Miles International Symposium Series
Number 11

Editors:

Roland F. Beers, Jr., M.D., Ph.D.
Miles Laboratories, Inc.
Elkhart, Indiana

Edward G. Bassett, Ph.D.
Miles Laboratories, Inc.
Elkhart, Indiana

Raven Press ■ New York

Raven Press, 1140 Avenue of the Americas, New York, New York 10036

Made in the United States of America

International Standard Book Number 0–89004–304–3
Library of Congress Catalog Card Number 78–52524
International Standard Serial Number 0363–4698

Preface

Pain, a sensory signal indicating an abnormality or danger to the integrity of man's well being, represents a major medical, social, and economic problem throughout the world. There is a long history of human effort to reduce the severity of pain, and thus suffering.

In an attempt to catalyze better communication between investigators studying the many facets of the cause, alleviation, and/or elimination of pain, Miles Laboratories sponsored the development of this volume and the symposium on which it is based, inviting internationally recognized leaders of pain research to participate in the Eleventh Miles International Symposium.

Of interest to both clinicians and investigators, this volume features significant scientific discoveries of the past decade in the field of pain and its relief. In-depth discussions of the mechanisms involved at both the molecular and neurophysiological levels follow many of the presentations. Highlighted are the neurophysiological models of pain, the biochemical basis of pain, the role of endogenous substances with analgesic action, and the molecular mechanism of analgesic compounds and their relationship to physical dependence and other undesirable side effects.

We are hopeful that this volume and the symposium on which it is based provide a forum for interdisciplinary exchange and stimulate the contributors to plan collaborative efforts having new research and clinical aims. This volume will be of interest to both clinical and research workers in the many areas that touch on the underlying basis and treatment of pain.

Roland F. Beers, Jr.
Edward G. Bassett

Acknowledgments

Under the General Chairmanship of Dr. Roland F. Beers, Jr., the Program Committee consisting of Drs. Julián E. Villarreal (Chairman), John J. Bonica, Kenneth L. Casey, H. O. J. Collier, Sergio H. Ferreira, and H. W. Kosterlitz organized the 3-day conference on which this volume is based for the discussion of the most recent multidisciplinary approaches to the problems of pain. Coordinator of the Symposium was Dr. Edward G. Bassett. The conference was held at The Johns Hopkins Medical Institutions and was attended by a large number of physicians, investigators, and other professionals in the medical and allied disciplines.

This Symposium and Proceedings are dedicated to the memory of Dr. Maurice Seevers. We are especially grateful to Walter Ames Compton, M. D., Chief Executive Officer and Chairman of the Board of Miles Laboratories, Inc., for his tribute to Dr. Seevers and again express our appreciation for his continued support of and interest in these Symposia.

The editors extend grateful thanks to the contributors for assisting in the prompt publication of their manuscripts. The discussions included in this volume have been edited by the Session Chairmen. Within the time allotted for editing, it was not possible for each discussant to proofread his remarks; if error or misunderstanding of remarks has resulted, the Editors take full responsibility.

Contents

Contributors

Huda Akil
*Department of Psychiatry and Behavioral
Sciences
Stanford University School of Medicine
Stanford, California 94305*

Jack D. Barchas
*Department of Psychiatry and Behavioral
Sciences
Stanford University School of Medicine
Stanford, California 94305*

Roland F. Beers, Jr.
*Miles Laboratories, Inc.
Elkhart, Indiana 46515*

Julia Bläsig
*Department of Neuropharmacology
Max-Planck-Institut für Psychiatrie
D-8000 München 40, Federal Republic of
Germany*

John J. Bonica
*Department of Anesthesiology
University of Washington School of Medi-
cine
Seattle, Washington 98195*

J. Timothy Cannon
*Department of Psychology
University of California, Los Angeles
Los Angeles, California 90024*

Kenneth L. Casey
*Departments of Neurology and Physiology
University of Michigan
Ann Arbor, Michigan 48109*

Antonio Castro
*Instituto Miles de Terapéutica Experimen-
tal
México, D.F., México*

Loris A. Chahl
*Department of Physiology
University of Queensland
St. Lucia, Queensland, 4067 Australia*

C. Richard Chapman
*Departments of Anesthesiology, Psychiatry
and Behavioral Sciences, and Psychology
University of Washington School of Medicine
Seattle, Washington 98195*

H. O. J. Collier
*Miles Laboratories, Ltd.
Stoke Poges
Slough SL2 4LY, England*

Walter Ames Compton
*Miles Laboratories, Inc.
Elkhart, Indiana 46515*

Stephen G. Dennis
*Department of Psychology
McGill University
Montreal, Quebec, Canada*

Ronald Dubner
*Neurobiology and Anesthesiology
Branch
National Institute of Dental Research
National Institutes of Health
Bethesda, Maryland 20014*

Sergio H. Ferreira
*Department of Pharmacology
Faculty of Medicine of Ribeirão
Preto
14.100 Ribeirão Preto
São Paulo, Brazil*

Wilbert E. Fordyce
Department of Rehabilitation Medicine
University of Washington School of Medi-
cine
Seattle, Washington 98195

Avram Goldstein
Addiction Research Foundation
Palo Alto, California 94304

Louis S. Harris
Department of Pharmacology
Medical College of Virginia
Richmond, Virginia 23298

Ronald L. Hayes
Neurobiology and Anesthesiology Branch
National Institute of Dental Research
National Institutes of Health
Bethesda, Maryland 20014

Albert Herz
Department of Neuropharmacology
Max-Planck-Institut für Psychiatrie
D-8000 München 40, Federal Republic of
Germany

Friedrich Hoffmeister
Institut für Pharmacologie
Bayer AG
D-5600 Wuppertal 1, Federal Republic of
Germany

John Hughes
Department of Biochemistry
Imperial College of Science and Technol-
ogy
London SW7 2AZ, England

D. R. Jasinski
Division of Research
National Institute on Drug Abuse
Addiction Research Center
Lexington, Kentucky 40583

Frederick W. L. Kerr
Department of Neurologic Surgery
Mayo Clinic
Rochester, Minnesota 55901

Werner A. Klee
Laboratory of General and Comparative
Biochemistry
National Institute of Mental Health
National Institutes of Health
Bethesda, Maryland 20014

H. W. Kosterlitz
Unit for Research on Addictive Drugs
Marischal College, University of Aberdeen
Aberdeen AB9 1AS, Scotland

John C. Liebeskind
Department of Psychology
University of California, Los Angeles
Los Angeles, California 90024

Don M. Long
Department of Neurosurgery
The Johns Hopkins University School of
Medicine
Baltimore, Maryland 21205

David J. Mayer
Department of Physiology
Medical College of Virginia
Virginia Commonwealth University
Richmond, Virginia 23298

Fedor Medzihradsky
Department of Pharmacology
The University of Michigan
Ann Arbor, Michigan 48109

Ronald Melzack
Department of Psychology
McGill University
Montreal, Quebec, Canada

R. Alan North
Department of Pharmacology
Loyola University Stritch School of Medi-
cine
Maywood, Illinois 60153

Leif Olgart
Departments of Pharmacology and End-
odontics
Karolinska Institutet
S-104 01 Stockholm 60, Sweden

Donald D. Price
Anesthesiology and Neurobiology Branch
National Institute of Dental Research
National Institutes of Health
Bethesda, Maryland 20014

D. E. Richardson
Department of Psychiatry and Behavioral
Sciences
Stanford University School of Medicine
Stanford, California 94305

Rüdiger Schulz
Department of Neuropharmacology
Max-Planck-Institut für Psychiatrie
D-8000 München 40, Federal Republic of
Germany

Federigo Sicuteri
Department of Clinical Pharmacology
University of Florence
50134 Florence, Italy

Charles B. Smith
Department of Pharmacology
The University of Michigan
Ann Arbor, Michigan 48109

Henry H. Swain
Department of Pharmacology
The University of Michigan
Ann Arbor, Michigan 48109

Julián E. Villarreal
Instituto Miles de Terapéutica Experimen-
tal
México, D.F., México

Stanley J. Watson
Department of Psychiatry and Behavioral
Sciences
Stanford University School of Medicine
Stanford, California 94305

William D. Willis, Jr.
Marine Biomedical Institute
University of Texas Medical Branch at
Galveston
Galveston, Texas 77550

James H. Woods
Department of Pharmacology
The University of Michigan
Ann Arbor, Michigan 48109

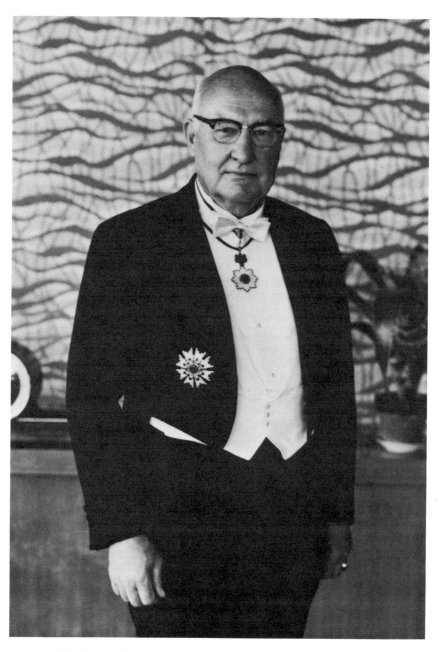

Maurice H. Seevers, Ph.D., M.D. October 3, 1901 to April 20, 1977.

Mechanisms of Pain and Analgesic Compounds,
edited by R. F. Beers, Jr., and E. G. Bassett.
Raven Press, New York © 1979.

1. Memorial to Dr. Maurice Seevers

Walter Ames Compton

Miles Laboratories, Inc., Elkhart, Indiana 46515

It is a pleasure once again to have the opportunity to express our appreciation to The Johns Hopkins University as our host, on the occasion of the 11th Miles International Symposium. Speaking principally on behalf of the Symposium attendees, I should also like to express our thanks to the Chairman of the Program Committee, Dr. Julian Villarreal, and to the speakers.

I have the honor to pay tribute to an old friend of many of us, the late Dr. Maurice Seevers. I was privileged to be his close friend for more than a quarter of a century and to enjoy his association as a consultant to, and member of the Board of, Miles Laboratories for most of those years.

For 29 years, he was Professor and Chairman of the Department of Pharmacology at the University of Michigan Medical Center, the oldest department of pharmacology in the United States. The juxtaposition of this Symposium on which this volume is based with the Annual Program of the Committee on Problems of Drug Dependence makes it especially appropriate that we have chosen to honor Dr. Seevers' memory. Certainly, few men living or of those who have gone before him have done more to advance our understanding of drugs for the relief of pain and the related problems of drug tolerance and dependence. Although his achievements in these difficult fields inevitably fell short of his own rigorously set goals, through his leadership, research, and brilliant teaching, he contributed uniquely to the development of pharmacology into the mature and highly respected discipline it is today.

In this brief chapter, it would be nearly impossible to construct for you an adequate characterization of Mose, as he was known to all his good friends. Some individuals can be compressed to an illuminating vignette, but the intellect of this man, the published works of his own research, the scope of his activities and services to professional societies and governments, his struggles to obtain proper recognition of his chosen field of pharmacology, and the international honors and distinctions given him all demand cataloging in detail, and yet this is manifestly impossible here. As evidence of his capabilities as a teacher, he has left a legacy of more than 150 pharmacologists who either trained under him directly or passed through his department as students, fellows, or staff members.

On hearing of Dr. Seevers' death, the moving testimony of Dr. Eikichi Hosoya,

1

one of his close friends and recently retired as Professor of Pharmacology at Keio University Medical School in Tokyo, was well summarized as follows: "That in his more than twenty visits to Japan Doctor Seevers had personally visited nearly all of the medical schools and universities of Japan; that for over a 20-year period he annually invited one or two young pharmacologists from Japan to the Department of Pharmacology at Ann Arbor to undertake extended study of the most modern pharmacology under ideal circumstances; thus, more than 30 budding pharmacologists were given this background, while somewhat briefer orientations at Ann Arbor were accorded to substantially every established pharmacologist of the country" (2). For these, for his contributions to education in Japan, and especially for his services as a consultant to the Japanese government in problems of narcotic drug addiction and its control, he was decorated with the Third Class Rising Sun Medal and the Second Class Order of the Sacred Treasure, joint distinctions possessed by few.

I am tempted to continue with a short review of his biography since it tells much about him. He was born in Topeka, Kansas, at the beginning of the century. It was shortly after receiving his bachelor's degree in 1924 at Washburn College that he dedicated the remainder of his life to an academic career in pharmacology. That preoccupation continued literally until the terminal weeks of his illness, only briefly disturbed by misgivings during the thirties when, as he put it, pharmacology was in the doldrums.

His first postgraduate work was at the University of Chicago with the famed Dr. A. L. Tatum, who was then resident pharmacologist in a combined Department of Pharmacology and Physiological Chemistry. While awaiting entry to Medical School at the University of Chicago, he took an elective course in pharmacology from Dr. Tatum in the spring of 1925, during which time there soon developed an association of mutual respect that resulted in an invitation to become Dr. Tatum's laboratory assistant. It was here that his studies on narcotic dependence began, in a combined laboratory and animal room approximately 20 × 30 feet in size, where it was his assignment to inject dogs and monkeys with morphine. This association was to continue until 1942 when Dr. Seevers accepted the Chair in Pharmacology at the University of Michigan. He had received his Ph.D. degree at the University of Chicago in 1928 and during 1929, while a medical student at Rush Medical School, he simultaneously served as Instructor in Pharmacology at Loyola University. In the meantime, Dr. Tatum had moved to the University of Wisconsin and, after receiving his M.D. degree, Dr. Seevers followed him there to become Assistant Professor of Pharmacology.

His early fortuitous association of morphine with primate experimentation was to color all the rest of his life and, indeed, one of his most important contributions was to be the establishment of a colony of morphine-dependent monkeys at the University of Michigan with the developed capability of self-administration of their medication; from these studies came the first really well-defined observations of physical dependence on narcotic drugs. He had a genuine feeling of liking and interested preoccupation in the character exhibited by monkeys. I recollect well visiting an island in Japan with him where an exceptional species of monkeys had long been permitted total freedom as the primary inhabitants of the island. It was an eerie feeling as we moved about the island among them, and, responsive to Mose's discourse, began to feel that we were actually visiting in their community and on occasion to a degree on their terms! We especially found this to be the case if carrying fruit, when we received a preemptory demand from one of the larger males to hand it over!

His first papers on the use of monkeys as the preferred animal model for a predictive test for physical dependency of an unknown narcotic analgesic issued in 1933, but this program moved into high gear after he had come to Michigan to succeed C. W. Edmunds, A. R. Cushny, and J. J. Abel as Chairman of the Department of Pharmacology in 1942. Shortly after World War II, one of the first commitments of the National Research Council's reorganized Committee on Drug Addiction and Narcotics was to support Dr. Seevers' procedure for dependence potential determination. Time does not permit detailed iteration of the whole story but as Julian Villarreal, our Symposium Program Chairman, said in his presentation address of the First Nathan E. Eddy Memorial Award to Dr. Seevers, ". . . through this research we can begin to say with some assurance that we now have an understanding of the main outline of what brings about the peculiar madness of the addict who tends to destroy himself and his social world by compulsive self-intoxication." Although the medical profession in particular and society at large have yet to cope effectively with the problems of drug addiction, Dr. Seevers and his intellectual progeny have placed in our hands the means to define the physical dependence potential of new analgesics at the preclinical level.

A review of Dr. Seevers' contributions as a scientist–statesman is illuminating and, in a way, may well be even more far reaching than his functions as a research scientist. We have left to us some extraordinarily interesting writing by Dr. Seevers appearing in a review of the history of the American Society for Pharmacology and Experimental Therapeutics and the Journal of the Society; it is highly appropriate that we make mention of this here, since the Society and its Journal were in such large measure the contribution of the great John Jacob Abel of this University some 70 years ago. Throughout Seevers' narrative runs the constant thread—the effort to give definition to the substance of pharmacology as a major and critical discipline of the medical sciences.

What are termed the basic medical sciences have had throughout the entire history of medicine a difficult interface with clinical medicine, but pharmacology, since it deals with direct application to therapy, has perhaps always had the greatest problem. The age-old facile assertion by the clinician that the proper role of pharmacology is, in the classical sense, in the laboratory (and may it be said the equally too ready dismissal of clinicians by the Ph.D.s as not qualified to have useful opinions in basic medical science!) was, amid considerable controversy, brought into proper perspective through the genius and determination of Dr. Abel, by the very title of the Journal of the Society that conjoined pharmacology and experimental therapeutics. As Dr. Seevers pointed out in the 1930s—an era of therapeutic nihilism, you will recall—the very ongoing existence of pharmacology as a profession was in question. However, as by a fresh seabreeze, this fog was dispelled with the discovery of the sulfonamides, the new concept of antibiosis, and the subsequent development of penicillin which opened the unprecedented age of "wonder drugs." There was an imperative demand for new concepts of research, teaching, and clinical application of the discipline of pharmacology. He wrote several papers that seem to be especially pertinent to these issues. I shall quote him rather extensively in the hope that it may prompt some of us to reread them. Although these papers were written some years ago, it is extraordinary how they speak to some of our current problems in governmental administration, university and medical school curricula, and indeed to some of the other most basic aspects of modern medical practice. The first of these papers is to be found in a review (1) of the first 60 years of the American Society for Pharmacology and Experimental Therapeutics. In the chapter entitled "Projection to the Future," Dr. Seevers reviews the vicissitudes of pharmacology and the problems of the pharmacologist over these years and engages in some effort to define basic principles that may help in similar problems of the future. I shall quote a few paragraphs verbatim knowing that the flow of his logic and prose will be enjoyed.

> Let me say this. If pharmacology is submerged it will be in institutions where the pharmacologist, even though medically trained, identifies pharmacology only in laboratory terms. It is not likely to happen where pharmacology occupies an important position in the basic and clinical teaching of medical students throughout their educational program; where clinical pharmacology conducts training programs at the postdoctoral level and is recognized as a bridge between general pharmacology and clinical medicine; where the clinical pharmacologist is trained in both; where he is formally and physically associated with both; where he interprets laboratory findings in clinical terms and serves as a coordinator in all things of a clinical–pharmacological nature. In the long run, it may be that this type of cooperative activity will be a principal reason why general pharmacology as an independent discipline will survive in medical schools.
>
> Unless pharmacology continues to assume the role of principal interpreter of the effects of chemicals and drugs *in man,* it will have abandoned its heritage, since this is its only function that is unique.
>
> In order to bring perspective to medical and public health problems concerning drugs, information from all sources, subcellular to the whole organism, must be evaluated with a minimum of bias. Often the pertinent information is found only in indigenous medicine. Often the picture must be constructed primarily from witnesses from the past. Competence for such reconstruction requires a broad background in the laboratory with more than a passing knowledge of the clinic, a 'composite' pharmacologist, if you please.
>
> *This* is pharmacology.

And in another and very timely area of observation:

The broad nature of the subject matter of pharmacology lends itself with particular ease to encroachment by many kinds of pseudoscience and pseudoscientists. Unfortunately there is a substantial group of individuals, some scientists, even in 'high places,' practicing what, for lack of a better term, I will designate 'pseudopharmacology.' This includes those who lack the background or the desire to bring perspective to the problems of drug action. It includes the hypercritical as well as the uncritical and those who purposely distort facts to support what they consider a worthy end.

Many of the most difficult public health problems (alcoholism, drug dependence, tobacco smoking, air and stream pollution, pesticides, food additives, over-the-counter drugs), involving as they do the total population, become the special province of a whole array of 'experts'—well-meaning but scientifically ignorant reformers; commentators and writers in communications media who misinterpret facts to fit their own bias or create spectaculars; politicians who find this a rich potential for popular appeal; scientists who do not limit their pronouncements to their own area of competence, including (here) even some pharmacologists!

I can best illustrate what I mean by 'pseudopharmacology' as practiced by scientists by citing a few examples: inflation of inconsequential data by disguising them as hypotheses; acceptance of data obtained with gadgetry even if they conflict with observations of behavior; extrapolation of data obtained by chronic administration of unrealistic doses in small animals to prediction of drug or chemical toxicity in man; ignoring long-time human experience in favor of arbitrary margins of safety in animals as a measure of safety in man;—and many more. Pseudopharmacology of scientist or lay origin weakens the integrity, devaluates the importance, and dilutes the effectiveness of pharmacology as a biomedical discipline. It not only confuses the public but may glamorize the hazard it purports to expose. If pharmacology is to achieve its greatest stature in the future, pharmacologists in responsible positions must be willing as individuals to sacrifice their own private and research time to combat these hazards to pharmacology and the public health (4).

Doctor Seevers' Chairman's address (3) before the Section on Experimental Medicine and Therapeutics at the 102nd Annual Meeting of the American Medical Association, entitled "Perspective Versus Caprice in Evaluating Toxicity of Chemicals in Man," is very much in keeping with specific problems of the present day. As the title indicates, he points out with rigorous, but constructive, logic the problems of the area where law and science must somehow find a common meeting ground in defining and protecting the public welfare. The article is in part philosophical and I will not attempt to quote extensively from it, contenting myself with listing what he called certain irrefutable principles on which evaluation of human toxicity must be based. To briefly touch on a few:

(a) Every chemical substance has a nontoxic and toxic dose for man; that is, no chemicals must be poisons and all chemicals can be poisons.

(b) The use of every chemical substance by man, whether it be as food, drug, cosmetic, insecticide or for any purpose is a potential hazard. There are only very few exceptions. The risk may be very small or very great, depending on the nature of the chemical, the conditions of use, the degree and duration of exposure, and the condition of the person.

(c) The toxicity of chemicals for man can be ultimately determined only by experiments on man.

(d) The use of every chemical substance in man involves a calculated risk. The degree of risk is calculated by balancing the toxicity of the chemical under conditions of use against its benefits to man whether these benefits are direct or indirect. Minimal risk is encountered when the dose or extent of exposure is calculated to be tolerated by the weakest member of the population.

(e) The greater the benefit of the chemical substance in man, the greater the justification for the increase in risk in its use.

His role as a scientist–statesman may be seen in a very abbreviated listing of some of the many groups and organizations to which he contributed. In the American Medical Association, he was Chairman of the Section of Experimental Medicine and Therapeutics, member of the Council on Pharmacy and Chemistry, member of the Committee on Alcoholism and Drug Dependence, and Chairman of the Committee on Tobacco and Health. He was on the Board of Scientific Councilors of the National Heart Institute, was on the Surgeon General's Committee on Smoking and Health, was Chairman on Behavioral Pharmacology, and American Coordinator of the US–Japan Cooperative Science Program on Drug Abuse; was Consultant to the Minister of Public Health, Thailand, and Consultant to the Minister of Health and Welfare of Japan. I have already mentioned his contributions to medical education in Japan and especially to all of the departments of pharmacology in substantially all of the medical schools of Japan. I was with him on one occasion when our train was not permitted to stop at a station where there was one of these medical schools nearby. A delegation from the school was down at the station knowing that he was going through on that train, standing in the rain and bowing as he went by to express their appreciation to him.

In this discussion, I am all too conscious of the omission of myriads of data on the man and especially the impossibility of listing the many great scholars who were his associates; I can only hope that my excerpts from a few of his papers might entice the reader to seek out others. As with all great teachers, his work continues since his students serve in academic institutions, pharmaceutical companies, governmental agencies, and laboratories in Mexico, in Japan, as well as in the United States. I think of all of the great lectures he gave, the "First Nathan B. Eddy Memorial Award Lecture" (5), is outstanding in that it provided the opportunity to view in informed detail the profile of one of the great scientists of our time as seen through the eyes of an illustrious contemporary in the same field. Both he and Dr. Eddy found great difficulty in accepting the concept of methadone maintenance in management of drug addiction, and both of them condemned out of hand any notion that usefulness can be found in the European concept of so-called "heroin maintenance"; one quote from this lecture well underlines both his and Dr. Eddy's concern:

> It is obvious that the goals of yesterday have been obscured in the current social clamor and political pressure for instant solutions to the drug problem. Having basked in the light of the idealistic goals which served as a basis for the establishment of this Committee (on Problems of Drug Dependence), I am impelled to express the

hope that future scientists will not accept as scientific achievement compromises which offer temporary or inadequate solutions to the opiate problem; but will continue the search which Eddy pioneered.

The lecture brilliantly outlines the still existing problems of drug dependence and the penetrating questions raised in this lecture are still with us today; for example,

When this search was initiated, the term 'addiction,' in the scientific sense, generally implied chronic compulsive use based upon the euphorigenic properties of the drug, leading to, and associated with, the development of physical dependence. But generally the hypothesis was expressed almost exclusively in terms of physical dependence, partly because this was one parameter which could be examined in the laboratory. With the passage of time, the goal just as distant, and the development of many new classes of dependence-producing substances which were euphorigenic but lacked the capacity to induce physical dependence, the original goal became somewhat obscured and certain puzzling questions arose. Should the primary goal be to eliminate physical dependence or to abolish the euphorigenic properties? Are euphoria and potent analgesia dependent variables and thus inseparable? Would elimination of physical dependence alone in this class of drugs destroy the dependence-producing properties? These questions and many more are still alive.

With the proliferation of psychoactive substances it became increasingly clear, and beyond any doubt, that any substance which has euphorigenic properties, however slight, and of whatever nature, will be exploited for this effect to the point of strong dependence by a few individuals. And for a few unfortunates, even drug-induced dysphoria is preferred to the status quo. Clearly these facts are not compatible with the goal of finding an analgesic which is devoid of dependence-producing properties in the absolute sense.

Unless one subscribes to the view that the nature of man will change significantly in the foreseeable future these facts also require acceptance of the corollary, that at best, society can only expect to reduce dependence to an irreducible minimum.

As I begin to close, I find that I have failed to comment on the very human side of his character. His blistering criticism and use of blunt talk when greatly disturbed by an important issue are well known to all his friends. Equally known are his total lack of any sense of self-importance and his great gentleness. In the same vein, I must note one of Dr. Seevers' greatest achievements. This was his marriage while at the University of Wisconsin in 1936 to Frances Hebl.

In concluding this memorial to Dr. Seevers, I sincerely hope that the papers you are about to read will contribute significantly to our knowledge of pain and its relief. Moreover, it is Miles' hope that this Symposium will help inspire continued adherence to the high principles of experimental pharmacology personified by Dr. Seevers, which he labored so long to establish.

REFERENCES

1. Chen, K. K., Ed. (1976): *The American Society for Pharmacology and Experimental Therapeutics: The First Sixty Years.* Judd & Detweiler, Washington, D.C.
2. Hosoya, E. (1978): Lamentation. *Folia Pharmacol. Jpn.,* 74:164.

3. Seevers, M. H. (1953): Perspective versus caprice in evaluating toxicity of chemicals in man. *JAMA*, 153:1329–1333.
4. Seevers, M. H. (1969): Projection to the future. In: *The American Society for Pharmacology and Experimental Therapeutics: The First Sixty Years*, edited by K. K. Chen, pp. 207–220. Judd & Detweiler, Washington, D.C.
5. Seevers, M. H. (1974): The Nathan B. Eddy Memorial Award. *Bull. Prob. Drug Dependence*, 36:21–28.

Mechanisms of Pain and Analgesic Compounds,
edited by R. F. Beers, Jr., and E. G. Bassett.
Raven Press, New York © 1979.

2. Introduction

Roland F. Beers, Jr.

Miles Laboratories, Inc., Elkhart, Indiana 46515

Pain, the subject of this volume, can be said to be a universal condition of man's existence responsible for a major share of his suffering. It has influenced the cultural characteristics of his societies dating back to prehistoric times and has been a determining factor in man's behavior.

Society's attitude toward pain as a necessary, but undesirable, condition of man's existence is reflected in the origin of the word pain, namely, payment by punishment for an act of transgression. In the absence of any rational understanding of the origins or relief of pain, man has turned to the supernatural through supplication, prayer, sacrifice, and other forms of "payment" as a form of restitution for the moral failure of his actions. By the same token, society has used pain and the threat of pain to coerce its members to conform to a code of ethical behavior. Various forms of corporal punishment have been used throughout the history of man.

This moral interpretation of the meaning of pain has influenced the response of the individual toward pain or the threat of pain and has determined, to a certain extent, the permissible forms of behavior in which pain is used as a coercive or persuasive force in interpersonal relationships. It has also influenced the ethical behavior of the clinician beginning with the Hippocratic oath. But, most important from the perspective of this volume has been the effect of social and psychological aspects of pain on the nature and success of pain research and therapy.

The difficulties in identifying and separating social, psychological, and physiological phenomena originate from the subjective nature of pain. It cannot be observed or measured directly by the investigator or clinician, but must be inferred by its effects on the subject's behavior. In animal models, this transduction system usually consists of some form of muscular activity: the tail flick, writhing, limping, etc.

The ability of man to translate the pain symptom into a language or symbol provides the data base for most clinical studies. Critical in clinical studies is the awareness of the investigator of the frequency and ease with which the patient in the translation process can introduce serious bias into the nature and degree of intensity of the pain symptom. For example, pain can be used by the patient to manipulate his environment through appeals to the empathy and sympathy of others.

Probably one of the most important psychological aspects of pain is the belief structure of the patient. Critical to the success of most psychotherapeutic procedures is a conviction by the patient of the validity of the particular model used by the therapist. Pain therapy falls within this category. Thus, the success of acupuncture or of chiropractic procedures in the face of orthopedic or neurosurgical failures contains a strong element of the patient's will to succeed based on his belief in the integrity of the models used by such therapists.

I would caution against any pejorative classification of such phenomena as placebo artifacts. The ultimate value of any therapeutic procedure for the relief of a symptom such as pain must be based on the patient's assessment of the relief of suffering, not on whether the rationale behind the therapeutic procedure conforms to the beliefs of the clinician. Treatment of a symptom is not equivalent to treatment of a pathological process. The latter may be successful without the active and conscious participation of the patient; the former always requires cooperation from the patient if for no other reason than to indicate the status of the pain symptom.

Pain is a symptom in a set of symptoms and signs identified as a syndrome representing an interacting system of pathophysiological and pathopsychological processes. The total system includes not only the patient, but his environment both present and past as well as the projected future. Pain can assume a variety of roles in this system that to a large extent determine the response of the patient and both the rationale and means for alleviation, abolition, or prevention by the clinician. Thus, although pain is usually considered a sensory signal indicating an abnormality or danger to the integrity of the patient, and as part of the essential sensory apparatus required for the survival of the species, in fact, because of the involvement of the higher brain centers, this negative feedback role is an oversimplification of the function of pain. Indeed, pain may replace the original etiological agent for pain and thus become self-perpetuating. Depending on the nature of the syndrome, the diagnostic and therapeutic approach may range from a simple "technological fix" with a suitably active pharmacological agent, which could be an analgesic, a sedative, or a tranquilizer, to a complex psychotherapeutic regime as represented by the pain clinics. The lesson to be learned in the history of man's coping with pain is the multifactorial nature of the syndrome associated with pain and the necessity to treat pain as a part of a system manifested in the syndrome. The importance of a systems approach to the problems of pain is exemplified in the nature both of the character of research on pain and of the therapeutic and preventive measures employed in coping with pain.

A frequent consequence of any expedient approach to the pain problem is not only an inability to treat successfully the total syndrome of the patient, but also the introduction of additional pathological processes including iatrogenic and drug-dependent problems.

Of particular relevance to this volume is the complexity and frequent inadequacy of clinical models used for studying the etiology, mechanism, and modulation or abolition of pain. These limitations result from the practical and often theoretical inability to isolate, as a simple variable, the pain symptom from the total syndrome. Those agents used to imitate or modulate the pain symptom for the purpose of gaining an understanding of the mechanism of pain are themselves multifactorial and produce undesired "artifacts." Moreover, some of the simplest, such as temperature or galvanometric stimulation, represent the real clinical situation only in the most superficial manner.

This multifactorial nature of the syndrome with pain as a major symptom precludes any simple therapeutic solution to all but the most transient conditions. However, the multifactorial character of pain should provide opportunities for a variety of therapeutic approaches that extend beyond pharmacological or surgical and are considered in some of the contributions to this volume.

The preoccupation of the clinical investigator with "placebo" effects of particular therapeutic measures reflects on the one hand the belief that the pain symptom must be isolated as a single controllable variable subject to modulation if one is to assess successfully the efficacy of a particular therapeutic approach. On the other hand, this also reflects a failure to acknowledge that the "placebo" effect is frequently a pseudonym for one's ignorance of the dynamics of pain as a process and of the effect of a variety of unknown and, therefore, uncontrollable variables acting on this process.

The investigator is faced with the same kinds of problems as are the clinicians. I mentioned earlier the artifactual nature of galvanic-induced pain which presumably has minimal inflammatory- or tissue injury-induced pain and should be a suitable model for measuring pure analgesic activity. Moreover, the investigator can vary both the intensity and duration of pain. A major deficiency in this model is that very fact. Both the threshold and tolerance of pain are strongly influenced by the patient's knowledge of its temporary nature. Thus, if he knows he can discontinue the stimulus at will, his capacity to endure the intensity and duration of pain will be considerably greater than if he had no such control. Complicating this problem even further are the psychological impacts of informed consent procedures.

In stressing the importance of a systems or holistic approach to the study of pain as a means of finding appropriate therapeutic procedures, I am acknowledging the risks of partial solutions that leave the patient permanently disabled. These are analogous to Lewis Thomas's halfway technologies that leave the patient with little or no autonomy or independence. Nowhere has this been more apparent than in the field of analgesia and in the problem of drug dependency. The hazards of trying to reduce this to a physiological problem with the label of physical dependence has been stressed before. Psychological dependence may, for the particular patient, be a more serious problem than physical dependence because of the adverse impact this has on the treatment of the associated syndrome. Of course, there is also the paradoxical difference in moral interpretation of physical and psychological dependence seen recently in the attempts to reduce alcoholism to a nonbehavioral problem of which the patient is innocent of any guilt or responsibility.

At the extremes, pain has both a biochemical and psychological component, but neither can be satisfactorily studied without considering the fact that the biochemical processes of pain have psychological components that affect the biochemistry and vice versa. The exciting breakthroughs during the last few years at the molecular level with receptor sites promise major advances in our understanding of the biochemical processes of pain. But, we are also witnessing similar advances of the psychological level. Neither group of investigators can afford to ignore the contributions and insights of the other, especially if their findings challenge cherished beliefs.

It is fitting, therefore, that we begin this volume with a review of pain seen as a clinical problem.

Mechanisms of Pain and Analgesic Compounds,
edited by R. F. Beers, Jr., and E. G. Bassett.
Raven Press, New York © 1979.

3. Introduction to Section A: Recent Clinical Contributions to the Understanding of Mechanisms of Pain and Pain Relief

John J. Bonica

Department of Anesthesiology, University of Washington School of Medicine, Seattle, Washington 98195

It is most appropriate to begin this section with the clinical aspect of pain, because in the final analysis the primary and ultimate goal of all the efforts of biomedical research is to prevent human disease. In the case of pain, it is human suffering of millions of Americans and people everywhere.

For this section, we have selected five of the dozens and, indeed, hundreds of aspects of clinical pain that could be considered.

I feel fortunate in having been successful in enlisting the contributions of four colleagues who, through their research, have contributed significantly to our understanding of the mechanisms of pain and pain relief.

Mechanisms of Pain and Analgesic Compounds,
edited by R. F. Beers, Jr., and E. G. Bassett.
Raven Press, New York © 1979.

4. Important Clinical Aspects of Acute and Chronic Pain

John J. Bonica

*Department of Anesthesiology, University of Washington School of Medicine,
Seattle, Washington 98195*

INTRODUCTION

In this brief chapter, I plan to mention some clinical aspects of acute and chronic pain that have emerged from recent research or have contributed to the understanding of mechanisms of pain and pain relief. I shall not attempt a complete review of the vast literature and will include only some of the most important key references.

We all appreciate that during the past two decades there has been an impressive surge of interest in pain research, and a vast amount of new information has been acquired (6,13). Although some of the studies have been done to satisfy pure scientific curiosity, most have been stimulated by the interest and desire to solve questions posed by clinical observations of human pain. One of the most important spin-offs has been to bring into sharper focus and thus appreciate a point I made a quarter of a century ago: that it is important to differentiate acute from chronic pain and to consider them separately (4). This is based on the fact that the etiology, mechanisms, physiopathology, function, diagnosis, and therapy of acute pain differ considerably from those of chronic pain.

ACUTE PAIN

Acute pain consists of a constellation of unpleasant perceptual and emotional experiences and certain associated autonomic, psychological, and behavioral responses. Invariably, acute pain and these associated responses are provoked by noxious or tissue-damaging stimulation produced by injury or disease: It is rare that acute pain is caused primarily by psychological factors. Usually, acute pain has important biological functions: It warns the individual that something is wrong and prompts him or her to seek medical counsel and is used by the physician as an important diagnostic aid. Moreover, the physiological and psychological responses usually help to preserve homeostasis, although, as I point out later, in many instances this is not the case.

It is important to note that most of the old and new knowledge concerning pain has been acquired about *acute pain* experimentally induced in laboratory animals or human volunteers. As a result of these experiments, we have acquired a great deal of knowledge about nociceptor–afferent systems in the periphery, the anatomy and physiology of the dorsal horn and ascending pathways and of the trigeminal system, and the anatomic, physiological, and biochemical substrates of descending control systems. It is also important to appreciate that certain clinical problems with acute pain have stimulated much of the past and current research. I will only mention a few examples. Acute dental pain, which constitutes an important national health problem, has stimulated much of the research in the mechanism and physiopathology of pain in the trigeminal system (9,21). The need to better prevent pain during surgical operations has stimulated studies on the effects of narcotic analgesics, anesthetics, and related drugs on the dorsal horn and other sites in the neuraxis involved in nociception (25). The problem of pain of parturition and the need to develop better methods for its control have prompted recent definitive studies of the mechanisms and pathways involved (8). Postoperative pain and the associated physiological and psychological responses have been the subject of numerous studies by psychologists, physiologists, and anesthesiologists (11,15). Moreover, the problem of effectively relieving this pain, as well as the acute pain of injury, has stimulated intense research by chemists and pharmacologists. Finally, as will be stressed by Chapman *(this volume),* the introduction of acupuncture analgesia has been one of the most important stimuli for recent pain research (30). Much of the new information derived from these and other studies are summarized in this volume.

To better appreciate the clinical implications of the new knowledge and the role clinician problems have had in stimulating pain research, it is desirable to mention briefly some aspects of acute pain. After being subjected to various peripheral, local, segmental, and supraspinal-modulating influences, nociceptive impulses from the periphery pass to various parts of the neuraxis and provoke segmental, suprasegmental, and cerebral cortical responses. Segmental autonomic (nocifensive) reflex responses include skeletal muscle spasm, vasospasm, inhibition of gastrointestinal and genitourinary activity, and other visceral functions. The suprasegmental responses usually consist of an increase in ventilation and hypothalamic activity with consequent increase in circulation and endocrine function. Cortical responses represent the net effects of highly complex interactions among various neural systems and their biochemical substrates and psychological factors. Through the interaction of the ascending and descending neural systems and neocortical processes, the individual is provided perceptual and discriminative information about the noxious stimuli that is analyzed against the background of past experience, learning, personality, cultural, and environmental factors, among others. Based on analysis and through sensory, motivational, and cognitive processes, the individual has the emotional experience we call pain. Usually, this pain initiates cerebral cortical responses consisting of psychodynamic mechanisms that produce the affective reactions of anxiety and apprehension and operant responses characteristic of overt behavior, such as verbalization (screaming, moaning), grimacing, posturing, prompt withdrawal of the injured part, or a combination of these.

Clinical Implications

In addition to warning the individual and helping the practitioner, the pain and associated responses usually are beneficial because they help to maintain homeostasis. The usefulness of reflex skeletal muscle spasm, inhibition of gastrointestinal and genitourinary tract function, and stimulation of circulation, respiration, and endocrine function to help the organism cope with the disease or injury are too well known to warrant discussion. However, what is not amply appreciated is that, not infrequently, the segmental, suprasegmental, and cortical responses become abnormal and are deleterious to the organism. I will briefly mention four examples.

In the postoperative period, persistent noxious stimulation from the operative site often causes abnormal reflex responses consisting of skeletal muscle spasm and splinting, ileus and decrease in urinary function, and a concomitant increase in the circulation, cardiac workload, and oxygen consumption (11). Moreover, the severe pain often provokes anxiety (15) which, in turn, increases the sympathetic tone and also causes conscious or involuntary immobility. These may be responsible for pulmonary and gastrointestinal complications that increase morbidity and, in critical patients, may prove fatal. Clinical studies have shown that incidence and severity of pain are markedly increased by anxiety caused by fright, uncertainty, and a feeling of helplessness that is often present in the uninformed patient (15,16). Other studies have shown that the anxiety and, consequently, the degree of pain and reflex responses can be markedly reduced by providing the patient with ample information before the operation by strong suggestion and by using other manipulations to help the patient use coping skills (15,17). In nearly all cases, the postoperative pain is managed with narcotics which most frequently are given in insufficient amounts because of the misconceptions of physicians and nurses that these drugs cause undue respiratory depression and have the risk of addiction. Consequently, the patient's apprehension and anxiety are increased and this, in turn, increases the pain and associated reflex responses. Since pain antagonizes the respiratory depression of narcotics, and because the use of these drugs for only a few days precludes any risk of addiction, they should be administered in sufficient amounts to provide adequate relief. In some instances, even large doses of narcotics will not adequately relieve the pain and reflex responses, whereas regional analgesia produces complete pain relief and obviates the development of the reflexes (11).

A second example is the pain and reflex and cortical responses consequent to acute myocardial infarction. Although initially the pain is useful because it prompts the patient to obtain medical help, unless it is promptly relieved, it may aggravate the myocardial physiopathology. Persistent noxious stimuli provoked by myocardial ischemia markedly increase sympathetic tone and thus increase heart rate, stroke volume, and cardiac output and, consequently, myocardial oxygen consumption (44). Since in all patients with myocardial infarction there is impairment of oxygen delivery to the myocardium by the fixed coronary arteriosclerotic lesion, increasing its consumption will aggravate the discrepancy between supply and demand. In addition, animal studies have shown that myocardial ischemia may produce segmental reflex coronary vasoconstriction which further impairs the delivery of oxygen to the myocardium (22,44). This will be a critical factor and may preclude survival if the reflex vasoconstriction involves collateral vessels that are not involved in the lesion and would otherwise be crucial to provide perfusion of the myocardium. Suprasegmental reflexes also stimulate autonomic centers in the hypothalamus and consequently increase general sympathetic tone and catecholamine release, a response that is markedly aggravated by anxiety (38,44). Thus, the combined effects of segmental and suprasegmental reflexes and anxiety greatly increase the workload of the heart and its oxygen consumption in the presence of an already compromised coronary circulation and thus markedly increase the discrepancy between oxygen supply and demand. One or more of these responses may be a critical factor that may cause death of the patient. It is, therefore, essential to relieve *promptly* the pain and decrease the aforementioned reflex responses. This relief can be achieved by administering narcotic analgesics intravenously in sufficient incremental doses to provide *adequate* relief. Even more effective is interruption of nociceptive and efferent pathways with a cervicothoracic sympathetic block or segmental epidural block that not only relieves the pain, but prevents the aforementioned responses (12). Moreover, there is some old and new evidence that complete interruption of afferent sympathetic fibers to the heart, as can be achieved with these procedures, will decrease mortality from myocardial infarction (19,28).

The third example of the deleterious effects of pain and reflex responses pertain to some cases of severe accidental injury. It is well known that under certain conditions such as massive injury, the reflex and cortical responses are excessive and, instead of normalizing the organism, they initiate and maintain the vicious circle of shock. In such instances, there is a persistent, grossly excessive vasoconstriction that produces tissue hypoxia and consequent biochemical and metabolic disturbances and toxic products that, in turn, produce new nociceptive stimulation and widespread deleterious effects that further aggravate the physiopathology. The vasoconstriction is most marked in the splanchnic vascular bed, and the resultant intestinal ischemia causes hypoxic tissue damage and consequent release of toxic substances [e.g., the myocardial depressant factor (MDF)] that depress the cardiovascular system, particularly the myocardium. A number of studies have shown that block of nociceptive and sympathetic pathways either prior to or soon after the injury will prevent or promptly eliminate the abnormal secretory responses, as well as pain, with consequent improvement in cardiovascular function (12).

The final example of the deleterious effects of pain and reflex responses involves the pain of labor. Human studies in unpremedicated primigravidas in labor have shown that the pain of uterine contraction causes a 5 to 20-fold increase in ventilation and a significant increase in cardiac output and blood pressure. The pain-induced hyperventilation, in turn, produces a severe respiratory alkalosis that decreases cerebral and uterine blood flows (5). Moreover, recent studies in pregnant ewes have shown that the pain and the concomitant increase in sympathetic tone increase catecholamine release which directly reduces uterine blood flow by causing uterine vasoconstriction (36,43). The combined effects of hyperventilation and catecholamine release in reducing uterine blood flow are likely to impair placental blood gas exchange and, consequently, compromise the condition of the fetus. If the fetus is already at risk because of obstetric complications, the pain-induced reduction in uterine blood flow may be the critical factor that precludes survival of the neonate. Human studies have shown that administration of moderate doses of narcotics partially relieved the pain and thus decreased the magnitude of the deleterious effects on ventilation, circulation, and uterine blood flow (5,27), whereas regional analgesia in the form of continuous epidural block will completely relieve the pain and the consequent deleterious effects on the mother and fetus (5,23).

CHRONIC PAIN

I have already mentioned some of the differences between acute and chronic pain. First, in contrast to the acute type, pain, in its chronic, persistent, and pathological form has no biological function. It is a malefic force that often imposes severe emotional, physical, economic, and social stresses on the patient, family, and society (7,10). Second, as will be stressed by Fordyce *(this volume)*, psychological and environmental factors play a prominent role in the etiology and the development of chronic pain behavior (24,37). Moreover, because we know much less about the mechanisms and physiopathology of chronic pain, its diagnosis and therapy are much more difficult than is the case with acute pain. Finally, the physiological, affective, and behavioral responses to chronic pain are quite different than those to acute pain. When pain due to disease or injury persists, in most patients the autonomic reflex responses decrease progressively and, in a short time, disappear, whereas in some they become excessive and constitute a new source of noxious stimulation (e.g., causalgia and other reflex sympathetic dystrophies).

Many patients with chronic pain undergo a progressive physical deterioration caused by disturbance in sleep, appetite, and often by excessive medication, all of which contribute to general fatigue and debility. Moreover, their pain threshold and pain tolerance decreases, probably in part, due to depletion of endorphins (39). The anxiety of acute pain not infrequently is replaced by reactive depression, hypochondriasis, somatic preoccupation with disease conviction, somatic focusing, and a tendency to deny life problems unrelated to their physical problem (7,24,33,37). This cluster of psychological factors, which Pilowsky, Chapman, and Bonica (33) have labeled "abnormal illness behaviors," is characteristic of chronic pain, whether due to somatic or psychological factors. Some patients with pain due to known but unremovable pathology (e.g., arthritis, cancer) cannot give meaning or purpose to the pain and become depressed and develop feelings of hopelessness and despair (37). These factors, like sleeplessness, spiral to greater proportion as the patient goes from one doctor to another and one clinic to another. Each time he or she experiences hopefulness and then disappointment, and gradually increasing bitterness and resentment toward the doctors. Many patients become more and more preoccupied with the pain and gradually lose interest in social activities. The pain becomes a central focus and dominates their lives. Eventually, the world of many patients with chronic pain centers around home, doctor's office, and pharmacy (37).

Behavioral changes are produced by medication prescribed in high dosage that may lead to intoxication and by environmental factors. Some patients with chronic pain, especially that due to the environmental and emotional factors, manipulate their families, persons at work, and their physicians to prescribe multiple drugs and one useless operation after another (37). In addition to withdrawal from all social activity, many of these patients diminish their physical activities and spend much of the time in bed or lying down.

Most of these patients are exposed to a high risk of iatrogenic complications including narcotic addiction, drug toxicity, and, not infrequently, to multiple useless and, at times, mutilating operations (7,10). A significant number of these patients turn from physicians and dentists to quacks who often provide no relief and sometimes do harm.

The social effects of chronic pain are equally devastating. Many patients with chronic pain become estranged from their families, lose their jobs, and some become so discouraged and desperate as to commit suicide. Nelson Hendler, a psychiatrist at The Johns Hopkins University, has reported that "70 percent of these people (with chronic pain) get divorced and 20 percent attempt or contemplate suicide" (31). As a concrete example, I cite the case of the late William Pawley, a highly respected diplomat and multimillionaire, whose life ended tragically on January 8, 1977 in Miami when he committed suicide because (as he wrote in his suicide note) he could not endure any longer the relentless pain and agony of postherpetic neuralgia (3).

Magnitude of the Problem

Chronic intractable pain must be considered a disease state of its own, which is the most frequent cause of disability and consequently constitutes a very serious national and world economic, as well as health, problem. Although accurate statistics are not available, data from a variety of sources prompt me to *speculate* that chronic pain syndromes cost the American people between $40 to 50 billion annually (7,9,10). Costs include those of hospital and health services, loss of work productivity, compensation payments, and, in some instances, litigation costs. This speculation is based, in part, on the following considerations:

(a) It has been estimated that 7 million Americans are partially or totally disabled because of low back pain and in excess of 250 million workdays are lost (18). The health services, together with the loss of work productivity, cost the American people an estimated $12 billion.

(b) Of 26 million Americans afflicted with arthritis, nearly 6 million are disabled, not so much by the mechanical dysfunction, but by pain. Recent estimates by the Arthritis Foundation suggest that the total economic impact on the American people is in excess of $13 billion (42).

(c) Severe or disabling headaches afflict 20% of males and 35% of females, and of these one-third have migraine (18). It is estimated that all types of headaches cause loss of approximately 180 million workdays and prompt patients to purchase over $1 billion of over-the-counter pills with a total cost of approximately $10 billion.

(d) Chronic pain to other musculoskeletal neurological, visceral, and psychological disorders costs in excess of $10 billion.

(e) Many of the patients that have been seen at the University of Washington Pain Center have had an average of four to six operations (one had 42!) for their pain, have expended over $40,000 for health care, which, together with the loss of work productivity, amounts to over $125,000 for each of such patients with very complex pain problems.

Reasons for Inadequate Management of Chronic Pain

Why do the deficiencies exist that seriously detract from our otherwise outstanding biomedical achievements? Many reasons can be grouped into three major categories: (a) voids in our knowledge of chronic pain mechanisms; (b) inadequate application of the knowledge currently available; and (c) problems of communication. Although I have discussed these issues before (10), they deserve reemphasis.

Lack of Knowledge

There still exist great voids in our knowledge of the mechanisms and pathophysiology of chronic pain syndromes. Unfortunately, most of the information acquired during the past 1½ centuries from studies of acute pain has not been as beneficial to patients with chronic pain as one might anticipate or as many people believe. This less-than-optimal payoff from the many research efforts in turn has been due to the fact that, until recent years, little attention has been paid to the application of new knowledge and technology to the study of chronic pain syndromes. In the past, many basic scientists working in the isolation of the animal laboratory were not concerned with clinical pain. As a result of the fragmented, independent research efforts on artificially induced acute pain, hypotheses and concepts were developed that, although reasonable for the times and the scientific data available, were not relevant to chronic pain. Moreover, the predominant concern with anatomic and physiological research on pain—consequent to the widespread assumption that pain was a purely sensory experience—caused emotional and psychological factors to be relegated secondary roles or considered by-products of the sensation and also discouraged psychological research. Consequently, we have had little information on the *exact* mechanism of chronic headache, of chronic pain associated with postherpetic neuralgia and causalgia, of chronic pain associated with arthritis, and of that due primarily to psychological and environmental factors. To be sure, many speculations have been proposed, but hard scientific supporting data are lacking.

Another reason for the voids in our knowledge of chronic pain has been the lack of sufficient scientifically trained persons working on this problem. Related to this has been the meager amount or total lack of funds for research or research training in this field. A computer print-out of the amount of funds spent by the National Institutes of Health (NIH) on pain-related research, for the years 1971 to 1974, revealed an average of $3.5 million annually; but less than 25% of this amount was spent on studies of the mechanisms and physiopathology of pain. These figures represent 0.012 and 0.003%, respectively, of the total NIH annual budget. The expenditures are significantly less than those budgeted for certain chronic disease states that afflict less than 10,000 Americans annually.

Inadequate Application of Current Knowledge

The second major group of reasons for the deficiencies in managing chronic pain has been the improper or inadequate applications of knowledge currently available. The reasons for this include: (a) the lack of organized teaching of medical students and physicians and other health professionals in managing patients with chronic pain; (b) the progressive trend toward specialization; and (c) the inability, or unwillingness, of some practitioners to devote the necessary time and effort to care for these patients. I know of no medical, dental, or other health professional schools that have a formal course in the basic principles of managing patients with chronic pain. I believe that this is due to the teachers' lack of appreciation of the differences between acute and chronic pain as a clinical entity. Consequently, students are taught how to use pain as a diagnostic tool and how to apply the same methods used for treating acute pain to the management of patients with chronic pain. This invariably results in failures, drug toxicity, useless (and, at times, mutilating) operations, and other iatrogenic disorders mentioned earlier.

The recent progressive trend toward specialization has been conducive to each specialist viewing pain in a narrow, "tubular" fashion. Thus, the anesthesiologist has attempted to treat all patients with chronic pain with nerve blocks, the neurosurgeon by cutting pain pathways, the orthopedic surgeon by removing disks, the internist by using drugs, and the psychiatrist by traditional psychotherapy. This type of "tubular" vision is particularly likely to occur when a specialist practices alone and sees these patients in isolation. These factors preclude viewing the pain problem within the perspective of the many diagnostic and therapeutic strategies that may be applicable to the particular problem in choosing which are best for the particular patient.

The inability or unwillingness of many health professionals to spend several hours in the initial work-up of the patient is probably due to the pressure of their clinical practice and lack of interest in, and knowledge of, chronic pain syndromes. Consequently, a correct diagnosis is not made and the patient is started on a course of therapy that usually ends up in drug toxicity and other iatrogenic complications and in an endless series of experiences of hopefulness, disappointments, frustrations, and hopelessness characteristic of many chronic pain patients. We have found that most of the patients seen in our multidisciplinary clinic facility could have been spared the prolonged suffering and disability if, at the initial contact, the physician could have spent more time to do a proper work-up of the patient or if the patient had been referred to someone who could do so.

Communications

A matrix common to all of the above-mentioned causative factors has been the poor and, indeed, at times total lack of communication among investigators and between this group and clinicians. The usual mechanism of disseminating new information—publications in highly specialized journals limited to specific fields and meetings generally limited to a specific group—until recently precluded cross-fertilization of ideas and dissemination of information among the various basic science groups and clinicians. The poor interaction among basic scientists of different disciplines has impaired the application of new, vitally important information acquired by biochemists, for example, to the pain research programs of neurophysiologists or other scientific disciplines. Moreover, it has impaired the interaction and collaboration between basic and clinical scientists that is essential to solve clinical problems. This has also resulted in a great lag in the clinical application of new information that is useful and pertinent to the care of patients with chronic pain. Other major communication problems include the lack of an international standard terminology for pain syndromes, no epidemiological data on pain as a disease state, and the lack of national and international pain data banks or data pools—essential requisites to optimal communication and evaluation of old and new methods of therapy.

Recent Trends

Fortunately, during the past decade or so, several developments have taken place that hold the promise of helping to rectify some of these deficiencies. One development has been an impressive surge of interest among some basic scientists in studying the mechanisms of chronic pain syndromes and collaborating with clinical investigators and practitioners to begin to solve some of the major problems. Time will not permit mention, let alone discussion, of all the recent efforts of basic scientists in elucidating the mechanisms and physiopathology of chronic pain. The development and subsequent publication of the "gate control" hypothesis by Melzack and Wall (29) were stimulated by their desire to explain a number of chronic pain syndromes in the light of new physiological and psychological evidence that showed that then-prevailing "specificity" and "pattern" theories had major weaknesses. Notwithstanding the fact that subsequent studies showed some deficiencies in the Melzack–Wall hypothesis, its publication must be considered a milestone in pain research; it provoked hundreds of laboratory and clinical studies, prompted the reintroduction of electrical stimulation as a therapeutic modality, and encouraged much greater collaboration among basic scientists, clinical scientists, and practitioners.

To answer questions pertaining to mechanisms, or explain puzzling responses to therapy and other aspects of chronic pain, a number of scientists have developed animal models with induced chronic pain states. Examples of these include: the rat animal model to study nerve fiber activity of neuromata by Wall and Gutnik (41); Perl's study (32) of sensitization of nociceptors produced by persistent stimulation and information as obtained in chronic pain states; the animal model developed by Anderson et al. (2) to study denervation phenomena and central pain states, trigeminal neuralgia, and other postherpetic neuralgia; and the animal model developed by Loeser and Ward (25a) to study the mechanisms of denervation hypersensitivity.

Another area of increased interest shown by basic and clinical scientists has entailed studies in patients during the course of neurosurgical operations (14,26). These have included physiological studies of pain perception that are amply discussed by Mayer and Price *(this volume)* and also clinical studies of pathological pain states that followed operations, accidental injury, disease, or neoplasm (14,26). One of the most important benefits of these studies has been the realization that surgical interruption of nociceptive pathways, whether in the periphery (as achieved by neurotomy or rhizotomy) or in the neuraxis (as achieved by cordotomy or mesencephalic tractotomy), for chronic pain states produces relief that is of limited duration. Still another important area of collaborative research in humans pertains to the recently discovered antinociceptive system. Some basic scientists, in collaboration with neurosurgeons, are studying the efficacy of chronic stimulation of the periaqueductal and periventricular gray matter in relieving pain produced by neoplastic disease (1,34,35). Others are intensively studying changes in the endorphins and other biochemical substrates of nociception in patients with chronic pain (39).

One of the most productive series of recent investigations done in the past decade or so has been carried out by psychologists and psychiatrists in patients with chronic pain. These studies and the studies of patients with experimentally induced pain has helped to emphasize the importance of (a) learning, (b) personality, (c) perceptual, affective, motivational, and emotional factors on the individual's total pain experience, and (d) the role of culture and the environment in influencing the patient's pain behavior and in helping to clarify the psychodynamics of anxiety, depression, hypochondriasis, and other emotional and affective consequences of chronic pain. Since Fordyce and Chapman *(this volume)* discuss in detail some of the most important aspects of this line of research, I will make no further comments except to stress the critically important impact these studies have had on our understanding of chronic pain behavior and in effecting marked improvement in the management of these patients.

Another recent development that is especially gratifying to me is the recent surge of interest in the multidisciplinary concept in the diagnosis and therapy of chronic pain states. This concept, which I first advocated and practiced nearly 30 years ago (4), implies that effective management of some patients with complex chronic pain problems is often possible only through the coordinated and concerted efforts of several physicians from different disciplines who contribute their individualized knowledge and skill for the common goal of making a correct diagnosis and planning the most effective therapeutic strategy. In addition to providing more efficient and better care to patients with chronic pain, this type of facility has greatly enhanced exchange of information and cross-fertilization of ideas, and it has been found to be a better milieu for teaching and training of clinicians. Moreover, it has served to stimulate the interest of basic scientists in research of chronic pain, and has encouraged multidisciplinary, collaborative laboratory and clinical research.

Another gratifying development of the past several years is the surge of interest by several of the National Institutes of Health to significantly increase their support for research specifically targeted at pain. At the present time, pain research is being given high priority by the National Institute of Dental Research, the National Cancer Institute, the National Institute of General Medical Sciences, and the National Institute of Drug Abuse. Recently, the National Institute of Neurological and Communicative Disorders and Stroke has appointed a panel to suggest strategies for pain research during the next decade. Another development is the recent appointment of an intra-NIH committee (20) composed of senior staff from various institutes to formulate plans to encourage development of major pain research projects in specific areas, particularly cancer.

Several other recent developments show the promise of correcting the aforementioned deficiencies regarding communication and transfer of knowledge to the care of patients. These developments include the progressive increase in the number of regional, national, and international meetings, symposia, and conferences dealing with pain research or therapy or both. In addition to the dissemination of information to the audience who attend these meetings, in many instances the proceedings have been, and continue to be, published as monographs so that the new information becomes available to a much greater audience. This Miles Symposium is an excellent example of this type of activity. The Second World Congress on Pain (13a) was the largest gathering of scientists and health professionals interested in pain research or therapy, or both, ever held; its scientific program provided a comprehensive review of new information on some of the most important aspects of acute and chronic pain. Finally, the founding of the International Association for the Study of Pain (IASP) and the initiation of the publication of the journal *Pain* in 1974 and the subsequent development of a number of chapters of the IASP since then must be considered one of the most important, if not the most important, developments in the field of pain research and therapy.

FUTURE NEEDS AND DIRECTIONS

These very recent developments are encouraging, but we must do much more in the future. A challenge to the biomedical scientific community, health professionals, and society as a whole is to organize, mount, and support a multipronged program consisting of: (a) an intensive campaign to make the public, the Congress, and the biomedical community appreciate the importance and magnitude of the problem; (b) develop and carry out greatly expanded research and research training efforts; (c) activation of teaching programs for students and practitioners; and (d) improvement of communication systems. The ultimate goal of all these efforts would be to improve the care of patients with chronic pain.

Research Program

Of these programs, more extensive and intensive laboratory investigation—and, even more important, collaborative research—must be one of the first offensives for, without more knowledge, even the well-informed health professional will have to continue to use empirical therapy in many patients. The future course of research on problems of pain must take a very different direction from that of the past. For one thing, we must exploit the vast amount of scientific knowledge and technology in all of the scientific disciplines and bring them to bear on the problem of pain in a collective and collaborative fashion. For another, in addition to continuing experimental laboratory research, we must study pathological pain states in patients. These two latter objectives require the interested, concerted, and well-coordinated efforts of neurophysiologists, biochemists, psychologists, pharmacologists, anatomists, and virtually every other type of basic scientist, clinical investigator, and clinician from different disciplines. Medical specialists who might be involved in such comprehensive investigative efforts include neurologists, neurosurgeons, anesthesiologists, psychiatrists, psychologists, and oncologists, among others.

The critical need for this type of multidisciplinary approach to pain research, which I first suggested in 1953 (4), was reemphasized by Professor Patrick Wall at the 1973 International Symposium on Pain held in Seattle: "In the challenge of pain, the clinician and basic scientist must play an interdependent role. It is the job of the clinician to collect and describe the phenomena of pain; the signs, symptoms, and pathology of patients—and organize and present the facts in terms of questions and see to it that the basic scientist understands the facts. He must be ready to collect more facts and to check theories against facts. The basic scientist must grapple with the entirety of the real facts and not just select the easy and convenient phenomena and ignore or deny the uneasy ones." (40).

The important ingredients of a multidisciplinary pain research center or institute include the following:

(a) Recruitment of a critical mass of basic and clinical scientists from different disciplines who have a special interest and expertise in their particular field and are willing to work as members of well-coordinated research teams.

(b) A director with leadership qualitites of a scientist, clinician, and administrator.

(c) Ample space and funds for technical and administrative personnel, equipment, etc.

(d) An optimal environment, preferably in a university health center with strong basic sciences and clinical departments and which affords interaction with the multidisciplinary pain therapy centers.

(e) Effective research training programs enabling it to become a national and regional resource.

Educational Programs

A second line of attack is to mount more effective educational programs for better patient care which should include: (a) formal courses in medical, dental, and other health professional schools, including special courses on pain and elective rotation on the "pain service"; (b) postgraduate programs for physicians and other health professionals; (c) opportunities for physicians and health professionals to work in a pain center; and (d) better sources of information, including books and journals. Through these and other mechanisms we should be able to encourage students and physicians to improve the care of patients with chronic pain by learning the basic principles of diagnosis and therapy, and by encouraging the development of a multidisciplinary, diagnostic, and therapeutic pain clinic or center.

Better Communication

Finally, there is a critical need for improvement of communication among all of the various disciplines and people involved in managing patients with chronic pain problems. This can be effected by the type of interdisciplinary meeting we held that preceded the publication of this volume. The World Congress on Pain and the various national and regional meetings of the chapters of the IASP should help improve communication. The journal *Pain,* which is helping to diffuse information among members of the IASP who represent numerous disciplines, should be supplemented with review articles in journals published by each discipline on aspects of pain not known to that particular specialty. Other critically important needs include the development and universal adoption of a taxonomy on pain and pain syndromes, of uniform record systems for various pain syndromes, and computer data banks that will facilitate storage and retrieval of information. These methods will enhance dissemination of scientific information, diffusion of epidemiological data, and the results of the efficacy of therapeutic modalities—essential requisites for the optimal care of patients with chronic pain.

REFERENCES

1. Adams, J. E. (1976): Naloxone reversal of analgesia produced by brain stimulation in the human. *Pain,* 2:161–166.
2. Anderson, L. S., Black, R. G., Abraham, J., and Ward, A. A., Jr. (1971): Neuronal hyperactivity in experimental trigeminal deafferentation. *J. Neurosurg.,* 35:444–452.
3. Anonymous (1976): Obituary of William Pawley. *Miami Herald,* January 11, 1976.
4. Bonica, J. J. (1953): *The Management of Pain.* Lea & Febiger, Philadelphia.
5. Bonica, J. J. (1972): Maternal respiratory changes during pregnancy and parturition. In: *Parturition and Perinatology,* edited by G. F. Marx, pp. 1–19. F. A. Davis, Philadelphia.
6. Bonica, J. J. Ed. (1974): *Advances in Neurology, Vol. 4: Proceedings of the International Symposium on Pain.* Raven Press, New York.
7. Bonica, J. J. (1974): New progress against pain. *U.S. News & World Report,* 77(27):46–49.
8. Bonica, J. J. (1975): The nature of pain of parturition. *Clin. Obstet. Gynecol.,* 2:499–516.
9. Bonica, J. J. (1975): Problems of Pain and Pain Research. Presented to the Advisory Council of the National Institute of Dental Research.
10. Bonica, J. J. (1976): Introduction of the First World Congress on Pain: Goals and objectives of IASP and the World Congress. In: *Advances in Pain Research and Therapy, Vol. 1: Proceedings of the First World Congress on Pain,* edited by J. J. Bonica and D. Albe-Fessard, pp. xxvii–xxxix. Raven Press, New York.
11. Bonica, J. J. (1978): Pathophysiology of pain. *Hosp. Pract.,* 13 (Special Report):4–14.
12. Bonica, J. J. (1979): Special methods of cardiac pain relief. In: *Proceedings of the National Conference on Cardiac Pain,* edited by J. J. Bonica. Warner-Chilcott, Morris Plains, N.J. *(in press).*
13. Bonica, J. J., and Albe-Fessard, D., Eds. (1976): *Advances in Pain Research and Therapy, Vol. 1: Proceedings of the First World Congress on Pain,* edited by J. J. Bonica and D. Albe-Fessard. Raven Press, New York.
13a. Bonica, J. J., Liebeskind, J., and Albe-Fessard, D., Eds. (1979): In: *Advances in Pain Research and Therapy, Vol. 3: Proceedings of the Second World Congress on Pain.* Raven Press, New York *(in press).*
14. Cassinari, V., and Pagni, C. A. (1969): *Central Pain: A Neurosurgical Survey.* Harvard University Press, Cambridge.
15. Chapman, C. R. (1978): Psychologic aspects of pain. *Hosp. Pract.,* 13 (Special Report):15–19.
16. Chapman, C. R., and Cox, G. B. (1977): Anxiety, pain, and depression surrounding elective surgery: A multivariate comparison of abdominal surgery patients with kidney donors and recipients. *J. Psychosom. Res.,* 21:7–15.
17. Chapman, C. R., and Cox, G. B. (1977): Determinants of anxiety in elective surgery patients. In: *Stress and Anxiety, Vol. 4,* edited by C. B. Speilberger, pp. 269–290. John Wiley & Sons, New York.
18. Chen, T. C. (1978): Reports on epidemiology of various chronic pain syndromes to Panel on Pain to the National Institute of Neurological and Communicative Disorders and Stroke.
19. Cox, W. V., and Robertson, H. F. (1936): The effect of stellate ganglionectomy on the cardiac function of intact dogs and its effect on the extent of myocardial infarction and on cardiac function following coronary artery occlusion. *Am. Heart J.,* 12:285–300.
20. DHEW–National Institutes of Health Report of the Interagency Committee on New Therapies for Pain and Discomfort, July 11, 1978.
21. Dubner, R., and Beitel, R. E. (1976): Peripheral neural correlates of escape behavior in rhesus monkey to noxious heat applied to the face. In: *Advances in Pain Research and Therapy, Vol. 1: Proceedings of the First World Congress on Pain,* edited by J. J. Bonica and D. Albe-Fessard, pp. 155–160. Raven Press, New York.

22. Feigl, E. O. (1975): Control of myocardial oxygen tension by sympathetic vasoconstriction in the dog. *Circ. Res.*, 37:88–95.
23. Fisher, A., and Prys-Roberts, C. (1968): Maternal pulmonary gas exchange. A study during normal labour and extradural blockade. *Anaesthesia*, 23:350–356.
24. Fordyce, W. E. (1976): *Behavioral Methods for Chronic Pain and Illness.* C. V. Mosby, St. Louis.
25. Heavner, J. E., and de Jong, R. H. (1974): Modulation of dorsal horn throughput by anesthetics. In: *Advances in Neurology, Vol. 4: Proceedings of the International Symposium on Pain,* edited by J. J. Bonica, pp. 179–185. Raven Press, New York.
25a. Loeser, J. D., and Ward, A. A., Jr. (1967): Some effects of deafferentation on neurons of the cat spinal cord. *Arch. Neurol.,* 17:629–636.
26. Loeser, J. D., Ward, A. A., Jr., and White, L. E., Jr. (1968): Chronic deafferentation in human spinal cord neurons. *J. Neurosurg.,* 29:48–50.
27. Marx, G. F., Macatangay, A. S., Cohen, A. V., and Schulman, H. (1969): Effect of pain relief on arterial blood gas values during labor. *NY State J. Med.,* 69:819–822.
28. McEachern, C. G., Manning, G. W., and Hall, G. E. (1940): Sudden occlusion of coronary arteries following removal of cardiosensory pathways. *Arch. Intern. Med.,* 65:661.
29. Melzack, R., and Wall, P. D. (1965): Pain mechanisms: A new theory. *Science,* 150:971–979.
30. Murphy, T. M., and Bonica, J. J. (1977): Acupuncture analgesia and anesthesia. *Arch. Surg.,* 112:896–902.
31. Neff, P. N. (1976): Management of chronic pain: Medicine's new growth industry. *Med. World News,* ·17:54.
32. Perl, E. R. (1976): Sensitization of nociceptors and its relation to sensation. In: *Advances in Pain Research and Therapy, Vol. 1: Proceedings of the First World Congress on Pain,* edited by J. J. Bonica and D. Albe-Fessard, pp. 17–28. Raven Press, New York.
33. Pilowsky, I., Chapman, C. R., and Bonica, J. J. (1977): Pain, depression and illness behavior in a pain clinic population. *Pain,* 4:183–192.
34. Richardson, D. E., and Akil, H. (1977): Pain reduction by electrical brain stimulation in man. I. Acute administration in periaqueductal and periventricular sites. *J. Neurosurg.,* 47:178–183.
35. Richardson, D. E., and Akil, H. (1977): Pain reduction by electrical brain stimulation in man. II. Chronic self-administration in the periventricular gray matter. *J. Neurosurg.,* 47:184–194.
36. Rosenfeld, C. R., Barton, M. D., and Meschia, G. (1976): Effects of epinephrine on distribution of blood flow in the pregnant ewe. *Am. J. Obstet. Gynecol.,* 124:156–163.
37. Sternbach, R. A. (1974): *Pain Patients: Traits and Treatment.* Academic Press, New York.
38. Strange, R. C., Vetter, N., Rowe, M. J., and Oliver, M. F. (1974): Plasma cyclic AMP and total catecholamines during acute myocardial infarction in man. *Eur. J. Clin. Invest.,* 4:115–120.
39. Terenius, L., and Wahlstrom, A. (1975): Morphine-like ligand for opiate receptors in human CSF. *Life Sci.,* 16:1759–1764.
40. Wall, P. D. (1974): The future of attacks on pain. In: *Advances in Neurology, Vol. 4: Proceedings of the International Symposium on Pain,* edited by J. J. Bonica, pp. 301–308. Raven Press, New York.
41. Wall, P. D., and Gutnik, M. (1974): Properties of afferent nerve impulses originating from a neuroma. *Nature (Lond.),* 248:740–743.
42. Wilson, C. H., Jr. (1978): Arthritis prevalence in the United States. Presented at the Annual Meeting of the Arthritis Foundation, New York City, May 30, 1978.
43. Wright, R. G., Schneider, N., Levinson, G., Roizin, M. S., and Wallace, L. (1978): The effect of maternal stress (pain) on plasma catecholamines and uterine blood flow in the pregnant ewe. In: *Abstracts of Scientific Papers of Annual Meeting of the American Society of Anesthesiologists.* Chicago, Ill.
44. Zanchetti, A., and Malliani, A. (1974): Neural and psychological factors in coronary disease. *Acta Cardiol. Suppl.,* 20:69–89.

Mechanisms of Pain and Analgesic Compounds,
edited by R. F. Beers, Jr., and E. G. Bassett.
Raven Press, New York © 1979.

5. Neural Mechanisms Subserving Pain in Man

David J. Mayer and *Donald D. Price

*Department of Physiology, Medical College of Virginia, Virginia Commonwealth University, Richmond, Virginia 23298 and *Anesthesiology and Neurobiology Branch, National Institute of Dental Research, National Institutes of Health, Bethesda, Maryland 20014*

INTRODUCTION

Considerable data obtained within the last 10 years from animal studies have led to important inferences about mechanisms of pain. However, there are important reasons for directly studying pain mechanisms in man. Humans are uniquely capable of describing the several dimensions of pain experience that presumably are related to neurophysiological mechanisms. Qualitatively similar data from animals are impossible to collect, and those data available about pain experience in animals must be inferred from behavioral data that are typically time-consuming to collect. Finally, human pain mechanisms are of greatest interest, since our ultimate concern is with understanding and controlling our own pain.

This chapter reviews and synthesizes information from studies which have direct bearing on pain mechanisms in man. These studies include, for the most part, those in which man is the experimental subject but those in which correlations have been made between human psychophysical response and neuronal responses of mammalian species, especially primates, are also included.

PRIMARY AFFERENT TRANSMISSION
OF NOCICEPTIVE INFORMATION

Human Psychophysics

Psychophysical studies on pain are critical in identifying neurons and neural mechanisms that subserve pain in man (1,31–33,68). The quantitative study of pain sensation, like any sensation, begins with an approach that correlates the subject's evaluation of some aspect of the sensations experienced, such as pressure and intensity, with the stimuli that evoke them. The latter are measured in physical units (i.e., mcal/cm^2). There are two kinds of theoretical strategies that are used in relating psychophysical and neurophysiological studies of pain

(65). In the first, a functional category of neurons, usually primary afferents, are stimulated by natural stimuli and the experimental conditions are designed so as to selectively activate only that category of neurons. If pain is evoked by identical stimulus conditions, then it is possible to infer that activity in this identified category of neurons is sufficient to evoke pain. A second strategy is to correlate responses of neurons to controlled noxious stimulation with human psychophysical responses to the same stimuli. The more these two types of responses co-vary under different stimulus conditions, the stronger is the case that a given category of neurons participates in pain. However, since the neural data are usually obtained from mammalian species other than man, an added assumption for both of the above strategies is that neurons and neural mechanisms of pain are generally similar among different mammalian species. This assumption is easier to make for primate species.

Of all the methods used to produce pain experimentally, that of heat-induced pain has been of the greatest value (33). Heat-induced pain can be controlled, quantitatively administered, and produced in such a manner so as to produce little or no tissue damage. The following discussion briefly summarizes some of the major findings derived from studies of heat-induced pain.

The threshold for thermally evoked pricking pain occurs at skin temperatures of 44 to 45°C, regardless of the rate of temperature increase used to arrive at these temperatures (31–33). This independence between threshold intensity and rate differs markedly from the sense of warmth, the perceived intensity of which is very much dependent on the rate of temperature increase (31–33). Moreover, the threshold intensity required for heat-induced pain exhibits much less spatial summation than that observed for warmth (33). The constancy of heat-induced pain raises the question of whether the threshold for reflex avoidance responses to pain are similar. Hardy (31) has shown that the threshold for the heat-induced flexion reflex in spinal man averages 44.1 ± 0.75°C, and this endpoint, like that for pain, is independent of the rate of temperature increase. The similar parametric requirements for heat-induced pain and flexion reflex support the hypothesis that both are subserved at least in part by common neural mechanisms. The stability of these thresholds under specific experimental contexts should not be misconstrued as indicating that they are unmodifiable. The threshold of heat-induced pain is influenced by the immediate past history of thermal stimulation and includes such factors as the number, duration, and intensities of previous stimuli. For example, long duration, low intensity, and noxious heat stimuli can evoke primary hyperalgesia, which is accompanied by a lowering of pain threshold and an augmentation of the intensity of suprathreshold pain (3,4,33).

Studies of suprathreshold heat-induced pain have shown that there is a monotonic and approximately linear relationship between perceived pain intensity and skin temperature over a 45 to 50°C range (1,33). These ratio scales of thermal pain have been obtained by magnitude estimation procedures, including the method of direct magnitude estimation and that of just noticeable differences.

However, the number of discriminable intensity differences over this range, 21 just noticeable differences, is much less than that for warmth (33). Studies of thermally induced pain indicate that, like other sensory modalities, there are sensory–discriminative aspects of pain.

Studies of first and second pain have been particularly useful in identifying primary afferents, central pathways, and neural mechanisms involved in pain (44,63,68). When a brief noxious stimulus is applied to the distal part of an extremity, an initial sharp, well-localized pain is followed 1 to 2 sec later by a burning or throbbing pain. The latter is less well localized, often long outlasts both the stimulus and the arrival of incoming impulses that evoke it, and becomes more intense with repeated application of the stimulus. Reaction times and compound action potential recordings obtained in such studies have unequivocally demonstrated that first and second pain are related to conduction of impulses in Aδ and C afferents, respectively (68,77). Second pain reliably increases in magnitude after ischemic or pressure blockade of all the myelinated afferents in a nerve (44,68), thereby indicating a central interaction between input over myelinated and unmyelinated afferents.

There are several features of experimentally induced second pain and of other types of pain evoked by selective stimulation of C afferents that provide important information for understanding mechanisms of chronic and pathological pain (44,54,63,77). Prolonged temporal summation and the capacity to outlast the stimulus are characteristics shared by experimentally induced second pain and by some pathological pain states such as postherpetic neuralgia and causalgia. Thus, Noordenbos (58) has observed three distinct characteristics of certain pathological pains: slow temporal summation, irradiation of pain to surrounding areas, and after-responses. All of these characteristics can be demonstrated for either second pain or heat-induced pain in normal human subjects and lead us to suspect that some of the major characteristics of pathological pain states represent exacerbations of existing physiological mechanisms. Further evidence for this hypothesis is presented.

Primary Cutaneous Afferents

The nociceptive receptors that signal impending tissue damage are not uniformly sensitive. They fall into several categories depending on their responses to mechanical, thermal, and chemical stimulation and on the conduction velocities of the axons that supply them (3,4,61,65). Although nociceptive afferents have been shown to innervate several types of tissue, those innervating the skin have been most extensively studied and are strongly implicated in pain mechanisms. Their essential characteristics are summarized below.

Aδ high-threshold mechanoreceptive afferents that respond only to intense mechanical stimuli and conduct between 4 and 40 m/sec have been described in the skin of the cat and in monkey extremities (61,65). Many respond only to stimulus intensities that produce overt tissue damage, others give threshold responses to nondamaging pressure applied to the skin ($< 1g/cm^2$). Most importantly, all primary mechanoreceptive afferents respond to noxious or potentially damaging skin stimuli with the highest impulse frequency. They are particularly sensitive to excitation by sharp objects but are relatively insensitive to heat. Therefore, they seem well adapted for transmitting information that is related to the localized pricking pain produced by mechanical stimuli. So far, primary afferents of this type have not been identified in human nerves.

Aδ heat nociceptive afferents conducting between 3 and 20 m/sec have recently been identified in the limb and facial skin of monkeys (23,24,68). Like Aδ high-threshold mechanoreceptive afferents, these afferents respond to intense mechanical stimulation. However, unlike the Aδ high-threshold mechanoreceptive afferents, Aδ heat nociceptive afferents respond monotonically to increases in receptive field skin temperature. These responses accelerate positively, the steep portion of the curve occurring in the 45 to 53°C range. Threshold temperatures for these afferents are usually below noxious or painful levels (40 to 44°C), but highly noxious skin temperatures (> 50°C) evoke maximum responses. The role of these neurons in signaling pain is clearly established. They are the only myelinated primary afferents innervating the skin of the extremities that can be reliably activated by noxious heat. Thus, heat-induced first pain, the latency of which corresponds to the activity in the small myelinated Aδ fibers, must be initiated by impulse in the Aδ heat afferents. Neither this first pain nor the responses of the Aδ heat afferents outlast the duration of the heat stimulus. Both the intensity of the first pain in man and the responses of the Aδ heat afferents in monkeys are progressively reduced during brief repeated application of heat stimuli to the same spot on the hand (68). Therefore, the characteristics of heat-induced first pain can be largely accounted for by the response characteristics of Aδ heat nociceptive afferents. Recently it has been shown that these afferents excite neurons of origin of the spinothalamic tract of monkeys (67). Therefore, Aδ heat nociceptive afferents have central connections consistent with a role in pain. However, direct confirmation of their functional role in man awaits their identification and analysis in human nerves.

C polymodal nociceptive afferents form an extremely important group of peripheral fibers since they constitute 80 to 90% or more of the C fiber population of primates (65,76,78). They innervate the skin of the monkey (3–5) and man (76,78) and are characterized by their responses to noxious mechanical, noxious heat, and chemical irritant stimuli. Some also respond to intense cold (< 10°C). These polymodal nociceptive afferents have several important properties such as sensitization to repeated applications of low-intensity noxious stimuli and response suppression by high-intensity noxious stimuli (3–5). They respond with their highest frequency to two or more forms of intense cutaneous stimuli, but also respond weakly to mechanical (1 to 10 g) and thermal (38 to 43°C) stimuli that are clearly not painful to human observers. They may, therefore, provide some information about nonpainful sensations.

There is little doubt that C polymodal nociceptive afferents signal tissue damage and contribute directly to pain sensations in man. Brief heat pulses evoke distinct first and second pain (68). Except for the very small population of C warm afferents that respond to noxious heat (3–5), polymodal nociceptive afferents are the predominant C afferent group activated by this stimulus in primates and are the peripheral population most likely accountable for heat-induced second pain.

Like the responses of Aδ heat nociceptive afferents, those of C polymodal afferents became progressively reduced in monkeys during a train of 3-sec interpulse interval (68) heat pulses. When an identical train of heat pulses was applied to the hands of human observers, second pain increased in intensity (68). Thus, second pain summation occurs when the afferents evoking it are partially suppressed and must be critically dependent on prolonged summation in the central nervous system. This explanation is supported by the observation that second pain is increased to an even greater extent when the location of the probe on the skin changes between successive heat pulses so that different receptors are activated with each stimulus. These observations are consistent with a study by Collins et al. (17), in which the exposed sural nerve was electrically stimulated in awake humans. They found that a single volley in C afferents (A's were blocked by cold) did not evoke any sensation but that repetitive stimulation at 3 per sec evoked mounting, burning pain.

The duration of second pain also extends beyond the arrival of incoming C fiber impulses. Experimentally induced second pain, some forms of chronic pain, and some pathological pain states are all characterized by summation and sensations outlasting stimulation (58,63,68).

C polymodal nociceptive afferents excite many of the same spinothalamic tract neurons that are activated by Aδ heat nociceptive afferents (67). Therefore, they have central synaptic connections adapted to play a role in pain mechanisms.

NOCICEPTOR TRANSDUCER MECHANISMS

As discussed above, it appears that distinct classes of primary afferent neurons carry information about noxious stimuli to the central nervous system. It is appropriate to ask what is the mechanism(s) involved in the initial excitation of the peripheral terminals of these fibers by noxious stimuli. At present, little information is available concerning the direct effects of noxious stimuli on the terminations of nociceptive afferents. There is, however, considerable evidence from studies in man that tissue-destructive stimuli release chemical substances that can lower pain threshold or directly produce pain. Such a process may be of considerable importance in natural pain states resulting from tissue-destructive stimuli.

Within 15 to 30 sec after injury to human skin, an area of several centimeters surrounding the site begins to show reddening (vasodilatation), and this response becomes maximal after 5 to 10 min. The reddened area is called a flare, and the region of skin where it is present shows a lowered pain threshold (6). Considerable effort has been expended to determine the critical event leading to the flare and the nature of the chemical substance underlying it.

Of critical importance in determining the events leading to flare, has been the demonstration that the afferent innervation to the area must be intact and it is probably the C fibers that are important (11,44). Destruction of the peripheral nerve innervating the region prevents the reaction (11,45). The possible involvement of autonomic and efferent innervation has been eliminated. The response is still present after sympathectomy but absent after section of the dorsal root distal to the dorsal root ganglion (11). Interestingly, section of the dorsal root proximal to the ganglion does not abolish the response (11). Since this procedure leaves the peripheral nerve intact, it demonstrates that the afferent fibers need not enter the cord in order to produce the response.

Stimulation of a peripheral nerve after section of the dorsal root proximal to the ganglion continues to elicit vasodilatation in the distribution of the nerve and, if the adjacent dorsal roots are intact, can elicit pain (25). This observation indicates that activation of primary afferent neurons—not injury to the terminals from the noxious stimulus—is critical for the vasodilatation. Also, this and other observations strongly suggest that the release of some chemical from the branches of peripheral primary afferent terminals is crucial to production of flare and hyperalgesia. More direct evidence for the existence of a chemical resulting from peripheral nerve activation, which can cause pain, derives from the work of Chapman et al. (10). They showed that the perfusate taken from the area of vasodilatation produced pain when injected into a remote area of skin.

These observations have led to a search for the chemical substance or substances involved. The discovery of such a substance would have obvious implications for the management of inflammatory pain and would probably provide important clues as to the nature of the transduction process. However, the search for the critical substance has not been successful, although some progress has been made in pointing to the type of substance involved. A large number of endogenously occurring substances capable of producing pain on injection into human skin have been described. These include histamine, acetylcholine, 5-hydroxytryptamine, K^+, ATP, Substance P, and various plasma kinins (11,40). Some can be eliminated as the algogenic substance involved in the flare response on firm experimental grounds. Histamine can be eliminated since antihistamines do not block the vasodilatation and hyperalgesia resulting from antidromic nerve stimulation (11). Similarly, the antidromic vasodilatation is neither blocked by atropine nor potentiated by eserine (37), making acetylcholine an unlikely candidate. Although ATP can be liberated by antidromic nerve stimulation, it seems unlikely to be of critical importance since the amount released is quite small compared to the amount needed to produce vasodilatation (36). Potassium appears to require concentrations above physiological levels to produce pain (47). The evidence implicating 5-hydroxytryptamine and Substance P is inconclusive. On the other hand, Chapman et al. (11) have provided strong evidence for the involvement of a bradykinin-like substance in the vasodilatation and hyperalgesia resulting from antidromic nerve stimulation and painful stimuli. The substance can be collected in amounts adequate to produce pain when reinjected into the skin. It appears to be a polypeptide, since it is relatively stable and is destroyed by chymotrypsin. The polypeptide itself is probably not released from the nerve terminals since its activity is greatly increased following 3-min incubation with globulin, indicating that the proteolytic enzyme capable of forming the polypeptide is in the extracellular fluid at that time. Thus, the substance actually released from the nerve is likely to be either a proteolytic enzyme activator or the enzyme itself. That the vasodilatation is due to this substance and that the substance is not a secondary consequence of vasodilatation is supported by the observation that no such substance is released during the vasodilatation of reactive hyperemia.

CENTRAL CONNECTIONS OF NOCICEPTIVE AFFERENTS

Extensive progress has been made in the last few years in our knowledge of anatomical organization and connections of primary nociceptive afferents. Although some of this work was done in cats (29) and in monkeys (43), the results serve to partly explain some of the failures to control human pain by surgical means. It is now clear that nociceptive afferents terminate mainly within the uppermost laminae of the dorsal horn (29,43) where they directly synapse onto neurons of origin of ascending nociceptive pathways (14,66,67,80). Given such a direct and simple relationship between first and second order nociceptive neurons, one may question why dorsal root rhizotomy is such a poor means of controlling pain. Several factors can be invoked to explain the return of pain following rhizotomy.

(a) Sensation at any given point on the skin appears to depend partly on input over several adjacent dorsal roots. Using the method of analysis of isolated dermatomes of awake monkeys, Denny-Brown and co-workers (18,19) have found that the zone of sensibility that remains when one dorsal root is isolated by cutting three adjacent roots on either side depends on input from dorsal roots as far as five spinal segments away.

(b) The rostral–caudal extent of innervation from single dorsal root afferents is far greater than previously thought (21). The most distant synapses made by these afferents are normally ineffective for exciting dorsal horn neurons but become effective once dorsal horn neurons are denervated of their primary source of afferent input. Moreover, drastic central changes are produced by peripheral denervation that might account for the observation that dorsal horn neurons become hyperresponsive and more spontaneously active after rhizotomy (48).

(c) Although most nociceptive afferents enter the spinal cord via dorsal roots, Coggeshall and colleagues (15,16) have shown that some enter through ventral roots, a finding that is at variance with the law of Bell and Magendie. This recently discovered fact is consistent with an older clinical observation that stimulation of ventral roots sometimes evokes pain (25,27).

CENTRAL TRANSMISSION OF NOCICEPTIVE INFORMATION: SPINAL CORD AND TRIGEMINAL NOCICEPTIVE NEURONS

It has often been suggested that pain perception and nociceptive reflexes are not directly and simply related to activity evoked in "pain" receptors but depend on several integrative mechanisms of central neurons (51–53) (e.g., the evident lack of a simple one-to-one relationship between C polymodal nociceptive responses and second pain). The objective of this section is to account for some aspects of pain perception that cannot be explained by the responses of primary afferent neurons. This explanation focuses on the characteristics of spinothalamic tract and trigeminothalamic tract neurons that could be involved in pain. There are three distinct types of such neurons found in primates that could convey information about tissue injury (65–67).

Wide dynamic range neurons exist within laminae I–VI of the dorsal horn but are most concentrated in laminae IV–VI (62,63–67,69,70,80). They receive synaptic excitatory effects from large, myelinated (Aβ), low-threshold mechanoreceptive afferents (LTM), Aδ high-threshold mechanoreceptive afferents (HTM), and C polymodal nociceptive afferents. As a result of this extensive convergence, these cells respond with increasingly higher frequencies of impulse discharge to touch, firm pressure, and noxious pinching. The responses of many of these cells are monotonic functions of increases in skin temperature within the noxious range (44 to 52°C), similar to the perceived magnitude of pain intensity over this same temperature range (1).

The responses of these wide dynamic range neurons to noxious stimuli of brief duration show a clear analogy to first and second pain. Brief noxious stimuli evoke a brief-latency, high-frequency impulse discharge that is related to the impulse input from myelinated A fibers and a delayed, lower frequency discharge related to the impulse input from C fibers (67,68). The first response, like first pain, does not outlast the arrival of the peripheral impulses but with each successive stimulus, either decreases in magnitude or stays the same. The delayed response, like second pain, long outlasts the arrival of incoming C impulses and increases in frequency and duration with each successive stimulus. This summation, like second pain, occurs only if the interstimulus interval is 3 sec or less. Thus, it is evident that C fiber impulses activate central facilitatory mechanisms in the dorsal horn.

The second type of dorsal horn spinothalamic neuron is relatively specific for responses to intense mechanical and thermal stimuli and is located primarily in the marginal layer (66,67,71). It receives excitatory synaptic effects from HTM, Aδ heat nociceptive afferents, and C polymodal nociceptive afferents. As a result of these inputs, this type of neuron responds to firm pressure and pinch with an increasingly higher frequency of impulse discharge. Some also respond to noxious skin temperatures. Responses to brief noxious stimuli are very similar to those of wide dynamic range neurons and therefore show parallels to first and second pain.

The third type of dorsal horn spinothalamic neuron, also found mainly in the marginal layer, is unequivocally specific for responses to noxious skin stimuli (66,67). It appears to receive input from only Aδ HTM since it responds only to noxious mechanical stimulation of the skin or to electrical stimulation of the Aδ afferents. Its responses do not outlast the stimulus, nor do they summate with repeated application. Therefore, like the Aδ HTM, this type of neuron is likely to be related to the first pain evoked by a needle prick.

The impulse discharge frequencies evoked in both *wide dynamic range* and *nociceptive-specific* neurons by skin stimulation are not simple direct functions of impulses in primary afferents, but are subject to local inhibitory and facilitatory mechanisms and to strong descending controls (for reviews, see refs. 49,53). The complexity of input–output functions of these neurons is further increased by the observation that some spinothalamic tract neurons send collateral axons to medial brainstem structures; these have been proposed to be critical for the affective–motivational component of pain (52,67).

Their numerous parallels to human psychophysical responses to controlled noxious stimuli and the anatomy of their input–output relationships strongly implicate both wide dynamic range and nociceptive-specific neurons in pain. However, a question remains as to whether wide dynamic range neurons or nociceptive-specific neurons are necessary and/or sufficient inputs for pain perception. This question might be partly answered by selective stimulation of either of these two neuronal populations in awake humans. That this could be done, in principle, was suggested by Willis et al. (2,26,80), who showed that conduction velocities of nociceptive-specific neurons are substantially slower than those of wide dynamic range neurons. Therefore, electrophysiological properties such as electrical thresholds and refractory periods are likely to differ between these two neuronal classes. With these considerations in mind, two studies were conducted in parallel. The first examined pain evoked by electrical stimulation of the anterolateral quadrant of awake humans undergoing percutaneous cordotomy (50). Parameters of threshold, frequency, and refractory period of stimulated axons were examined. The second study (69) compared these parameters with those required to antidromically activate functionally identified dorsal horn neurons projecting in the monkey anterolateral quadrant (ALQ). Inferences could then be made about which class of nociceptive neurons were sufficient to produce pain. In the context of this analysis, important observations were made about neural coding mechanisms of pain.

In the first study, it was found that pain could be evoked by ALQ stimulation in all 18 subjects. Pain thresholds ranged from 120 to 1,000 μA (at 50 Hz; 0.2 msec pulses), but the majority of thresholds were below 300 μA. Further analysis of threshold data revealed that the higher thresholds (> 300 μA) were probably the result of marginal placements within the ALQ (50). This conclusion was arrived at by correlating the duration of lesion current necessary to produce complete contralateral analgesia with the ALQ-evoked pain threshold. For all patients with a pain threshold below 300 μA, complete analgesia resulted from a 5 sec, 500 μA radio frequency lesion, whereas in no patient with a threshold above 300 μA did complete analgesia occur with this duration of lesion.

The refractory periods of the stimulated axons were analyzed by the double-pulse technique originated by Deutsch (20). This procedure involves delivering pulse-pairs, the independent variable being the interpulse interval. The interpulse interval is varied over the range of expected neuronal refractory periods (e.g., 0.5 to 4.0 msec), and some behavior is measured as a function of the interpulse interval. If the behavior being observed is mediated by a relatively homogeneous neuronal population, it will increase in a quantal fashion when the interpulse interval surpasses the refractory period of the neural population that is stimulated. Pain evoked by ALQ stimulation was found to be mainly between 1.0 to 1.5 msec.

In the second study, it was found that electrical shocks applied to the rhesus monkey C_1–C_2 ALQ by a cordotomy electrode antidromically activated contralateral L-7 dorsal horn neurons. Electrical shocks of less than 300 μA intensity activated laminae IV–VI wide dynamic range neurons, which could be excited by sensitive mechanoreceptive and by nociceptive afferents. The refractory periods of these neurons were mainly between 1.0 to 1.5 msec. In contrast, both the electrical antidromic thresholds and refractory period values were higher for dorsal horn nociceptive-specific neurons. Thus, the electrical thresholds and refractory periods of wide dynamic range neurons but *not* nociceptive-specific neurons parallel those of ALQ-evoked pain in man. The authors of the two studies concluded that pain may be signaled by the combined output of nociceptive-specific and wide dynamic range neurons, but that activation of the latter is a sufficient condition to evoke pain.

Two critical assumptions in their analysis are that the same physiological types of nociceptive dorsal horn neurons are found in both monkeys and humans and that the electrophysiological differences between nociceptive-specific and wide dynamic range neurons' axons are present in both species. These assumptions are indirectly supported by several lines of evidence. For one, it is becoming increasingly clear that the types and organization of nociceptive neurons in the spinal cord are very similar for rat, cat, monkey, and man (28,59,64–69,80), the responses of these neurons to standardized noxious stimuli are similar across these species, and, as shown above, parallel psychophysical responses of humans to similar stimuli (65–68). The anatomy of the dorsal horn neurons giving rise to ALQ axons is similar for monkey and man (41,75). In both species, anterolateral cordotomy results in retrograde chromatolysis of cells in layer I, most of which have small diameters in coronal section and are likely to be nociceptive-specific neurons (41,75). Chromatolysis of larger cells of nucleus proprius is also observed, many of which are probably wide dynamic range neurons (41,75). These anatomical observations fit with physiological results that indicate that nociceptive-specific neurons give rise to slow conducting axons and wide dynamic range neurons give rise to fast conducting axons (69,80). Thus, there is considerable indirect support for the assumptions in Price and Mayer's analysis (69).

In the context of determining which types of spinal cord ALQ neurons are sufficient to evoke pain, several observations were made that have direct bearing on pain mechanisms in man. First, it is of considerable significance that pain evoked by ALQ stimulation was similar to that evoked by naturally occurring stimuli. Most of the reports were burning pain, but descriptions of dull aching pain, cramping, and sharp pain were also given. These types of pain were evoked by 50 Hz trains of regularly spaced pulses, a pattern that is not likely to be generated by natural stimuli. Therefore, it is unlikely that pain is subserved by some special temporal pattern that depends on the exact intervals of impulses in spinal cord nociceptive neurons. However, the intensity of pain was found to be dependent on the overall frequency in ALQ neurons over a range of 5 to 100 Hz (50). A linear relationship was found between stimulation frequency and percentage of subjects reporting pain. One hundred percent of subjects reported pain at 25 Hz and none reported pain at 5 Hz. Wide dynamic range neurons responded to graded noxious heat with a frequency of 5 to 25 Hz over a skin temperature range of 44 to 46.5°C (67), the range over which most human heat pain threshold values are distributed (33). In contrast, the frequency of nociceptive-specific responses extend between 5 and 25 Hz over a skin temperature range of 46 to 48°C (67). These temperature values evoke suprathreshold pain in most human subjects (33). Thus, pain appears critically dependent on overall frequency in wide dynamic range neurons.

The above studies also support the concept that central spatial summation is especially critical for pain. When the frequency was held constant (50 Hz), it was found that the perception of ALQ-evoked pain invariably required larger stimulus intensities and presumably activation of a larger number of ALQ axons than that required for perceptions of tingle, warmth, or cooling (50). The amount of spatial summation was critical since stimulus intensities just sufficient to evoke tingle would do so even when stimulus frequencies extended up to 500 Hz. In contrast, when stimulus intensities were increased to activate a critical number of axons, much lower frequencies (5 to 25 Hz) evoked pain. These results fit well with other lines of evidence indicating heat pain requires central spatial summation (18,19,67).

Although it was not stated in their original report (50), ALQ-evoked pain was clearly aversive, although certainly tolerable (Price and Mayer, *unpublished observations*). Behavioral responses and reports indicating that the pain was unpleasant (i.e., "bad," "hurts") were given without provocation or suggestion. Since the currents and frequencies were adjusted so as to activate mainly the axons of wide dynamic range neurons, these indications of aversion are significant. They lead to the inference that wide dynamic range neurons activate central mechanisms related to the affective–motivational dimension of pain as well as the central mechanism related to sensory discrimination. The observation that the same wide dynamic range neuron projects to both VPL and medial brainstem (see above) lends support to such an inference.

BRAIN PROCESSING OF NOCICEPTIVE INFORMATION

Beyond the level of the efferents emanating from the spinal cord dorsal horn and the homologous components of the trigeminal system, detailed information concerning the processing of nociceptive information has been scant and controversial. Several factors have been responsible for this situation in the human studies to be discussed.

(a) The types of studies that can be done are obviously limited by ethical and practical considerations. For example, although the information yield might be great from single unit recording studies, these have been few due to the time involved, the need to apply repeated peripheral noxious stimuli, and the necessity of recording from control structures not involved in the normal invasive procedures.

(b) Probably the most common disease process leading to stereotactic invasion of the human brain for pain relief is carcinoma, yet the typically short survival time of these patients renders interpretation of results difficult. On the other hand, patients with long survival times are often afflicted with pain syndromes of idiopathic, psychogenic, or central origin, and observations made on them may not accurately reflect normal processing of nociceptive information.

(c) The evaluation of results of lesioning procedures has not utilized consistent criteria for designated success and failure, making comparison of results between studies difficult.

(d) Postlesion sensory testing has not been consistently utilized, and when it has been done, is typically cursory and qualitative. Thus, a wealth of valuable information about human pain physiology has been lost.

(e) Direct histological verification, particularly of stimulation and recording sites, is difficult to achieve.

Medulla and Pons

Information about the neural processing of pain at this level of the neuraxis derives principally from attempts to interrupt spinothalamic fibers for the relief of shoulder and neck pain. A careful review of this work has been given by White and Sweet (79). As would be expected, destruction of the spinothalamic tract at the medullary level produces results qualitatively similar to those resulting from anterolateral cordotomy. In a review of nine studies by different investigators, Birkenfled and Fisher (7) reported complete relief of pain in 41 of 50 patients and partial relief in four. Thus, results at the medullary level also appear to be quantitatively similar to those at the spinal level. As with anterolateral cordotomy, medullary tractotomy typically results in at least temporary analgesia to acute pain on the contralateral body surface (79). It seems reasonable to conclude, then, that little significant divergence of nociceptive information occurs at the medullary level in man. No attempt has been made to evaluate the effects of destruction in man of those more medial pontobulbar structures in the vicinity of the nucleus reticularis gigantocellularis, which have been implicated in the neural processing of pain in animals.

Stimulation of medullary structures in conscious humans has been restricted to attempts to verify electrode placement within the spinothalamic tract. Pain does result from stimulation of the tract (79), thus supporting the conclusion that the nature of pain pathways does not change significantly at this level.

Mesencephalon

At the mesencephalic level, important information about neural processing of pain in man is derived from neurosurgical procedures attempting to alleviate pain by severing either spinothalamic pathways or spinoreticular connections.

Studies at this level begin to reveal a divergence of pain pathways with important theoretical and practical significance.

Spinothalamic tractotomy at the mesencephalic level is a procedure that has been, for the most part, abandoned because of the high incidence of deleterious side effects (79). Those cases which have been reported are highly instructive. Analysis of the review presented by White and Sweet (79) reveals that this procedure can produce at least temporary relief of clinical pain although the probability of success, even when the lesion is correctly placed, is lower than at more caudal levels (12/20 cases). Recurrence of pain within a short period after surgery appears likely. Analgesia to acute pain over at least some portion of the body again is less likely than with tractotomy at medullary or spinal levels (13/20 cases), and the analgesia is more likely to quickly recede. Of particular interest are reports (22,79) that the quality of pain sensation to acute noxious stimuli sometimes changes. Pinprick and thermal stimuli can result in reports of deep, diffuse, and poorly localized pain after tractotomy.

Examination of the effects of more medial midbrain destruction and stimulation, although not without overlapping effects of spinothalamic tractotomy, is more revealing in the complimentary effects observed. Destruction of the midbrain periaqueductal gray matter alone had been done only for the relief of pain of central origin. The procedure seems effective for the relief of this type of pain (74), but its effect on chronic pain of peripheral origin remains unknown. The suffering aspect of central pain has been reported to be affected by this procedure (74). Of particular interest is the observation that lesions restricted to the mesencephalic periaqueductal gray matter do not appear to interfere with localization or detection of acute noxious stimuli, although the sensory sequelae of this lesion have not been analyzed in detail (74).

The most striking effect of electrical stimulation of periaqueductal structures in man is the elicitation of an emotional complex of unpleasantness and fear that often results in the subject not allowing further stimulation (57,74). At higher stimulation intensities, reports of frankly painful sensations occur. The pain is typically diffuse, deep, and localized to midline structures, particularly the face (56,57,74). This is in contrast to midbrain spinothalamic stimulation which produces sharp, well localized pain referred to the contralateral body surface (56).

In summary, the available evidence from studies in man suggest that a divergence of neural processing of nociceptive information occurs at least as caudal as the mesencephalic level. The lateral mesencephalic structures continue to carry information more concerned with the sensory–discriminative aspects of pain, whereas the most medial structures appear to be preferentially involved with the emotional and motivational aspects of the sensation. It is important to point out that this separation is certainly not an exclusive one. In fact, it is this overlap of function that probably leads to the unpredictable results of surgical interventions at this level as well as at more rostral levels of the neuraxis. It should also be mentioned that there is clear evidence that medial mesencephalic structures are importantly involved not only in the afferent transmission of nociceptive information, but also in the centrifugal control of this system (38, 49,72). Thus, studies of this area in man are likely to produce complex results and should be interpreted with caution.

Diencephalon

The specialization of neural systems mediating different aspects of the total pain experience is perhaps even more clear from studies of thalamic structures in man. Lesions of the specific sensory nuclei of the thalamus (VPL and VPM) result in, at best, mediocre relief of chronic pain, and this relief is usually transient (79). The procedure is no longer commonly utilized (8). White and Sweet (79) report a case similar to the phenomenon discussed above for midbrain lesions in which a specific sensory nucleus lesion resulted in the disappearance of localized pain but was replaced by diffuse, aching pain. Some loss of sensibility to pinprick occurs, but this typically is incomplete, and the peripheral field involved is generally smaller than with spinothalamic tractotomies at more caudal levels (79).

Electrical stimulation of the ventrobasal complex in man typically produces sensations of tingling and numbness but rarely frank reports of pain (56,79). On the other hand, Halliday and Logue (30) and Hassler (35) have reported that electrical stimulation of a restricted region in the most ventral aspect of the nucleus ventrocaudalis results in specific, localized pains referred to the contralateral body. The reports of pain seem similar to those reported from stimulation of the spinothalamic system at more caudal levels. The latter suggest a thalamic specialization for the coding of sensory–discriminative aspects of pain in man.

It appears that destruction of a variety of medial thalamic structures can have at least a temporary beneficial effect on chronic pain in man. These structures include the Cm-Pf complex, nucleus limitans, anterior thalamic nuclei, dorsomedial nuclei, and the pulvinar. The results of these interventions are, however, highly variable. Overall, it appears that Cm-Pf, nucleus limitans, and pulvinar lesions are most effective, but the advantage of any one of these over the others is controversial [e.g., compare White and Sweet (79) and Laitinen (42)]. It also may be that the size of the lesion is critical since enlargement of the lesion can improve the result of an initial smaller lesion (79), and combined medial and lateral lesions appear more effective than either alone (55). These lesions do not appear to alter the response to acute noxious stimuli, although this has not typically been systematically explored.

Stimulation of these thalamic structures does not typically produce pain, but reports of discomfort are common (79). However, stimulation of intralaminar structures (Cm-Pf and nucleus limitans) has been reported to produce pain with a burning (73) or aching (35) quality and has been referred to large portions of the contralateral and even ipsilateral body surface. Interestingly, one of these groups (39) has recorded from neurons in the human thalamus. They found 20/80 neurons in the Cm-Pf complex that responded to pinprick but not light touch or joint rotation. No neurons in the dorsal medial nucleus responded in this way.

The Cerebral Cortex

The role of the cerebral cortex in the elaboration of input from several sensory systems has been worked out in considerable detail. Such is not the case with pain. It is clear that the specific somatosensory projection areas are not critical for the relatively normal perception of both chronic and acute pain. SI lesions have consistently had no effect on chronic or acute pain and may even result in hyperpathia (34,79). Lesions of SII cortex or SI + SII cortices do not result in the lack of appreciation of either chronic or acute pain (34,79), although some hypalgesia has been reported with SII lesions (35). Electrical stimulation of somatosensory cortex typically does not produce reports of pain (46,79), although Penfield and Boldrey (60) elicited very weak pain sensation from 11 of 426 stimulation sites. Thus, it can be concluded that the cortical projection areas of the specific thalamic nuclei do not code even the sensory–discriminative dimension of pain with the same specificity as at lower levels of the spinothalamic system. This conclusion does not exclude the possibility that other cortical areas participate in the elaboration of noxious inputs, and a few recent electrophysiological studies suggest this may be so. These experiments have attempted to stimulate selectively nociceptive afferents. Chatrian et al. (12,13) have used tooth pulp stimulation and Carmon et al. (9) have used a laser beam to excite heat nociceptors. These stimuli are synchronous and result in cortical-evoked potentials that can be recorded over somatosensory cortex but are maximal at vertex. Such a result suggests widespread cortical involvement in the processing of this information. The pain-related components have a latency of less than 300 msec, eliminating the involvement of C fibers. In the experiment by Carmon et al. (9), the evoked potential is unlikely to be elicited by prepain sensations since stimuli that give rise only to a sensation of warmth do not result in an evoked potential. Whether these potentials are related to the perceptual aspects of pain or to a more global variable (such as arousal) remains to be demonstrated.

ACKNOWLEDGMENT

Portions of this work were supported by Public Health Service grant DA-00576 to David J. Mayer.

REFERENCES

1. Adair, E. E., Stevens, J. C., and Marks, L. E. (1968): Thermally induced pain: The dol scale and the psychophysical power law. *Am. J. Psychol.,* 81:147–164.
2. Applebaum, A. E., Beall, J. E., Foreman, R. D., and Willis, W. D. (1975): Organization and receptive fields of primate spinothalamic tract neurons. *J. Neurophysiol.,* 38:572–586.

3. Beitel, R. E., and Dubner, R. (1976): The response of unmyelinated (C) polymodal nociceptors to thermal stimuli applied to the monkey's face. *J. Neurophysiol.*, 39:1160–1175.
4. Beitel, R. E., and Dubner, R. (1976): Fatigue and adaptation in unmyelinated (C) polymodal nociceptors to mechanical and thermal stimuli applied to the monkey's face. *Brain Res.*, 112:402–406.
5. Beitel, R. E., and Dubner, R. (1976): Sensitization and depression of C-polymodal nociceptors by noxious heat applied to the monkey's face. In: *Advances in Pain Research and Therapy, Vol 1: Proceedings of the First World Congress on Pain,* edited by J. J. Bonica and D. Albe-Fessard, pp. 149–153. Raven Press, New York.
6. Bilisoly, F. N., Goodell, H., and Wolff, H. G. (1954): Vasodilatation, lowered pain threshold and increased tissue vulnerability. *AMA Arch. Intern. Med.*, 94:759–773.
7. Birkenfled, R., and Fisher, R. G. (1963): Successful treatment of causalgia of upper extremity with medullary spinothalamic tractotomy: Case report and review of the literature. *J. Neurosurg.*, 20:303–311.
8. Bouchard, G., Mayanagi, Y., and Martins, L. F. (1977): Advantages and limits of intracerebral stereotactic operations for pain. In: *Neurosurgical Treatment in Psychiatry, Pain and Epilepsy,* edited by W. H. Sweet, S. Obrador, and J. G. Martin-Rodriguez, pp. 693–697. University Park Press, Baltimore.
9. Carmon, A., Mor, J., and Goldberg, J. (1976): Evoked cerebral responses to noxious thermal stimuli in humans. *Exp. Brain Res.*, 25:103–107.
10. Chapman, L. F., Goodell, H., and Wolff, H. G. (1959): Augmentation of the inflammatory reaction by activity of the central nervous system. *Arch. Neurol.*, 1:557–572.
11. Chapman, L. F., Ramos, A. O., Goodell, G., and Wolff, H. G. (1961): Neurohumoral features of afferent fibers in man: Their role in vasodilatation inflammation and pain. *Arch. Neurol.*, 4:617–650.
12. Chatrian, G. E., Canfield, R. C., Knauss, R. A., and Lettich, E. (1975): Cerebral responses to electrical tooth pulp stimulation in man: An objective correlate of acute experimental pain. *Neurology (Minneap.)*, 25:747–757.
13. Chatrian, G. E., Farrell, D. R., Canfield, R. C., and Lettich, E. (1975): Cerebral evoked potentials in a case of congenital insensitivity to noxious stimuli. *Arch. Neurol.*, 32:141–145.
14. Christensen, B. N., and Perl, E. R. (1970): Spinal neurons specifically excited by noxious or thermal stimuli: Marginal zone of the dorsal horn. *J. Neurophysiol.*, 33:293–307.
15. Clifton, G. L., Vance, W. H., Applebaum, M. L., Coggeshall, R. E., and Willis, W. D. (1974): Responses of unmyelinated afferents in the mammalian ventral root. *Brain Res.*, 82:163–167.
16. Coggeshall, R. E., Applebaum, M. L., Fazen, M., Stubbs, T. M., and Sykes, M. T. (1975): Unmyelinated axons in human ventral roots, a possible explanation for the failure of dorsal rhizotomy to relieve pain. *Brain,* 98:157–166.
17. Collins, W. F., Nulsen, F. E., and Randt, C. T. (1960): Relation of peripheral nerve fiber size and sensation in man. *Arch. Neurol.*, 3:381–385.
18. Denny-Brown, D., Kirk, E. J., and Yanagisawa, N. (1972): The tract of Lissauer in relation to sensory transmission in the dorsal horn of spinal cord in the Macaque monkey. *J. Comp. Neurol.*, 151:175–200.
19. Denny-Brown, D., and Yanagisawa, N. (1973): The function of the descending root of the fifth nerve. *Brain,* 96:783–814.
20. Deutsch, J. A. (1964): Behavioral measurement of the neural refractory period and its application to self-stimulation. *J. Comp. Physiol. Psychol.*, 58:1–9.
21. Devor, M., Merrill, E. G., and Wall, P. D. (1977): Dorsal horn cells that respond to stimulation of distant dorsal roots. *J. Physiol.*, 270:519–531.
22. Drake, C. G., and McKenzie, K. G. (1953): Mesencephalic tractotomy for pain: Experience with six cases. *J. Neurosurg.*, 10:457–462.
23. Dubner, R., and Beitel, R. E. (1976): Peripheral neural correlates of escape behavior in rhesus monkey to noxious heat applied to the face. In: *Advances in Pain Research and Therapy, Vol 1: Proceedings of the First World Congress on Pain,* edited by J. J. Bonica and D. Albe-Fessard, pp. 155–160. Raven Press, New York.
24. Dubner, R., Gobel, S., and Price, D. D. (1976): Peripheral and central trigeminal "pain" pathways. In: *Advances in Pain Research and Therapy, Vol 1: Proceedings of the First World Congress on Pain,* edited by J. J. Bonica and D. Albe-Fessard, pp. 137–148. Raven Press, New York.
25. Foerster, O. (1927): *Die Leitungsbahnen des Schmerzegefuhls und die chirurgische Behandlung der Schmerzzustande.* Urban und Schwarzenberg, Berlin.

26. Foreman, R. D., Beall, J. E., Applebaum, A. E., Coulter, J. D., and Willis, W. D. (1976): Effects of dorsal column stimulation on primate spinothalamic tract neurons. *J. Neurophysiol.*, 39:534–546.
27. Frykholm, R., Hyde, J., Norlen, G., and Skoglund, C. R. (1953): On pain sensations produced by stimulation of ventral roots in man. *Acta Physiol. Scand. [Suppl]*, 106:455–469.
28. Giesler, G. J., Menetrey, D., and Besson, J-M. (1976): Response properties of dorsal horn neurons to noxious and non-noxious stimuli in the spinal rat. In: *Advances in Pain Research and Therapy, Vol 1: Proceedings of the First World Congress on Pain*, edited by J. J. Bonica and D. Albe-Fessard, pp. 105–110. Raven Press, New York.
29. Gobel, S., and Binck, J. M. (1977): Degenerative changes in primary trigeminal axons and in neurons in nucleus caudalis following tooth pulp extirpations in the cat. *Brain Res.*, 132:347–354.
30. Halliday, A. M., and Logue, V. (1972): Painful sensations evoked by electrical stimulation in the thalamus. In: *Neurophysiology Studied in Man*, edited by G. G. Somjen, pp. 221–230. Excerpta Medica, Amsterdam.
31. Hardy, J. D. (1953): Thresholds of pain and reflex contraction as related to noxious stimuli. *J. Appl. Physiol.*, 5:725–739.
32. Hardy, J. D., Harold, G., Wolff, H. G., and Goodell, H. (1948): Studies on pain: An investigation of some quantitative aspects of the dol scale of pain intensity. *J. Clin. Invest.*, 27:380–386.
33. Hardy, J. D., Wolff, H. G., and Goodell, H. (1952): *Pain Sensations and Reactions.* Williams & Wilkins, Baltimore.
34. Hassler, R. (1960): Die zentralen Systeme des Schmerzes. *Acta Neurochir.*, 8:354–364.
35. Hassler, R. (1970): Dichotomy of facial pain conduction in the diencephalon. In: *Trigeminal Neuralgia*, edited by R. Hassler and A. E. Walker, pp. 123–138. W. B. Saunders, Philadelphia.
36. Holton, P. (1959): The liberation of adenosine triphosphate on antidromic stimulation of sensory nerves. *J. Physiol.*, 145:494–504.
37. Holton, P., and Perry, W. L. M. (1951): On the transmitter responsible for antidromic vasodilatation in the rabbit's ear. *J. Physiol.*, 114:240–251.
38. Hosobuchi, Y., Adams, J. E., and Linchitz, R. (1977): Pain relief by electrical stimulation of the central gray matter in humans and its reversal by naloxone. *Science*, 197:183–186.
39. Ishijima, B., Yoshimasu, N., Fukushima, T., Hori, T., Sekino, H., and Sano, K. (1975): Nociceptive neurons in the human thalamus. *Confin. Neurol.*, 37:99–106.
40. Keele, C. A. (1970): Chemical causes of pain and itch. *Annu. Rev. Med.*, 21:67–74.
41. Kerr, F. W. L. (1975): Neuroanatomical substrates of nociception in the spinal cord. *Pain*, 1:325–356.
42. Laitinen, L. V. (1977): Anterior pulvinotomy in the treatment of intractable pain. In: *Neurosurgical Treatment in Psychiatry, Pain and Epilepsy*, edited by W. H. Sweet, S. Obrador, and J. G. Martin, pp. 669–672. University Park Press, Baltimore.
43. LaMotte, C. (1977): Distribution of the tract of Lissauer and the dorsal root fibers in the primate spinal cord. *J. Comp. Neurol.*, 172:529–561.
44. Landau, W., and Bishop, G. H. (1953): Pain from dermal, periosteal, and fascial endings and from inflammation. *Arch. Neurol. Psychiatry*, 69:490–504.
45. Lewis, T., Harris, K. E., and Grant, R. T. (1927): Influence of the cutaneous nerves on various reactions of the cutaneous vessels. *Heart*, 14:27–47.
46. Libet, B. (1973): Electrical stimulation of cortex in human subjects and conscious sensory aspects. In: *Handbook of Sensory Physiology*, edited by A. Iggo, pp. 743–790. Springer-Verlag, Berlin.
47. Lindahl, O. (1961): Experimental skin pain induced by injection of water soluble substances in humans (20 subjects). *Acta. Physiol. Scand. [Suppl.]*, 51:75–78.
48. Loeser, J. D. (1974): Dorsal rhizotomy: Indications and results. In: *Advances in Neurology, Vol 4: International Symposium on Pain*, edited by J. J. Bonica, pp. 615–619. Raven Press, New York.
49. Mayer, D. J., and Price, D. D. (1976): Central nervous system mechanisms of analgesia. *Pain*, 2:379–404.
50. Mayer, D. J., Price, D. D., and Becker, D. P. (1975): Neurophysiological characterization of the anterolateral spinal cord neurons contributing to pain perception in man. *Pain*, 1:51–58.
51. Melzack, R. (1973): *The Puzzle of Pain.* Basic Books, New York.
52. Melzack, R., and Casey, K. L. (1968): Sensory, motivational, and central control determinants

of pain: A new conceptual model. In: *The Skin Senses,* edited by D. R. Kenshalo, pp. 423–439. Charles C Thomas, Springfield, Ill.

53. Melzack, R., and Wall, P. D. (1965): Pain mechanisms: A new theory. *Science,* 150:971–979.
54. Mendell, L. M. (1966): Physiological properties of unmyelinated fiber projections to spinal cord. *Exp. Neurol.,* 16:316–332.
55. Mundinger, F., and Becker, P. (1977): Long-term results of central stereotactic interventions for pain. In: *Neurosurgical Treatment in Psychiatry, Pain and Epilepsy,* edited by W. H. Sweet, S. Obrador, and J. G. Martin-Rodriguez, pp. 685–692. University Park Press, Baltimore.
56. Nashold, B. S., Jr., Wilson, W. P., and Slaughter, G. (1974): The midbrain and pain. In: *Advances in Neurology, Vol 4: International Symposium on Pain,* edited by J. J. Bonica, pp. 191–196. Raven Press, New York.
57. Nashold, B. S., Wilson, W. P., and Slaughter, D. G. (1969): Stereotactic midbrain lesions for central dysesthesia and phantom pain: Preliminary report. *J. Neurosurg.,* 30:116–126.
58. Noordenbos, W. (1959): *Pain.* Elsevier, Amsterdam.
59. Pearson, A. A. (1952): Role of gelatinous substance of spinal cord in conduction of pain. *Arch. Neurol. Psychiatry,* 68:515–519.
60. Penfield, W., and Boldrey, E. (1937): Somatic motor and sensory representation in the cerebral cortex of man as studied by electrical stimulation. *Brain,* 60:398–418.
61. Perl, E. R. (1968): Myelinated afferent fibers innervating the primate skin and their response to noxious stimuli. *J. Physiol. (Lond.),* 197:593–615.
62. Pomeranz, B., Wall, P. D., and Weber, W. V. (1968): Cord cells responding to fine myelinated afferents from viscera, muscle and skin. *J. Physiol. (Lond.),* 199:511–532.
63. Price, D. D. (1972): Characteristics of second pain and flexion reflexes indicative of prolonged central summation. *Exp. Neurol.,* 37:371–387.
64. Price, D. D., and Browe, A. C. (1975): Response of spinal cord neurons to graded noxious and non-noxious stimuli. *Exp. Neurol.,* 48:201–221.
65. Price, D. D., and Dubner, R. (1977): Neurons that subserve the sensory–discriminative aspects of pain. *Pain,* 3:307–338.
66. Price, D. D., Dubner, R., and Hu, J. W. (1976): Trigeminothalamic neurons in nucleus caudalis responsive to tactile, thermal, and nociceptive stimulation of the monkey's face. *J. Neurophysiol.,* 39:936–953.
67. Price, D. D., Hayes, R. L., Ruda, M., and Dubner, R. (1978): Spatial and temporal transformation of input to spinothalamic tract neurons and their relation to somatic sensation. *J. Neurophysiol. (in press).*
68. Price, D. D., Hu, J. W., Dubner, R., and Gracely, R. (1977): Peripheral suppression of first pain and central summation of second pain evoked by noxious heat pulses. *Pain,* 3:57–68.
69. Price, D. D., and Mayer, D. J. (1975): Neurophysiological characterization of the anterolateral quadrant neurons subserving pain in *M. mulatta. Pain,* 1:59–72.
70. Price, D. D., and Wagman, I. H. (1970): The physiological roles of A and C-fiber input to the dorsal horn of *M. mulatta. Exp. Neurol.,* 29:373–390.
71. Rexed, B. (1952): The cytoarchitectonic organization of the spinal cord in the cat. *J. Comp. Neurol.,* 96:415–496.
72. Richardson, D. E., and Akil, H. (1977): Pain reduction by electrical brain stimulation in man. II. Chronic self-administration in the periventricular gray matter. *J. Neurosurg.,* 47:184–194.
73. Sano, K., Yoshioka, M., Ogashiwa, M., Ishijima, B., and Ohye, C. (1966): Thalamolaminotomy: A new operation for relief of intractable pain. *Confin. Neurol.,* 27:63–66.
74. Schvarcz, J. R. (1977): Periaqueductal mesencephalotomy for facial central pain. In: *Neurosurgical Treatment in Psychiatry, Pain and Epilepsy,* edited by W. H. Sweet, S. Obrador, and J. G. Martin-Rodriguez, pp. 661–667. University Park Press, Baltimore.
75. Smith, M. C. (1976): Retrograde cell changes in human spinal cord after anterolateral cordotomies. Location and identification after different periods of survival. In: *Advances in Pain Research and Therapy, Vol 1: Proceedings of the First World Congress on Pain,* edited by J. J. Bonica and D. Albe-Fessard, pp. 91–98. Raven Press, New York.
76. Torebjörk, H. E. (1974): Afferent C units responding to mechanical, thermal and chemical stimuli in human non-glabrous skin. *Acta Physiol. Scand.,* 92:374–390.
77. Torebjörk, H. E., and Hallin, R. G. (1973): Perceptual changes accompanying controlled preferential blocking of A and C fibre responses in intact human nerves. *Exp. Brain Res.,* 16:321–332.

78. VaHees, J., and Gybels, J. M. (1972): Pain related to single afferent C fibers from human skin. *Brain Res.,* 48:397–400.
79. White, J. C., and Sweet, W. H. (1969): *Pain and the Neurosurgeon. A Forty-Year Experience.* Charles C Thomas, Springfield, Ill.
80. Willis, W. D., Trevino, D. L., Coulter, J. D., and Maunz, R. A. (1974): Responses of primate spinothalamic tract neurons to natural stimulation of hindlimb. *J. Neurophysiol.,* 37:358–372.

Mechanisms of Pain and Analgesic Compounds,
edited by R. F. Beers, Jr., and E. G. Bassett.
Raven Press, New York © 1979.

6. Current Status of Neuroaugmentation Procedures for Chronic Pain

Don M. Long

Department of Neurosurgery, The Johns Hopkins University School of Medicine, Baltimore, Maryland 21205

INTRODUCTION

The past 10 years have brought dramatic changes in the therapy of chronic pain. Prior to that time, interest in the problem of chronic pain was limited primarily to neurosurgeons who carried out destructive procedures, anesthesiologists who performed nerve blocks, and a few individuals who proposed comprehensive multidisciplinary programs for the evaluation and treatment of such patients. Information about pain was primarily procedure oriented whether these procedures were surgical, percutaneous, or psychotherapeutic. There was little understanding about the differences between acute pain, cancer pain, and chronic pain of benign origin. In 1965, the publication (26) of the "Gate" theory of pain perception kindled an interest in pain research and therapy that is burgeoning today. The concept of neuroaugmentation grew out of the attempts to apply the Gate theory of pain to clinical practice. Shealy and Sweet (44,51) independently developed a concept of implantable neural stimulators in an attempt to apply the principles of the Gate theory to the treatment of chronic pain. Sweet and Wepsic's efforts (48,49) focused on the peripheral nervous system, whereas Shealy and co-workers (44,47,49) chose to attempt to stimulate the spinal cord. Experiences with implantable stimulators led to the concept of transcutaneously applied afferent stimulation. The possibility of stimulation at other nervous system levels for pain control naturally followed these initial pioneering efforts.

Those individuals interested in applying and investigating these devices joined together early to form a national study group. This study group has continued to function to the present time although the format has changed. Regular meetings have been held to discuss the various forms of electrical stimulation and to exchange information concerning the techniques being employed. Since the initial enthusiasm for neuroaugmentation, the use of these devices has been limited to a relatively small number of neurosurgeons interested in the problem of chronic pain, and the approach has been reasonably uniform.

It is of interest that the concept of a comprehensive multidisciplinary pain program originated and popularized by J. J. Bonica was not to have a major impact on pain therapy in the United States until the wave of enthusiasm that accompanied the development of the various implantable stimulators for chronic pain. Much of the success in the development of pain treatment programs in the United States in the past 10 years can be related to the increased understanding of chronic pain that has paralleled the experience with the use of neuroaugmentation devices. Most individuals seriously involved in the explorations of these therapeutic techniques have come to understand Bonica's thesis that chronic pain is an extremely complicated phenomena and that patient selection is probably the most important aspect of neuroaugmentation.

This chapter attempts to outline important factors in patient selection as currently practiced at The Johns Hopkins Pain Treatment Center and briefly summarizes the current status of neuroaugmentation procedures in the therapeutic armamentarium for chronic pain.

PATIENT SELECTION

The first important aspect of patient selection is accurate diagnosis, which means that the underlying disease state causing the pain must be clearly defined. This should include an accurate physical diagnosis with all underlying factors, an accurate psychological diagnosis, and complete social and vocational history to elucidate factors that may be important in the way the patient perceives and reacts to the pain. The diagnostic criteria must be rigorous. Such euphemisms as chronic low back syndrome must be avoided. If the diagnosis of herniated lumbar or cervical disk is made, then the selection criteria must be strict. When lumbar or cervical spondylolysis is diagnosed as the cause of the patient's pain, then the relationships must be clear-cut and the therapy specifically designed to correct a specific problem that is clearly causing the pain. Operations on lumbar disks without clear-cut indications are unwarranted. Operations for lumbar or cervical spondylolysis should be carried out only when stringent physical criteria are met and complete psychiatric evaluations have been performed. These criteria must be particularly strict in the case of third party liability or when an industrial accident is the root of the problem.

The evaluation of the psychiatric and psychosocial problem that these patients have must be equally rigorous (46). It is especially important to remember that the patient suffering from the "failed back" syndrome who has been subjected to multiple operations may very well have had a psychiatric cause of the pain in the first place, and this has only been complicated by the addition of multiple surgical procedures. The original operation may have been unwarranted and, therefore, it is unlikely that the subsequent procedures would have an effect on the patient's pain.

The psychological evaluation should include a complete psychosocial history. Remarkable social problems often are at the root of chronic pain syndromes and before any therapy is undertaken, it is necessary to elucidate their nature in detail. Complete psychological testing is equally important. At The Johns Hopkins Pain Treatment Center, we currently utilize a special battery of tests:

the Hendler Pain Perception Test; the Adjective Check List; the California Psychological Inventory; the Melzack Pain Questionnaire; the Symptom Check List; the Minnesota Multiphasic Personality Inventory; and the Folstein Mini-Mental Examination. A complete psychiatric evaluation is important, and then the examining physician's assessment of the pain, its anatomical distribution, and character will be helpful. There are several important facts to remember. Virtually all patients with chronic pain have chronic anxiety states and become depressed. These states do not indicate an underlying psychiatric disturbance, but may simply result from the pain itself. Furthermore, the classic conversion-V of the Minnesota Multiphasic Personality Inventory may be nothing more than a patient who has begun with scales elevated and has had satisfactory therapy of the center scale which is depression. Far from being an abnormality, it represents the first step to therapy in an otherwise typical patient with chronic pain.

At The Johns Hopkins Medical Institutions, these psychiatric and psychosocial evaluations are now synthesized to provide a rating of each patient. We currently employ a purely arbitrary patient classification in order to guide the choice of therapy. The first classification is termed *objective,* which consists of patients who have a demonstrable somatic pain generator and whose behavior and psychiatric evaluation is appropriate to that cause of pain. These are patients who may be candidates for interventional procedures. The second category of patients are termed the *exaggerated pain response.* These people may have a somatic pain generator, but their response to the pain is greatly exaggerated. Most patients with industrial commission problems fall, in our experience, in this class. The disability and reports of pain are completely out of character with anything that can be observed or discovered by physical examination. The third class we employ is termed *affective* or *psychiatric.* These patients appear to have pain as an expression of psychiatric disease. Obviously, such patients are not candidates for interventional procedures in the treatment of pain.

Patients are further categorized according to the four stages of development of chronic disease. These stages in pain appear to be similar to those which occur in life-threatening diseases. The first or acute stage occurs immediately after the painful process begins. Patients in this phase are generally anxious to find a magic cure and do not wish to hear any explanation of the process that will not lead to cure usually without any effort on their part. They are particularly prone to accept advice for surgery during this phase and often go from physician to physician seeking the one who has the easy answer for them. The second, or subacute phase, is characterized by hostility and anger. These patients are resentful of both their disability and the medical profession for not curing them and usually are embroiled in a social–vocational problem that feeds this hostility. It is particularly important to determine this phase, for these individuals become very litigious. The third stage is characterized by depression. It is in this phase that the patients present with a full-blown pain neurosis. They become seriously depressed, exhibit severe chronic anxiety, and abuse drugs. It is unlikely that the patients or physicians can determine the value of any therapy for pain unless this stage is successfully treated. The fourth and final stage is that of acceptance. During this stage, patients have come to grips with their disability and are able to understand and accept rational treatment programs.

The first aim of patient selection is to identify those patients with objective pain problems that require treatment. Patients with exaggerated pain responses are rarely candidates for any interventional procedure, and those with affective disorders are certainly not likely to benefit from any interventional technique. The application of interventional procedures to a patient who is not yet able to accept the disease and its treatment is inappropriate.

The second aim of patient selection is to bring the patient selected as a potential candidate for a procedure to the optimal state for having the procedure done. This requires manipulation and elimination of such things in the patient's environment as drug abuse, habituation, and addiction. As long as the patient remains addicted to a narcotic, it is not possible for either the physician or the patient to determine the level of pain. While no definitive studies have been done, except with implantable brain stimulators, it also appears likely that the use of narcotics will interfere with the techniques of neuroaugmentation. Habituation to other drugs such as diazepam (Valium ®) is equally disruptive. The discomfort that results from withdrawal symptoms will seriously interfere with the ability of the pain team to determine how much pain an individual patient has and whether a specific treatment is helpful.

The next aim of this phase of treatment is to improve activity levels by establishing a reasonable goal for an individual patient. If a patient's goals are unreasonable, either too high or too low, the therapy may either disappoint him (although it has, in fact, been very successful) or he may not function at a level that the success of therapy should allow. For most patients, it is also necessary to carry out extensive psychotherapy during this period of time. Most have had their lives so disrupted by the pain that a great deal of effort should be expended in the therapeutic aspects of the problem. In many cases, even patients with objective pain problems can be taught to accept the disability, to minimize it by their own activities and thought processes, so that the need for further interventional procedures will be obviated.

Following the complete psychiatric evaluation of these patients and the establishment of an adequate diagnosis, it is obvious that a specific procedure should be employed, if available, rather than carrying out a neuroaugmentative procedure. However, in most instances, no specific procedures are available. In this case, the next step should be a careful trial of transcutaneously applied afferent stimulation. When transcutaneous stimulation is satisfactory, then no other procedures should be utilized. The Johns Hopkins Program does not use this method as a predictor for success of an implantable stimulator. In the event that it is not completely satisfactory for pain relief, then percutaneous stimulation of the area of the nervous system where implant might be used is carried out to determine if there is satisfactory relief of pain before implantation is undertaken. The technical aspects of these temporary stimulations are discussed in more detail in a later section.

The implantation of a neuroaugmentation device is undertaken only after the complete psychiatric assessment is available, and all secondary aspects of the pain neurosis are under satisfactory therapy. Implantations are not used when transcutaneous electrical stimulation is satisfactory, and permanent implants are not employed until the temporary devices give evidence that excellent pain control will be obtained.

SPECIFIC TECHNIQUES OF NEUROAUGMENTATION

Transcutaneous Electrical Stimulation of the Nervous System

Electrical stimulation for the relief of pain is an ancient technique. Taub and Kane (50) have reported the use of the electric fishes to provide pain relief in Greek and Roman days. Soon after electricity was harnessed to be controllable, medical applications appeared. The history of electrical stimulation from 1750 through 1900 is a curious mix of experimentation, accurate scientific reporting, and charlatanism. In this century, electrical stimulation has been used for the relief of postoperative abdominal pain and ileus, pain of peripheral nerve injury origin, trigeminal neuralgia, and labor pain. Nevertheless, there was little clinical use of the technique at the time that the Gate theory of pain was published (21,22,43). Interest was rekindled in transcutaneous electrical stimulation primarily by those individuals searching for predictive techniques to improve the utilization of implanted neuroaugmentation devices. However, early experience of several investigators indicated that transcutaneously applied electrical stimulation might be of real benefit as a treatment modality. Two firms produced well-designed electrical stimulators using modern engineering principles and following the prototype designed by Hagfors. Long and Carolan (22) first reported the results of a large patient survey utilizing transcutaneous stimulation as the major treatment modality. Shealy, Ebersold, and Picaza all reported large groups of patients who were able to utilize transcutaneous electrical stimulation for pain relief (6b,35,43). Nathan and Rudge (32) reported a success rate of approximately 40% for the relief of postherpetic neuralgia and the thalamic syndrome. The majority of these early studies (5,19,22) are surveys of large numbers of patients. The problem of control for any pain treatment modality is a difficult one. These studies represent the application of a technique to a large number of patients suffering from what would have previously been intractable pain. Given all diagnoses and all psychiatric and drug abuse problems, the overall success rates reported were approximately one-third of patients achieving good pain relief. Long and Carolan (22) reviewed 104 patients after 1 year of stimulator use and found that there was no apparent fall away in pain relief. Hundreds of articles on transcutaneous stimulation have been written.

It is now appreciated that the control of psychiatric and drug problems in patients with chronic pain and the application of the techniques to those patients with primarily somatic pain problems greatly improve results. Long has now carried out a study of 300 consecutive patients in the context of a chronic pain treatment program, and the results are seen in Table 1. It is obvious that when patients are carefully selected with elimination of those patients whose problems are compounded by serious psychiatric difficulties, or who continue to misuse medications and exhibit significant symptoms of pain neurosis, the success rates of the technique are greatly improved. Patients with pain of peripheral nerve injury origin, amputation stump pain, neuroma pain, postherpetic neuralgia, and mild forms of phantom limb syndrome appear to be the best candidates for this procedure. Patients with pain complaints who are least likely to succeed in obtaining relief with transcutaneous electrical stimulation include those with pain of major exaggerated or psychogenic components, the central pain states, and metabolic peripheral neuropathies.

Success of transcutaneous electrical stimulation in pain relief is significantly greater in patients who do not fall in the category of the pain neurotic. When pain is not complicated by psychiatric factors, drug misuse or abuse, and multiple operations, significantly greater results can be expected. Although the use of transcutaneous electrical stimulation in routine physical therapy appears to be increasing, there are few specific papers that detail the value of the technique.

The third area in which transcutaneous electrical stimulation appears to have significant merit is in the relief of postoperative pain. Postoperative pain was

TABLE 1. *Efficacy of transcutaneous electrical stimulation[a]*

No. of patients	Diagnosis or modality	Relief in treatment period (%)		
		1 day	3 days	1 month
50 ⎫ Blind	TNS[b]	94	67	—
50 ⎬ crossover	Subliminal TNS	37	11	—
50 ⎭ study	Batteryless TNS	8	0	—
175	Multiple low back procedures	80	45	35
40	Multiple cervical procedures	80	40	33
11	Phantom limb pain	94	80	70
20	Neuroma, peripheral nerve pain	94	90	80
22 pain of muscle	Acute spinal pain	87	87	—
20 spasm origin	Chronic spinal pain (1 operation or less)	85	85	85
12	Postherpetic neuralgia	75	48	48

[a] 300 Patients in a comprehensive pain treatment center with satisfactory relief—50% or more.

[b] Transcutaneous neural stimulation.

first treated by Hymes and associates (14). Their retrospective analysis of cases indicated a significant reduction in narcotic usage and elimination of ileus as a complication in patients undergoing thoracotomy and laparotomy with the use of transcutaneous electrical stimulation. Prospective studies by now clearly demonstrate that postoperative pain can be controlled effectively with transcutaneous electrical stimulation. Currently, the major drawbacks are the lack of both completely satisfactory prepackaged sterile electrodes and trained personnel to apply the techniques. Relief of pain and reduction in the complications of ileus and atelectasis appear to be well demonstrated (14).

Percutaneous Stimulation of the Nervous System

Percutaneous electrical stimulation of the nervous system is used in a predictive fashion. Stimulation of the peripheral nerves or the spinal cord can be used to determine the value of an implantable stimulator. Percutaneous stimulation of the peripheral nerves is carried out in exactly the same fashion that would be utilized for conventional nerve block. The patient is prepared in the same way, but instead of the usual needle and injection technique, an electrode system is placed near the nerves. A percutaneous cordotomy electrode and 17 gauge thin-walled needle is perfectly satisfactory. Care must be taken not to deliver a large electrical current through the needle since its tip represents a point source. The needle is placed near the nerve to be stimulated, but not in it. Any convenient nerve stimulator can then be used. Strength of stimulation is increased until paresthesias are elicited and stimulation is continued for a variable period of time. Usually, stimulation is kept at less than 45 min, although longer stimulations at low current level are perfectly acceptable. The patient should achieve pain relief during stimulation without temporary loss of neurological function. If the stimulation is carried out long enough or at high enough levels, it is possible to produce analgesia, complete anesthesia, or complete paralysis of nerve function. Usually, this does not occur with less than 45 min of stimulation. The best predictor for the success of an implantable peripheral nerve stimulator is relief that persists several hours beyond the stimulation.

Percutaneous stimulation of the spinal cord is equally simple. Its only purpose is to predict the value of an implanted spinal cord stimulator for pain relief (12). The patient is prepared as for any spinal or epidural puncture and the procedure is carried out with the patient in the prone position, using fluoroscopy for control of electrode placement. Aseptic technique is used and an epidural puncture is made in any convenient location that will allow passage of the electrode into the appropriate area of the spinal cord. Since the usual candidate for the spinal cord stimulator suffers from lumbar arachnoiditis, it is most common that the puncture is made in the L-1 L-2, L-2 L-3 area. Using fluoroscopic control, the electrode is passed through the needle and directed into the midline over the dorsum of the spinal cord. A monopolar system can be used with a single electrode and an externally placed ground; it is also possible to pass two electrodes to allow bipolar stimulation. Following accurate placement of the electrode using fluoroscopic control, stimulation is carried out to make certain that it is felt in the area where the pain is located. The electrode is then manipulated until adequate stimulation is perceived by the patient. The parameters of stimulation are usually less than 10 V with a pulse width of 1 msec or less and a frequency of 60 to 100 Hz. When the electrode is accurately positioned, the needle is withdrawn and the electrode sutured in place with a single stitch through the skin. The stimulator can then be used for several days with the patient ambulating in whatever fashion would usually precipitate the pain. This allows an accurate assessment of whether a stimulator will be of lasting value in pain relief. After the stimulation trial is over, the electrode is simply pulled out and the trial discontinued. In our initial trials, 26 of 31 patients achieved 6 months of pain relief following permanent spinal cord stimulator implantation after percutaneous stimulation suggested that the permanent procedure would be of value. A later study (34) carried out at 2 years indicates that 40 to 50 patients so chosen have achieved pain relief when their stimulators are functional.

It must be stressed that percutaneous stimulation of peripheral nerves and the spinal cord is a diagnostic test at this point. Its purpose is to predict the success or failure of implantable stimulating devices. It appears that good pain relief obtained with percutaneous stimulation techniques predicts a good result for an implantable stimulator. However, it is not certain that long-term pain relief will be obtained with an implantable device. No one has attempted the negative correlation of the success of implantable devices in patients who fail to achieve success with percutaneous techniques.

IMPLANTABLE PERIPHERAL NERVE STIMULATORS

Sweet and associates (47,48,51) were the first to suggest long-term stimulation of peripheral nerves for the control of pain. The first commercially available stimulators utilized for the relief of nerve injury pain were implanted by Long in 1969 (20). Picaza et al. (35) was the first to attempt the relief of pain by stimulation of nerves remote from the area of pain. The initial successes with this technique were promising (6a). Campbell and Long (4) have recently reviewed all of their personal data from peripheral nerve implants for pain relief, and these data are summarized in Table 2. Although only a few researchers have utilized this technique, the available data certainly indicate that the implantation of a stimulator on a peripheral nerve for pain secondary to injury of that nerve is an effective technique (27). The best results have been obtained with pain of ulnar nerve origin. Sciatic stimulation has been slightly less successful. Only a few stimulators have been placed on median and peroneal or tibial nerves, but the results appear to be satisfactory. Brachial plexus stimulation has been less useful, but has been employed primarily for less well-defined pain states than peripheral injury. Review of the available data indicates that the majority of brachial plexus stimulators have been put in place for causalgia-

TABLE 2. *Satisfactory relief with implantable peripheral nerve stimulators*

Site (no. of implants)	Results
Ulnar 5	5 Excellent
Median 2	1 Excellent
	1 Removed
Brachial plexus 10	3 Excellent
	1 Satisfactory
	3 Failures
	2 Initial successes; failure after 2 years
	1 Excellent, but side effects unpleasant
Sciatic 17 [a]	4 Satisfactory
	13 Failures

[a] All were done for pain remote from nerve; procedure has now been discontinued. Excellent relief initially (6 months), then gradual failure.

like syndromes secondary to unusual injury of the upper extremity. Many of these patients have been helped by the implanted stimulator, but the results are not as dramatic as with straightforward peripheral nerve injury (4).

The implantable peripheral nerve stimulator consists of a cuff electrode attached to a small radiofrequency remote receiver. The surgical procedure is generally carried out under general anesthesia. The electrode must be implanted proximal to the site of injury or origin of pain. A straightforward exposure of the nerve sufficient to allow the cuff electrode to be easily placed around the nerve is all that is necessary. The lead wire is tunneled subcutaneously to a convenient place for the radioreceiver. For upper extremity implant, the subclavicular space is usually chosen, whereas posterior iliac fossa is most commonly used for lower extremity implants. The patient controls the degree of stimulation be an external power supply coupled to the implanted slave by means of an antenna attached to the skin with an adhesive disk. This general system is in use for all of the implantable devices and only the electrode configurations vary significantly.

Use of the electrical stimulators for pain remote from the distribution of the peripheral nerve has not been proven to be of long-term value. Such techniques appear to relieve pain very satisfactorily initially, but there is a gradual disappearance of effectiveness, and within 6 months, the pain relief is generally dissipated. The same appears to be true in employing sciatic nerve stimulation for intractable sciatica. In this case, the stimulator is placed distal to the area of injury of the nerve. Such patients usually suffering from traumatic neuritis secondary to disk herniation and surgery will routinely respond to the temporary stimulation of the sciatic nerve at the notch. Implantation of a peripheral nerve stimulator in the same area will also relieve these patients for a significant period of time. However, it is our experience that this relief of pain will gradually fail and, except in unusual circumstances, the sciatic nerve stimulator is no longer used for this type of patient (4).

There are several interesting points in regard to use of these stimulators. The first observation is that the duration of pain relief often far exceeds the time of stimulation. It is not unusual for such a patient to achieve long-lasting pain relief with a short period of stimulation often lasting only a few hours. Another interesting characteristic of this phenomenon is that it usually increases with time. After such patients have had a stimulator in place for 6 to 12 months, it is common for them to use it less and less in order to achieve pain relief (1). However, most such patients continue to require some stimulation even though it may be at irregular intervals. The third interesting point is the failure of peripheral nerve stimulation to relieve pain when applied distal to the area of pain. This certainly suggests that the beneficial effects of peripheral nerve stimulation on pain are local and not central (15).

STIMULATION OF THE SPINAL CORD

Stimulation of the spinal cord for relief of pain was introduced by Shealy et al. in 1967 (28,44,45). He first carried out a series of implants using a prototype for stimulation of the posterior surface of the spinal cord. Initial success in patients with intractable pain complicating terminal malignancy encouraged Shealy to treat chronic pain of benign origin. A number of other investigators began to evaluate these devices in the treatment of chronic pain. A national study group was formed under the auspices of one of the manufacturers, and careful evaluation of the results was undertaken.

The initial implantable devices were passive radiofrequency receivers that could be implanted subcutaneously and attached to a variety of electrode forms, which could be placed over the dorsal surface of the spinal cord. Both monopolar and bipolar systems were available and the electrode design varied greatly. All utilized a remote external power supply coupled to the implanted device by means of an antenna applied to the skin. A laminectomy was required to implant the device over the dorsal surface of the spinal cord. Virtually every anatomical placement over the entire length of the spinal cord was employed. Electrodes were placed in the subdural, intradural, and extradural locations. After Shealy, Nashold and Friedman (31) were the first to report an extensive experience with these devices. The national study group continued its evaluation of efficacy from its origin in 1970 until December 1973 when an international symposium[1] was held to study the efficacy of the devices implanted up to that period of time. Virtually, all of the researchers (2,6,8,13,16–18,23,30,33,36,39,49) who had treated a significant number of patients participated in the conference. Shealy (24) presented data suggesting that the total relief of pain occurred in 15% of patients and that satisfactory relief was achieved in 31%. Long and Erickson (23) reported similar data with complete relief of pain occurring in 19% and satisfactory relief in 30%. Burton's figures (2) were somewhat better with satisfac-

---

[1] Minneapolis Pain Seminar, December 6–8, 1973.

tory relief of pain occurring in 58%. Review of the data by Burton and Hosobuchi et al. also reported satisfactory relief of pain in slightly more than 50% of the patients (24). A summary of the data available at that time indicated that the so-called dorsal column stimulation by the techniques then in use provided satisfactory relief of pain in slightly over 50% of patients (24).

However, there are several important factors that must be elaborated upon. First is the fact that this was a completely unselected group of patients. There was little understanding of the psychodynamics of chronic pain, few psychiatrists were interested in the problem, and the importance of drug addiction was not appreciated at the time. It is probable that a significant number of the patients who were treated with a dorsal column stimulator would now be rejected as candidates for such a device. However, it is possible to make this statement only after significant advances in the understanding of chronic pain have been made. At the time, these multiple factors that influenced the success of any pain treatment were not known. The second major factor relates to the technique employed. A success rate of slightly over 50% in patients for whom there is no other therapy available is respectable, but the major operation required to achieve this success rate and the complications of this operation discouraged most of the investigators in the field from continuing this form of spinal cord stimulation. Fortunately, just at the time that these data were becoming available, a major technical breakthrough occurred (1,3). Flexible wire stimulating electrodes that could be implanted percutaneously for efficacy trials became available. It was soon possible to implant permanent electrodes by the same percutaneous technique, thus obviating the need for a major operation. When percutaneous epidural electrodes became available, a success rate of 50% or greater was suddenly much more acceptable. It is one thing to achieve a success rate of 50% with an operation requiring general anesthesia and laminectomy, but it is completely different when the same or a better success rate can be achieved with a minor procedure that can be done under a local anesthesia and for which no significant complications resulting in major neurological deficit have yet been reported.

The new epidural technique was quite different from the implantation of a dorsal column stimulator via laminectomy. In this situation, the patient does not require an anesthetic and is positioned on an operating table with fluoroscopic control available. Tuohy needles are inserted into the epidural space at two levels (usually at L-1 L-2 and L-2 L-3) and flexible wire electrodes are slipped into the epidural space and positioned in the midline so that good stimulation of the entire painful area can be obtained. Any temporary electrical stimulator can be used to satisfactorily position the electrodes. An incision is then made around the needles, the needles withdrawn, and a temporary portion of the electrode brought out through a separate stab wound. The permanent electrode is sutured into position and the wound closed so that the only portion which is externalized is the temporary portion that will later be discarded. A temporary electrical stimulator can then be attached and the patient is allowed to ambulate to be certain that electrode position is proper. If pain relief is satisfactory and the position of the electrodes appears to be optimal, it is possible to complete the procedure after several days. Again, under local anesthesia, a lateral flank incision is made in the posterior iliac space and the electrodes exposed. The temporary portions are disconnected from the electrodes and the radio receiver is implanted and attached. North et al. (34) have reported on the results of 31 patients treated with these systems; 23 to 26 of them could be considered to have achieved satisfactory pain relief. Burton (1) has also presented similar data with the use of epidural electrical stimulation. The major problems with the epidural technique appear to be a slightly increased risk of infection when the temporary externalization is utilized and the propensity of the electrodes to move. In the series reported by North et al., it was necessary to revise the electrode system 36 times. Each revision requires hospitalization and a minor operative procedure. This technical problem must be solved if the epidural stimulators are to achieve widespread success (37,38).

Several investigators have attempted to stimulate other surfaces of the spinal cord for pain relief. D. Erickson *(unpublished observations)* has reported the placement of stimulators on the anterior surface of the spinal cord in the cervical region usually through a transdiscal approach. Preliminary results in a few patients were encouraging, but no long-term follow-ups are available for discussion. Larson and associates (18) have utilized electrode placements both in front of and behind the cord. None of the published data indicates that the success rate is significantly higher than that enjoyed by epidural electrical stimulation, and the procedures are much more complex (18).

There is now sufficient experience in human implantations to estimate some of the problems and risks. The original potential complications related to the acute implantation of dorsal column stimulators have been discussed (7a). Although the list is impressive in its length, the total number of complications reported by most authors is small. Epidural electrical stimulation has potential hazards, but, to date, infection has been the only significant complication. There has been no reported incidence of neurological deficit from the implantation of the device. The major problem with epidural electrical stimulation clearly is the potential for movement of the electrodes, which occurs with enough regularity that it will limit the applicability of this technique for the treatment of chronic pain until the movement problem can be solved. Another major area of difficulty is the mechanical and electrical failures of the devices. These failures are not common early after implantation, but within a few years they seem to occur more and more frequently. The most likely problem appears to be a break in the electrode with subsequent corrosion of the system by body fluid (3).

As yet, there is no evidence that long-term stimulation of the nervous system is detrimental. Peripheral nerve, spinal cord, and brain stimulators have now been implanted for many years and there are no reports of late complications or deterioration of neurological function. Nevertheless, the long-term effects still have not been completely studied and will not be for many years. It is important that these patients be followed to ensure that no late untoward effects occur. It is not yet certain what percentage of these devices may fail because of the many manufacturing changes that have occurred over their years of use (3,7a).

The reported information concerning efficacy is difficult to synthesize. In the early days, these devices were used for pain of many origins without, what would now be considered, adequate psychiatric evaluation or control of habituating drugs. The importance of the psychiatric aspects of chronic pain and the influences of drugs were simply not understood at that time. In this completely unselected group of patients (many of whom would now be rejected as candidates for stimulator implant or at least would have other techniques employed before stimulator implantation), the results are still reasonable. It appears that slightly over 50% of such patients with otherwise untreatable chronic pain can be relieved by dorsal column stimulation. Improved methods of patient selection and the application of the experience of many years with the devices have allowed some investigators to achieve significantly greater results than these. Burton (1–3) has reported a success rate of slightly greater than 70%. North et al. (34) originally reported 26 of 31 patients achieving satisfactory relief with epidural electrical stimulation. The average follow-up of this report was less than 1 year. Subsequent evaluations at 2 years indicate that those patients who have functional stimulators continue to achieve excellent pain relief. The complicating factor has been the need for revision. Failure has been frequent enough in some patients to significantly reduce the effectiveness of the pain relief and the attractiveness of the technique because of the need for repeated hospitalization and revisions of the system. If these technical problems can be solved, it appears that epidural electrical stimulation can be a very valuable technique when applied to patients who have been carefully selected and whose ancillary pain problems have received adequate attention (24).

BRAIN STIMULATION

The most exciting technique for relief of intractable pain is long-term stimulation of the brain via stereotactically implanted electrodes. The origins of chronic brain stimulation for the relief of pain originated in the Gate Control Theory, the pioneering work of Delgado, and the ablative procedures carried out by many investigators. With this foundation in neurosurgery, it is not surprising that attempts to stimulate the brain for pain relief emerged almost simultaneously with the advent of dorsal column, stimulation (7). Several investigators (9–11, 24,29,40–42) independently began explorations of stimulation throughout the thalamus for pain relief. Hosobuchi et al. (10) were first to describe satisfactory pain relief from stimulation within the sensory portions of the thalamus and in the internal capsule. Richardson and Akil (40–42) first described stimulation in the medial posterior thalamus in areas now known to be related to the opiate receptor system. Published reports are still sparse, but a recent survey of the major investigators working in the field indicates that over 150 such implants have been utilized. The overall success rate appears to be 60 to 80% (24).

The stimulators are identical to those employed for all other implantable techniques, except in electrode configuration. The electrode is a flexible wire that can be inserted with any standard stereotactic technique. There are four stimulating points on the tip of the electrode so that the different combinations of stimulating points can provide different electrical fields and activate different areas of the brain. Standard stereotactic techniques are employed. Instead of inserting a lesion-making electrode, however, the flexible stimulating electrode is passed into the desired target point. It is fixed to the periosteum and a temporary portion is externalized. In general, the side opposite the pain is chosen. For widespread pain problems or bilateral pain, the dominant side is generally used. It is then possible to stimulate the chosen target area using different electrode pairs over an extended period of time to be certain that pain relief exists.

There are three target areas currently employed for pain relief. The first is sensory radiation in the posterior limb of the internal capsule. The electrode position is chosen to provide paresthesias in the distribution of the pain. The second is the ventrobasal complex of the thalamus. Again, an appropriate area of the thalamus is chosen to provide stimulation in the painful area. The sensory thalamus is often utilized when face pain is the underlying problem. The third is in the region of the posterior commissure in the medial thalamus–periaqueductal gray region. This target area corresponds to the opiate receptor system described by Snyder (45a). In general, stimulation in the specific sensory system is chosen for deafferentation pain states, whereas stimulation in the opiate receptor system is utilized for other kinds of pain (7,9–11,40–42). However, G. Gucer and D. M. Long *(unpublished observations)* have achieved satisfactory pain relief in patients with thalamic syndrome following stimulating in the opiate receptor system.

It appears that thalamic stimulation is virtually the only therapy that is likely to be of value for the thalamic syndrome, otherwise intractable phantom limb pain, anesthesia dolorosa, pain of paraplegia, and related deafferentation syndromes. Its place in less exotic pain problems has not yet been defined. Theoretically, stimulation in the opiate receptor system should be an excellent technique for relief of cancer pain. A small number of patients with intractable pain from lumbar arachnoiditis have been successfully treated and it seems likely that the technique can be expanded to include many more categories of pain than have been treated to date. The mechanism of action of thalamic stimulation is certainly not fully known; it appears that stimulation in sensory pathways is different from stimulation in the opiate receptor–catecholamine system. In the former system, there may very well be a gating phenomenon. However, in the latter it seems likely that the effect is chemical (9,40–42). Several factors make this probable. First, the pain relief obtained by stimulation in the opiate receptor system often requires some time to develop. Pain relief can be fatigued by overstimulation. Narcotic intake appears to obviate the success of the technique, and analgesia obtained by thalamic stimulation can be reversed by naloxone. Furthermore, it has been reported that stimulation in the posterior thalamus increases third ventricular concentration of enkephalin. Although none of these data are conclusive, they certainly suggest that the pain relief obtained by stimulation in the opiate receptor system is a chemically mediated phenomenon (25).

The overall success rate of brain stimulation appears to be excellent. A minimal number of complications have occurred, although the possibility of serious complications certainly exists with passage of electrodes into critical areas of the brain. Brain stimulation is a valuable technique for the treatment of deafferentative pain states for which no other therapy exists. It appears likely that this will be one of the most valuable techniques of pain therapy.

DISCUSSION

Afferent stimulation for the relief of chronic pain has now been in use for almost 10 years. Its use has been widespread for 5 to 7 years, and a great deal of information is now available (24). There is little question that transcutaneous electrical stimulation is a valuable treatment modality for many pain states. Its use in postoperative pain certainly appears to warrant wider utilization. The technique is gradually being expanded into other acute pain states, particularly those which traditionally require physical therapy. A broad, although still largely anecdotal, experience indicates success in the treatment of the acute low back and acute cervical syndromes. Implantable stimulators for peripheral nerve stimulation are also very valuable. Their use appears to be limited to pain of peripheral nerve injury origin. Even the unusual pain states that are generally thought to come from peripheral nerve injury, such as the reflex sympathetic dystrophies or causalgia-like syndrome, are not always relieved by peripheral nerve stimulation. Fortunately, it is possible to predict with reasonable certainty whether an implantable stimulator will be valuable with the use of temporary percutaneous stimulation. No published data currently available substantiates the original belief that peripheral nerve stimulation was of value in the relief of pain remote from the distribution of the nerve being stimulated.

Spinal cord stimulation is a complex subject that is difficult to analyze. Many variables must be considered in deciding about the value of the technique. A review of the literature suggests that an overall success rate of slightly greater than 50% was obtained by the use of spinal cord stimulation in the form of the initial dorsal column stimulator. However, in considering the value of the technique, it must be remembered that the dorsal column stimulator was implanted into patients for whom no other pain therapy was available. Another important factor was the lack of appreciation of the deleterious psychiatric effects of chronic pain. Furthermore, no one understood the problems of narcotic addiction in interpreting the results of therapy. A combination of factors have now rejuvenated spinal cord stimulation as a treatment for chronic pain. Much improved psychiatric evaluation is available and the psychiatric effects of chronic pain are much better understood. Narcotic addiction is now recognized as a relative contraindication to implantation of a stimulator, and it is possible to test a patient by temporary percutaneous stimulation of the spinal cord. When all of these factors predict a good result, pain relief is achieved more than 80% of the time on a short-term basis. There are significant technical factors with the spinal epidural stimulator that make it difficult to obtain optimal function in every patient consistently, but the technique still is very valuable, particularly for patients suffering from arachnoiditis and related problems. Whether there will be a decline of efficacy with time is not yet known.

With the dorsal column stimulator, there was an apparent decrease in efficacy. However, it is not possible to state with certainty whether this represented plasticity within the nervous system or tolerance to stimulation. There were so many uncontrolled factors in the original studies with the dorsal column stimulator that it is simply not possible to state the cause of the apparent decline in efficacy over 3 to 5 years. Studies are currently under way with epidural stimulation that should answer this question.

The stimulation within the thalamus is efficacious, particularly for a group of patients with deafferentative syndromes for whom virtually nothing else is available. The number of investigators working in this field has been small, but results obtained by them are good, varying between 60 and 80%. Brain stimulation clearly should be limited to a highly selected group of patients and carried out only by those individuals with the capabilities for complicated stereotactic surgery. Nevertheless, it appears to be one of the most successful techniques of neuroaugmentation and clearly deserves wider application.

The effects of neuroaugmentation procedures on the disordered physiology of the patient in chronic pain are still not well understood. There are no concrete data that allow anything more than theorizing, except with brain stimulation in medial thalamus. The best data currently available suggest that stimulation in the medial thalamus activates a naturally occurring opiate-like substance within the brain for the control of pain. Even this information is preliminary and not universally demonstrable.

Perhaps the most important result of neuroaugmentation in the past 3 years has been the greatly improved understanding of the chronic pain process. When the implantable stimulators were first utilized in pain treatment, little was known about the psychiatry of chronic pain. The effects of narcotics on stimulator function and on the assessment of pain in general were certainly not well understood, and very few comprehensive pain programs were available for patient referral. Now, it is evident that the neuroaugmentation procedure should be utilized in patients that have been completely evaluated and carefully screened through comprehensive pain evaluation and treatment. In The Johns Hopkins Pain Treatment Program, it is the practice to carry out accurate diagnosis, complete psychiatric assessment, and implement the full pain treatment program before making a decision for any interventional procedure. Neuroaugmentation procedures are used in a small number of patients and only after careful patient selection. It is quite obvious that a neural stimulator is not appropriate therapy for pain that is largely psychiatric in origin, and those patients should be directed to proper psychiatric therapy. Likewise, neuroaugmentation is not appropriate to the exaggerated or operant pain problems. Appropriate treatment within the context of the Pain Treatment Program is necessary, but in general it would be inappropriate to employ neuroaugmentation procedures beyond transcutaneous electrical stimulation.

SUMMARY

Neuroaugmentation techniques have been employed for almost 10 years and have been in common usage for 7 years. Transcutaneous electrical stimulation is efficacious in many pain problems, particularly those that relate to peripheral nerve injury. Postoperative pain can be controlled effectively with transcutaneous electrical stimulation and it is a useful adjunct in physical therapy techniques. Percutaneous stimulation techniques are utilized to predict the effectiveness of implantable peripheral nerve or spinal cord stimulators. The peripheral nerve stimulators are highly effective for pain of peripheral nerve injury origin when patients are chosen by preliminary percutaneous stimulation techniques. The original dorsal column stimulators required laminectomy for implantation and have been largely abandoned. They have been replaced by epidural stimulating electrodes that can be implanted percutaneously to allow the patients to be tested thoroughly for efficacy before committal to an implanted device. The success of epidural stimulation has been excellent. Multiple technical factors continue to be a problem, but the technique is very useful in the intractable low back cripple. Brain stimulation has generally been reserved for the most difficult problems, particularly deafferentation syndromes. The thalamic stimulators have been very effective and the field is currently being expanded. Neuroaugmentation devices were first the subject of a great wave of enthusiasm after their introduction, but an almost equal disenchantment followed and now they appear to be reaching their potential place in the therapeutic armamentarium (38).

Neuromodulation should be employed in the context of a comprehensive pain management program. Careful patient selection should limit the application of a technique to those patients with somatic objective pain problems whose secondary features are of chronic pain. Before an implantable stimulator is used, depression and anxiety must be treated; insomnia must be eliminated as well as narcotic addiction or optimal results are not likely to be obtained. When these stimulators are employed in the context of a comprehensive pain management program, results are gratifying, and the data currently available suggest that 60 to 80% of patients with otherwise intractable pain can be satisfactorily relieved.

REFERENCES

1. Burton, C. V. (1977, 1978): Safety and clinical efficacy of implanted neuroaugmentive spinal devices for the relief of pain. *Appl. Neurophysiol.,* 40:2–4; 175–184.
2. Burton, C. V. (1975): Dorsal column stimulations: Optimization of application. *Surg. Neurol.,* 4:171–179.
3. Burton, C. V. (1975): Implanted devices for electronic augmentation of nervous system function. *Med. Instrum.,* 9:221–223.
4. Campbell, J. N., and Long, D. M. (1978): Transcutaneous electrical stimulation for pain: Efficacy and mechanism of action. In: *Seminars in Psychiatry,* edited by R. L. Katz. Grune & Stratton, New York *(in press).*
5. Cauthen, J. C., and Renner, E. (1975): Transcutaneous and peripheral nerve stimulation for chronic pain states. *Surg. Neurol.,* 4:102–105.
6. Clark, K. (1975): Electrical stimulation of the nervous system for control of pain. *Surg. Neurol.,* 4:164–167.
6a. Davis, R., and Lentini, R. (1975): Transcutaneous nerve stimulation for treatment of pain in patients with spinal cord injury. *Surg. Neurol.,* 4:100–101.
6b. Ebersold, M. J., Laws, E., Stonnington, H., and Stillwel, G. (1975): Transcutaneous electrical stimulation for treatment of chronic pain. *Surg. Neurol.,* 4:96–99.
7. Fields, H., and Adams, J. E. (1973): Pain after cortical injury relieved by electrical stimulation of the internal capsule. *Brain,* 67:169–178.
7a. Fox, J. L. (1974): Problems encountered with neuropacemakers. *Surg. Neurol.,* 2:59–64.
8. Hoppenstein, R. (1975): Electrical stimulation of the ventral and dorsal columns for relief of chronic intractable pain. *Surg. Neurol.,* 4:187–199.
9. Hosobuchi, Y., Adams, J. E., and Linchitz, R. (1977): Pain relief by electrical stimulation of the central gray matter in humans and its reversal by naloxane. *Science,* 197:183–186.
10. Hosobuchi, Y., Adams, J. E., and Rutkin, B. (1973): Chronic thalamic stimulation for the control of facial anesthesia dolorosa. *Arch. Neurol.,* 29:158–161.
11. Hosobuchi, Y., Adams, J. E., and Rutkin, B. (1973): Chronic thalamic and internal capsule stimulation for control of central pain. *Surg. Neurol.,* 4:91–93.
12. Hosobuchi, Y., Adams, J. E., and Weinstein, P. R. (1972): Preliminary percutaneous dorsal column stimulation prior to permanent implantation: Technical note. *J. Neurosurg.,* 37:242–245.
13. Hunt, W. E., Goodman, J. H., and Bingham, W. G. (1975): Stimulation of the dorsal spinal cord for treatment of intractable pain. *Surg. Neurol.,* 4:153–157.
14. Hymes, A. C., Raab, D. E., Yonehiro, E. G., Nelson, G. D., and Printy, A. L. (1974): Acute pain control by electrostimulator: A preliminary report. In: *Advances in Neurology, Vol. 4: Proceedings of the International Symposium on Pain,* edited by J. J. Bonica, pp. 761–767. Raven Press, New York.
15. Ignelzi, R. J., and Nyquist, J. (1976): Direct effect of electrical stimulation on peripheral nerve evoked activity: Implications in pain relief. *J. Neurosurg.,* 45:159–165.
16. Krainick, J. U., and Thoden, U. (1974): Experience with dorsal column stimulation (DCS) in the operative treatment of chronic intractable pain. *J. Neurosurg. Sci.,* 18:187–189.
17. Krainick, J. U., Thoden, U., and Riechert, T. (1974): Spinal cord stimulation in post-amputation pain. *Surg. Neurol.,* 4:167–171.
18. Larson, S., Sances, A., Cusick, J., Meyer, G., and Swiontek, T. (1975): A comparison between anterior and posterior spinal implant systems. *Surg. Neurol.,* 4:180–187.
19. Loeser, J., Black, R., and Christman, A. (1975): Relief of pain by transcutaneous stimulation. *J. Neurosurg.,* 42:308–314.
20. Long, D. M. (1973): Electrical stimulation for relief of pain from chronic nerve injury. *J. Neurosurg.,* 39:718–722.
21. Long, D. M. (1974): External electrical stimulation as a treatment of chronic pain. *Minn. Med.,* 57:195–198.
22. Long, D. M., and Carolan, M. T. (1974): Cutaneous afferent stimulation in the treatment of chronic pain. In: *Advances in Neurology, Vol. 4: Proceedings of the International Symposium on Pain,* edited by J. J. Bonica, pp. 755–759. Raven Press, New York.
23. Long, D. M., and Erickson, D. (1975): Stimulation of the posterior columns of the spinal cord for relief of intractable pain. *Surg. Neurol.,* 4:134–142.

24. Long, D. M., and Hagfors, N. (1975): Electrical stimulation in the nervous system: The current status of electrical stimulation of the nervous system for relief of pain. *Pain,* 1:109–123.
25. Mayer, D. J., and Price, D. D. (1976): Central nervous system mechanisms of analgesia. *Pain,* 2:379–404.
26. Melzack, R., and Wall, P. D. (1965): Pain mechanisms: A new theory. *Science,* 150:971–979.
27. Meyer, G. A., and Fields, H. L. (1972): Causalgia treated by selective large fiber stimulation of peripheral nerve. *Brain,* 95:163–168.
28. Mortimer, J. T., Shealy, C. N., and Wheeler, C. (1970): Experimental non-destructive electrical stimulation of the brain and spinal cord. *J. Neurosurg.,* 32:553–559.
29. Nashold, B. S. (1974): Central pain: Its origins and treatment. *Clin. Neurosurg.,* 21:311–322.
30. Nashold, B. S. (1975): Dorsal column stimulation for control of pain: A three year follow-up. *Surg. Neurol.,* 4:146–148.
31. Nashold, B. S., and Friedman, H. (1972): Dorsal column stimulation for control of pain: Preliminary report on 30 patients, *J. Neurosurg.,* 36:590–597.
32. Nathan, P. W., and Rudge, P. (1974): Testing the Gate-Control theory of pain in man. *J. Neurol. Neurosurg. Psychiatry,* 37:1366–1372.
33. Nielson, K. D., Adams, J. E., and Hosobuchi, Y. (1975): Phantom limb pain: Treatment with dorsal column stimulation. *J. Neurosurg.,* 42:301–307.
34. North, R., Fischell, T., and Long, D. M. (1977–1978): Chronic stimulation via percutaneously inserted epidural electrodes. *Appl. Neurophysiol.,* 40:184–191.
35. Picaza, J. A., Cannon, B., Hunter, S., Boyd, A., Guma, J., and Maurer, D. (1975): Pain suppression by peripheral nerve stimulation. II. Observations with implanted devices. *Surg. Neurol.,* 4:115–26.
36. Pineda, A. (1975): Dorsal column stimulation and its prospects. *Surg. Neurol.,* 4:157–164.
37. Ray, C. D. (1977): Neuroaugmentation: What lies ahead? In: *Current Concepts in the Management of Chronic Pain,* edited by D. LeRoy, pp. 155–169. Symposia Specialists, Miami.
38. Ray, C. D. (1977): New electrical stimulation methods for therapy and rehabilitation. *Orthoped. Rev.,* 6(10):29–39.
39. Ray, C. D., and Maurer, D. D. (1975): Electrical neurological stimulation systems: A review of contemporary methodology. *Surg. Neurol.,* 4:82–90.
40. Richardson, D. E., and Akil, H. (1977): Pain reduction by electrical brain stimulation in man. I. Acute administration in periaqueductal and periventricular sites. *J. Neurosurg.,* 47:178–183.
41. Richardson, D. E., and Akil, H. (1977): Pain reduction by electrical brain stimulation in man. II. Chronic self-administration in the periventricular gray matter. *J. Neurosurg.,* 47:184–194.
42. Richardson, D. E., and Akil, H. (1977): Long-term results of periventricular gray self-stimulation. *J. Neurosurg.,* 1:199–202.
43. Shealy, C. N. (1974): Transcutaneous electrical stimulation for control of pain. *Clin. Neurosurg.,* 21:269–277.
44. Shealy, C. N., and Mortimer, J. T. (1971): Dorsal column electroanalgesia. In: *Neuroelectric Research, Electroneuroprosthesis, Electroanesthesia and Nonconvulsive Electrotherapy,* edited by D. V. Reynolds and E. A. Sjoberg, pp. 146–150. Charles C Thomas, Springfield, Ill.
45. Shealy, C. N., Mortimer, J. T., and Hagfors, N. R. (1970): Dorsal column electroanalgesia. *J. Neurosurg.,* 32:560–564.
45a. Snyder, S. H., Pasternak, G. W., and Pert, C. B. (1976): Opiate receptor mechanisms. In: *Handbook of Psychopharmacology,* edited by L. L. Iverson, S. D. Iverson, and S. H. Snyder, pp. 329–360. Plenum Press, New York.
46. Sternbach, R. A. (1974): Psychological aspects of pain and the selection of patients. *Clin. Neurosurg.,* 21:323–333.
47. Sweet, W. H. (1968): Lessons on pain control from electrical stimulation. *Trans. Stud. Coll. Physicians Phila.,* 35:171–184.
48. Sweet, W. H., and Wepsic, J. G. (1968): Treatment of chronic pain by stimulation of fibers of primary afferent neuron. *Trans. Am. Neurol. Assoc.,* 93:103–105.
49. Sweet, W. H., and Wepsic, J. G. (1974): Stimulation of the posterior columns of the spinal cord for pain control: Indications, technique and results. *Clin. Neurosurg.,* 21:278–310.
50. Taub, A., and Kane, A. (1975): A history of local electrical analgesia (abstract). *Abstracts of the First World Congress on Pain,* p. 173.
51. Wall, P. D., and Sweet, W. H. (1967): Temporary abolition of pain in man. *Science,* 155:108–109.

Mechanisms of Pain and Analgesic Compounds,
edited by R. F. Beers, Jr., and E. G. Bassett.
Raven Press, New York © 1979.

7. Contribution of Research on Acupunctural and Transcutaneous Electrical Stimulation to the Understanding of Pain Mechanisms and Pain Relief

C. Richard Chapman

Departments of Anesthesiology, Psychiatry and Behavioral Sciences, and Psychology, University of Washington School of Medicine, Seattle, Washington 98195

INTRODUCTION

The control of pain remains one of the great problem areas of contemporary medicine in spite of many years of intensive research in this field. Recently, increasing attention has been given to methods of pain control that do not depend on the use of opiate or other analgesic drugs. In the early 1970s, demonstration of pain control during surgery with only acupunctural stimulation by Chinese physicians provoked curiosity and excitement among investigators in several western countries. The result has been a period of investigation of what might be best termed stimulation-induced analgesia (SIA). This term incorporates pain control procedures such as electrical acupunctural stimulation and transcutaneous electrical stimulation (TES). The purpose of this chapter is to review the developing literature on SIA, to describe the procedures for pain measurement currently used in laboratory research, and to evaluate the contributions of this work to current understanding of pain and its control.

SIA RESEARCH BY OTHERS

Most investigations of the efficacy of acupunctural stimulation have used psychophysical methods for the measurement of pain. The first psychophysical reports were those of Chinese investigators who induced pain in human volunteers using potassium iontophoresis dolorimetry and recorded the pain thresholds over time in various parts of the body while applying electrical acupunctural stimulation to sites in the hands and legs (35). They observed a gradual increase in pain threshold over time which seemed to reach a stable state after 30 to 40 min. Although complete analgesia was not obtained, the pain threshold did increase to 160 to 190% of its original value. These Chinese researchers have also studied the roles of humoral and neurological factors in mediation of the analgesic effects.

Cutaneous Dolorimetry

American research on cutaneous experimental pain and the analgesic effects of acupuncture has been somewhat disconcerting. Li et al. (26) compared the effects of acupuncture and hypnosis on pain induced near the supraorbital nerve in human volunteers. In a carefully controlled study, they determined the level of stimulation at which subjects experienced minimal sensation, minimal pain, and maximal or intolerable pain. Acupuncture had no significant effects on these measures, although significant differences were evident under hypnosis. Acupuncture also failed to affect blood pressure, pulse rate, EKG, respiration rate, and EEG. In contrast, Stacher and associates (37) used electrical stimulation of the skin to induce pain in the thyroid area, measuring pain tolerance and pain threshold under control and acupunctural conditions. Traditional acupuncture elevated the pain threshold and was significantly more effective in doing this than was acupuncture at nonspecific points. However, pain tolerance did not rise significantly more under "real" acupuncture than under nonspecific site acupuncture. Since both studies were carefully designed, there is no apparent explanation for this discrepancy.

Stewart et al. (38) used a multiple locus contact heat stimulation system to induce pain in volunteers who experienced control conditions, acupunctural electrical stimulation (2.5 Hz) at true acupuncture sites, and similar stimulation at nonacupuncture sites. The duration of the mounting heat stimulus was their primary dependent variable. They observed that acupuncture was more effective than suggestion in raising the overall body pain threshold. Pain tolerance also increased significantly but the difference between true acupuncture and pseudoacupuncture failed to achieve significance. The authors noted that both genuine and pseudoacupuncture needles were located in the same dermatomes.

Radiant heat also has been used to study the effects of acupuncture in the skin. Berlin et al. (7) used radiant heat dolorimetry to create cutaneous pain in the forearms of volunteers. Ignoring sensory pain threshold to radiant heat, which has been a highly controversial issue in American analgesia research, they measured the duration of time that subjects would accept a continuous heat stimulus before terminating it because of pain. Response latencies to painful stimuli were increased significantly by acupunctural stimulation, and sites not considered acupuncture points had less effect on response time. They cautioned that the effects, while significant, were small, and that it was not possible to separate physiological changes from those in attitude or emotional set that might affect response latency.

The issue of bias in response set raised by Berlin and associates (7) has caused substantial controversy in sensory psychophysics where verbal reports or human judgments are generally used as dependent measures. If judgments are accepted at face value as indications of sensory experience, systematic distortions may arise. For example, pain threshold values may increase or decrease substantially as a function of instructional set or of the attitudes or beliefs held by the experimental subject. The biases maintained by subjects are not necessarily held as conscious performance strategies, and it may be difficult for the experimenter to detect the presence of bias contamination. By reanalyzing the data collected by Day et al. (20), Chapman (8) demonstrated that response bias was an important influence in their data. Day and co-workers used themselves as experimental subjects, and their data reveal that their negative attitudes toward experimental outcome determined the measures of pain threshold that they obtained during psychophysical testing.

Clark and Yang (19) attempted to account for response bias by using Sensory Decision Theory (SDT) methodology to evaluate the responses of volunteers to radiant heat testing during acupunctural stimulation. Following Chinese procedures for analgesia of the forearm, they compared perception in the acupunctured and in the untreated arm. No decrease in sensory sensitivity was evident, but a significant increase in response bias was observed in the acupunctured limb during electrical stimulation. Critics have suggested that the failure of Clark and Yang to demonstrate sensory changes with acupuncture might be due to procedural factors that limited the precision of measurement (24,29).

Dental Dolorimetry

Although the data collected in studies using cutaneous stimulation have been conflicting, reports involving dental stimulation have been largely positive. Mumford and Bowsher (32) found a small increase in the dental pain threshold after acupuncture. Andersson and Holmgren in Sweden (6,25) induced pain in the laboratory by stimulating the tooth pulp electrically in a manner similar to that used by Mumford and Bowsher. They examined pain threshold over time and reported a gradual increase in pain threshold with acupunctural stimulation of the hands and cheeks that was similar in pattern to the result observed by the Chinese with potassium iontophoresis of the skin. Unlike the Chinese, however, they administered acupunctural stimulation to facial sites in the neurological segment used for dolorimetric testing in addition to sites in the hands that were unrelated to the innervation of the test area. Stimulation of the hands alone resulted in a trivial increase of dental pain threshold, whereas stimulation of the hands and cheeks together, or the cheeks alone, resulted in a substantial analgesic effect. Consistent with the Chinese observations, the Swedish researchers found that the effect decayed gradually after the removal of the needles. Andersson and Holmgren have repeatedly replicated their findings.

Studies investigating the impact of acupuncture on experimental pain have also demonstrated the effects of TES delivered to acupuncture sites. Andersson and associates (4,5) have repeatedly demonstrated that electrical stimulation can reduce the ability of subjects to detect and discriminate among painful dental shocks in the laboratory. The history of the use of electrical stimulation has been reviewed by Taub (39), who has also discussed the theoretical rationale for early work on transcutaneous electrical analgesia. Taub has provided evidence that, at least in some situations, electrical stimulation may cause a blockade of primary afferent fibers rather than a gating out of noxious sensory input at the spinal cord due to the modulating effect of large fiber activity on that of small fibers. The efficacy of TES for the management of patients with chronic pain has been demonstrated and discussed by Loeser et al. (27). Electroanalgesia, electroanesthesia, and electronarcosis have been investigated in Europe at numerous laboratories (36,40). The data available to date strongly suggest that electrical stimulation may be a potentially valuable means of modulating pain clinically and that it deserves further investigation under controlled laboratory conditions.

SIA INVESTIGATIONS IN OUR LABORATORY

Over the past 3 years, we have systematically attempted to: (a) determine whether acupuncture and related treatments can modify the perception of nociceptive sensory input in normal humans; (b) provide information about the parameters critical to the induction of acupuncture analgesia effects; and (c) obtain information that will help to elucidate the mechanism or mechanisms underlying acupunctural analgesia. The following information provides a description of our procedures and experiments, as well as an overview of our findings.

Characteristics of Electrical Stimulation for Analgesia

Electrical Parameters

In all of our work, a Model 626 acupuncture stimulator manufactured in the People's Republic of China has been used to provide SIA. We have used this 9-V source to deliver pulses ranging in intensity from 6 to 18 mA, and stimulation has always been carried out at 2 to 3 Hz. This stimulator produces a biphasic spike wave. These electrical parameters are similar to those employed by Chinese physicians who use acupunctural stimulation to control the pain associated with major surgery, as observed by a United States study group comprised of scientists and clinicians (1).

Stimulation Sites

We have studied the effects of acupunctural SIA techniques to determine their ability to modify the perception of painful tooth stimulation. Both distal sites in the hands and sites in the second division of the trigeminal nerve have been used in our laboratory studies. When distal sites were employed, we inserted an acupuncture needle cathode bilaterally into the web between the thumb and the first finger approximately 2 cm deep. This site is traditionally known as "hoku." An electrode taped to the palmar surface of the first finger served as an anode. Facial acupuncture sites located 1 cm lateral to the ala of the nose (1 cm deep) and on the lower border of the zygomatic arch, proximal to the infraorbital plexus (2 cm deep), were employed. Only sites ipsilateral to the tooth being tested were used.

For TES procedures we used exactly the same loci, and standard EKG electrodes filled with conductive jelly were taped to the acupuncture sites.

Induction Time

Before beginning testing for analgesia, we allowed subjects 15 to 20 min of induction time (i.e., SIA stimulation at a predetermined criterion level). When distal sites were employed, we requested that subjects accept enough stimulating current to cause noticeable twitching in the fingers and thumb. Subjects undergoing facial acupuncture were asked to gradually increase the stimulating current until it reached a level of intensity high enough to create an illusion of "pounding" in the bicuspid ipsilateral to the needles.

Dolorimetric Methodology

Dental Stimulation

Our research has been carried out entirely with human subjects, and we have studied the ways in which response to induced dental pain is modified by SIA treatments. We have found that tooth pulp electrical stimulation provides a highly reliable and safe way of creating experimental pain in man. This method has been used by Swedish investigators (4,5), English researchers (31–33), and others (16,17), in addition to ourselves (9,12,14,15,23). When the tooth is shocked by electrical current, subjects experience a sensation that they commonly liken to the pain of biting frozen food or the pain of clinical dental work. It has been demonstrated by Mumford and Bowsher (31–33) that there is minimal adaptation to dental stimulation and little or no change in dental sensitivity over repeated trials. This is a decided advantage over most other methods of creating pain in the laboratory since, in many circumstances, subjects tend to adapt to cutaneous electrical shocks, and repeated radiant heat stimulation of an area of skin results in a sensitization of polymodal nociceptors unless the skin is carefully and slowly cooled between trials. Furthermore, dental stimulation yields a relatively pure pain experience, whereas other methods involve a mixture of pain and other somatosensory sense modalities. Anderson et al. (2,3) have asserted that "there is little evidence that sensations other than pain can be aroused by stimulating intradental receptors."

Equipment

Our dolorimetry system employs a Grass S-44 stimulator with a stimulus isolation unit and a constant current unit. In addition, a current-sensing instrument is used to measure the current flow through the electrodes. The tooth, generally a central or lateral upper incisor that is healthy and without fillings, is stimulated via a 4-mm conductive rubber electrode (cathode) that is held by the subject against the dried dental surface. The anode is a standard EKG electrode taped to the cheek. A 10-msec (5 msec when evoked potentials are recorded) square wave pulse is employed. Stimulus intensity is controlled by varying current.

Methods of Measuring Sensitivity to Pain

Psychophysical Methods

Most of our studies have employed psychophysical methods to evaluate the human pain response (i.e., verbal responses to painful dental shocks have been recorded and evaluated in a statistical model to yield measures of sensitivity to pain). The most basic measure employed is the well-known pain threshold, but we have also used magnitude estimation procedures in which the subject gives category judgment responses to varying levels of dental shock. The methodology used in most studies has been that of SDT (22). The advantage of using the rather complex SDT methodology is that the statistical model yields two types of measures: an index of sensory sensitivity to painful stimulation and a relatively independent measure of response bias or willingness to report the stimulation as painful. Very often, subjects given placebo analgesic treatments report that they feel less pain when, in fact, their ability to perceive painful stimuli has not really been changed. When SDT methods are used, this tendency is measured as response bias and measures of sensory sensitivity remain invariant (11,13,15,18). We have used this methodology to help separate the physiological changes in perception that are caused by SIA (losses in ability to feel pain) from the psychological changes that lead subjects to act as though they are perceiving less pain when they are not actually analgesic.

Cerebral-Evoked Responses

Most recently, we have been measuring certain characteristics of the cerebral-evoked response to painful dental stimulation. These measures are recorded from vertex with reference to inion using standard EEG electrodes, with an EKG electrode taped to the zygomatic arch as ground. Excellent pioneering work in this area by Chatrian et al. (16,17) shows that the phenomenon is most robust when assessed at these loci. We sampled a 600-msec period beginning 100 msec before the onset of the 5-msec dental shock. The complex waveform that resulted from the summation of 192 trials is illustrated in Fig. 1. The principal components of interest are those that are generally termed late components (i.e., they occur later than 80 to 100 msec after the stimulus). In the figure, the three major components of the waveform are identified as C_1, C_2, and C_3. The peak-to-peak amplitude of each of these components correlates

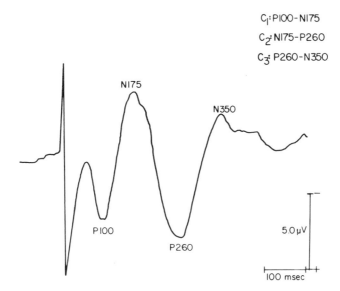

C_1: P100-N175

C_2: N175-P260

C_3: P260-N350

FIG. 1. Cerebral-evoked response waveform from one subject undergoing 192 trials of 5-msec dental electrical stimuli. 600 msec of EEG are represented. The first 100 msec are background EEG and at 100 msec the tooth shock artifact is evident. Slow wave components are labeled as C_1, C_2, and C_3.

highly with both the subjective strength of the painful stimulus and the amount of current delivered to the tooth (23). Peak latencies are highly stable and thus far we have observed them to remain invariant with SIA, although 33% nitrous oxide analgesia alters the latency of the peak at N175.

In general, analgesic treatments reduce the peak-to-peak amplitudes of the major components of the evoked response. Figure 2 shows the effect of 33% nitrous oxide in a typical subject. Chapman and Benedetti (9a) recently examined the effects of 33% nitrous oxide on the cerebral-evoked responses of 12 subjects and then injected subjects with either 0.4 mg naloxone or saline under double-blind conditions. A partial reversal of the analgesia obtained with gas inhalation was observed following the injection of 0.4 mg naloxone, but saline had no effect. The reversal involved only the component labeled C_1 in Fig. 1.

Preliminary work reported by Chapman et al. (10) demonstrated that 0.1 mg of the opiate fentanyl significantly reduced the peak-to-peak amplitudes of the evoked potential waveform to a strong pain stimulus. Injection of the narcotic antagonist naloxone (0.4 mg) reversed the peak-to-peak amplitudes of the waveform that had been reduced by the narcotic. A representative set of waveforms illustrating this effect is presented in Fig. 3. These phenomena must be interpreted cautiously, because the reduction in peak-to-peak amplitude could reflect the sedative properties of the drug rather than its analgesic qualities. Work in progress is designed to answer this question.

One of the fundamental measurement issues of concern in evoked potential

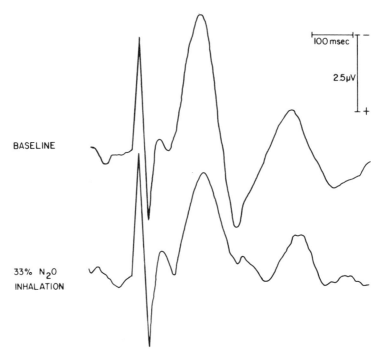

FIG. 2. Effects of 33% nitrous oxide–oxygen inhalation on the cerebral-evoked response of a typical subject.

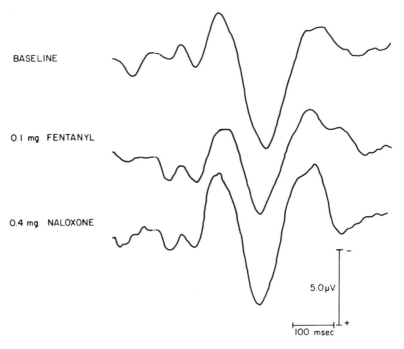

FIG. 3. Reduction of evoked response waveform amplitudes with injection of 0.1 mg fentanyl and reversal of this effect with injection of 0.4 mg naloxone.

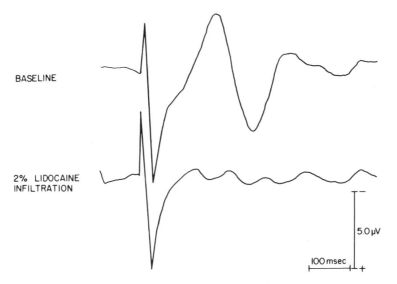

BASELINE

2% LIDOCAINE
INFILTRATION

5.0 μV

100 msec

FIG. 4. Evoked response waveform to "strong pain" before and after local infiltration of lido-caine.

research is that of validity of measurement. It is assumed that the evoked response is the result of the activation of nociceptors in the dental pulp. It is possible that electrical stimulation of the tooth could result in the activation of receptors in other tissues or produce a stimulus artifact that would result in an evoked potential measure closely related to stimulus intensity. To determine whether this hypothesis is valid, Gehrig and Chapman (21) tested subjects who received local infiltration in the area of the test tooth. Six subjects were injected with 2% lidocaine, whereas another six subjects received a similar injection of normal saline, and these procedures were carried out under double-blind conditions. Subjects receiving the local anesthetic infiltration showed a dramatic reduction in peak-to-peak amplitude of the waveform following injection. In essence, their evoked response waveforms were completely destroyed, leaving only the random variation of a normal EEG trace. No change was seen in the saline subjects. Figure 4 shows a typical example of a subject who was measured under base-line conditions to a strong pain dental stimulus and assessed again after local infiltration of lidocaine. The data, which reveal a significant reduction in amplitude ($p < 0.02$) for the lidocaine subjects as opposed to the saline subjects, indicate that nerve block eliminates the evoked response.

Laboratory Demonstrations of SIA

Psychophysical Findings

Our initial study (14) was concerned with acupunctural analgesia as reported by physicians in the People's Republic of China for the control of pain during surgery. In order to study acupunctural analgesia in the laboratory, we divided human volunteers into three groups: a control group, a group that received acupuncture, and a group that received 33% nitrous oxide inhalation. The latter group was intended to serve as an analgesic standard against which the effects of acupuncture could be evaluated. The subjects in each group underwent a series of base-line measures followed by a series of test measures during which they received the treatment assigned to them. A SDT task employing four levels of dental shock was involved. On each trial, the subject rated the shock he experienced as: nothing, possible sensation, very faint pain, prepain sensation, mild pain, or moderate pain, strong pain.

Both measures of sensory sensitivity to painful dental shock and response bias for reporting pain were obtained. The data revealed that both acupuncture and nitrous oxide caused a partial loss of pain sensibility. In addition, both groups showed changes in response bias such that they became more reluctant to report strong tooth shocks as painful. Although the sensory losses due to acupuncture were statistically significant, they were small in magnitude; many of the apparent analgesic changes in subjective reports were due to response bias, which reflected a psychological rather than physiological change in response to acupuncture.

In a second study, we attempted to replicate these findings and to extend our research in new directions (15). We used four groups of subjects who received proper acupuncture, incorrect acupuncture for which needles were placed in the hands at a site considered inappropriate by acupuncturists, TES at a proper acupuncture site, and a control group. Acupuncture was carried out exactly as described above.

We observed that the subjects in all three of the treatment groups gave reduced judgments of pain magnitude after receiving treatment. SDT analysis indicated that acupuncture and TES subjects showed small, but statistically significant, sensory losses after treatment as well as a change in response bias similar to that observed in a previous study. In this respect, the second study replicated the first and extended the findings to TES. Those subjects who received acupuncture in the wrong sites on the hands failed to show a significant sensory loss, but they showed the same shift in response bias as the other subjects (i.e., they tended to report the stimuli as less painful). It is clear from these studies that there is a substantial psychological component to the treatment effect associated with acupuncture in our experimental setting. It is interesting to note that TES and acupuncture were roughly equivalent.

Having observed during visits to the People's Republic of China that the Chinese often insert acupuncture needles into the same neurological segments in which the surgical incision is to be made (1), we decided to study the effects of intrasegmental SIA in the laboratory. Work by Andersson and associates in Sweden (4,5) has suggested that this is an important consideration since electrical stimulation in the second trigeminal division of subjects undergoing tooth pulp testing results in a large increase in the pain threshold. We attempted to replicate and extend Andersson's findings by studying the effects of electrical acupunctural stimulation delivered at facial acupuncture sites. Employing both pain threshold and SDT measures, we observed a mean increase to 187% of original value in pain threshold over 20 min of stimulation, which replicated closely the reports of Andersson et al. After threshold measures were completed, subjects performed a SDT task using several levels of painful tooth shock. Analysis of data from this task showed that the observed threshold increases reflected relatively pure sensory loss with no significant response bias. Thus, intrasegmental acupunctural stimulation was shown to have almost a pure sensory effect, whereas stimulation in the hands was largely a psychological effect. In a latter unpublished study, we were able to demonstrate that TES performed at the same sites yielded approximately the same analgesic response.

Cerebral-Evoked Response Measures of SIA

We have recently begun to investigate the effects of SIA on the cerebral-evoked response to painful tooth stimulation. Since we observed that stimulation of facial acupuncture points has a good effect on sensory sensitivity to pain, we sought to examine the effects of electrical acupuncture on the brain-evoked response. Because other analgesic treatments reduce the amplitudes of the evoked response, we have predicted that acupunctural stimulation will have a similar effect. Of course, not all subjects respond analgesically to acupuncture, but we normally observe good response in 75% or more when psychophysical measures are employed. The following data demonstrate the effects of acupuncture on 11 volunteers.

All subjects received 192 tooth pulp shocks at a level they considered to be "strong pain," and this served as a base-line measure. Twenty minutes of acupunctural stimulation was carried out, as in previous studies, using facial sites. With stimulation continuing, new measures were collected for 192 trials to determine whether acupuncture affected the waveform. The results are shown in Table 1.

TABLE 1. *Effects of acupunctural stimulation on the amplitudes* (μV) *of the cerebral-evoked response to a painful dental stimulus*

		C_1	C_2	C_3
		P100–N175	N175–P260	P260–N350
Base line	$\bar{\chi}$	4.313	7.013	5.673
	SE	0.964	1.361	1.408
Electrical acupuncture	$\bar{\chi}$	2.660	5.440	4.538
	SE	0.704	1.366	1.267
Statistical significance	t-test $df = 10$	2.319[a]	2.687[a]	1.875

[a] $p < 0.05$.

Subjects showed significant reductions in waveform amplitude at P100–N175 (component C_1) and at N175–P260 (component C_2), but not at P260–N350 (C_3), although some reduction was evident. We have previously observed similar amplitude decreases in response to 33% nitrous oxide (12 subjects) and in response to 0.1 mg fentanyl. The data presented here support our psychophysical studies in showing that electrical acupuncture stimulation can modify the perception of pain in man.

Steps Toward Finding a Mechanism for SIA

One theoretical explanation for the observation described above and also for the phenomena demonstrated in Chinese operating rooms, when acupuncture is used for surgical analgesia, is provided by the endomorphine hypothesis. Recent isolation in vertebrates of morphine-like substances that are produced endogenously suggests that humans may be able to modulate pain experience by producing several types of polypeptides that have certain similarities to opiates. These substances are thought to bind to specialized receptors in the periaqueductal gray areas of the brain and to trigger an antidromic inhibitory process that blocks nociceptive input from the periphery via the dorsolateral funiculus.

In order to test the hypothesis that SIA releases endogenous opiates, we designed an experiment in which naloxone, a morphine antagonist, would be injected after the establishment of an analgesic state in laboratory subjects (9). We reasoned that naloxone would block the effects of an endogenous opioid and hypothesized that such an injection would destroy TES-induced analgesia.

We tested two groups of subjects repeatedly over time. Both groups received TES analgesia delivered at facial acupuncture sites. Base-line measures were collected as well as measures following 20 min of TES and those following the injection 0.4 mg of either naloxone or normal saline. A double-blind design was employed so that half the subjects received an injection of normal saline, whereas the remainder received 0.4 mg naloxone. TES continued during and after the injection.

Both groups of subjects demonstrated an analgesic effect after 20 min of TES as measured by changes in verbal report. Following injection, those who received saline showed a slightly increased analgesia, but those who received naloxone showed a statistically significant partial reversal of analgesic effect. These findings are consistent with the hypothesis that an endogenous morphine-like substance is released by acupunctural stimulation, since naloxone may have acted as an antagonist of such a substance. Because the reversal of analgesia was only partial, we believe that at least two mechanisms are at work in SIA. One is probably an endomorphine release in response to stress, whereas the other is yet still unspecified. Gate Control Theory (30) could provide an explanation by postulating that the large fiber stimulation of SIA closes the gate against the small fiber input generated by the tooth pulp stimulation. Of course, it is possible that our effects would have been more complete if we had used a higher dosage of antagonist.

Our findings are consistent with those reported by Pomeranz et al. (34), who studied response to acupuncture in animals and with those of Mayer et al. (28), who investigated the effects of acupuncture on man. Both investigators found that SIA was partly reversed by injection of the morphine antagonist naloxone.

CONCLUSIONS

In our laboratory, SIA treatments clearly modify the perception of laboratory-induced dental pain in healthy human volunteers. In most instances, the analgesia produced involves both a loss of sensory ability to feel pain and a change in attitude toward reporting the stimulation as painful. The sensory effects of SIA are apparently complex and appear to involve both peripheral mechanisms of pain modulation and the release of endogenous opiate-like substances centrally. Our data indicate that this approach to pain modulation is a viable one that merits further laboratory and clinical research.

ACKNOWLEDGMENT

This work was supported by a grant from the National Institute of Dental Research, no. DE-04004.

REFERENCES

1. American Acupuncture Anesthesia Study Group (1976): *Acupuncture anesthesia in the People's Republic of China.* National Academy of Sciences, Washington, D.C.
2. Anderson, D. J. (1975): Pain from dentine and pulp. *Br. Med. Bull.,* 31:111–114.
3. Anderson, D. J., Hannam, A. G., and Matthews, B. (1970): Sensory mechanisms in mammalian teeth and their supporting structures. *Phys. Rev.,* 50:171–195.
4. Andersson, S. A., Erickson, T., Holmgren, E., and Lindqvist, G. (1973): Electroacupuncture and the pain threshold. *Lancet,* 2:564.
5. Andersson, S. A., Erickson, T., Holmgren, E., and Lindqvist, G. (1973): Electroacupuncture: Effect on pain threshold measured with electrical stimulation of teeth. *Brain Res.,* 63:393–396.
6. Andersson, S. A., and Holmgren, E. (1975): On acupuncture analgesia and the mechanism of pain. *Am. J. Chin. Med.,* 3:311–334.
7. Berlin, F. S., Bartlett, R. L., and Black, J. D. (1975): Acupuncture and placebo: Effects on delaying the terminating response to a painful stimulus. *Anesthesiology,* 42:527–531.
8. Chapman, C. R. (1975): Psychophysical evaluation of acupunctural analgesia: Some issues and considerations. *Anesthesiology,* 43:501–506.
9. Chapman, C. R., and Benedetti, C. (1977): Analgesia following transcutaneous electrical stimulation and its partial reversal by a narcotic antagonist. *Life Sci.,* 21:1645–1648.
9a. Chapman, C. R., and Benedetti, C. (1979): Nitrous oxide effects on cerebral evoked potential to pain: Partial reversal with a narcotic agonist. *Anesthesiology (in press).*
10. Chapman, C. R., Benedetti, C., and Butler, S. H. (1977): Cerebral response measures of stimulation-induced and opiate-induced dental analgesia in man: Attempted analgesia reversal with narcotic antagonist. In: *Pain in the Trigeminal Region,* edited by D. J. Anderson and B. Matthews, pp. 423–433. Elsevier/North-Holland Biomedical Press, Amsterdam.
11. Chapman, C. R., and Butler, S. H. (1978): Effects of doxepin on perception of laboratory-induced pain in man. *Pain,* 5:253–262.
12. Chapman, C. R., Chen, A. C., and Bonica, J. J. (1977): Effects of intrasegmental electrical acupuncture on dental pain: Evaluation by threshold estimation and sensory decision theory. *Pain,* 3:213–227.

13. Chapman, C. R., and Feather, B. W. (1975): Effects of diazepam on human pain tolerance and pain sensitivity. *Psychosom. Med.,* 35:330–340.
14. Chapman, C. R., Gehrig, J. D., and Wilson, M. E. (1975): Acupuncture compared with 33 percent nitrous oxide for dental analgesia. *Anesthesiology,* 42:532–537.
15. Chapman, C. R., Wilson, M. E., and Gehrig, J. D. (1976): Comparative effects of acupuncture and transcutaneous stimulation on the perception of painful dental stimuli. *Pain,* 2:265–283.
16. Chatrian, G. E., Canfield, R. C., Knauss, T. A., and Lettich, E. (1975): Cerebral responses to electrical tooth pulp stimulation in man: An objective correlate of acute experimental pain. *Neurology (Minneap.),* 25:745–757.
17. Chatrian, G. E., Canfield, R. C., Lettich, E., and Black, R. G. (1974): Cerebral response to electrical stimulation of tooth pulp in man. *J. Dent. Res.,* 53:1299.
18. Clark, W. C. (1974): Pain sensitivity and the report of pain: An introduction to sensory decision theory. *Anesthesiology,* 40:272–287.
19. Clark, W. C., and Yang, J. C. (1974): Acupunctural analgesia? Evaluation by signal detection theory. *Science,* 184:1096–1098.
20. Day, R. L., Kitahata, L. M., Kao, F. F., Motoyama, E. K., and Hardy, J. D. (1975): Evaluation of acupuncture anesthesia: A psychophysical study. *Anesthesiology,* 43:507–517.
21. Gehrig, J. D., and Chapman, C. R. (1979): Cerebral evoked potentials response to tooth stimulation as a measure of pain: Effects of nerve block and placebo on evoked response. In: *Advances in Pain Research and Therapy, Vol. 3: Proceedings of the Second World Congress on Pain,* edited by J. J. Bonica, J. Liebeskind, and D. Albe-Fessard. Raven Press, New York *(in press).*
22. Green, D. M., and Swets, J. A. (1974): *Signal Detection Theory and Psychophysics.* Robert E. Kruger, New York.
23. Harkins, S. W., and Chapman, C. R. (1978): Cerebral-evoked potentials to noxious dental stimulation: Relationship to subjective pain report. *Psychophysiology,* 15:248–252.
24. Hayes, R. L., Bennett, G. J., and Mayer, D. J. (1975): Acupuncture, pain, and signal detection theory. *Science,* 189:65–66.
25. Holmgren, E. (1975): *Effects of Conditioning Electrical Stimulation on the Perception of Pain.* Doctoral dissertation. University of Göteborg, Göteborg, Sweden.
26. Li, C. L., Ahlberg, D., Lansdell, H., Gravitz, M. A., Chen, T. C., Ting, C. Y., Bak, A. F., and Blessing, D. (1975): Acupuncture and hypnosis: Effects on induced pain. *Exp. Neurol.,* 49:272–280.
27. Loeser, J. D., Black, R. G., and Christman, A. (1975): Relief of pain by transcutaneous stimulation. *J. Neurosurg.,* 42:308–314.
28. Mayer, D. J., Price, D. D., and Rafii, A. (1977): Antagonism of acupuncture analgesia in man by the narcotic antagonist naloxone. *Brain Res.,* 121:368–372.
29. McBurney, D. H. (1976): Signal detection theory and pain. *Anesthesiology,* 44:356–358.
30. Melzack, R., and Wall, P. D. (1965): Pain mechanisms: A new theory. *Science,* 150:971–979.
31. Mumford, J. M. (1963): Pain threshold of normal human anterior teeth. *Arch. Oral. Biol.,* 8:493–501.
32. Mumford, J., and Bowsher, D. (1973): Electro-acupuncture and pain threshold. *Lancet,* 2:667.
33. Mumford, J. M., and Bowsher, D. (1976): Pain and protopathic sensibility: A review with particular reference to the teeth. *Pain,* 2:223–243.
34. Pomeranz, B., Cheng, R., and Law, P. (1977): Acupuncture reduces electrophysiological and behavioral responses to noxious stimuli: Pituitary is implicated. *Exp. Neurol.,* 54:172–178.
35. Research Group of Acupuncture Anesthesia–Peking Medical College, Peking (1977): Effect of needling positions in acupuncture on pain threshold of human skin. *Chin. Med. J. [Engl.],* 3:151–157.
36. Smith, R. H. (1963): *Electrical Anesthesia.* Charles C Thomas, Springfield, Ill.
37. Stacher, G., Wancura, I., Bauer, P., Lahoda, R., and Schulze, D. (1975): Effect of acupuncture on pain threshold and pain tolerance determined by electrical stimulation of the skin: A controlled study. *Am. J. Chin. Med.,* 3:143–149.
38. Stewart, D., Thomson, J., and Oswald, I. (1977): Acupuncture analgesia: An experimental investigation. *Br. Med. J.,* 1:67–70.
39. Taub, A. (1974): Percutaneous local electrical analgesia. *Minn. Med.,* 57:172–175.
40. Wageneder, F. M., and Shuy, St., Eds. (1970): *Electrotherapeutic Sleep and Electroanaesthesia.* Excerpta Medica, Amsterdam.

Mechanisms of Pain and Analgesic Compounds,
edited by R. F. Beers, Jr., and E. G. Bassett.
Raven Press, New York © 1979.

8. Principles of Operant Conditioning in Pain Research and Therapy

Wilbert E. Fordyce

Department of Rehabilitation Medicine, University of Washington School of Medicine, Seattle, Washington 98195

INTRODUCTION

The objectives of this chapter are to show that in chronic pain the focus is on patient behavior; to show that behavior is not simply an extension or reflection of underlying nociception, or even of underlying suffering; to describe a behavioral perspective of chronic pain; and to illustrate a data base for such a perspective.

OBSERVATIONS AND DISCUSSION

A Behavioral Perspective—What Is It?

Lazarus (3) has said that only a devotee of extrasensory perception would take the position that we can understand a person without looking at his/her behavior. The first essential to a behavioral perspective is recognition that behavior has significance in its own right. To understand a person we must observe and measure his/her behavior. Traditional views have tended to characterize behavior as under the control of motivational or personality factors within the person; that to understand the behavior, one must understand those underlying factors. In short, behavior is an extension or reflection of processes "within the black box." There is, however, an abundance of evidence to indicate that behavior of people cannot be understood solely in terms of inferences about underlying processes. The principle source of evidence is the observation, confirmed by countless controlled studies, that behavior is subject to influence by contingent reinforcement occurring within the environment. Reinforcement has an effect which, while presumably leading to alterations within the black box, can only be understood by analysis of existing contingency arrangements in the environment. This analysis provides the essential basis for the observation that behavior has significance in its own right, for behavior is inevitably linked to the environment in which it occurs and has varying degrees of independence from personality or motivational factors within the organism.

There is a second feature to a behavioral perspective. If one carries out some form of intervention or treatment, the criterion for assessing whether there has been an effect is change in behavior. A treatment that does not result in a behavioral change, whatever other effects it might bring about, has done nothing of confirmable merit. This is not simply a doctrinaire assertion as to the importance of behavior. The point draws our attention to the distinction between inferences about underlying states of the person perhaps drawn from verbal reports asserting there is "suffering" and the behavior of the person. True, verbal reports are also behavior but their significance to the point being made is that, in this example, they refer to alleged underlying states and do not necessarily relate to what the person will or will not do.

A third defining characteristic of a behavioral approach is the emphasis on operationalizing the measures of behavior. Rather than relying on subjective judgments or some kind of observer ratings, behavioral methods dictate that there be measurement of the actions of people: what they do. This point has particular relevance to this volume because of the concern with measurement in the context of clinical pain. From a behavioral perspective, there is a commitment to measurement and what is measured is what people do irrespective of what they may report about pain and suffering.

"Pain" as Pain Behavior

When discussing pain, acute or chronic, clinicians typically use the term "pain" when in fact they are talking about or basing their comments on "pain behavior." And they are often quite unaware of that semantic error. In order to clarify this issue, we must go back to some basic definitions. The conceptualization and associated definitions used here are the work of John D. Loeser, a colleague of mine at the University of Washington, to whom a special note of gratitude is extended.

Without belaboring the point, it can now be accepted that there is a neurosensory system we can label as a pain system. Thermal or mechanical stimuli (nociception) impinging on appropriate receptors activate Aδ and C fibers which, in turn, enter the spinal cord and proceed to subcortical centers wherein, in response, there is experienced a sensation we identify as "pain." The sensation of "pain" is possible without nociception, as in tic doloureux, and nociception is possible without the sensation of "pain" as in the soldier who is wounded but does not become aware of that fact until hours after life-threatening combat. The linkage between nociception and the sensation of "pain" is less than perfect, although somewhat close.

The clinical pain problem is not, however, that "pain sensation." That sensation activates fibers leading to higher centers which, in turn, generate negatively toned affective responses we label as "suffering." Yet, the clinician does not, in the strict sense, observe "suffering." "Suffering" in turn generates behaviors: pain behaviors. Those pain behaviors (e.g., moaning, grimacing, limping, talking about or describing pain, requesting medications or a diagnostic procedure, and curtailing activities) are the observable phenomena of chronic pain; they are the basic data with which the clinician deals.

To summarize, the conceptual sequence is: nociception → sensation of "pain" → suffering → pain behavior. As one progresses through that conceptual sequence, there is an increasing vulnerability to the influence of, or intrusion from, factors other than nociception. That is, "pain" as a sensation has potential independence from nociception. "Pain" may occur in the absence of nociception or may not occur in the presence of nociception. But it is even more the case, as one opens the "Pandora's box" of higher nervous centers, that the cross currents of those higher centers enter in to warp, influence, or distort "suffering." For example, to a person already depressed it is difficult to discriminate between "pain" and "depression." Each may be perceived as the other. One consequence is that a person may be experiencing depression but label it as pain. This perceptual or labeling error is enhanced further by the tendency for our language to equate "pain" and "suffering." We may talk about the former when, were we being more precise in our use of language, we would be referring to the latter. The loss of a loved one, for example, often is referred to as "the *pain* of heartbreak."

We are forced to conclude, therefore, that "suffering" is by no means inevitably linked to "pain" and, antecedent to that—nociception, although a person may behave as if he/she were suffering in ways ordinarily attributable to nociception.

The linkage between nociception and pain behavior is even more loose. We may suffer and not display suffering-like pain behavior. We may also display pain behaviors or suffering-like behaviors without "suffering."

Both suffering and pain behaviors, mediated by higher nervous centers, are subject to influence by a variety of factors, some quite foreign and unrelated to nociception and "pain." Prior experience, current affective states, and prevailing environmental contingencies all can and do influence both suffering and pain behavior.

As clinicians, we deal in the context of chronic pain, with two sets of information. We are confronted with and observe pain behavior. We may, as circumstances dictate, *infer* that those pain behaviors are an extension of underlying suffering, although there are alternative explanations of which we must be mindful. We may also infer that the inferred suffering has been elicited by the sensation of pain which, in turn, occurs because of nociception. Again, however, there are highly tenable alternative explanations as to why the pain behaviors and the inferred suffering may be occurring.

The second set of information available to the clinician is the history of previous trauma and, perhaps, of treatment interventions for the reported pain problem, and whatever "physical findings" may derive from the medical work-up—information on the state of the organism. That second set of information bears directly on the question of nociception but it does not describe current nociception. The information may, with varying degrees of reliability or precision, provide a basis for *inferring* that there is, currently, nociceptive input. It might be said that those data provide a basis for speculation or hypothesizing as to the presence of currently active nociception. The data do not, however, demonstrate or confirm either the presence of nociception or, if present, establish that the nociception accounts well for the observed pain behaviors. This is not to suggest that this speculation or inference is always highly questionable. Indeed, the evidence may be most compelling. It must be remembered, however, that it is an inference or speculation and not a statement of facts.

In problems of acute or recent onset pain, the linkage between "physical findings" data and the pain behaviors observed is probably rather tight. The major exceptions are likely to relate to people with extensive prior histories of extended episodes of pain behavior. In such cases, some cue or stimulus in the environment in lieu of persisting nociception may reinvoke a previously well-established, well-articulated repertoire of pain behaviors not recently expressed.

In problems of chronic pain, the opportunity is certain for other factors to have begun to exert an influence (e.g., prior experience, emotional/affective problems or states, and contingent environmental reinforcement). How much those factors will have exerted lasting distortion on the linkage between speculated nociception and observed pain behavior remains to be clarified in each case. It should also be evident that clarification of the question of distortion is not to be found solely in appraisal of physical findings. Concomitantly, there must be appraisal of the role of prior experience, emotional/affective problems, and the environmental contingencies prevailing for that person in regard to his/her expressions of pain behaviors or their alternatives: well behaviors (1).

To summarize, in the clinical setting, clinicians speak of "pain" when their observations are limited to pain behaviors and physical findings. They are assuming the pain behaviors observed are linked to suffering, that the inferred suffering is linked to a sensation of "pain," and that sensation is linked to nociception, which they are, in turn, inferring from their physical findings. Unfortunately this three-phase inference is fraught with risk of error. Pain behaviors are, like all other behavior, subject to influence by a variety of factors, some of which are quite unrelated to nociception, "pain," or suffering. In all cases of chronic pain, the question must be asked as to what factors are maintaining the pain behaviors. Moreover, it must be remembered that those behaviors are quite capable of occurring and continuing to occur because of contingent environmental reinforcement, as well as other possible factors (2).

Empirical Data for a Behavioral Perspective

One form of pain behavior often central to appraisal of a pain problem is the patient's activity or exercise tolerance. A housewife who reports she is unable to vacuum a rug or to make more than one bed without resting is often judged thereby to have a significant pain problem that, among other consequences, limits her activities. There is an alleged pain-related limitation of exercise tolerance.

The matter of exercise tolerance in the context of chronic pain was studied by Fordyce et al. *(in preparation)*. First, a series of 77 chronic pain patients, all receiving prescribed exercises in physical therapy were studied. During the study, all subjects were instructed to "exercise to tolerance," operationally defined as "Do as many (sit-ups, let-backs, pelvic tilts, etc.) as you can before pain, weakness, or fatigue cause you to want to stop. You decide when to stop."

If this particular pain behavior, exercise tolerance, is linked intimately to nociception, pain sensation, and suffering, the number of repetitions of exercises performed should be essentially randomly distributed across the set of patients. Looking at the last digit of the number of repetitions completed, for example, there should be an approximately equal probability that people will quit on a number ending in 1 (e.g., 11, 21, 31), 2 (12, 22, 32), etc. The results from a total of 442 exercise sets across these 77 subjects is shown in Fig. 1. Chance would have been approximately 20% for each last digit combination of 1–6, 2–7, 3–8, 4–9, 5–0. As shown in the figure, the findings were that subjects ended on a multiple of 5 fully 50% of the time. Such a finding would be inexplicable if one assumed the pain behavior was directly linked to nociception. Obviously other factors entered into exercise tolerance in this study.

A second project was then carried out. The question now raised concerned the influence on exercise tolerance, as defined previously, if people had minimal information about how much exercise had been performed. In the first study, it was a simple matter for people to count how many repetitions of each exercise they had completed. In the second study, that counting was made more difficult by the use of an apparatus designed to obfuscate the amount of work completed. Three examples will illustrate this procedure, although several additional exercise

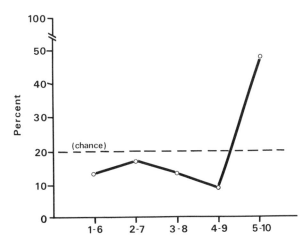

FIG. 1. Exercise tolerance values as proportion of 442 exercise trials involving 77 patients in whom the number of repetitions of exercises ended in 1 or 6 (e.g., 11 or 16, 21 or 26), 2 or 7, 3 or 8, etc.

patterns were also studied. A fixed bicycle was equipped such that there was no speed or distance indicator. Moreover, electronically controlled programs changed the axle ratio in an essentially random fashion every few seconds, on an irregular schedule (e.g., 4 sec at ratio x, 6.5 sec at ratio y, 5 sec at ratio z, 4.5 sec at ratio w, etc.). Independently and asynchronously, electronically controlled equipment changed the drag on the axle in another random schedule for time intervals and amounts of change. As a second example, patients walked on a treadmill for which the speed varied in an electronically controlled, near random manner. As a third example, a series of exercises were prescribed in which subjects reclined on an exercise table and exerted force with one or both arms or one or both legs against a bar attached by cables to weights suspended behind their heads. They were instructed to exert force against the bar sufficient to keep a light lighted. The light, in turn, was connected to an electronically controlled program by which the weights attached to the bar could be varied. For example, while reclining and pushing against the bar suspended above the chest, 25 lbs of force might be required to light the light for 6 sec, followed by a requirement of only 18 lbs for 9 sec, 26 lbs for 8 sec, 12 lbs for 5.5 sec, etc. As the load on the bar lightened, subjects nearly always eased the amount of force exerted, only to have to increase it again seconds later by some varied amount. It clearly was difficult for people to judge precisely how much work they had done. Moreover, they could not wear a timepiece and there was no clock in the room.

It was necessary to calculate the amount of work performed in strictly relative values, as measured by the distance into the electronic programs the subjects progressed before stopping. The amounts performed across the prescribed set of exercises was pooled for each subject individually. That is, the distance into the electronic program progressed by subject no. 1 for exercise A was pooled with exercises B, C, D, etc., yielding a single value. Subjects performed four sessions, usually on consecutive days. the amount performed the first day was given an arbitrary value of 1, and the amounts completed on successive days was calculated as a ratio of the first day.

In this study, there was an experimental and a control group. The experimental group consisted of 20 chronic pain patients being seen in the beginning phases of evaluation. They were not yet in treatment, so the effects to be shown can hardly be accounted for as effects of treatment. The control group comprised 14 young adults who responded to an advertisement to complete an exercise program. Controls were screened to eliminate subjects reporting a problem of acute or chronic pain. Controls were given the same instructions: exercise to tolerance. Exercises were chosen or prescribed by a physician according to the nature of the pain problem and general medical status of the patients under evaluation. Exercises were randomly assigned to the control group.

If the pain behaviors of exercise tolerance were under control of internal factors (nociception–"pain"–suffering), the absence of environmental feedback as to amount of work performed should be essentially irrelevant. The results are shown in Fig. 2. It should be remembered that the values shown are relative. The amount each person did in his/her first session forms the base value of 1, and his/her subsequent performances were ratios of that. The findings reported in Fig. 2 (upper portion) show first that the experimental and control groups did, relatively, almost the same amount of work. Had the chronic pain patients' exercise tolerance pain behavior been under control of internal factors, one would expect quite different results from those obtained by people reporting no underlying "pain" problem. Second, in the case of both groups, there was a steady increase in amount performed such that, by the fourth session, mean values for all subjects were twice those recorded in the first session. A third curve is also shown in Fig. 2 for comparative or reference purposes, a performance curve obtained from a different set of chronic pain patients exercising to tolerance in the typical physical therapy fashion, as in the first study. Their performances were calculated in similar fashion to subjects of the second study. Amounts done in the first session were pooled and given the arbitrary value of 1; subsequent session values were calculated as a ratio of the first session.

It is evident from Fig. 2 that, under the conditions of this study, the potential impact of social or environmental feedback in the form of information about amount of exercise performed has considerable effect. The linkage of exercise tolerance to suffering, "pain," and nociception clearly is loose. The fact that under conditions of minimal feedback both experimental and control subjects increased so rapidly, and more rapidly than did the reference group exercising with feedback, further emphasizes the point.

The results of these studies are taken to support the inference that pain behaviors, in the context of chronic pain, and in this instance, exercise tolerance, are demonstrably influenced by factors unrelated to alleged or inferred nociception.

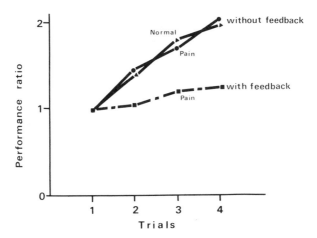

FIG. 2. Exercise tolerance with and without feedback. Amount performed during trial 1 was given a value of 1. Subsequent trials are shown as a ratio of trial 1.

A third study has recently been completed (Fordyce et al., *in preparation*) which bears further on the sensitivity of pain behaviors to diverse environmental influences and, accordingly, on the hazards of relying on patient verbal report as a reliable source of information about suffering, "pain," or nociception. The study explored the relationship between directly observed pain behaviors during exercise being performed by chronic pain patients in evaluation and amount of exercise performed.

Twenty-five chronic pain patients, all being seen on an in-patient basis for evaluation of their pain problems, were assigned a set of physical therapy exercises on physician prescription. They were instructed to exercise to tolerance, as previously defined. The amounts performed on the four most frequently prescribed exercises were recorded: riding a fixed bicycle, climbing flights of stairs, walking measured laps, and partial sit-ups. In each case and during each exercise session, a physical therapist was in attendance. The therapist recorded both amounts of exercise performed and also each visible or audible expression of pain or distress emitted by the patient while exercising.

The amount of exercise performed for each exercise could be expected to vary in range, mean, and dispersion. Therefore, each subject's distribution of amounts performed on each of the four exercises studied, across the sessions (which ranged from 4 to 15 for the 25 subjects), was transformed into a common scale (T scores) having a mean of 50 and a standard deviation of 10. Thus, each subject had four T-score distributions and all subjects' performances were transformed to this common scale (mean 50; SD 10). This permitted averaging the amount done across four exercises and across subjects.[1]

These patients were in the early phases of evaluation and not yet the benefiting recipients of treatment beyond that inherent in the evaluation process and these early exercise trials. Were exercise tolerance linked closely to nociception–"pain"–suffering, one would expect a positive relationship between reported distress and exercise performance. One major reason bringing patients such as these to a pain evaluation process is that their pain problems are both distress productive and an intrusion into their lives, thereby limiting their activities. In short, generally and typically, they will have been reporting that their pain problems impose constraints on what they can do and, correspondingly, that their "pain"–suffering is related to activity, as in exercise.

The findings, as shown in Fig. 3, are quite to the contrary. The two curves shown depict a clearly ascending amount of exercise performed across an extended series (sessions 4 to 15) of trials and concomitant, clearly descending rate of emission of pain behaviors. The correlation coefficient between these two sets of observations, exercise performed and pain behaviors emitted, is $r = -0.37$, $N = 278$, $p = .001$.

There are a number of possible reasons why patient performance increased

[1] The reference curve shown in Fig. 2 and relating to the previous study is the amount these subjects did in their first four sessions, but where the mean T score for the first session was assigned the value of 1 and subsequent sessions a ratio of that.

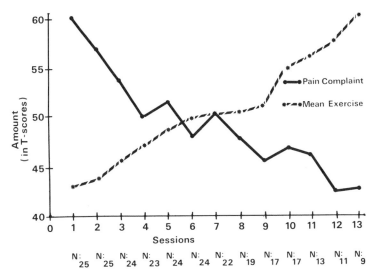

FIG. 3. Exercise–complaint relationship. Exercise values are based on the four most commonly prescribed exercises: riding fixed bicycle, climbing flights of stairs, walking laps, partial sit-ups. Means and standard deviations were calculated for each subject across exercise trials. Those values were transformed to a common scale (T scores) with mean of 50 and SD of 10. Values shown are means of each subject's mean T score across the four exercises. Numbers diminish because subjects had unequal number of trials. Complaint values are means across subjects for each exercise session.

and they will be considered briefly below. The major point for the moment is, however, the further indication from this study of the loose linkage between pain behaviors, including verbal report, and nociception. Were that linkage tight, the correlation between these two curves should have been positive. The data show that the correlation is neither positive, nor even zero order, but negative.

It would be our expectation that were this study repeated using recent onset or acute pain subjects, the findings would be in the opposite direction, namely, a positive correlation between amount performed and pain behavior emitted. The findings reported here emphasize the importance of the distinction between acute and chronic pain. Moreover, the data add further support to the inference that, in chronic pain, pain behaviors are subject to influence by a variety of factors and cannot be seen simply as an extension or visible/audible expression underlying suffering, "pain," and nociception.

The question as to why performance increased is tangential to the purpose of this chapter and so receives only brief consideration. Most of the subjects in study no. 3 became addicted to pain medications and were on a regimen that was rapidly reducing their previously rich ingestion of narcotics or analgesics. That could be one factor accounting for ascending performance. Another probably significant factor is that the therapist was always present when they were performing. That, in turn, it is speculated, could have had two correlated effects. One is that the mere presence of a health-care professional might in itself elicit a desire by patients to do well in order to win approval. About that possibility, however, one might reason that patients could use the opportunity of therapist presence to further "document" or "authenticate" their pain problems by limiting performance when permitted to work to their own decision as to tolerance. The other therapist effect that seems to us to have probable significance is that the therapist avoided trying to caution patients to limit themselves. To the contrary, her posture was one of neutrality, neither praising performance nor encouraging additional effort. By her social nonresponsiveness, she was also implicitly sanctioning the safety of proceeding with further effort. She expressed no alarm, no cautions, no fears that exercise would be harmful or painful.

CONCLUSION

This chapter has sought to draw attention to the importance of recognizing that the methods by which pain patients communicate their pain consist of behavior. Those pain behaviors cannot be understood simply as automatic extensions of some underlying state of the organism (e.g., nociception and the sensation of pain).

Each of the three studies described lend support to the inference that pain behaviors are subject to influence by factors quite unrelated to nociception.

There are a number of implications to these findings and the perspective set forth in this chapter. Perhaps most important of all is to note that clinicians talk about "pain" as if they were describing, or, at the least, implying some underlying state of suffering–"pain"–nociception, when in fact they are talking about something else, namely, pain behavior. Until that semantic error is recognized and avoided, there will continue to be needless confusion and the not infrequent implementation of inappropriate diagnostic and treatment procedures.

A second implication is that the analysis of chronic pain requires careful study of patient behavior and of the spectrum of factors which influence that behavior. In problems of acute pain, these factors will likely not yet have had much opportunity to exert influence and therefore the distinction is less important. Such an analysis, including although not restricted to a behavioral analysis, requires expertise not falling within the preparation of the average practicing physician. This observation provides basis for the statement that, just as war has been noted to be too important to be left to generals, in somewhat the same vein, chronic pain is too important to be left solely to traditional medical perspectives.

ACKNOWLEDGMENT

This project was supported, in part, by Rehabilitation Services Administration grant no. 16–P–56818.

REFERENCES

1. Fordyce, W. E. (1976): *Behavioral Methods in Chronic Pain and Illness.* C. V. Mosby, St. Louis.
2. Fordyce, W. E., Fowler, R. S., Lehmann, J. F., DeLateur, B. J., Sand, P. L., and Trieschmann, R. B. (1973): Operant conditioning in the treatment of chronic pain. *Arch. Phys. Med. Rehabil.,* 9:399–408.
3. Lazarus, A. (1977): Has behavior therapy outlived its usefulness? *Am. Psychol.,* 32:550–554.

Mechanisms of Pain and Analgesic Compounds,
edited by R. F. Beers, Jr., and E. G. Bassett.
Raven Press, New York © 1979.

9. Discussion

Moderator: John J. Bonica

R. J. Schneider: Dr. Mayer, we found what may be an effect on the arousal of anterolateral quadrant stimulation, that is, an ongoing, evoked activity of the somatosensory cortex. Others have observed a similar effect. Would you comment on how they relate to the sensory discriminative versus effective components of pain?

D. J. Mayer: I really did not have a chance to talk about it in any detail. There have been a number of cortical evoked potential studies using, presumably, peripheral stimuli of some sort that evoke only pain, for example, the work of Chatrian and that of Dr. Chapman, as well as your own.

In almost all of these studies, the evoked potentials are of such a latency that one would have to say only Aδ fiber input is being measured. Thus, their relationship to pain of pathological origin, which is probably more related to C fiber input, is most likely questionable, and I would recommend to those working in that field to examine later-evoked potentials that may be relatable to C fiber input. I think the interpretation of these kinds of studies is very difficult—that is, teasing out the variables of whether it is a sensory discriminative aspect of pain or the motivational affective component of pain that is involved, or a more general variable such as arousal or tension that is being measured in these studies.

Nevertheless, I think it is a very promising approach and I hope that people like you and others will continue such studies. Perhaps we will be able to find some objective correlate or pain that can be recorded in the cerebral cortex and is involved in almost all behaviors.

J. N. Johannessen: Dr. Long, in regard to your classification procedure for the efficacy of transcutaneous stimulation, I recently read of a study that used injection of a local anesthetic as a predictor for the success of acupuncture. Have you tried that approach as a predictor of the success of transcutaneous stimulation?

D. M. Long: No, I have not. We are now in the process of validating the testing that allows us to categorize our patients. We also have some validation in other procedures that is interesting; for instance, in a study using a denervation technique—which we believe is a radiofrequency destruction of the medial branch of the posterior primary ramus—we had 150 patients who fell into the objective category and met our other criteria for undergoing this procedure. At a 1-year follow-up of these patients, the success rate in relieving their back pain was 80%.

In a comparable series of patients who fell into our so-called "exaggerated pain group"—those exhibiting pain behavior without an apparent significant organic cause—and subjected to exactly the same procedures, the success rate was zero; we did not even achieve a placebo response. We predict that the validation is going to show that this categorization is correct, but other kinds of interventional procedures to help the validation have not been attempted.

J. J. Bonica: I would like to interject a comment. I wish you could find a word better than "exaggerated" because, as a matter of fact, the patient has real pain that, in my opinion, is an unpleasant perceptual or emotional experience felt in the brain. I think that the people will get the impression that it is exaggerated willfully, that the patient is making this up and it is not real. The fact of the matter is that the pain is real.

D. M. Long: That is a good point. We are not at all implying that this is malingering or exaggeration which is deliberate on the patient's part. As I said, those categories are purely empiric at this point and I would welcome a suggestion as to a more appropriate term.

W. E. Fordyce: Dr. Long, what you are observing is pain behaviors. The question is: Are those pain behaviors under the control of an antecedent stimulus as in the form of nociception? If they are, then that is what Skinner, many years ago, termed respondent. It is an action of the organism responding to an antecedent stimulus. In this context, I would call that respondent pain.

If, instead, those pain behaviors are not under the control of antecedent stimulus in the form of nociception but appear to be related to other factors such as, but not limited to, contingent environmental reinforcement, it seems to me that one can categorize that situation as a problem of operant pain. The behavior is the same. The suffering, as Dr. Bonica pointed out, is the same. The difference is the factors that influence it.

J. J. Bonica: We just got the new terminology. . . .

J. N. Johannessen: It just occurred to me that the exaggerated group may present some form of pain that would be selected out by prior testing of the patients with intrathecal injection of a local anesthetic.

A second comment directed to Drs. Long and Chapman is an observation by an occasional reader of the literature on acupuncture and transcutaneous stimulation. It seems to me that people do not stress often enough the importance of the subjective effect of the stimulation, be it acupuncture or transcutaneous stimulation.

I think, as Dr. Mayer pointed out, that you can distinguish activity in different nerve fiber groups according to subjective sensation. In many reports of acupuncture technique, a manual stimulation that is reported as being some sort of dull, painful sensation to the patient is used. In other studies, an electronic stimulator is used—producing more of a vibrational feeling or tingling sensation—that I think is probably distinguishable from a painful sensation.

I think you see the same effect in transcutaneous stimulation in that while sometimes using the dorsal column or large fiber stimulation—versus the intense transcutaneous stimulation that Melzack reports as being helpful in pain patients—it seems more advantageous to use subjective reports of what the patient was perceiving while undergoing stimulation. Although the mechanisms may be a bit different, I think it would aid in clarifying the situation.

C. R. Chapman: I can only agree with your comment. I think that is a very good observation and hereafter I will make a point of doing so.

W. A. Check: Dr. Long, as the effects of dorsal column stimulation are known to wear off after several years, could the 60 to 90% results you observe at 1 month following transcutaneous nerve stimulation continue for 2 to 3 years?

D. M. Long: The problem of accommodation of dorsal column-stimulated patients is very difficult because this group of patients was chosen because of their complaint of pain—long before anyone except Drs. Fordyce and Bonica were aware of the topics we have been discussing this morning. The patients were not well selected and the psychological factors were not controlled. At the time, we did not even know that one should eliminate drugs before treating these patients. So, much of this apparent fall-away of efficacy may be due to patient selection, not to any plasticity of the nervous system.

A second point is that we did study the same group of patients over a 1-year period, and if the efficacy at 1 month was compared to that at 1 year, there was no statistically significant change.

W. A. Check: Dr. Long, you stated that use of these physical stimulation procedures should be confined to people with objective pain. In a practical sense, when people come to your pain clinic and you decide whether to try these procedures, what operational criteria do you use for classification?

D. M. Long: Our technique employs, first, a physical diagnosis whenever possible and, second, a complete psychiatric and psychological characterization, using a pain perception battery. The third classification is really the evaluation by the full staff of the pain treatment center and, after all the data are studied, we believe that interventional procedures are warranted.

We may use diagnostic interventional procedures to help in making that decision, but the point that I was really making is that it is unlikely that one of these implantable electrical stimulators is valid therapy for a patient who has primarily an operant problem, as Dr. Fordyce has mentioned. It is not, however, appropriate for a patient who has primarily a psychiatric problem with an expression of pain.

What I am trying to say is that things which are done for somatic or respondent pain are different than what we do for operant pain—we use the term "psychiatric" pain as well—but I am really talking about psychiatric disease with pain as a complaint. Those so afflicted are not candidates for surgical procedures. Much of the patient's trouble began with a failure to employ this characterization and was further complicated by six operations piled one on top of another on a patient whose problem was operant to begin with.

A. Ganz: I direct this question to both Drs. Fordyce and Chapman and perhaps to Dr. Bonica. Do we need to establish such a great distinction between acute and chronic pain? It appears to me that chronic pain is an opportunity for development of the operant or behavioral effects. There are some situations in which acute pain can be a disease as well as a symptom and others where chronic pain can also have some symptomatic aspects.

From a practical viewpoint, I think you have to treat both the pathophysiological or the sensory problems as well as the behavioral problems. This is why I question the need for making that sharp distinction.

J. J. Bonica: In my opinion, our past failures have been due to the fact that we have not recognized the distinction between these two types of pain. There is a little question about the basic mechanisms; whether it is acute or chronic pain, both the nervous system and the mind are involved. I think, however, that in the acute process there is usually an acute disease that may be due to accidental injury; very rarely do you see a patient who has pain without demonstrable pathology in the acute process.

In chronic pain, in contrast, there is a significant population of patients who do not have so-called organic pathology or somatic input. The failure to differentiate these pain types has caused millions of patients to be subjected to drug toxicity, useless operations, and so forth.

Moreover, I believe that the systems that we have elucidated from laboratory studies of acute pain in both humans and animals are probably not as predominant as those in the chronic pain patient. It is my speculation that after you cut the anterolateral segments of the spinal cord and have interrupted the primary pathway for acute pain, the pain comes back. How do you explain it?

It is most likely, I think, that other afferent systems come into play—this is part of nature, the plasticity of the nervous system. Perhaps I have overstated the differences, but this was done purposely to bring them to the attention of the physicians and others who examine pain—whether it is acute or chronic—as an acute process, and treat it as such. Pain in the jaw from a toothache is an acute process, and one has to approach it differently than pain that has existed for several years. The latter will involve many more complex psychological, behavioral, and environmental factors. I hope that partially answers your objection to the dichotomy or the separation of pain types.

C. R. Chapman: I think that this differentiation has been tremendously useful at the clinical level. It has been a functional dichotomy, but dichotomies always oversimplify things. As basic scientists, what we need to deal with is the notion of a continuum ranging from acute to chronic pain with a great many things that fall in the gray area between these two poles.

Migraine headaches, for example, are neither acute or chronic but because they recur, they are not chronically there. So recurrent pains are left out of our classification and are a little difficult to deal with.

J. J. Bonica: Not of mind. They are chronic because they last for a long period of time even though they are not continuous.

C. R. Chapman: That supports my earlier point.

It is going to be important for us to develop the concept and to work out the details of a continuum on which we evaluate these things. I am interested in perceptual processes that surround the pain experience; they are altogether different when the pain is relatively novel than when it is very familiar, recurrent, and continuously present.

W. E. Fordyce: I also want to underscore what Dr. Bonica said and reemphasize that the problem in dealing with chronic pain is that so often people fail to sufficiently consider what I hear called operant pain. They start with the assumption that it is nociception and proceed from there, often leading people down a blind alley.

I would like to underscore that the terms are not mutually exclusive. One rarely sees, using the terminology I employ, the problem being characterized as purely operant pain. Similarly, in chronic pain, one rarely sees the problem as purely respondent pain.

J. J. Bonica: That is the view of the psychologist. I can attest to the fact that I am a respondent, chronic pain sufferer who has had pain for a number of years. After they put my artificial hips in, the pain markedly decreased. I feel better and do not have any of the problems my colleagues talked about. That chronic pain is usually a behavioral problem is overstating the situation. There are many patients who have chronic pain of arthritis, of cancer, and pain of many other conditions that are respondent pain and obviously require a different approach to the problem. I think conditioning of those patients would be partially or completely fruitless.

D. M. Long: I wish to add that the reason we have the categorization described earlier is purely practical. It enables us to choose patients who are likely to respond to interventional procedure appropriately and to direct others into behavioral conditioning or into psychotherapy or whatever is the appropriate therapy for their pain. It is simply that kind of practical clinical tool.

A. Taub: Dr. Fordyce, I would like to voice an objection to the continued use of "operant" and "respondent" in referring to pain—pain being an experience. If you want to append "behavior," I will accept that.

Can you give us a practical paradigm by which you can detect to what degree a particular patient in a clinical setting—not an artificial laboratory setting— is manifesting respondent or operant pain behavior. Specifically, how would you go about it?

W. E. Fordyce: I am sorry I must disagree, Dr. Taub, with your comment. In chronic pain you are not observing pain as an experience; you are strictly observing pain behavior and you are inferring a pain experience. That is the basis of my disagreement.

A. Taub: I agree with you in that we cannot observe an experience; you are always observing behavior. When you say operant and respondent, you are talking about behavior, not about pain; pain is an experience.

W. E. Fordyce: Absolutely. I fully agree with that. As to the distinction between operant and respondent pain, I cannot do it justice in such a short time. Let me make two quick generalizations. In treatment of chronic pain, it is important, in addition to doing the medical work-up of the problem, that one should also do behavioral analysis. This behavioral analysis should have at least the following components. The first is a record of what the person does, such as through the use of diary forms by which they note when they are up and when they are down, when they are moving around, and so forth. The second part of it is the asking, in a variety of ways, two general questions:

First, what good things happen when I hurt that otherwise would not? Two examples of this are PRM medications—I have to hurt to get a fix—that are pain contingent and attention, which often is pain contingent.

Second, what bad things do not happen when I engage in pain behavior that otherwise would happen? Putting that another way, what potentially aversive events, like a dissatisfying job or having to do something I do not want to do, do I effectively avoid by engaging in pain behavior? It corresponds very roughly to secondary "gain" although that is probably a less precise term.

R. W. Houde: I would like to emphasize the point that you made regarding the fact that not all chronic pain is without underlying pathology. Also, I am concerned with what is judgmentally stated as exaggerated pain.

I understand that if you are going to intervene by electrical stimulation techniques, the patient is withdrawn from medication, this being a necessary condition for treating the patient. How do you know that these patients truly do not have some underlying pathology that is really responsible for their complaint?

D. M. Long: Our technique for using any of the stimulators, except the transcutaneous stimulators, requires that the patient enroll in our chronic pain treatment program, during which time a psychiatric and physical evaluation and appropriate diagnosis is made. Furthermore, the patient must be withdrawn from medication. The withdrawal from narcotics is a standard part of the program and we make no exceptions to it. He must have his depression, sleeplessness, chronic anxieties—all the concomitants of chronic pain—treated. After all of these things are under control, we make a decision as to whether an interventional procedure appears to be indicated.

One type of patient with which we deal would experience pain from an industrial accident, have no physical abnormalities at the time of the accident, and none since. He would show normal, or virtually normal, profile after X-ray, neurological, and associated examinations. As far as we can determine, this is a normal patient who says his back hurts so much he cannot go to work. He is the one who is likely to fall into our exaggerated classification.

By contrast, the patient in whom we might implant an electrical stimulator has undergone an average of six operations on the back, has demonstrable arachnoiditis, and a significant neurological deficit.

These two categories have little, if any, overlap. Maybe we are wrong in not using these devices to help more of the less seriously injured patients, but that has been my choice to date.

J. J. Bonica: I just wish to add that in our own program we find many patients, as Dr. Fordyce has indicated, who are intoxicated from nonnarcotic drugs. For example, we had a lady who was taking 125 pills a day, which had been prescribed by no less than seven physicians. She was so confused and intellectually dulled that we simply could not begin the work-up—let alone start therapy. When we withdrew the drugs, as a part of our program, the patient later said, "You know, my pain isn't so bad after all." Situations involving multiple drug intake and drug toxicity represent a very serious problem with chronic pain patients.

R. W. Houde: Although it is unquestionably recognized that the drugs are strong reinforcers of behavior, it is also recognized that with narcotics (in particular, good analgesics) tolerance develops with repeated administration. I simply cannot understand why reduction or the withdrawal of a drug is a necessary condition for a patient with objective signs of pain scheduled for electrical stimulation. You would not proceed further if your psychological testing disqualifies the patient from your program.

D. M. Long: Once we have decided that the electrical stimulators or any other kind of interventional procedure may be indicated, we rarely do a destructive procedure. That problem has a very different answer than that of deciding to limit this procedure to those patients who appear to have a real respondent pain problem. There are two purposes for this course of action. First, while patients are addicted—it has been our experience that their response to therapy is unpredictable—we cannot trust their statements because they cannot distinguish between pain and the need for the drug. When they need the drug, their pain is worsened. If you are using a therapy during that period of time, you simply cannot trust what patients say about the temporary stimulation.

Second, there is reasonable evidence—anecdotal and not proven—that the drugs interfere with the effectiveness of the electrical stimulation: If patients have been implanted with a thalamic stimulator, they will achieve excellent pain relief. However, if they are given narcotics, pain relief disappears.

We are not as certain about this reversal in cases of spinal cord stimulation, but we have a number of patients who return to the use of narcotics for their own purposes and lose the efficacy of the dorsal column stimulator, only to have efficacy return as soon as they withdraw from narcotics. I cannot prove this to be the case for anything except the pain stimulation, but since there is enough chance of interference, I like to have them off narcotics so we can assess the effectiveness of the technique before we commit them to an implant.

R. W. Houde: Has that been well documented? Do you have a published reference to it?

D. M. Long: Papers on brain stimulation studies by Richardson and by Adams and Hosobuchi have appeared in *Science* in the past year. We have yet to publish these data because we are still in the process of evaluating the effects of these stimulations with and without naloxone and with and without narcotics. We feel this is a correct interpretation and want the narcotic eliminated prior to the use of any forms of—except TNS—electrical stimulation.

J. J. Bonica: During the intermission one of the members of the audience asked me why I did not stress how to better provide, primarily with narcotics, good relief to a patient with acute and chronic pain. It has been both my personal experience as a postoperative patient and my observation of patients throughout the world that postoperative, posttraumatic, and postburn pain are treated inadequately because of the misconception of the physician and the nurse. I might also blame our system wherein giving small or large doses of narcotics for a short period of time means either the individual is an addict or has a low pain threshold.

The fact is that these drugs are effective and should be used to provide good pain relief. If one titrates the needs of the patient with the drug dosage, one finds that side effects, particularly respiratory depression, do not occur. Thus, I would like to plead for wider usage of narcotic drugs for patients with acute pain.

In patients with *chronic* pain, however, the story is different and calls for prolonged narcotic therapy. If there are other methods that would be more effective, it would be a disservice to the patient. On the other hand, as Dr. Houde believes, although the patient becomes incapacitated, as a last resort he can be returned to usefulness by the use of repeated, controlled doses of narcotics. I think I share his views that this should be done. Unfortunately, it is not done in this country.

More importantly is the fact that patients with inoperable recurrent cancer pain are treated abominably in this country and many other countries. I recently attended a meeting in Venice at which the message was loud and clear: Throughout the world, except for a few centers in Great Britain and America, cancer pain is inadequately relieved because—again—doctors and nurses feel that 50 mg of demerol or 10 mg of morphine should do it. If that treatment does not do it, that is too bad. The fact is that physicians treating these patients find that it is often necessary to administer up to 100 mg of morphine orally every 4 hr in order to obtain relief. If you titrate the patient after this regimen, you find that the patient is rehabilitated: He is not depressed and is much more alert than he would be without the drug.

Again, I plead for adequate pain relief in cancer patients. If narcotic therapy is selected, sufficiently high dosages should be given. There are other therapeutic modalities that might be more effective, but unfortunately we do not have enough time to discuss them.

A. Wikler: Dr. Chapman, in the tooth pulp stimulation experiment you described, was the sensation evoked in the patient the threshold sensation? Was that a tap followed by an ache? What was the sensation that the patient reported?

C. R. Chapman: After one shocks a tooth electrically, a very small range of prepain sensation is experienced by some, but not all, subjects. It is felt as a very subtle tingling immediately followed by a brief ache. It is rather like biting into very cold ice cream. Almost anything you do to the tooth produces a similar sort of experience.

A. Wikler: To which of these two sensations do you think the evoked potential—the N175–P260 part of the curve—was related?

C. R. Chapman: Let me emphasize that these are very late evoked responses. They probably reflect some sort of activity in association cortex or at least integration of the experience. I do not think it is a matter of nerve impulses arising at some central location to indicate that pain occurred, but rather than appreciation or interpretation of these impulses. We are doing some work on what we call far-field, as opposed to near-field, evoked responses that occur in the first 10 or 20 msec.

A. Wikler: I was surprised to see that fentanyl reduced the magnitude of the N175–P260 segment. I express surprise because many years ago the Addiction Research Center studies on pain thresholds to radiant heat or electrical stimulation of teeth produced no consistent results. In our 1950 or 1952 study, we found that morphine had no effect at all on the ability of subjects to estimate the intensities of electrically delivered shocks of known wattage and fixed durations to the skin; but it very profoundly affected the subject's overestimation of the intensity of the shock. We deliberately increased the patient's fear and anxiety about the procedure, and morphine corrected the error. Examining another group of patients, in which the fear and anxiety was minimized, morphine had no effect whatever on the ability to estimate the intensity of the shock. This is why I am surprised that fentanyl, which acts like morphine, reduced the magnitude of the N175–P260 segment.

C. R. Chapman: As I indicated, there is a large psychology literature on evoked somatosensory responses in the late waves. These waves are related not to the arrival of information from the periphery but to the subject's appreciation or meaning of the stimulus. I think that is the point you are making. It is a psychological and not simply a sensory component that we are looking at.

I am sorry there was insufficient time in my presentation to mention that we do not really know yet whether fentanyl is reducing that evoked response due to its analgesic or sedative properties. We have to clarify the action of fentanyl in the experiments so that we can be firm in our conclusions.

With regard to your comments about why our effect is more clear than in early studies, both radiant heat stimulation and electrical shock methods involve a very large range of sensations between the thresholds of detection and pain. The tooth pulp work encompasses a very tiny range and gives us considerably more precision than if we used the other methods.

Mechanisms of Pain and Analgesic Compounds,
edited by R. F. Beers, Jr., and E. G. Bassett.
Raven Press, New York © 1979.

10. Introduction to Section B: An Overview of the Neurological Significance of Pain

Kenneth L. Casey

*Departments of Neurology and Physiology, University of Michigan,
Ann Arbor, Michigan 48109*

Pain has been considered a major clinical problem since the beginning of medicine. Pain has also been regarded as one of the major somatic and visceral senses and, as such, important in the study of information processing in nervous systems. The study of pain mechanisms adds to our understanding of how sensory events are identified, distinguished from one another, and localized in time and space. Contemporary research into the neural mechanisms of pain has further emphasized that pain is a problem of major significance in neurobiology because it touches on a wide range of some of the most fundamental questions in neuroscience.

RECEPTOR ACTIVATION

The perception of somatic pain is common to a variety of physically distinct stimuli: thermal, mechanical, or chemical, which damage, or threaten to damage, tissue. This suggests the presence of a class of cutaneous nociceptors that respond to any form of stimulus energy of sufficient intensity. It is now well established that there are, in cutaneous and deeper tissues, nociceptors that generate action potentials in finely myelinated and unmyelinated afferent nerve fibers (2). Since all noxious stimuli threaten tissue damage, the question arises as to the mechanism by which nociceptors are activated. The physical and biochemical steps by which noxious stimuli specifically activate these receptors are not known. Since most of the experimental work has been on cutaneous afferents, much less is known about the nature of stimuli that excite deep or visceral nociceptors. If current research directions prove fruitful, however, continued investigation may lead to a greatly improved understanding of the biochemical and biophysical steps interposed between a noxious stimulus, the local chemical changes induced in tissue, and the resulting electrophysiological events leading to the generation of propagated action potentials. The significance of these advances would clearly extend well beyond the field of pain research.

SEGMENTAL REFLEX ORGANIZATION

As an acute event, activation of nociceptors by events that damage, or threaten to damage, tissue results in protective action to preserve tissue integrity or at least prevent further damage. Localized, segmental reflexes are engaged at spinal and brainstem levels to withdraw the body from the offending stimulus. By studying the neurophysiology of these intrinsic, unlearned responses, much has been learned about the functional segmental and intersegmental organization of the somatic nervous system and how its input and output is modulated by drugs and by suprasegmental neural activity. Acute nociceptive input also elicits reflex responses from the autonomic nervous system, resulting in increased sympathetic discharge. These adaptive responses may also be accompanied by global endocrine changes such as an increased secretion of ACTH, cortisol, and epinephrine. Noxious stimuli thus provide a useful means for investigating the determinants and mechanisms of autonomic and neuroendocrine as well as somatic motor activity.

It is now well established that nociceptive afferents activate distinct groups of spinal cord or trigeminal nuclear neurons, some responding exclusively to noxious stimuli and others showing a graded range of response to innocuous and noxious stimuli (13). At the first central synapse, it becomes clear that the central transmission of signals from nociceptors is strongly dependent on excitatory and inhibitory influences generated from adjacent segmental neurons, presynaptic and postsynaptic interactions among other afferent fibers, and suprasegmental neurons with descending projections (12). A major problem for present and future research is to analyze the anatomy, physiology, and chemistry of local segmental circuits and the effect of extrasegmental influences on their operation.

SUPRASEGMENTAL FUNCTIONS

Acute and chronic pain is characterized by the presence of more complex, suprasegmentally organized behaviors aimed at escaping or avoiding noxious stimuli. Like all strongly goal-directed behaviors, these are initiated by motivational mechanisms that, in highly complex and organized nervous systems, are usually assumed to be associated with an affective internal state. Pain is not simply the detection of tissue damage; it is an experience that includes the distinctly aversive or unpleasant quality typically associated with tissue-damaging events (4). Of course, aversive experiences are not uniquely associated with tissue damage; unpleasant sights, sounds, and odors are common. Noxious, tissue-damaging stimuli, however, are the type most frequently accompanied by an unpleasant or negative affective state and aversive motivation to escape, attack, or withdraw. It is as though the afferent activity generated by nociceptors has an especially strong input to the neural mechanisms generating these internal states and the resulting behaviors. This distinguishes pain from other senses and lends special significance to the investigation of pain mechanisms. It is likely that an understanding of pain mechanisms will progress along with further insight into the neural determinants of affective state.

Although motivational and affective states are of interest in themselves, they are of equal importance as necessary states for the learning of new behaviors. Under especially strong motivational circumstances, such as those established by noxious stimuli, permanent learning may take place in a single trial. Learning often occurs in the presence of positive, rather than negative, reinforcement, but the activation of nociceptive afferents provides a functionally and anatomically distinct, readily accessible means of engaging a neural system that is a fundamental part of establishing learning.

The central pathway for pain is not known. The ventral and lateral spinothalamic tracts, which contain the axons of nociceptive dorsal horn neurons, terminate in at least three regions of the thalamus (6). Collateral projections from these tracts also terminate at several levels of the brainstem reticular formation where nociceptive responsive cells have also been recorded (3). To this already substantial amount of neural tissue may be added the neurons activated via the polysynaptic reticular substance of the spinal cord, for there is clinical and experimental evidence that these cells may mediate some aspect of pain (1). Finally, there continues to be considerable uncertainty as to the role of the cerebral cortex in pain sensation. Some anatomical and clinical evidence, for example, would suggest that a relatively specific nociceptive cortical region may exist (7). To sort out the functional significance of these different projection systems and to relate their activities to some aspect of pain is a prodigious task that will require many more years of work in all phases of neuroscience. It is likely, for example, that combined behavioral, neurophysiological, and neurochemical approaches will have to be developed for experiments with the awake, behaving animal since anesthesia significantly alters the pain-related responses of many central neurons.

CENTRAL CONTROL MECHANISMS

The modulation of nociceptive reflexes and pain perception emphasizes the functional significance of CNS control systems that regulate sensory and motor activities. There are few, if any, circumstances in which the effect of selective attention mechanisms is more dramatically demonstrated than in those instances in which normally painful tissue damage is ignored, even though anesthetic or analgesic agents have not been administered. Inattention to otherwise painful events is commonly observed in athletic events, war combat, religious rituals, hypnosis, or similar conditions in which the brain appears to be attending to other events, but is somehow filtering out an input that is normally highest in the hierarchy of engaging attentional mechanisms and reflexive action. The brain appears to have switched to a unique mode of operation, and occurrence of this switch is indicated by the lack of response to noxious stimulation. Shift of attentional focus is, of course, a continually recurring event throughout the normal life of any higher organism. The neural mechanisms involved, however, are more likely to be most active when noxious stimuli are ignored than when attention is shifted away from innocuous somatic, auditory, or visual events.

The current high level of research interest in sensory control systems in the CNS was rekindled in large part by the experimental observation that an apparently selective and profound analgesia could be induced by focal electrical stimulation within selected regions of the brain and brainstem (9,10). The subsequent observation that such analgesia shows cross-tolerance with morphine and is reversed by naloxone (8) is especially significant in view of the recently discovered opiate receptors (11) and endogenous opiate peptides in the brain (5). Among many other possibilities, these exciting findings provide the opportunity to study pain mechanisms by producing controlled analgesia by a variety of methods. The significance of these findings, however, extends beyond an understanding of the mechanisms of pain and analgesia. Continued research on the mechanisms of pain modulation is likely to continue to provide further insight into the mechanisms by which the brain regulates many other sensory and reflex processes.

The investigation of pain mechanisms, then, goes well beyond adding essential details to our knowledge of sensory processing and somesthesis. It leads into studies of the molecular mechanisms of receptor activation; somatic, autonomic, and neuroendocrine reflex organization; the neural basis of motivation, affect, and accompanying emotional states; the neural events providing a necessary condition for learning; and the determinants of attentional control over sensory and motor processes.

Significant advances in our understanding of pain mechanisms have been made in recent years. The new knowledge acquired has often contributed to other areas of neuroscience and has provided a new basis for the consideration of new therapeutic approaches. There is little doubt that, with the proper resources, future research will supply the new knowledge that is necessary for continued progress in many areas of basic and clinical neuroscience.

ACKNOWLEDGMENT

These studies were supported by grants NS–12015 and NS–12581 from the National Institutes of Health.

REFERENCES

1. Basbaum, A. I. (1973): Conduction of the effects of noxious stimulation by short-fiber multisynaptic systems of the spinal cord in the rat. *Exp. Neurol.,* 40:699–716.
2. Burgess, P. R., and Perl, E. R. (1973): Cutaneous mechanoreceptors and nociceptors. In: *Handbook of Sensory Physiology, Vol. II, Somatosensory System,* edited by A. Iggo, pp. 29–78. Springer-Verlag, New York.
3. Casey, K. L. (1969): Somatic stimuli, spinal pathways, and size of cutaneous fibers influencing unit activity in the medial medullary reticular formation. *Exp. Neurol.,* 25:35–36.

4. Casey, K. L., and Melzack, R. (1967): Neural mechanisms of pain: A conceptual model. In: *New Concepts in Pain and Its Clinical Management,* edited by E. L. Way, pp. 13–32. F. A. Davis, Philadelphia.

5. Hughes, J. (1975): Isolation of an endogenous compound from the brain with pharmacological properties similar to morphine. *Brain Res.,* 88:295–308.

6. Jones, E. G., and Burton, H. (1974): Cytoarchitecture and somatic sensory connectivity of thalamic nuclei other than the ventrobasal complex in the cat. *J. Comp. Neurol.,* 154:395–432.

7. Jones, E. G., and Burton, H. (1976): Areal differences in the laminar distribution of thalamic afferents in cortical fields of the insular, parietal and temporal regions of primates. *J. Comp. Neurol.,* 168:197–247.

8. Mayer, D. J., and Price, D. D. (1976): Central nervous system mechanisms of analgesia. *Pain,* 2:379–404.

9. Mayer, D. J., Wolfle, T. L., Akil, H., Carder, B., and Liebeskind, J. C. (1971): Analgesia from electrical stimulation in the brainstem of the rat. *Science,* 174:1351–1354.

10. Reynolds, D. V. (1969): Surgery in the rat during electrical analgesia induced by focal brain stimulation. *Science,* 164:444–445.

11. Snyder, S. H., Pert, C. B., and Pasternak, G. W. (1974): The opiate receptor. *Ann. Intern. Med.,* 81:534–540.

12. Wall, P. D. (1967): The laminar organization of dorsal horn and effects of descending impulses. *J. Physiol.,* 188:403–423.

13. Willis, W. D. (1976): Spinothalamic system: Physiological aspects. In: *Advances in Pain Research and Therapy, Vol. 1: Proceedings of the First World Congress on Pain,* edited by J. J. Bonica and D. Albe-Fessard, pp. 215–223. Raven Press, New York.

Mechanisms of Pain and Analgesic Compounds,
edited by R. F. Beers, Jr., and E. G. Bassett.
Raven Press, New York © 1979.

11. Segmental Circuitry and Ascending Pathways of the Nociceptive System

Frederick W. L. Kerr

Department of Neurologic Surgery, Mayo Clinic, Rochester, Minnesota 55901

INTRODUCTION

The structural features of the central nervous system, although inherently fascinating, assume their full significance only when their functional roles are understood. Conversely, physiological observations that are not closely tied to underlying circuitry often rest on an uncertain base; when structural and functional observations are in close accord, inferences regarding both are more likely to be correct.

In this summary of current concepts of the circuitry and transmission pathways underlying nociception, I have attempted to correlate structural and functional data wherever possible, recognizing that much is necessarily oversimplified in view of the still limited knowledge we possess regarding the complex circuitry of each of the nuclei involved in the integrative processes, of the ancillary pathways involved in relay of nociceptive input to higher centers, and of the role of the cerebral cortex in pain mechanisms, to name but a few areas that remain poorly understood.

An important caveat the reader should bear in mind in regard to any discussion of anatomical or neurophysiological aspects of pain is that, in most instances, correlation between such data and the experience of pain is fraught with subtle difficulties. In neurophysiological investigations, in which efforts are made to correlate firing characteristics of single units in the central nervous system with pain, several fundamental issues must be considered. Thus, the fact that a central neuron fires at progressively higher frequency as a stimulus to the peripheral receptive area passes from nonnoxious to progressively more intense and finally overtly noxious levels neither guarantees nor negates that that particular neuron is relaying a message which at higher levels in the neuraxis will be interpreted as pain. For example, a segmental neuron responding in this manner may simply be an interneuron in the flexor reflex pathway. Alternatively, there is no certainty that, because a central neuron connected to a peripheral mechanoreceptor discharges at higher frequencies when the receptive field is stimulated at supramaximal intensities, it is relaying nociceptive information to higher centers. It is quite possible that its central connections are to autonomic centers concerned with the vasomotor cardioaccelerator or pupillodilator responses characteristically observed during noxious stimulation; furthermore, even if its central connections are with neurons in the somesthetic pathway, it may feed into a neuron pool whose activation is not related to the experience of pain (i.e., it may be concerned with purely mechanoreceptor activities). The implication is that a relay neuron at a lower level in the neuraxis may discharge at frequencies over and above those reached when the peripheral mechanoreceptor is maximally activated. This could be due to activation of other mechanoreceptor afferents with overlapping peripheral and central fields or to central convergence from nociceptor afferents or the relay neuron, neither of which need imply nociceptive relay by the latter.

On the other hand, a central neuron that does not respond at low or intermediate stimulus intensities, that is, nonnoxious (determined by psychophysical tests), but begins to respond at stimulus intensities that are clearly within the noxious range, may or may not be in the pathway to conscious appreciation of pain. Again, it might be in the reflex pathways (somatic or autonomic) referred to earlier. It is therefore necessary to establish not only the response characteristics of neurons under scrutiny, but also the target site to which they project.

Finally, if the psychophysical correlate of pain can also be added to the preceding postulates, such that the firing pattern of the neuron correlates well with the behavioral responses observed, the level of confidence is further enhanced. It is well to note that even then one is dealing with degrees of probability but not certainty.

Obviously, it is rarely possible to assemble such a complex battery of tests during single unit recordings in order to provide substantive evidence that one is in fact dealing with a "pain neuron." The preceding comments may, however, serve to focus more attention on some of the frequently overlooked difficulties inherent in drawing conclusions in regard to the complex problem of pain from single neuron recording techniques.

Relating structural (histological or electron microscopic) observations to nociception has presented still greater difficulties since, among other limitations, functional correlates have been lacking in the past and more or less cautious extrapolations from other experimental or clinical studies have been required.

The recent development of intracellular labeling techniques has improved this situation in a very significant manner, so that neurophysiologists and neuroanatomists now have a common meeting ground. Particularly noteworthy in this respect are the results obtained by other investigators (16,17,46,62,63,98).

Thus, neuroanatomy is undergoing an overt revolution and reorganization with correlation between structure and function becoming far closer than could have been anticipated even a decade ago.

SEGMENTAL CIRCUITRY

Since the general features of the distribution of primary afferents at the segmental level of the spinal cord have been the subject of a number of reviews in recent years (14,52,55,57,90), and as a result are well known, these may be dealt with in a rather cursory manner. Much new information has been acquired, however, in the past 2 to 3 years by several groups of investigators; this information requires careful consideration and critical analysis.

General

The separation into a lateral fine calibered and a medial large calibered division as the dorsal root enters the cord is well established (see reviews listed). It should be noted that all fibers of the lateral division are of small caliber, whereas the medial division contains a moderate number of small fibers. Also, the fibers of the lateral division may enter either into the Lissauer's tract, where they are said to run for up to two segments, or may pass directly from the root into the marginal zone and substantia gelatinosa. Fibers of the medial division continue ventrally along the medial border of the dorsal horn, where they divide into several branches; one of these branches enters the dorsal horn and reverses direction to run dorsally through part of the magnocellular nucleus just beneath the s. gelatinosa. Here a number of them bifurcate into an ascending and a descending branch that, overall, may extend for 1.5 to 1.7 mm (16). From these longitudinal branches, the candelabra-like tufts of endings (21) project into the gelatinosa to end at levels that are variously stated to either laminae III or II, as noted later in Fig.1; each of these complex tufts terminates in huge numbers of boutons. The total number of endings for the parent fiber, although as yet unknown, undoubtedly runs into the tens or perhaps hundreds of thousands.

OBSERVATIONS AND DISCUSSION

Excitatory Input

New Observations on the Distribution of Primary Afferents

Several issues of considerable interest have been raised in the past 2 to 3 years. First, it has been proposed (58–60,62,63,88) that the terminals of large primary afferents (PAs) end in lamina III without reaching lamina II. There is general agreement that fine PAs end in laminae I and II, and they may extend deeper in some instances; Rethelyi (88) has proposed that the only site of termination of unmyelinated PAs is lamina II.

This type of organization would then suggest rather strongly that laminae I and II are concerned primarily with nociceptive input, whereas nonnoxious input would be distributed in lamina III and perhaps deeper layers. That fine PA fibers distribute to the marginal zone and s. gelatinosa has been inferred since the studies of Cajal (21; Fig. 120 therein), although their precise sites of termination have been unknown until recently.

Rethelyi (88), using the Golgi–Kopsch technique, concluded that the fine fibers, which appeared to originate from unmyelinated primary afferents in dorsal roots, were distributed in narrow, longitudinally oriented lamellae and confined exclusively to the s. gelatinosa, to which they provided both "en passage" and terminal endings. This observation correlates well with the electrophysiological studies of Kumazawa and Perl (58,59), according to which gelatinosa neurons are specifically excited by PAs connected to polymodal nociceptors.

Further support for this point of view has been provided by Light and Perl (62), who applied horseradish peroxidase (HRP) to crushed dorsal roots of cat and monkey in which either the medial or the lateral division of the dorsal root had been transected. They found that in the former situation there was widespread labeling of the marginal zone and s. gelatinosa, whereas in the latter experiments, only the nucleus proprius contained HRP, thus providing a clear parallel with the study by LaMotte (60).

The issue remains controversial, however, since Yaksh et al. (108) have recorded the responses of over 300 s. gelatinosa neurons and found that the majority of these cells are activated by light mechanical stimulation of the skin and none responds to stimulation of unmyelinated fibers. That the unit responses they describe are in fact from neuronal somata and not simply recordings of fibers is clearly demonstrated both by their failure to follow at low stimulus frequencies and by significant variation in latency of individual responses.

Evidence has been presented recently by Cervero et al. (25,27,28) that both nonnociceptive-as well as nociceptive-driven gelatinosa units are present. That this possibility should be considered was indicated in the original diagram of synaptic circuitry of the dorsal horn I proposed (50,53), which forms the basis for a postsynaptic inhibitory balance theory for pain mechanisms. In this proposal, regardless of the noxious or nonnoxious nature of the PA input to gelatinosa cells, with the exception of the few elements that project to higher levels (see below), their output is regarded as inhibitory. The report by Denny-Brown and co-workers (35) provides behavioral evidence for the inhibitory role of gelatinosa neurons, and direct evidence that these neurons are inhibitory has been found by Wall and Yaksh (106).

Recent studies with HRP transport by Proshansky and Egger (82,83) indicate that at least some of the medially located, large PAs to the dorsal horn reach as far as lamina I, whereas Snyder (98) reported that these larger fibers are distributed mainly in lamina III, but also enter into lamina II; furthermore, Brown (16) (see below), using intracellular electrophoresis of HRP, has shown that some of the larger fibers (slowly adapting claw mechanoreceptors) are distributed from laminae II to V or VI. The obvious conflicts between the various groups of investigators remain to be resolved. Finally, Hamano et al. (43) report that PAs are often distributed to more than two laminae and that some supply only the medial, others the lateral, whereas yet others distribute in both areas of the dorsal horn.

Functional Neuroanatomy of PAs

The technique of intracellular electrophoretic extrusion of a cellular marker [pioneered by Stretton and Kravitz (99)], combined with physiological characterization of the properties of a PA neuron in terms of sensory modality, receptive field characteristics, threshold, conduction velocity, and chronaxie, is currently providing some of the most important information on the central distribution of PAs as well as those of higher order neurons. The introduction of HRP as the labeling agent (34,46,61,97) makes it possible to visualize, in histological sections, physiologically identified neurons and their processes with details equivalent to, or surpassing, the best Golgi preparations.

With this technique, Brown (16) has reported that each type of PA has a specific pattern of termination in the dorsal horn. This approach has been most successful with larger fibers and, occasionally, with those in the Aδ range; it

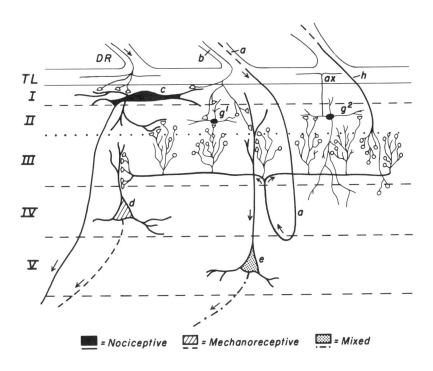

FIG. 1. A simplified diagram of some excitatory circuits as seen in a longitudinal section of the dorsal horn. A larger mechanoreceptor fiber (a) from skin after a retroflex course bifurcates into ascending and descending branches from which multiple tufts of terminal endings ascend and distribute mainly in lamina III with a variable extension into lamina II. These endings in the gelatinosa are in a position to provide great numbers of terminal contacts to dendrites of both deeper (laminae IV and V) and more superficial (laminae I and II) neurons. Nociceptive afferents (b) distribute in laminae I and II where they synapse on dendrites of marginal neurons and probably of gelatinosa cells. Note that dendrites of gelatinosa neurons may extend well beyond the lamina in which their soma lies (e.g., g²), and those of lamina V neurons may reach as far as lamina I; also, numerous other types of terminal distribution of large primary afferents occur, as described in the text. c, marginal neuron; d, mechenoreceptor neuron in lamina IV; DR, dorsal root; e, wide dynamic range neuron in lamina V; h, direct mechanoreceptor primary afferent.

is not applicable to C fibers at the present time, due to the technical problem of penetrating axons with micropipettes. Brown (16) has summarized the results obtained by his group and demonstrated that PAs connected to hair follicle receptors give rise to up to 11 collaterals from the longitudinally coursing bifurcation branches of PAs (Fig. 1) over a rostrocaudal distance of 1 cm or more; these terminals are restricted to laminae III and IV. Afferents from mechanoreceptors in hairy skin and from claw receptors, each having different patterns of termination are observed; these differ, in turn, from those of the hair follicle receptors.

Light and Perl (62,63) have been able to inject axons connected to mechanical nociceptors with conduction velocities as low as 7.5 m/sec; they report that these afferents have numerous terminals in the marginal zone and a few in the gelatinosa. Conversely, D-hair afferents were found to distribute mainly to laminae IV and V. Like Brown (16), they report that the PA axon of each identified type of receptor (G1, G2, type I and II slowly adapting mechanoreceptors, etc.) has a distinctive pattern of distribution in the dorsal horn.

Some Cytological Features

A basic feature that is often overlooked in evaluating input to the spinal gray is the extent of the dendritic arborization of neurons. Thus, even gelatinosa neurons, with somata measuring 5×10 μm, usually have dendritic expansions that extend for 100 to 200 μm or more and reach well into adjacent laminae. Cajal (21) had already described these cells as having dendritic arbors oriented radially as well as longitudinally in the s. gelatinosa, the longitudinally oriented processes being considerably longer; even a cursory examination of his illustrations shows that many gelatinosa neurons have dendrites that span both laminae II and III of the Rexed classification. Sugiura (100) also illustrates gelatinosa neurons whose somata lie in lamina II and show dendritic arbors that extend into lamina III (Fig. 2).

Thus, in a very real sense, arguments regarding absence of PA input to gelatinosa neurons in lamina II based on whether the PA fibers reach this lamina or not carry little weight, since, on the one hand, there is reasonable evidence that they do reach this level (lamina II) and, on the other, good evidence is available that even if they did not, the dendritic arborizations of many, if not all, lamina II cells would be readily accessible to them.

Input to the marginal zone (lamina I) from small PAs is generally accepted on the basis of Golgi studies (21,88,89,93,94,101) and electron microscopy (49). In a recent electron microscopic study, Narotzky and Kerr (73) showed that PAs established predominantly axodendritic contacts on marginal neurons. Since, as noted above, the input to the marginal zone is mainly or exclusively from small fibers, it seems reasonable to infer that this axodendritic input is

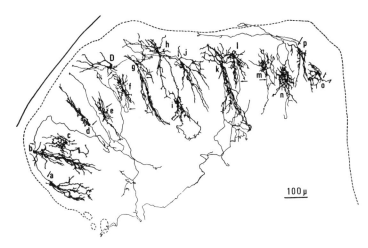

FIG. 2. The dendrites of gelatinosa neurons are seen extending well into deeper laminae; therefore, neurons in lamina II can be readily influenced by PAs ending in lamina III or deeper. (From Sugiura, ref. 100.)

predominantly nociceptive; this would be in good accord with the now classic study of Christensen and Perl (29).

In addition to activation of marginal and gelatinosa neurons (laminae I and II), there are other important elements whose relationship to primary input is much less apparent but no less important. I refer to the apical dendrites of neurons whose somata lie in lamina V and adjacent laminae IV and possibly VI. Again, Cajal (21) clearly illustrated neurons that he categorized as "giant cells of the center of the dorsal horn"; in his Fig. 148, the apical dendrite of such a neuron extends not only into the s. gelatinosa, but into the marginal zone and even into the Lissauer's t. These observations have been amply confirmed by Kenshalo and Willis (48), who have demonstrated cells in the same location with almost identical dendritic distribution (i.e., reaching laminae I and II), using the entirely different technique of retrograde transport of HRP from the thalamus. In studies currently underway in our laboratory (T. L. Yaksh, S. Yasuoka, and F. W. L. Kerr, *unpublished observations*) using intracellular microiontophoresis of HRP, we have also found neurons of lamina V with apical dendrites reaching lamina II, although not as far as the marginal zone as yet.

Finally, it should be noted that collateral branches frequently arise from axons shortly after their origin from the soma. This has been shown in a most elegant fashion by Brown (16) and by Rastad et al. (87) for neurons of origin of the spinocervical tract (Fig. 3). These collaterals provide a most profuse terminal arborization in the spinal gray at the segmental level; such neurons must, therefore, function both as local circuit neurons as well as projection

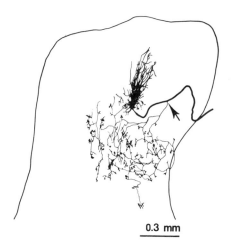

FIG. 3. Example of profuse distribution of an axonal collateral of a spinocervical tract neuron. (From Rastad et al., ref. 87.)

0.3 mm

neurons in long tracts. Insofar as the nociceptive system is concerned, Cajal (21) had noted that axons of marginal neurons give a few collaterals in the spinal gray; it will be of much interest to know whether, with the HRP technique, these collaterals will be found to give rise to a terminal arbor in the dorsal horn comparable to that of the spinocervical neurons discussed above. If this is so, they might well provide a nociceptive input to deeper lying neurons such as the "wide dynamic range" cells of lamina V, in addition to the direct input from PA fine fibers in laminae I and II proposed earlier. On the other hand, the local arborization may activate gelatinosa interneurons and provide an inhibitory feedback circuit in the way that Renshaw cells modulate motoneuron activity.

From the preceding summary, it seems evident that fine fibers distributed to the marginal zone and s. gelatinosa may be able to activate not only marginal and gelatinosa neurons, but also deep-lying neurons in the center of the dorsal horn via apical dendrites of the latter.

Another problem that remains to be resolved in regard to PAs is that of the organization and function of the glomeruli of the s. gelatinosa. The structural complexity (42) suggests that equally complex integrative processes must affect those primary endings that terminate in them.

Other Excitatory Input

The issue of afferent fibers in ventral roots has been reevaluated in much detail by Coggeshall et al. (30,31), and the possibility that they may convey nociceptive input and thus be responsible for some of the failures of dorsal rhizotomy has again been raised. Most reports of stimulation of ventral roots during operative procedures in conscious patients have been negative (107), because of the methods of stimulation employed; however, Frykholm et al.

(39) elicited deep-aching sensations by both mechanical and thermal stimulation of ventral roots but could not evoke pain by electrical stimulation, even at relatively high intensities. In a recent study, Light and Metz (64) traced ventral root afferents into the dorsal horn using the HRP transport method. Of particular interest is their observation that fine fibers appeared to distribute to the s. gelatinosa, whereas larger afferents gave profuse collateral arborizations to the nucleus proprius, before continuing into the dorsal column without contributing to the s. gelatinosa.

Inhibitory Circuits in the Dorsal Horn: Gelatinosa Neurons

The role of inhibition in nociception has been inferred for many years, but credit for bringing this factor to the attention of investigators is undoubtedly due to Melzack and Wall (70), who emphasized the major role it must play and on which they based their elegant Gate Control Theory to a major extent. That the theory has not withstood subsequent physiological testing (76) is of secondary significance in view of the impact that it has had on conceptual approaches to the problem of nociception.

The structural details of the inhibitory circuitry of the dorsal horn are still imperfectly understood, and in much of what follows, assumptions are made regarding function which will, no doubt, require revision as further evidence is obtained.

The first assumption is that gelatinosa neurons play a major role in segmental inhibitory processes, and the recent neurophysiological evidence discussed earlier substantiates this view. It does not follow, however, that gelatinosa neurons form a homogeneous population since, as noted elsewhere (52), at least some of the cells of this area send their axons to higher levels via the spinothalamic tract. In a recent study in which HRP was used to evaluate projections to the thalamus from the trigeminal spinal nucleus of the rat, a moderate number of gelatinosa neurons were found to project up to thalamic levels (40,41). The vast majority of these cells are, however, local circuit elements, as defined by Rakic (85); that is, their axons distribute near the cell body. It may be noted that this is in marked conflict with much of the classically accepted doctrine regarding gelatinosa neurons; thus, Cajal (21) concluded that short axon neurons were virtually nonexistent in either ventral or dorsal horn, although he noted that as a result of great perseverance, he was able to demonstrate a few such cells in the s. gelatinosa. Most gelatinosa neurons, according to Cajal, send their axons into the dorsolateral tract (of Lissauer) or to the fasciculi proprii that surround the dorsal horn. Szentagothai (101) concluded that these axons ran for as much as four to five segments in the Lissauer's t. before returning to the s. gelatinosa, where they could not be followed to their termination.

Kerr (52) and Narotzky and Kerr (73) investigated the pattern of degeneration that resulted from transection of Lissauer's t., inferring that most of the transected axons arose from gelatinosa neurons, in view of the unanimous agreement on this point in the literature, and that the remainder were extrinsic fibers corresponding to fine primary afferents located almost entirely in the medial half of the tract. Differentiation between PA degeneration and degeneration of intrinsic fibers (of gelatinosa neuron origin) was based on comparison with dorsal rhizotomy results, total Lissauer tractotomies, and partial (lateral) Lissauer tractotomies.

Of particular interest, and initially a source of considerable perplexity, was our inability to demonstrate degenerative changes in boutons of the marginal zone or s. gelatinosa following lateral Lissauer tractotomies—either single or double (i.e., at the rostral and caudal end of a segment), specimens being taken from the midpoint between the tractotomies. On the other hand, when specimens were obtained at distances of 3 mm or less from the incisions and in the absence of any evidence of vascular impairment, clear-cut evidence of degeneration of many of the axosomatic contacts on marginal cells was found. This suggested rather strongly that axons in the tract travel for very short distances, but the conclusion was so obviously in conflict with prevailing concepts, that initially we were reluctant to challenge the accepted viewpoint. However, excellent supportive evidence for this concept was provided by Wall *(personal communication)* who, with his associates Merrill and Yaksh, had been equally puzzled by finding that the compound action potential evoked by stimulation of the lateral part of Lissauer's t. could be followed for a distance of only some 3 mm (71). Furthermore, they had observed the striking similarity between the conduction characteristics of Lissauer's t. and the parallel fiber system of the cerebellar cortex.

Important structural confirmation regarding this point comes from the study by Sugiura (100). It has usually been difficult to trace the axons of gelatinosa neurons for any appreciable distance, but using a three-dimensional reconstruction method on Golgi-stained material from kittens, this investigator was able to follow the axon of a lamina II neuron for a distance of 1.2 mm in Lissauer's t., at which point it returned to the s. gelatinosa; the short course of the axon in the tract is thus in excellent accord with the preceding observations. Other lamina II neurons were found to send their axons into the deeper laminae of the dorsal horn before entering the adjacent fasciculus proprius and bifurcating into ascending and descending branches. It is also important to note that axons of most gelatinosa cells give rise to great numbers of collateral branches before entering Lissauer's t. or similar tracts (67). At least two consequences can be inferred from the latter finding: (a) Their sphere of influence in the s. gelatinosa is greatly enlarged and (b) efforts to evaluate their synaptic distribution by Lissauer tractotomies will result in the demonstration of only a part of the axonal system of such neurons.

Figure 4 illustrates, in a highly simplified manner, some of the principal inhibitory circuits for which either structural or neurophysiological evidence, or both, as discussed herein, is available. Gelatinosa neurons, which, as noted earlier, are activated by primary afferents, send their axons into Lissauer's t. where they run for short distances (approximately 2 to 3 mm) and return to lamina I where they establish axosomatic contacts with marginal neurons. Whether or not they contribute presynaptic contacts on PA endings in the s.

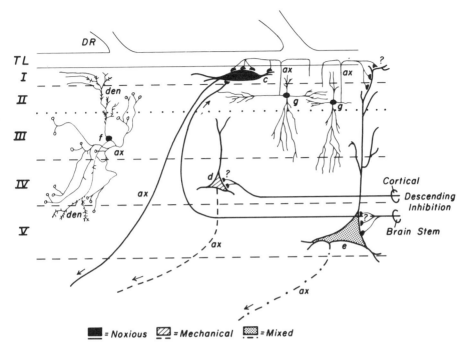

FIG. 4. Some inhibitory circuits shown in a schematic longitudinal section of the dorsal horn. Gelatinosa neurons (g) provide axosomatic contacts on marginal neurons and may also contact apical dendrites of deeper neurons. Note the very short course of their axons in the Lissauer's t. (TL). The deeper lying gelatinosa neurons (f) of layer III have numerous axonal collaterals that distribute in laminae II through V, while their dendrites span laminae I to V (see Fig. 5 in ref. 67.) ax, axon; c, marginal neuron; d, mechanoreceptor neuron in lamina IV; den, dendrites; DR, dorsal root; e, wide dynamic range neuron in lamina V. Possible but unproven connections are indicated by ?.

gelatinosa is unknown; in a limited study of this point, we did not find evidence for this type of organization, but more work is necessary before it can be excluded. In view of the prevailing uncertainty, presynaptic inhibitory contacts of gelatinosa cell origin are not diagrammed in the figure. Suprasegmental or descending inhibitory systems are indicated and discussed below.

Lamina III

Lamina III appears to contain a significant number of neurons whose axons do not reach Lissauer's t. or the fasciculi proprii. The Golgi study by Mannen and Sugiura (67) shows that at least some of these neurons have an axon that rapidly breaks up into an extremely complex arborization, which extends throughout lamina III and into adjacent laminae IV and II (Fig. 5). A short axon neuron of lamina III of the type described by Mannen and Sugiura (67) is included in the semischematic diagram (Fig. 4).

A possible role for these lamina III neurons is to provide the presynaptic

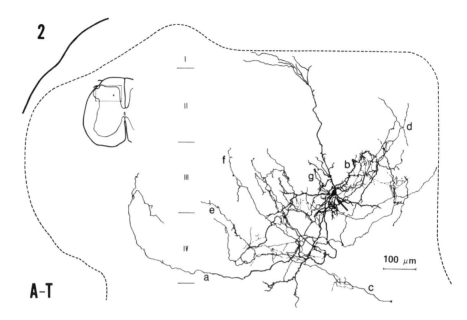

FIG. 5. A gelatinosa neuron whose soma is in lamina III, but whose dendrites *(dense outline)* span laminae I to IV, and part of V. The axonal arborization *(fine outline)* distributes widely in laminae III, IV, and part of II. The widespread extent of dendritic processes of these cells renders hypotheses of input to neurons based on laminar distribution of afferents in relation to the cell bodies virtually meaningless. (From Mannen and Sugiura, ref. 67.)

endings on PAs that, as noted earlier, are both frequent and of unknown origin. This is speculative at this time and will be difficult to test with any current technique.

Other Putative Inhibitory Systems

It has been noted that identified PA endings in the s. gelatinosa receive axoaxonic contacts in a high proportion of instances: spinal cord (86,90) and subnucleus caudalis of the trigeminal (49). In fact, such contacts are so prevalent that, when they were not seen, it seemed probable that it was due to the plane of section rather than to an actual absence of such boutons (49). The source of the presynaptic boutons is still uncertain. As noted above, Lissauer tractotomies suggest that they apparently do not stem from gelatinosa neurons; however, since quite abundant collateral arborizations arise from axons of these cells before they reach Lissauer's t. and axons of gelatinosa neurons in lamina III distribute locally, it is entirely possible that deeper lying gelatinosa neurons do, in fact, provide the axoaxonic contacts on PAs.

A recent observation of much interest is the report by Barber et al. (5) who, using immunocytochemical methods, have demonstrated glutamic acid decarboxylase (GAD), the enzyme mediating the synthesis of γ-aminobutyric acid

(GABA), in a high proportion of the presynaptic terminals on PAs in the s. gelatinosa. This does not resolve the issue of the cells of origin of the presynaptic elements, but gives strong supporting evidence for GABA-mediated inhibition of PAs.

Descending Inhibitory Systems

The structural and functional bases for inhibition of spinal cord interneurons by suprasegmental systems originating from areas ranging from the cerebral cortex to the low medulla has been reviewed in detail by Schmidt (95); therefore, comments are limited here to systems described recently.

Basbaum et al. (8), using anterograde transport of ^{3}H-leucine, demonstrated three descending pathways that originate from the reticular and raphe nuclei of the medulla. Of these systems, that which originates in the nucleus raphe magnus descends bilaterally in the dorsolateral white columns and distributes to laminae I, II, and III and to some extent to laminae V through VII; because of these endings in areas that are well-known sites of termination of PAs and also of the origin of spinothalamic systems, this system is of special interest in terms of nociceptive modulation. This is further reinforced by the fact that electrical stimulation of n. raphe magnus results in marked analgesia (78,84).

Striking specificity of inhibitory effects has been demonstrated by Coulter et al. (32), who showed that stimulation of the sensorimotor cortex inhibited low-threshold units of lamina IV, which projected via the spinothalamic system, but had no influence on high-threshold lamina V spinothalamic neurons. This type of connection is illustrated in Fig. 4, but the possibility of an interreacted segmental interneuron must be considered.

In pilot studies (F. W. L. Kerr, *unpublished observations*) of the synaptic organization of some of these descending systems, following hemisection at the spinomedullary junction area, degenerating boutons were found on marginal neurons, as illustrated in Fig. 6. These direct projections were present both on the soma and on the proximal dendrites of marginal neurons, ipsilaterally as well as contralaterally. Some may be endings of the raphe magnus system described by Basbaum (8) that, as noted, descends bilaterally in the dorsolateral columns. In view of the observations by Beall et al. (9) and Martin et al. (68), other sources of these endings that should be considered are the nuclei pallidus and obscurus of the raphe. The fact that we find both axodendritic and axosomatic endings in the descending projections and that degenerating boutons contain both spherical and flat vesicles suggests that the endings arise from at least two separate sources.

With these observations, it appears that most afferent input to marginal neurons has been established; this is summarized in Fig. 7. The excitatory input to these cells is mainly from small-calibered PAs (29,58,59) and terminates predominantly on dendrites (49,52,73), whereas the inhibitory input from gelatinosa neurons is mainly axosomatic (52,73).

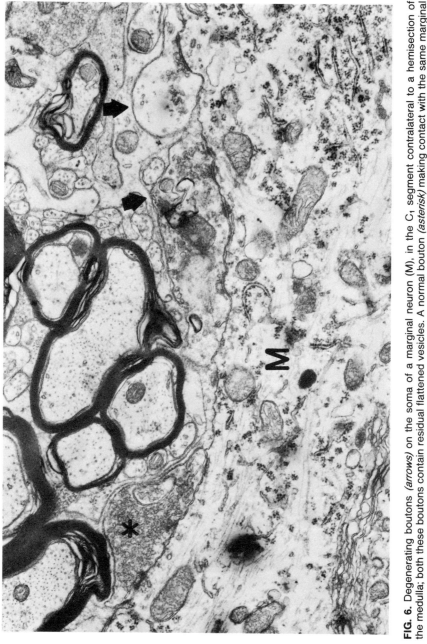

FIG. 6. Degenerating boutons *(arrows)* on the soma of a marginal neuron (M), in the C₁ segment contralateral to a hemisection of the medulla; both these boutons contain residual flattened vesicles. A normal bouton *(asterisk)* making contact with the same marginal neuron appears further to the left.

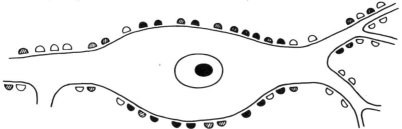

FIG. 7. Diagrammatic representation of synaptic input to marginal neurons.

In regard to the functional properties of the suprasegmental input, too little is yet known to draw any conclusions; it would seem more likely that it should be inhibitory, in view of the predominance of such action in descending pathways to the dorsal horn as described earlier, but this is only speculation.

Histochemical Correlations

A discussion of the structure of the dorsal horn of the spinal cord would be seriously flawed if the localization of peptides with putative neurotransmitter function and of pharmacological agents involved in pain mechanisms were omitted. The development of immunohistochemical techniques for the demonstration of peptides in CNS tissue by Hökfelt and associates (44,45), and the application of radioautography to the problem of localization of opiate and opiate-like substances by Atweh and Kuhar (4) and Pert et al. (79), have revealed a striking specificity of distribution of these agents.

Figure 8 is a composite diagram summarizing the localization of substance P and somatostatin based on the studies of Hökfelt and associates (44,45), of opiates by Pert et al. (79), and of enkephalin by Simantov et al. (96). A feature which is immediately apparent in this diagram is that active substances as different as opiates and peptides are localized or bound in a highly specific manner in the s. gelatinosa. To this feature should be added the previously discussed localization of GAD in the gelatinosa (5). The localization of these various substances is not completely lamina-specific, as indicated by the shading, but it is evident that lamina II and variable extents of laminae I and III are preeminently involved in each instance. Substance P and somatostatin are present in the dorsal root ganglia and in peripheral nerve fibers in addition to the localization in the s. gelatinosa (44,45). Pickel et al. (80) and Barber et al. (6), using the peroxidase–antiperoxidase electron microscopic immunohistochemical technique, reported that substance P is located in axon terminals in laminae I and II and appears to be associated with large, dense core vesicles. However, most boutons with dense core vesicles do not degenerate following dorsal rhizotomy

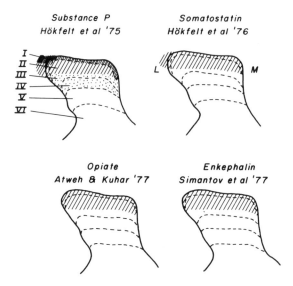

FIG. 8. The distribution in the dorsal horn of some putative neurotransmitters (which may be involved in nociceptive input) compared with that of opiates and the endogenous opiate-like peptide enkephalin. The specificity and similarity of distribution of those widely differing agents in the s. gelatinosa is evident. (Adapted from refs. 4,44,45,96.)

(49,86). Cuello et al. (33), using similar techniques, demonstrated that substance P was located in spherical vesicles in boutons in the s. gelatinosa; this is in good accord with the electron microscopic degeneration studies.

Opiates and enkephalin have virtually identical localization; this suggests that both substances are closely associated with the PA terminals. Whether they are located on the synaptic endings of the latter or are associated with the presynaptic endings on PAs, or even elsewhere, remains to be determined. However, the striking propinquity of opiates and enkephalin, with their marked analgesic actions, to substance P with its possible nociceptive transmitter function and to somatostatin and GABA (both of which are putative inhibitory transmitters), appears to provide a most esthetically pleasing, although not necessarily correct correlation between pharmacological actions, neuroanatomical circuitry, and neurophysiological observations.

ASCENDING PATHWAYS

Although there is no question that in the human the lateral spinothalamic tract (LSTT) is the major pathway for the relay of noxious input from the spinal cord to higher levels, it has been recognized for many years that it is not the only nociceptive projection system; suffice it to note that complete and bilateral anterolateral cordotomy in man does not abolish pain caudal to the lesion level, but, instead, elevates the pain threshold to a more or less marked degree. Increasing the stimulus intensity sufficiently will result in a "break-through" of pain that is of a particularly unpleasant "C fiber" type (see reviews 52,57,107). It is also necessary to note that, in addition to noxious and thermal sensations, the LSTT carries several other modalities, among which tactile and genital sensations are best known. More recently, Noordenbos and Wall (77a) reported on a patient in whom all but one anterolateral quadrant (ALQ) of the cord had been transected. She was able to recognize pressure and passive movement of the extremities and unpleasant dysesthesiae to pinprick and electrical stimulation below and ipsilateral to the transection; the spectrum of sensations carried in the ALQ is evidently considerably greater than believed heretofore.

Since the major features of the LSTT have been described repeatedly and reviewed elsewhere (14,15,52,69), comment will be limited to a brief summary of its main features and a more detailed account of recent findings. Other ascending pathways that may be involved in nociceptive transmission will be subsequently discussed.

LSTT

The LSTT system arises from neurons widely distributed throughout the spinal gray; thus, not only dorsal horn elements contribute, but cells in the intermediate and ventral gray as well (103). These investigators stimulated the tract just before it entered the thalamus and identified the spinal neuron somata by recording their antidromically evoked discharges. Although the functional role of most spinothalamic cells in the dorsal horn is reasonably well known, we have little or no information about the sensory modalities mediated by those whose cell bodies lie in the intermediate gray and in the ventral horn. The distribution and types of neurons giving rise to the spinothalamic tract have also been determined by retrograde transport of HRP (1,102); these findings are in good accord with the electrophysiological studies referred to above.

Until recently it has been assumed that the spinothalamic tract was either completely crossed or, that at most, a very minor proportion of it ascended ipsilaterally to the side of input. That ipsilateral spinothalamic projections may be somewhat more frequent than generally believed is suggested by the case of Noordenbos and Wall (77a) described earlier, and also by the findings of Kenshalo and Willis (48), who repeated earlier studies on retrograde transport of HRP from the thalamus and found that there were 24% of ipsilaterally projecting spinothalamic tract cells in the sacral cord and 5% in the lumbar enlargement of the macaque monkey. Following the studies of Bowsher (15) and of Mehler et al. (69), the course and connections of ascending fibers of the anterolateral quadrant have been established on a firm basis. This can be summarized briefly as follows: From the relay neurons in the dorsal horn, a predominantly crossed system of fibers, which maintains a good somatotopic lamination throughout, ascends in the ALQ of the cord. Part of this continues directly to the diencephalon where it bifurcates into a lateral and a medial branch. The lateral branch terminates in small bursts scattered throughout the n. ventralis posterolateralis with good somatotopic organization. The medial branch ascends beside the fasciculus habenulo-interpeduncularis and gives a discrete projection to the n. parafascicularis, passes around and in part through the n. centrum medianum without providing synaptic connections to it (69), and then distributes to the intra-and paralaminar nuclei. En route to the thalamus, the ascending system of the ALQ also gives rise to a large number of connections, among which are profuse projections to the reticular nuclei of the medulla, some to the pontine reticular nuclei (subceruleus dorsalis, ventralis, and processus pontis reticularis lateralis). In the mesencephalon, there is a clear-cut projection into the periaqueductal gray, to the suprageniculate nucleus, and to a portion of the medial geniculate nucleus usually referred to as the magnocellular division. However, the latter cells appear to represent a posterior prolongation of n. ventralis posterolateralis of the thalamus rather than a separate entity.

A mesencephalic projection that distributes to the n. cuneiformis, and that has not been described previously, was noted in study of the ventral spinothalamic tract (VSTT) (51); it also degenerates following transection of the ALQ and after midline sagittal myelotomy.

A major proportion of the projections to the reticular substance of the brainstem from the spinal cord that are so prominent after anterolateral cordotomy, are of ipsilateral origin, as shown by degeneration following extensive midline myelotomies (56). Most of these ipsilateral projections are probably not related to nociception but, as noted, some ipsilaterally conducted noxious sensation is present. The role of individual reticular relays in the brainstem remains to be determined; some may function as relays for nociception to higher levels, whereas others, particularly those at more caudal levels, may act as reflex centers concerned with vasomotor, cardiac, and respiratory rhythm changes.

Evidence has been accumulating from various independent disciplines in recent years that supports the concept of a cortical area for the representation of pain (57). Of particular interest is the report by Burton and Jones (20), who showed that the suprageniculate nucleus, which receives input from the LSTT, projects to the granular insular cortex.

VSTT

The existence of a separate spinothalamic tract in the anterior or ventral funiculus had been proposed early in the century, but the evidence was sufficiently tenuous that most modern investigators had justifiably disregarded it. In a recent study in the primate, in which the ventral funiculus was transected without impinging on the area occupied by the LSTT, Kerr (51) has shown that this ventral tract is present, shares most of the structural features of the LSTT including a significant projection to the n. cuneiformis in the mesencephalon, and has some additional connections that are absent in the LSTT. Since the transections were performed only in the cervical cord, it is not known whether it subserves input from forelimb, hindlimb, or both. Nothing is known about sensory modalities mediated by it, although it can be argued indirectly that, because it shares the connections of the LSTT in the mesencephalon and thalamus, it participates in pain mechanisms. In work currently under way, it appears that the cells of origin of this tract are located in laminae I, IV, V, VI, and VII (S. Yasuoka and F. W. L. Kerr, *unpublished observations*).

A Reappraisal and New Concept of the Spinothalamic System

Descriptions by Bowsher (15) and by Mehler et al. (69) of the ascending degeneration that resulted from transection of the ALQ of the spinal cord, in which profuse terminal and subterminal degeneration was observed in extensive parts of the medullary, pontine, and mesencephalic reticular formation, in addition to the projections to the paralaminar and ventroposterolateral (VPL) nuclei, provided the basis for the concept of a medial, phylogenetically old, spinothalamic system and a lateral neospinothalamic pathway. The medial pathway was believed to be a primitive system composed of unmyelinated fibers and to relay at one or several levels in the reticular core en route to the thalamus; this appeared to account in good part for the long delay in perception of second pain mediated by C fibers in peripheral nerves. The small myelinated fibers were believed to relay directly to the paralaminar nuclei as a somewhat more recent phylogenetic system or paleospinothalamic pathway that mediated pricking pain, temperature, and possibly touch. Finally, a group of the largest fibers in the LSTT projected directly to VPL and was considered to be the newest acquisition or neospinothalamic tract concerned mainly with discriminative aspects of touch (see reviews 11,12).

Several other observations, some recent and others of long standing, suggest that a reappraisal of this concept is appropriate. The belief that unmyelinated primary afferents project via higher order, unmyelinated fibers as an archispinothalamic system relaying in the reticular core is not supported by the study of Lippman and Kerr (65), who found no evidence for unmyelinated fibers in the area of the spinothalamic tract.

The profuse input from the ALQ to the medullary reticular nuclei seen after anterolateral cordotomy appears to be composed predominantly of ipsilateral or uncrossed fibers, as evidenced by the results of extensive midline myelotomies (56); in the latter, only a minor input to the n. reticularis gigantocellularis, paragigantocellularis dorsalis, and lateralis is seen. It has been shown that a number of neurons in these nuclei respond specifically to high-threshold peripheral stimulation (10,24); trained cats will avoid stimulation delivered to the medullary reticular formation by moving from one side of a test box to the other, which action terminates the stimulus (23,24). However, the animals did not manifest spitting, loud cries or screams, baring of teeth, or the other behavioral signs usually associated with noxious stimulation in this species (66).

The stimulation may then have been disagreeable (i.e., nauseating or have elicited vasomotor, gastrointestinal, or other visceral reactions that are readily evoked from this area), but not necessarily painful. The fact that neurons in this area are activated by high-threshold stimuli may indicate that they are in the pathway to conscious appreciation of pain, or they may be in the autonomic reflex pathway for vasopressor, cardioacceleratory, and other visceral concomitants of pain as discussed in the introductory paragraphs; the medullary reticular formation contains many neurons concerned with these visceral functions. It seems, therefore, that evidence for a nociceptive relay in the medulla is inconclusive at this time.

In the pontine area, there is virtually no terminal degeneration following midline myelotomies.

When the mesencephalic level is reached, input to the periaqueductal gray and the reticular formation is similar after anterolateral cordotomy, midline myelotomy, or transection of the ventral funiculus. The degeneration is seen as a fine low-density plexus of fibers distributed throughout the n. cuneiformis of Olszewski [i.e., that part of the reticular substance lateral and slightly ventrolateral to the central gray (51,56)]. In a single unit study of this area, Young and Gottschaldt (109) found 43 neurons that responded only to noxious cutaneous stimulation; 37 of the 43 cells had very widespread receptive fields involving both sides of the body including all four limbs and face, all showed little tendency to adapt, and latency of response was short, suggesting central conduction over myelinated fibers. Histologically, cells with these characteristics were shown to lie within the area Olszewski defined as n. cuneiformis. This area was one of the earliest to be correlated with behavioral activity indicative of pain. Thus, Magoun et al. (66), in both lightly anesthetized and in decerebrate unanesthetized monkeys and cats, showed that stereotaxically delivered electrical stimulation to this area produced clear-cut signs of noxious activation such as loud cries, screams, snarling faces, and, in the cat, spitting.

Further evidence that this area is involved in nociception has been provided by the observations of Nashold et al. (75) on stimulation of the periaqueductal gray and adjacent mesencephalic reticular area in man; the area from which painful responses were evoked corresponded to the n. cuneiformis and the adjacent periaqueductal gray.

Correlating the degeneration studies with the electrophysiological, animal behavioral, and human intraoperative results, it appears that a strong case can be made for an important spinothalamic relay for nociception in the n. cuneiformis. It is of much interest that Edwards and De Olmos (37), using anterograde transport of ^{3}H-leucine and radioautography, have shown that n. cuneiformis projects rostrally into the parafascicular, intra-, and paralaminar nuclei of the thalamus. These areas are recognized to be involved to a major degree with nociceptive mechanisms, thus forming a final link in the nociceptive pathway from spinal cord to thalamus. In the transition zone between mesencephalon and thalamus, the posterior group of nuclei of the thalamus (PO) zone of Poggio and Mountcastle (81) receives an important nociceptive input from the spino-thalamic system. Neurons showing not only wide spatial convergence, as evidenced by their extensive peripheral receptive fields, but also polymodal input (including input from nociceptors), were shown to be present by these investigations; their findings have been confirmed by Casey (22) and by others. Structurally the area is complex and includes the magnocellular nucleus of the medial geniculate body, the suprageniculate, and the limitans nuclei. It is in the medial part of this area, or nucleus PO medialis, that spinothalamic fibers are found to terminate. Burton and Jones (20), using the orthograde transport of tritiated amino acids, have shown that this area projects to the retroinsular cortex or area SII.

From the proceeding brief summary, alternative spinothalamic pathways from the cord to the thalamus and cortex are seen to exist (Fig. 9):

(i) A lateral system including (a) the pathway to n. ventralis posterolateralis and hence to SI, which is predominantly (or perhaps exclusively) concerned with tactile functions and discriminating abilities. In this respect, it has lemniscal properties; and

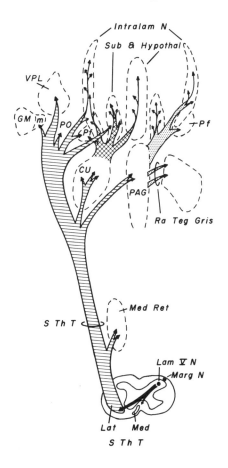

FIG. 9. A concept of the spinothalamic system as discussed in the text. Note, particularly, the pronounced "fanning" out of the system when it reaches the mesencephalon and that the relays from the n. cuneiformis and the periaqueductal gray distribute to the intra- and paralaminar thalamic nuclei and to the hypothalamus. Also, the periaqueductal gray projects to the n. cuneiformis (CU) as the radiatio tegmenti grisea of Weischedel (Ra Teg Gris). GM, medial geniculate nucleus, m, magnocellular division; Med Ret, medullary reticular nuclei; PAG, periaqueductal gray area; Pf, parafascicular nucleus; PO, posterior group of nuclei of the thalamus; S Th T, spinothalamic tracts; VPL, n. ventralis posterolateralis of thalamus; Lat and Med, lateral and medial spinothalamic tracts.

(b) a pathway relaying in PO and hence to SII, which is concerned mainly with nociception.

(ii) A medial system including (a) a possible relay in the rostral medullary reticular formation and hence to the thalamus (PO area?); (b) a relay via the periaqueductal gray and hence to the intralaminar nuclei of the thalamus; and (c) the relay via the n. cuneiformis and from there to the intralaminar nuclei. This concept has been summarized recently (54).

In view of the multiplicity of pathways available to nociceptive input at this rostral level, it is not surprising that attempts to suppress pain by stereotaxically placed lesions in the thalamus have met with very limited success.

The Spinocervical Tract

The spinocervical tract (SCT) arises from neurons located mainly in laminae IV and V (19) but also in VI and VII and ascends in the dorsolateral quadrant of the cord where it lies superficially, close to the dorsal horn. It relays in the lateral cervical nucleus which, in the cat, is a prominent cluster of large neurons located ventrolaterally to the dorsal horn in the C_1 and C_2 segments. The axons of these neurons cross the midline and join the opposite medial meniscus, running with it to reach the ventroposterior thalamus.

Although many SCT neurons are concerned with mechanoreceptor relay, Brown and Franz (18) reported that the great majority of these neurons are also activated by noxious heat; similarly, Cervero et al. (26) have shown that they respond to noxious stimulation of the skin. Thus, they have response properties similar to the wide dynamic range neurons discussed earlier, and could, on electrophysiological grounds, be regarded as candidates for an accessory "pain" pathway.

Whereas this occurs in the cat (in which these observations were made), and Kennard (47) concluded that in this animal most of the nociceptive pathways lie in the dorsal half of the spinal cord, the situation is distinctly different in the human. In the monkey, the lateral cervical nucleus and its associated tract is much less prominent than in the cat; its cells are rather inconspicuous, spindle-shaped elements, which lie close to the dorsal horn, and incoming SCT fibers form a very modest plexus around them (see review 77). Finally, in the human, the lateral cervical nucleus is either absent or represented by an occasional neuron. Thus, it can be concluded, that insofar as human pain problems are concerned, the SCT system is probably not a significant factor.

Conduction of Nociception by Other Pathways in the Cord

Of the fiber systems of the cord, at this point the dorsolateral quadrant (DLQ) (exclusive of the SCT), the fasciculi proprii, and the dorsal intracornual tract remain to be considered as possible routes for conduction of nociception.

DLQ

The DLQ has been studied from this point of view by Nijensohn and Kerr (77), who transected it and followed the ascending degeneration using the Nauta method. They concluded, on the basis of the connections that were demonstrated, that it was unlikely that it played any significant role in nociceptive relay. However, it is recognized that inferences regarding pain based on negative neuroanatomical evidence are by no means conclusive and that a variety of results based on different techniques, and all of which are in accord, must be assembled before persuasive evidence can be considered to have been acquired. For example, Moffie (72) has reported that in two patients a percutaneous cordotomy erroneously located in the DLQ had resulted in relief of intractable pain secondary to invasion by malignant tumors. The relief of pain by a lesion such as this is extremely difficult to reconcile with the integrity of the lateral spinothalamic system, since this is unquestionably the major nociceptive relay pathway. What could have occurred to so radically alter input over this major system, especially when somatic and visceral motor pathways, whose functional impairment would be immediately apparent, are reported to be intact? Conversely, although to a lesser degree, how can one explain the striking relief of pain and the associated thermanalgesia that ensues immediately after a well-performed spinothalamic cordotomy, if these accessory pathways are unaffected?

One possibility that must be considered is that significant interpersonal variations in the relative proportion of nociceptive relay between the main (LSTT) and ancillary tracts may be present. That very remarkable variations occur has been documented by French and Peyton (38) and by Voris (105) in their descriptions of thermanalgesia ipsilateral to spinothalamic cordotomies, and who concluded that the pathway was uncrossed in those instances. Such major anomalies of the nociceptive pathway are rare, but at least they provide a basis for considering anomalies of other types.

Fasciculi Proprii

Whether or not the fasciculi proprii may carry nociceptive messages is unknown at this time. The only suggestive evidence we have is the observation and the illustrations by Cajal (21), indicating that axons of marginal neurons enter these longitudinally running systems. It is worth keeping this possibility in mind when considering alternate pathways for pain.

Dorsal Intracornual Tract

Similarly, there is a possibility that the dorsal intracornual tract (i.e., the dense system of longitudinally running myelinated fibers that are so prominent in the center of the dorsal horn) may act as an accessory ascending pathway for nociception as discussed elsewhere (52). Basbaum (7) has suggested that in the rat nociception may be relayed via short axon neurons in the spinal gray.

The Dorsal Columns

The possibility that the dorsal columns may participate in the relay of pain to consciousness has been considered sporadically over the years. In operations on conscious human patients, Nashold and Friedman (74) reported that on stimulation of the dorsal columns at mild to moderate stimulus intensities, the subjects described thumping changing to vibratory sensations as frequency was increased; as the current intensity was raised, complaints of discomfort were elicited. The very real possibility of current spread to dorsal roots or their branches, or beyond the dorsal columns, must be remembered when higher current intensities are used.

PAs of the dorsal columns are well known to be concerned with mechanoreception and thus are not candidates for nociceptive relay. However, Uddenberg (104), using electrophysiological techniques, showed that a significant population of nonprimary afferent fibers was present. These findings were confirmed and extended by Rustioni (91,92) and by Angaut-Petit (2,3), who reported that 85% of these dorsal column fibers respond with increasing discharge frequency as stimulus strength is increased; this, however, does not guarantee that they are concerned with nociception or with its relay to consciousness, as discussed in the Introduction.

In conclusion, the role of the nonprimary afferents in the dorsal column remains unknown, and, although the possibility exists that they may relay nociception to consciousness, the likelihood appears to be small.

ACKNOWLEDGMENT

This study is based, in part, on work supported by grant NS-5995 from the National Institute of Neurological and Communicative Disorders and Stroke, the National Institutes of Health.

REFERENCES

1. Albe-Fessard, D., Levante, A., and Lamour, Y. (1974): Origin of spinothalamic tract in monkeys. *Brain Res.*, 65:503–509.
2. Angaut-Petit, D. (1975): The dorsal column system. I. Existence of long ascending postsynaptic fibres in the cat's fasiculus gracilis. *Exp. Brain Res.*, 22:457–470.
3. Angaut-Petit, D. (1975): The dorsal column system. II. Functional properties and bulbar relay of the postsynaptic fibres of the cat's fasiculus gracilis. *Exp. Brain Res.*, 22:471–493.
4. Atweh, S., and Kuhar, M. J. (1977): Autoradiographic localization of opiate receptors in rat brain. I. Spinal cord and lower medulla. *Brain Res.*, 124:53–67.
5. Barber, R. P., Vaughn, J. E., Saito, K., McLaughlin, B. J., and Roberts, E. (1978): GABAergic

terminals are presynaptic to primary afferent terminals in the substantia gelatinosa of the rat spinal cord. *Brain Res.,* 141:35–55.

6. Barber, R. P., Vaughn, J. E., Slemmon, J. R., Roberts, E., and Leeman, S. E. (1977): Substance P terminals from synaptic junctions in spinal cord. *Soc. Neurosci. Abstr.,* III:403.

7. Basbaum, A. I. (1973): Conduction of the effects of noxious stimulation by short-fiber multisynaptic systems of the spinal cord in the rat. *Exp. Neurol.,* 40:699–716.

8. Basbaum, A. I., Clanton, C. H., and Fields, H. L. (1978): Three bulbospinal pathways from the rostral medulla of the cat: An autoradiographic study of pain modulating systems. *J. Comp. Neurol.,* 178:209–224.

9. Beall, J. E., Martin, R. F., Applebaum, A. E., and Willis, W. D. (1976): Inhibition of primate spinothalamic tract neurons by stimulation in the region of the nucleus raphe magnus. *Brain Res.,* 114:328–333.

10. Benjamin, R. M. (1970): Single neurons in the rat medulla responsive to nociceptive stimulation. *Brain Res.,* 24:525–529.

11. Bishop, G. H. (1959): The relation of fiber size to sensory modality: Phylogenetic implications of the afferent innervation of the cortex. *J. Nerv. Ment. Dis.,* 128:89–114.

12. Bishop, G. H. (1962): Normal and abnormal sensory patterns. In: *Pain in Neural Physiopathology,* edited by R. G. Grenell, pp. 95–133. Hoeber, New York.

13. Bobilier, P., Seguin, S., Petitjean, F., Salvert, D., Touret, M., and Jouvet, M. (1976): The raphe nuclei of the cat brainstem: A topographical atlas of their efferent projections as revealed by autoradiography. *Brain Res.,* 13:449–486.

14. Boivie, J. J. G., and Perl, E. R. (1975): Neural substrates of somatic sensation. *Int. Rev. Sci. Neurophysiol.,* 13:303–411.

15. Bowsher, D. (1957): Termination of the central pain pathway in man: The conscious appreciation of pain. *Brain,* 80:606–621.

16. Brown, A. G. (1977): Cutaneous axons and sensory neurons in the spinal cord. *Br. Med. Bull.,* 33:109–116.

17. Brown, A. G., House, C. R., Rose, P. K., and Snow, P. J. (1976): The morphology of spinocervical tract neurones in the cat. *J. Physiol.,* 260:719–738.

18. Brown, A. G., and Franz, D. N. (1969): Responses of spinocervical tract neurons to natural stimulation of identified cutaneous receptors. *Exp. Brain Res.,* 7:231–249.

19. Bryan, R. N., Coulter, J. D., and Willis, W. D. (1974): Cells of origin of the spinocervical tract in the monkey. *Exp. Neurol.,* 42:574–586.

20. Burton, H., and Jones, E. G. (1976): The posterior thalamic region and its cortical projection in New World and Old World monkeys. *J. Comp. Neurol.,* 168:249–302.

21. Cajal, S. R. (1909): *Histologie du Systemè Nerveux de l'Homme et des Vertébrés, Vol. I.* Consejo Superior de Investigaciones Cientificas, Madrid.

22. Casey, K. L. (1966): Unit analysis of nociceptive mechanism in the thalamus of the awake squirrel monkey. *J. Neurophysiol.,* 29:727–750.

23. Casey, K. L. (1971): Escape elicited by bulboreticular stimulation in the cat. *Int. J. Neurosci.,* 2:29–34.

24. Casey, K. L., Keene, J. J., and Morrow, T. (1974): Bulboreticular and medial thalamic unit activity in relation to aversive behavior and pain. In: *Advances in Neurology, Vol. 4: Proceedings of the International Symposium on Pain,* edited by J. J. Bonica, pp. 197–205. Raven Press, New York.

25. Cervero, F., Ensor, D. R., Iggo, A., and Molony, V. (1977): Activity from single neurons recorded in the substantia gelatinosa Rolandi of the cat. *J. Physiol. (Lond.),* 269:35–36P.

26. Cervero, F., Iggo, A., and Molony, V. (1977): Responses of spinocervical tract neurones to noxious stimulation of the skin. *J. Physiol. (Lond.),* 267:537–558.

27. Cervero, F., Iggo, A., and Ogawa, H. (1976): Nociceptor-driven dorsal horn neurones in the lumbar spinal cord of the cat. *Pain,* 2:5–24.

28. Cervero, F., Molony, V., and Iggo, A. (1977): Extracellular and intracellular recordings from neurones in the substantia gelatinosa Rolandi. *Brain Res.,* 136:565–569.

29. Christensen, B. N., and Perl, E. R. (1970): Spinal neurons specifically excited by noxious or thermal stimuli: Marginal zone of the dorsal horn. *J. Neurophysiol.,* 33:293–307.

30. Coggeshall, R. E., Coulter, J. D., and Willis, W. D. (1974): Unmyelinated axons in the ventral roots of the cat lumbosacral enlargement. *J. Comp. Neurol.,* 153:39–58.

31. Coggeshall, R. E., and Ito, H. (1977): Sensory fibres in ventral roots L7 and S1 in the cat. *J. Physiol. (Lond.),* 267:215–235.
32. Coulter, J. D., Maunz, R. A., and Willis, W. D. (1974): Effects of stimulation of sensorimotor cortex on primate spinothalamic neurons. *Brain Res.,* 65:351–356.
33. Cuello, A. C., Jessell, T. M., Kanazawa, I., and Iversen, L. L. (1977): Substance P: Localization in synaptic vesicles in rat central nervous system. *J. Neurochem.,* 29:747–751.
34. Cullheim, S., and Kellerth, J. O. (1976): Combined light and electron microscopic tracing of neurones, including axons and synaptic terminals, after intracellular injection of horseradish peroxidase. *Neurosci. Lett.,* 2:307–313.
35. Denny-Brown, D., Kirk, E. J., and Yanagisawa, N. (1973): The tract of Lissauer in relation to sensory transmission in the dorsal horn of the spinal cord in the Macaque monkey. *J. Comp. Neurol.,* 151:175–200.
36. Duggan, A. W., Hall, J. G., and Headley, P. M. (1977): Suppression of transmission of nociceptive impulses by morphine: Selective effects of morphine administered in the region of the substantia gelatinosa. *Br. J. Pharmacol.,* 61:65–76.
37. Edwards, S. B., and De Olmos, J. S. (1976): Autoradiographic studies of the projections of the midbrain reticular formation: Ascending projections of nucleus cuneiformis. *J. Comp. Neurol.,* 165:417–432.
38. French, L. A., and Peyton, W. T. (1948): Ipsilateral sensory loss following cordotomy. *J. Neurosurg.,* 5:403–404.
39. Frykholm, R., Hyde, J., Norlen, G., and Skoglund, C. R. (1953): On pain sensations produced by stimulation of ventral roots in man. *Acta Physiol. Scand.,* 29 (Suppl. 106):455–469.
40. Fukushima, T., and Kerr, F. W. L. (1977): The organization of trigeminothalamic neurons as determined by horseradish peroxidase retrograde labelling. *Soc. Neurosci. Abstr.,* III:481.
41. Fukushima, T., and Kerr, F. W. L. (1979): Organization of trigeminothalamic tracts and other thalamic afferent systems of the brainstem of the rat. *J. Comp. Neurol.,* 183:169–184.
42. Gobel, S. (1974): Synaptic organization of the substantia gelatinosa in the spinal trigeminal nucleus of the adult cat. *J. Neurocytol.,* 3:219–243.
43. Hamano, K., Mannen, H., and Ishizuka, N. (1978): Reconstruction of trajectory of primary afferent collaterals in the dorsal horn of the cat spinal cord using Golgi-stained serial sections. *J. Comp. Neurol.,* 181:1–15.
44. Hökfelt, T., Elde, R., Johansson, O., Luft, R., Nilsson, G., and Arimura, A. (1976): Immunohistochemical evidence for separate populations of somatostatin-containing and substance P-containing primary afferent neurons in the rat. *Neuroscience,* 1:131–136.
45. Hökfelt, T., Kellerth, J-O., Nilsson, G., and Pernow, B. (1975): Experimental immunohistochemical studies on the localization and distribution of substance P in cat primary sensory neurons. *Brain Res.,* 100:235–252.
46. Jankowska, E., Rastad, J., and Westman, J. (1976): Intracellular application of horseradish peroxidase and its light and electron microscopical appearance in spinocervical tract cells. *Brain Res.,* 105:557–562.
47. Kennard, M. A. (1954): The course of ascending fibers in the spinal cord of the cat essential to the recognition of painful stimuli. *J. Comp. Neurol.,* 100:511–524.
48. Kenshalo, D. R., and Willis, W. D. (1978): Laminar distribution of spinothalamic cells in the primate lumbosacral spinal cord. *Anat. Rec.,* 190:433 (Abstr.).
49. Kerr, F. W. L. (1970): The organization of primary afferents in the subnucleus caudalis of the trigeminal: A light and electron microscopic study of degeneration. *Brain Res.,* 23:147–165.
50. Kerr, F. W. L. (1975): Pain: A central inhibitory balance theory. *Mayo Clinic Proc.,* 50:685–690.
51. Kerr, F. W. L. (1975): The ventral spinothalamic tract and other ascending systems of the ventral funiculus of the spinal cord. *J. Comp. Neurol.,* 159:335–356.
52. Kerr, F. W. L. (1975): Neuroanatomical substrates of nociception in the spinal cord. *Pain,* 1:325–356.
53. Kerr, F. W. L. (1976): Segmental circuitry and spinal cord nociceptive mechanisms. In: *Advances in Pain Research and Therapy, Vol. 1: Proceedings of the First World Congress on Pain,* edited by J. J. Bonica and D. Albe-Fessard, pp. 75–89. Raven Press, New York.
54. Kerr, F. W. L. (1978): A new concept of the spinothalamic system. *Anat. Rec.,* 190:443–444.

55. Kerr, F. W. L., and Casey, K. (1978): Pain. *Neurosci. Res. Program Bull.,* 16:1–207.
56. Kerr, F. W. L., and Lippman, H. H. (1974): The primate spinothalamic tract as demonstrated by anterolateral cordotomy and commissural myelotomy. In: *Advances in Neurology, Vol. 4: Proceedings of the International Symposium on Pain,* edited by J. J. Bonica, pp. 147–156. Raven Press, New York.
57. Kerr, F. W. L., and Wilson, P. R. (1978): Pain. *Annu. Rev. Neuroscience,* 1:83–102.
58. Kumazawa, T., and Perl, E. R. (1976): Differential excitation of dorsal horn substantia gelatinosa and marginal neurons by primary afferent units with fine (Aδ and C) fibers. In: *Sensory Functions of the Skin,* edited by Y. Zotterman, pp. 67–89. Pergamon Press, New York.
59. Kumazawa, T., and Perl, E. R. (1978): Excitation of marginal and substantia gelatinosa neurons in the primate spinal cord: Indications of their place in dorsal horn functional organization. *J. Comp. Neurol.,* 177:417–434.
60. LaMotte, C. (1977): Distribution of the tract of Lissauer and the dorsal root fibers in the primate spinal cord. *J. Comp. Neurol.,* 172:529–562.
61. Light, A. R., and Durkovic, R. G. (1976): Horseradish peroxidase: An improvement in intracellular staining of single, electrophysiologically characterized neurons. *Exp. Neurol.,* 53:847–853.
62. Light, A. R., and Perl, E. R. (1977): Differential termination of large-diameter and small-diameter primary afferent fibers in the spinal gray matter as indicated by labeling with horseradish peroxidase. *Neurosci. Lett.,* 6:59–63.
63. Light, A. R., and Perl, E. R. (1977): Central termination of identified cutaneous afferent units with fine myelinated fibers. *Soc. Neurosci. Abstr.,* III:486.
64. Light, A. R., and Metz, C. B. (1978): The morphology of the spinal cord efferent and afferent neurons contributing to the ventral roots of the cat. *J. Comp. Neurol.,* 179:501–516.
65. Lippman, H. H., and Kerr, F. W. L. (1972): Light and electron microscopic study of crossed ascending pathways in the anterolateral funiculus in monkey. *Brain Res.,* 40:496–499.
66. Magoun, H. W., Atlas, D., Ingersoll, E. H., and Ranson, S. W. (1937): Associated facial, vocal and respiratory components of emotional expression: An experimental study. *J. Neurol. Psychopathol.,* 17:241–255.
67. Mannen, H., and Sugiura, Y. (1976): Reconstruction of neurons of dorsal horn proper using Golgi-stained serial sections. *J. Comp. Neurol.,* 168:303–312.
68. Martin, R. F., Jordan, L. M., and Willis, W. D. (1977): Differential projections of cat medullary raphé nuclei in spinal cord white matter. *Soc. Neurosci. Abstr.,* III:504.
69. Mehler, W. R., Feferman, M. E., and Nauta, W. J. H. (1960): Ascending axon degeneration following anterolateral cordotomy: An experimental study in the monkey. *Brain,* 83:718–750.
70. Melzack, R., and Wall, P. D. (1965): Pain mechanisms: A new theory. *Science,* 150:971–979.
71. Merrill, E. G., Wall, P. D., and Yaksh, T. L. (1978): Properties of two CNS unmyelinated fibre tracts: The lateral Lissauer tract and the parallel fibers of the cerebellum. *J. Physiol. (Lond.) (in press).*
72. Moffie, D. (1975): Spinothalamic fibres, pain conduction and cordotomy. *Clin. Neurol. Neurosurg.,* 78:261–268.
73. Narotzky, R. A., and Kerr, F. W. L. (1978): Marginal neurons of the spinal cord: Types, afferent synaptology and functional considerations. *Brain Res.,* 139:1–20.
74. Nashold, B. S., and Friedman, H. (1972): Dorsal column stimulation for control of pain. *J. Neurosurg.,* 36:590–597.
75. Nashold, B. S., Wilson, W. P., and Slaughter, D. G. (1969): Sensations evoked by stimulation of the midbrain in man. *J. Neurosurg.,* 30:14–24.
76. Nathan, P. W. (1976): The gate-control theory of pain: A critical review. *Brain,* 99:123–158.
77. Nijensohn, D. E., and Kerr, F. W. L. (1975): The ascending projections of the dorsolateral funiculus of the spinal cord in the primate. *J. Comp. Neurol.,* 161:459–470.
77a. Noordenbos, W., and Wall, P. D. (1976): Diverse sensory functions with an almost totally divided spinal cord. *Pain,* 2:185–195.
78. Oliveras, J. L., Redjemi, F., Guilbaud, G., and Besson, J. M. (1975): Analgesia induced by electrical stimulation of the inferior centralis nucleus of the raphe in the cat. *Pain,* 1:139–145.
79. Pert, C. B., Kuhar, M. J., and Snyder, S. H. (1976): Opiate receptor: Autoradiographic localization in the rat brain. *Proc. Natl. Acad. Sci. USA,* 73:3729–3733.

80. Pickel, V. M., Reis, D. J., and Leeman, S. E. (1977): Ultrastructural localization of substance P in neurons in rat spinal cord. *Brain Res.,* 122:534–540.
81. Poggio, G. F., and Mountcastle, V. B. (1960): A study of the functional contribution of the lemniscal and spinothalamic systems to somatic sensibility. Central nervous mechanisms in pain. *Bull. Johns Hopkins Hosp.,* 106:266–316.
82. Proshansky, E., and Egger, M. D. (1977): Staining of the dorsal root projection to the cat's dorsal horn by anterograde movement of horseradish peroxidase. *Neurosci. Lett.,* 5:103–110.
83. Proshansky, E., and Egger, M. D. (1977): Morphology of endings of primary afferent collaterals to the spinal cord selectively stained by anterograde movement of HRP. *Soc. Neurosci. Abstr.,* III:506.
84. Proudfit, H. K., and Anderson, E. G. (1975): Morphine analgesia: Blockade by raphe magnus lesions. *Brain Res.,* 98:612–618.
85. Rakic, P. (1975): Local circuit neurons. *Neurosci. Res. Program Bull.,* 13:299–301.
86. Ralston, H. J. (1968): Dorsal root projections to dorsal horn neurons in the cat spinal cord. *J. Comp. Neurol.,* 132:303–330.
87. Rastad, J., Jankowska, E., and Westman, J. (1977): Arborization of initial axon collaterals of spinocervical tract cells stained intracellularly with horseradish peroxidase. *Brain Res.,* 135:1–10.
88. Rethelyi, M. (1977): Preterminal and terminal arborizations in the substantia gelatinosa of the cat's spinal cord. *J. Comp. Neurol.,* 172:511–528.
89. Rethelyi, M., and Capowski, J. J. (1977): The terminal arborization pattern of primary afferent fibers in the substantia gelatinosa of the spinal cord in the cat. *J. Physiol. (Paris),* 73:269–277.
90. Rethelyi, M., and Szentagothai, J. (1973): Distribution and connections of afferent fibres in the spinal cord. In: *Handbook of Sensory Physiology, Vol. 2,* edited by A. Iggo, pp. 207–253. Springer-Verlag, New York.
91. Rustioni, A. (1973): Non-primary afferents to the nucleus gracilis from the lumbar cord of the cat. *Brain Res.,* 51:81–95.
92. Rustioni, A. (1974): Non-primary afferents to the cuneate nucleus in the brachial dorsal funiculus of the cat. *Brain Res.,* 75:247–259.
93. Scheibel, M. E., and Scheibel, A. B. (1968): Terminal axonal patterns in cat spinal cord. II. The dorsal horn. *Brain Res.,* 9:32–58.
94. Scheibel, M. E., and Scheibel, A. B. (1969): Terminal patterns in cat spinal cord. III. Primary afferent collaterals. *Brain Res.,* 13:417–443.
95. Schmidt, R. F. (1973): Control of access of afferent activity to somatosensory pathways. In: *Handbook of Sensory Physiology, Vol. 2: Somatosensory System,* edited by A. Iggo, pp. 151–206. Springer-Verlag, New York.
96. Simantov, R., Kuhar, M. J., Uhl, G. R., and Snyder, S. H. (1977): Opioid peptide enkephalin: Immunohistochemical mapping in the rat central nervous system. *Proc. Natl. Acad. Sci. USA,* 74:2167–2171.
97. Snow, P. J., Rose, P. K., and Brown, A. G. (1976): Tracing axons and axon collaterals of spinal neurons using intracellular injection of horseradish peroxidase. *Science,* 191:312–313.
98. Snyder, R. L. (1977): Dorsal root projections to the lumbar spinal cord in the cat: A light and electron microscopic autoradiographic study. *Soc. Neurosci. Abstr.,* III:508 (Abstr. No. 1630).
99. Stretton, A. O. W., and Kravitz, E. A. (1968): Neuronal geometry: Determination with a technique of intracellular dye injection. *Science,* 162:132–134.
100. Sugiura, Y. (1975): Three dimensional analysis of neurons in the substantia gelatinosa Rolandi. *Proc. Jap. Acad.,* 51:336–341.
101. Szentagothai, J. (1964): Neuronal and synaptic arrangement in the substantia gelatinosa Rolandi. *J. Comp. Neurol.,* 122:219–240.
102. Trevino, D. L., and Carstens, E. (1975): Confirmation of the location of spinothalamic neurons in the cat and monkey by the retrograde transport of horseradish peroxidase. *Brain Res.,* 98:177–182.
103. Trevino, D. L., Coulter, J. D., and Willis, W. D. (1973): Location of cells of origin of the spinothalamic tract in the lumbar enlargement of the monkey. *J. Neurophysiol.,* 36:750–761.
104. Uddenberg, N. (1968): Functional organization of long, second-order afferents in the dorsal funiculus. *Exp. Brain Res.,* 4:377–382.

105. Voris, H. (1957): Variations in the spinothalamic tract in man. *J. Neurosurg.,* 14:55–60.
106. Wall, P. D., and Yaksh, T. L. (1978): The effect of Lissauer tract stimulation on activity in dorsal and ventral roots. *Exp. Neurol.,* 60:570–583.
107. White, J. C., and Sweet, W. H. (1955): *Pain and the Neurosurgeon,* 1st edition. Charles C Thomas, Springfield, Ill.
108. Yaksh, T. L., Wall, P. D., and Merrill, E. G. (1977): Response properties of substantia gelatinosa neurones in the cat. *Soc. Neurosci. Abstr.,* III:495.
109. Young, D. W., and Gottschaldt, K.-M. (1976): Neurons in the rostral mesencephalic reticular formation of the cat responding specifically to noxious mechanical stimulation. *Exp. Neurol.,* 51:628–636.

Mechanisms of Pain and Analgesic Compounds,
edited by R. F. Beers, Jr., and E. G. Bassett.
Raven Press, New York © 1979.

12. Physiology of Dorsal Horn and Spinal Cord Pathways Related to Pain

William D. Willis, Jr.

Marine Biomedical Institute, University of Texas Medical Branch at Galveston, Galveston, Texas 77550

INTRODUCTION

There is now a substantial body of evidence that nociception in the mammal depends on a set of specific nociceptive afferents in peripheral nerves. The organization of the central nociceptive pathways is still unclear. Certain ascending tracts, such as the spinothalamic tract in primates (including man), are likely to be critically important for transmission of nociceptive data to the brain. In addition, there are descending control systems originating in the brainstem that regulate the activity of the ascending pathways. The emphasis in this chapter is on the response properties of dorsal horn neurons that are activated by nociceptive afferents, especially of identified spinothalamic tract cells in the monkey which can be excited powerfully by stimuli known to activate specific nociceptors in skin and muscle.

RESPONSES OF DORSAL HORN INTERNEURONS TO NOXIOUS STIMULI

Early investigations of the response properties of interneurons of the dorsal horn revealed that these cells typically receive a convergent input from cutaneous mechanoreceptors and nociceptors (41,43). Because graded mechanical stimuli ranging in intensity from innocuous to noxious produced a graded response that was maximal only when the stimulus was noxious, cells of this kind were said to have a *wide dynamic range* (29). Some dorsal horn interneurons were found to respond best to mechanical stimuli in the innocuous range (42). However, most investigators failed to detect interneurons that are specifically responsive to noxious inputs [a notable exception being the work of Kolmodin and Skoglund (21)], until the report by Christensen and Perl (14). The latter study showed that there is a concentration of *nociceptive-specific* neurons in the dorsalmost layer of the cat dorsal horn (lamina I of Rexed or the marginal layer of earlier neuroanatomists). Figure 1A–C shows the responses of a cell in lamina I to a graded series of mechanical stimuli, whereas Fig 1D shows the locations of a number of lamina I cells that responded only to strong mechanical stimuli

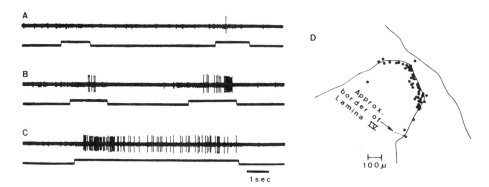

FIG. 1. Responses of a lamina I neuron in the cat spinal cord. **A:** Stroking the skin with a glass rod. **B:** Squeezing the skin with smooth-surfaced forceps. **C:** Squeezing the skin with serrated forceps. The locations of neurons responsive to strong mechanical stimuli or to strong mechanical stimuli and noxious heat are shown in **D.** (Modified from Christensen and Perl, ref. 14.)

or to both strong mechanical stimuli and noxious heat. These observations in the cat have been confirmed (11), and they have been extended to the monkey (23,36,45) and the rat (30). In addition, similar nociceptive-specific neurons have been found in deeper layers of the dorsal horn (30,35,36,45).

Recently, there have been a few reports of recordings from neurons located within the substantia gelatinosa (12,22,46). Some of these cells appear to be nociceptive specific (22), while many have a wide dynamic range of responsiveness (46).

CELLS OF ORIGIN OF THE SPINOTHALAMIC TRACT

Since it is not possible to specify what role interneurons play in nociceptive pathways unless the destinations of their axons are known, we chose to concentrate our attention on tract cells that belong to pathways thought to play a significant part in nociception. The spinothalamic tract is such a pathway in primates, including man (17,33). Spinothalamic tract cells can be identified by antidromic activation following stimulation in the thalamus (38).

Until recently, the locations of the cells of origin of the spinothalamic tract were known only from circumstantial evidence. We mapped the locations of these cells using electrophysiological techniques (38), but a more direct approach is by use of the horseradish peroxidase (HRP) retrograde labeling technique (25). Our results will be illustrated, but they are, in part, similar to the findings of other groups (1,37). The injections were made in regions of the thalamus known to receive spinothalamic tract terminals (20,28).

Figure 2 shows the results of an experiment in which HRP was injected into the lateral part of the thalamus in a region that included the ventral posterior

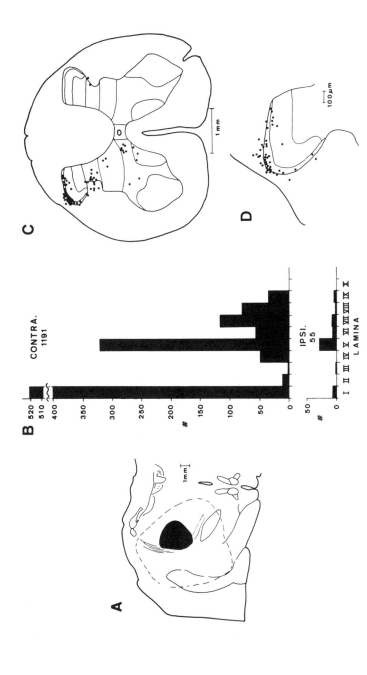

FIG. 2. Locations of spinothalamic tract cells that project to the lateral thalamus. The site of injection of HRP into the thalamus of a monkey is shown in **A**; the dashed line is the limit of spread of HRP, whereas the black area represents the region of greatest concentration of HRP that presumably approximates the zone of uptake. The histogram in **B** shows the distribution of HRP-labeled cells in segments L5–S1 of the spinal cord. Most of the cells were contralateral to the thalamic injection site (CONTRA.), but some were ipsilateral (IPSI.). The distribution of all of the cells in 15 consecutive alternate 50-μm sections in the lumbosacral enlargement is shown in **C**; the cells in the uppermost layers of the dorsal horn are shown in an expanded view in **D**.

lateral nucleus (Fig. 2A). The distribution of labeled spinothalamic tract neurons in the lumbosacral enlargement following this injection is shown in the histogram in Fig. 2B. Most of the cells were in laminae I and V on the side of the cord contralateral to the injection site. The locations of the cells at a representative level are shown in Fig. 2C. A more detailed view of the positions of the cells in the uppermost layers of the dorsal horn is shown in Fig. 2D. This evidence is in accord with previous observations that cells in laminae I and V can be labeled by HRP injected into the region of the ventral posterior lateral nucleus (1,37). It is also worth noting that some spinothalamic tract cells were found within the substantia gelatinosa.

Figure 3 shows the results of an experiment in which HRP was injected into the medial thalamus in an area that included the intralaminar nuclei. Two levels of the injection site are shown in Fig. 3A. The distribution of spinothalamic tract cells in the laminae of Rexed is shown in Fig. 3B. Although there were numerous spinothalamic tract neurons in laminae I and V, the majority of the cells were in laminae VI through VIII, in contrast to the previously described experiment in which HRP was injected laterally in the thalamus. A representative sample of spinothalamic tract cell locations is shown in Fig. 3C and D. These observations differ from those of Albe-Fessard et al. (1), who reported finding labeled cells just in the marginal zone in a monkey in which HRP was injected into the intralaminar nuclei.

The anatomical evidence indicates that there are numerous spinothalamic tract cells in the regions of the spinal cord known to contain both *nociceptive-specific* and *wide dynamic range* neurons. These regions include laminae I and V. The next question is whether spinothalamic tract neurons in these regions behave as if they carry nociceptive information.

NOCICEPTIVE RESPONSES OF SPINOTHALAMIC TRACT CELLS

Nociceptors transmit information centrally by way of either small myelinated (Aδ) or unmyelinated (C) afferent axons (5,9,15,19,24,34). If spinothalamic tract cells carry nociceptive information, it would be expected that they should be excited by volleys in Aδ and C fibers. That this is the case is illustrated in Fig. 4. The responses of a wide dynamic range spinothalamic tract cell are shown by the poststimulus histograms in Fig. 4A–C, whereas the afferent volleys recorded from the sural nerve and the cord dorsum potentials are shown in the insets. A scale over each histogram indicates the conduction velocities of afferent fiber groups that could be responsible for the responses, assuming monosynaptic excitation. The responses were apparently due to A$\alpha\beta$, A$\alpha\beta\delta$, and A + C fibers in Fig. 4A, B, and C, respectively.

In addition to evidence from volleys evoked by electrical stimulation of peripheral nerves, it is necessary to show that natural forms of noxious stimuli also cause responses before a central neuron can be said to convey nociceptive information. This is true because Aδ and C fibers arise from a heterogeneous assortment of receptors, which include mechanoreceptors and thermoreceptors in

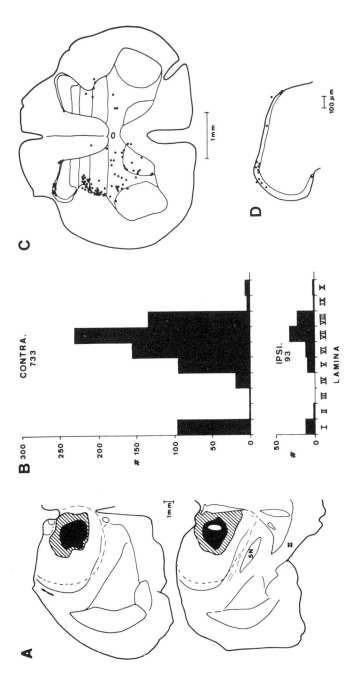

FIG. 3. Locations of spinothalamic tract cells that project to the medial thalamus in the monkey. The injection site is shown in **A** by drawings at two levels of the thalamus. The limits of spread of HRP are indicated by the dashed lines. The region of highest density of HRP is shown by the black area and that of intermediate density by the hatched area. The white oval in the lower drawing is the position of the habenulopeduncular tract. The histogram in **B** shows the distribution of labeled cells in the contralateral and the ipsilateral lumbosacral enlargement. The locations of cells in 15 consecutive alternate 50-μm sections are shown in **C**, and the locations of cells in the uppermost layers of the dorsal horn are represented in the expanded diagram in **D**.

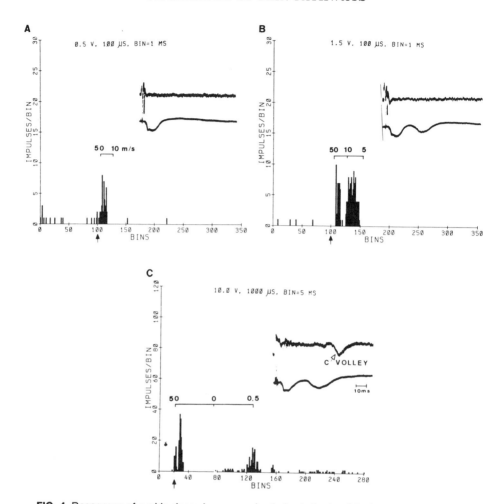

FIG. 4. Responses of a wide dynamic range spinothalamic tract cell in the neck of the dorsal horn to volleys in A and C fibers. The poststimulus time histogram **A** shows the response to a volley in fast myelinated fibers of the sural nerve. The ordinate is impulses per bin, and the abscissa is bins. The histogram was compiled from 10 stimulus repetitions. Stimulus parameters and bin width are indicated at the top and timing of stimulus indicated by an arrow. A conduction velocity scale shows the timing of central events that would be produced by monosynaptic excitation by different components of the afferent volley. The upper trace in the inset shows the afferent volley recorded from the sural nerve 38 mm proximal to the stimulating cathode. The lower trace is the sequence of cord dorsum potentials evoked by volley. **B:** The response to a volley in most of the myelinated fibers of the sural nerve. **C:** The response to A + C fibers (C volley indicated by open arrow in inset). Note that the bin width is 1 msec for **A** and **B**, but 5 msec for **C**. The time scale in the inset of **C** applies to all inset traces.

addition to nociceptors. We have been able to demonstrate that spinothalamic tract cells respond to several varieties of noxious stimuli (45). For instance, the cell illustrated in Fig. 4 was excited by noxious mechanical and thermal stimuli.

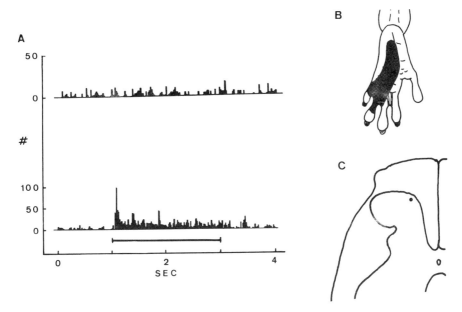

FIG. 5. Responses of a spinothalamic tract cell located in lamina I of the monkey spinal cord to intense mechanical stimulation. The receptive field and the location of the cell are indicated in the drawings at the right. The poststimulus time histograms show a failure of the cell to respond to pressure **(upper),** but a substantial response to a very intense mechanical stimulus **(lower).** (From Willis et al., ref. 45.)

Figure 5 shows the response of a spinothalamic tract cell located in lamina I to an intense mechanical stimulus (lower histogram) applied within the receptive field of the cell, but not to a moderately strong mechanical stimulus (upper histogram). This cell appeared to be nociceptive specific. Other spinothalamic tract cells showed a wide dynamic range of responsiveness. For example, the spinothalamic tract cell that yielded the responses illustrated in Fig. 6 was activated in a rapidly adapting fashion by a weak mechanical stimulus, the displacement of a single hair (upper histogram). However, when the skin was indented, the cell responded also in a slowly adapting fashion with a discharge rate that was graded with the intensity of the stimulus (middle and lower histograms). Such responses continued to increase as the mechanical stimulus was raised to damaging intensities.

A form of noxious stimulus that is more readily controlled than mechanical stimulation is noxious heat. We have been interested in comparing the responses of nociceptive-specific cells in lamina I to those of wide dynamic range cells following the application of noxious heat pulses to the skin. Figure 7 shows two sets of poststimulus time histograms. In each case, a series of heat pulses was applied, raising the skin temperature from an adapting level of 35°C to progressively higher levels of 43, 45, 47, and 50°C. The column of histograms on the left (I) represents recordings from a lamina I cell, whereas the column

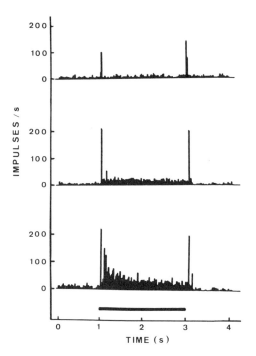

FIG. 6. Responses of a wide dynamic range spinothalamic tract neuron to grade mechanical stimuli. The uppermost histogram shows the response of the cell to movement of a single hair. The middle histogram shows the effect of skin indentation. The lower histogram is the result of a similar skin displacement starting from a position of greater static indentation. (Modified from Willis, et al., ref. 45.)

at the right (II) is from a wide dynamic range cell. The responses of the two cells were very similar, and so one can conclude that both kinds of spinothalamic tract cell are capable of conveying information concerning noxious heat stimuli to the brain.

Another form of noxious stimulus that can be controlled relatively well is the introduction of algesic chemicals into the arterial circulation of a limb (8, 13,26). It is known that algesic chemicals, like bradykinin, serotonin, or K^+, activate just group III and IV muscle afferents and not group I or II muscle afferents (31,32), whereas bradykinin and serotonin excite mechanoreceptors as well as nociceptors in skin (4). We simplified the interpretation of our findings by limiting the chemical stimuli to muscle afferents by denervating the hindlimb except for the nerves to the triceps surae muscles (18). Figure 8A–C shows the powerful excitatory effect of bradykinin, serotonin, and K^+ on spinothalamic tract cells. In addition, injection of hypertonic saline into muscle tissue produced a long-lasting increase in activity of spinothalamic cells (Fig. 8D). Such injections are painful in man (27). Some spinothalamic tract cells did not respond to the injection of algesic chemicals into the arterial circulation of the triceps surae muscles. A high proportion of the cells lacking a response was located in lamina I. Most of the cells that were excited were located in laminae V. Apparently, the receptive fields of some lamina I cells include skin but not muscle. If this is so, such neurons could signal well-localized pain, whereas

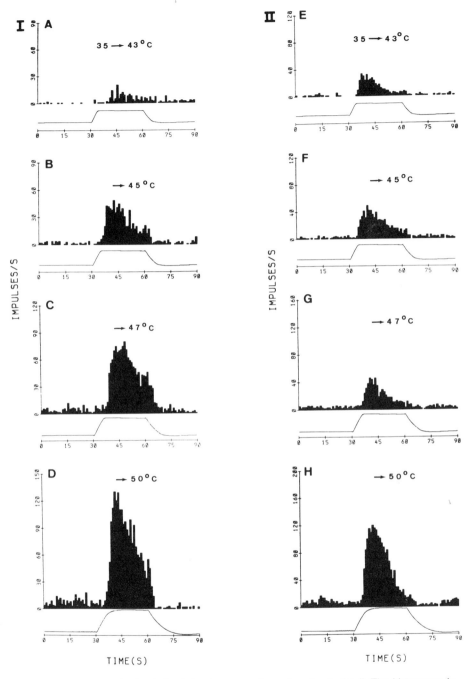

FIG. 7. Responses of spinothalamic tract neurons to noxious heat stimuli. The histograms in **I** represent the responses of a spinothalamic tract cell in the region of lamina I to a series of noxious heat stimuli applied to the receptive field with a Peltier effect thermal stimulator. **A–D** are the responses to changes in skin temperature from an adapting level of 35 to 43, 45, 47, and 50°C. The rate of temperature change was 2°C/sec. The histograms in **II** show the results of a similar series of noxious thermal stimuli on the activity of a wide dynamic range neuron located in the neck of the dorsal horn.

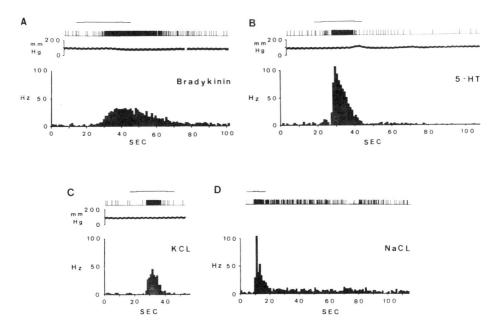

FIG. 8. Responses of a wide dynamic range spinothalamic tract neuron to injections of algesic chemicals. The effects of mechanical stimulation of the skin were determined before complete denervation of the skin. The cell responded to hair movement, but it had a much greater response to pinch. These responses disappeared when denervation was completed. Intraarterial injections of algesic chemicals resulted in a marked excitation of the neuron, as illustrated in **A** for bradykinin (26 μg), **B** for serotonin (135 μg), and **C** for KCl (0.1 meq). The cell was also excited by an intramuscular injection of 6% NaCl, **D**. (Modified from Foreman et al., ref. 18.)

spinothalamic neurons with receptive fields in both skin and muscle might participate only in poorly localized pain sensations.

OTHER NOCICEPTIVE PATHWAYS IN THE SPINAL CORD

There are several other pathways that convey nociceptive information to the brain, one of which is the spinocervical tract. This pathway has been studied best in the cat [reviewed by Brown (6)], but it exists also in the monkey (7) and probably in man (39). Many spinocervical tract neurons respond to noxious forms of stimulation [Fig. 9; also see (10)], and so this pathway could make a contribution to nociception. Another pathway that has responses very similar to those of the spinothalamic tract is the second order dorsal column pathway (2,3,40). Although neither of these pathways is likely to be primarily responsible for nociception in man, they might play some part in the return of pain sensation that frequently occurs after an initially successful cordotomy for the relief of pain (44). The spinoreticular [(16); however, see (20)] and spinotectal tracts may also contribute to nociception, although neither have been studied sufficiently to allow firm conclusions to be drawn.

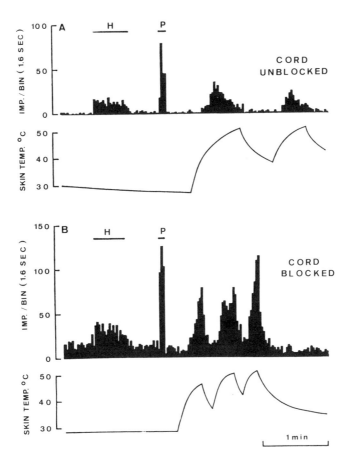

FIG. 9. Responses of a spinocervical tract neuron in the cat to innocuous and noxious stimuli. The innocuous stimulus was hair movement (H), whereas the noxious stimuli were pinprick (P) and noxious heat (indicated by upward deflexions in the temperature scale below the histograms). The responses at the top were with the spinal cord intact (anesthetized preparation), whereas the responses at the bottom were during cold block of the cord to eliminate tonic descending inhibitory controls. (From Cervero et al., ref. 10)

SUMMARY

It appears that there are at least two kinds of neurons in the dorsal horn that respond to noxious stimuli: the *nociceptive-specific* neuron and the *wide dynamic range* cell. The former are concentrated in lamina I and the latter in lamina V, although both cell types are present in both regions. Spinothalamic tract cells projecting to the lateral part of the thalamus are abundant in laminae I and V. Spinothalamic tract cells that project to the medial part of the thalamus also occur in these laminae, although more are located in deeper parts of the cord gray matter. Nociceptive-specific and wide dynamic range spinothalamic tract cells can be recognized on the basis of their responses to graded mechanical stimulation. However, both types of spinothalamic tract cells respond equally well to noxious heat stimuli. Spinothalamic tract cells, especially those located in lamina V, can also be excited by chemical stimulation of muscle nociceptors. Other tracts that may contribute to nociception include the spinocervical tract, the second order dorsal column pathway, the spinotectal tract, and the spinoreticular tract.

ACKNOWLEDGMENTS

The author wishes to thank Gail Silver for her expert technical assistance. The work in the author's laboratory was done in collaboration with Drs. J. D. Coulter, J. M. Chung, R. D. Foreman, D. R. Kenshalo, Jr., R. B. Leonard, R. A. Maunz, R. F. Schmidt, and D. L. Trevino. Support was from National Institutes of Health research grant NS-09743.

REFERENCES

1. Albe-Fessard, D., Boivie, J., Grant, G., and Levante, A. (1975): Labelling of cells in the medulla oblongata and the spinal cord of the monkey after injections of horseradish peroxidase in the thalamus. *Neurosci. Letters,* 1:75–80.
2. Angaut-Petit, D. (1975): The dorsal column system. I. Existence of long ascending postsynaptic fibres in the cat's fasciculus gracilis. *Exp. Brain Res.,* 22:457–470.
3. Angaut-Petit, D. (1975): The dorsal column system. II. Functional properties and bulbar relay of the postsynaptic fibres of the cat's fasciculus gracilis. *Exp. Brain Res.,* 22:471–493.
4. Beck, P. W., and Handwerker, H. O. (1974): Bradykinin and serotonin effects on various types of cutaneous nerve fibres. *Pflügers Arch.,* 347:209–222.
5. Bessou, P., and Perl, E. R. (1969): Response of cutaneous sensory units with unmyelinated fibers to noxious stimuli. *J. Neurophysiol.,* 32:1025–1043.
6. Brown, A. G. (1973): Ascending and long spinal pathways: Dorsal columns, spinocervical tract and spinothalamic tract. In: *Handbook of Sensory Physiology, Vol. II: Somatosensory System,* edited by A. Iggo, pp. 315–338. Springer-Verlag, New York.
7. Bryan, R. N., Coulter, J. D., and Willis, W. D. (1974): Cells of origin of the spinocervical tract in the monkey. *Exp. Neurol.,* 42:574–586.
8. Burch, G. E., and DePasquale, N. P. (1962): Bradykinin, digital blood flow, and the arteriovenous anastomoses. *Circ. Res.,* 10:105–115.
9. Burgess, P. R., and Perl, E. R. (1967): Myelinated afferent fibres responding specifically to noxious stimulation of the skin. *J. Physiol. (Lond.),* 190:541–562.
10. Cervero, F., Iggo, A., and Molony, V. (1977): Responses of spinocervical tract neurones to noxious stimulation of the skin. *J. Physiol. (Lond.),* 267:537–558.
11. Cervero, F., Iggo, A., and Ogawa, H. (1976): Nociceptor-driven dorsal horn neurones in the lumbar spinal cord of the cat. *Pain,* 2:5–24.
12. Cervero, F., Molony, V., and Iggo, A. (1977): Extracellular and intracellular recordings from neurones in the substantia gelatinosa Rolandi. *Brain Res.,* 136:565–569.
13. Coffman, J. D. (1966): The effect of aspirin on pain and hand blood flow responses to intra-arterial injection of bradykinin in man. *Clin. Pharmacol. Ther.,* 7:26–37.
14. Christensen, B. N., and Perl, E. R. (1970): Spinal neurons specifically excited by noxious or thermal stimuli: Marginal zone of the dorsal horn. *J. Neurophysiol.,* 33:293–307.
15. Croze, S., Duclaux, R., and Kenshalo, D. R. (1976): The thermal sensitivity of the polymodal nociceptors in the monkey. *J. Physiol. (Lond.),* 263:539–562.
16. Fields, H. L., Clanton, C. H., and Anderson, S. D. (1977): Somatosensory properties of spinoreticular neurons in the cat. *Brain Res.,* 120:49–66.

17. Foerster, O., and Gagel, O. (1931): Die Vorderseitenstrangdurchschneidung beim Menschen. Eine klinisch-patho-physiologisch-anatomische Studie. *Z. Gesamte Neurol. Psychiatr.,* 138:1–92.
18. Foreman, R. D., Schmidt, R. F., and Willis, W. D. (1977): Convergence of muscle and cutaneous input onto primate spinothalamic tract neurons. *Brain Res.,* 124:555–560.
19. Georgopoulos, A. P. (1976): Functional properties of primary afferent units probably related to pain mechanisms in primate glabrous skin. *J. Neurophysiol.,* 39:71–83.
20. Kerr, F. W. L., and Lippman, H. H. (1974): The primate spinothalamic tract as demonstrated by anterolateral cordotomy and commissural myelotomy. In: *Advances in Neurology, Vol. 4: Proceedings of the International Symposium on Pain,* edited by J. J. Bonica, pp. 147–156. Raven Press, New York.
21. Kolmodin, G. M., and Skoglund, C. R. (1960): Analysis of spinal interneurons activated by tactile and nociceptive stimulation. *Acta Physiol. Scand.,* 50:337–355.
22. Kumazawa, T., and Perl, E. R. (1978): Excitation of marginal and substantia gelatinosa neurons in the primate spinal cord: Indications of their place in dorsal horn functional organization. *J. Comp. Neurol.,* 177:417–434.
23. Kumazawa, T., Perl, E. R., Burgess, P. R., and Whitehorn, D. (1975): Ascending projections from marginal zone (lamina I) neurons of the spinal dorsal horn. *J. Comp. Neurol.,* 162:1–12.
24. LaMotte, R. H., and Campbell, J. N. (1978): Comparison of responses of warm and nociceptive C-fiber afferents in monkey with human judgements of thermal pain. *J. Neurophysiol.,* 41:509–528.
25. LaVail, J. H., and LaVail, M. M. (1974): The retrograde intra-axonal transport of horseradish peroxidase in the chick visual system: A light and electron microscopic study. *J. Comp. Neurol.,* 157:303–358.
26. Levante, A., Lamour, Y., Guilbaud, G., and Besson, J. M. (1975): Spinothalamic cell activity in the monkey during intense nociceptive stimulation: Intra-arterial injection of bradykinin into the limbs. *Brain Res.,* 88:560–564.
27. Lewis, T. (1942): *Pain.* Macmillan, New York.
28. Mehler, W. R., Feferman, M. E., and Nauta, W. J. H. (1960): Ascending axon degeneration following anterolateral cordotomy: An experimental study in the monkey. *Brain,* 83:718–750.
29. Mendell, L. M. (1966): Physiological properties of unmyelinated fiber projection to the spinal cord. *Exp. Neurol.,* 16:316–332.
30. Menétrey, D., Giesler, G. J., and Besson, J. M. (1977): An analysis of response properties of spinal cord dorsal horn neurones to nonnoxious and noxious stimuli in the spinal rat. *Exp. Brain Res.,* 27:15–33.
31. Mense, S. (1977): Nervous outflow from skeletal muscle following chemical noxious stimulation. *J. Physiol. (Lond.),* 267:75–88.
32. Mense, S., and Schmidt, R. F. (1974): Activation of group IV afferent units from muscle by algesic agents. *Brain Res.,* 72:305–310.
33. Morin, F., Schwartz, H. G., and O'Leary, J. L. (1951): Experimental study of the spinothalamic and related tracts. *Acta Psychiatr. Neurol.,* 26:371–396.
34. Perl, E. R. (1968): Myelinated afferent fibres innervating the primate skin and their response to noxious stimuli. *J. Physiol. (Lond.),* 197:593–615.
35. Price, D. D., and Browe, A. C. (1973): Responses of spinal cord neurons to graded noxious and non-noxious stimuli. *Brain Res.,* 64:425–429.
36. Price, D. D., and Mayer, D. J. (1974): Physiological laminar organization of the dorsal horn of *M. mulatta. Brain Res.,* 79:321–325.
37. Trevino, D. L., and Carstens, E. (1975): Confirmation of the location of spinothalamic neurons in the cat and monkey by the retrograde transport of horseradish peroxidase. *Brain Res.,* 98:177–182.
38. Trevino, D. L., Coulter, J. D., and Willis, W. D. (1973): Location of cells of origin of spinothalamic tract in lumbar enlargement of the monkey. *J. Neurophysiol.,* 36:750–761.
39. Truex, R. C., Taylor, M. J., Smythe, M. Q., and Gildenberg, P. L. (1965): The lateral cervical nucleus of cat, dog and man. *J. Comp. Neurol.,* 139:93–104.
40. Uddenberg, N. (1968): Functional organization of long, second-order afferents in the dorsal funiculus. *Exp. Brain Res.,* 4:377–382.
41. Wall, P. D. (1960): Cord cells responding to touch, damage, and temperature of skin. *J. Neurophysiol.,* 23:197–210.

42. Wall, P. D. (1967): The laminar organization of dorsal horn and effects of descending impulses. *J. Physiol. (Lond.),* 188:403–423.
43. Wall, P. D., and Cronly-Dillon, J. R. (1960): Pain, itch and vibration. *Arch. Neurol.,* 2:365–375.
44. White, J. C, and Sweet, W. H. (1969); *Pain and the Neurosurgeon. A Forty-Year Experience.* Charles C Thomas, Springfield, Ill.
45. Willis, W. D., Trevino, D. L., Coulter, J. D., and Maunz, R. A. (1974): Responses of primate spinothalamic tract neurons to natural stimulation of hindlimb. *J. Neurophysiol.,* 37:358–372.
46. Yaksh, T. L., Wall, P. D., and Merrill, E. G. (1977): Response properties of substantia gelatinosa neurones in the cat. *Soc. Neurosci. Abstr.,* III:495.

Mechanisms of Pain and Analgesic Compounds,
edited by R. F. Beers, Jr., and E. G. Bassett.
Raven Press, New York © 1979.

13. Pain Mechanisms in the Trigeminal System

Ronald Dubner and Ronald L. Hayes

Neurobiology and Anesthesiology Branch, National Institute of Dental Research, National Institutes of Health, Bethesda, Maryland 20014

INTRODUCTION

The classic notion that the caudalmost part of the trigeminal nucleus in the medulla is concerned with the transmission of nerve impulses or signals related to pain sensations has received considerable support from recent anatomical and physiological studies. As shown in Fig. 1, sensory messages from the mouth and face travel along peripheral nerve fibers that terminate in the trigeminal brainstem nucleus. This nucleus extends from the pons to the upper cervical segments of the spinal cord and can be further divided into subnuclei in the rostrocaudal direction. The caudal subdivision, called nucleus caudalis, is a layered structure, similar in lamination to the spinal cord dorsal horn (14,16). The marginal zone (layer I) and substantia gelatinosa (layers II and III) appear to receive exclusive input from small myelinated and unmyelinated axons whose receptor terminals are activated primarily by noxious (tissue-damaging) and thermal stimuli (8,15). This nociceptive input ultimately results in activation of layer I and deeper neurons (layers IV to VI) that project to the ventroposterior thalamus in primates. Nociceptive input also activates neurons in nucleus caudalis whose axons are confined to the rostrocaudal extent of the trigeminal brainstem nucleus. Their intranuclear axonal projections ascend and descend throughout the trigeminal nucleus in distinct fiber bundles (17). In addition, the activity of caudalis neurons is subject to considerable modulation of input from other brain areas including the cerebral cortex, midline brainstem raphe nuclei (Fig. 1), and other brainstem reticular zones (11). The earlier concepts of nucleus caudalis as only a relay station in the trigeminal pain pathway must be revised in light of the considerable modification of nociceptive information that can take place at this level of the trigeminal system.

Although nucleus caudalis appears to be a major site for the filtering and modulation of noxious input, there is evidence that other levels of the trigeminal brainstem nucleus play a role in nociception. Recent studies suggest that nucleus caudalis exerts a modulating influence on pain transmission at more rostral subdivisions of the nuclear complex via ascending intranuclear connections (5,28). In addition, tooth pulp pathways, a major source of pain signals, appear

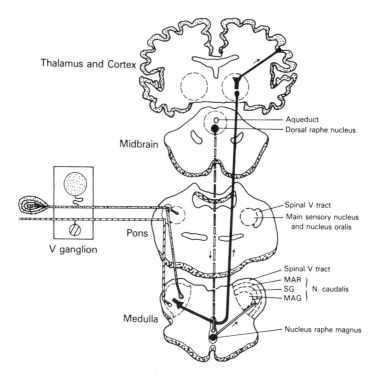

FIG. 1. Diagram of trigeminal nociceptive pathways. Both large-diameter (neuron with specialized receptor ending and large trigeminal ganglion cell body) and small-diameter (neuron with free nerve ending and small trigeminal ganglion cell body) afferents project to trigeminal nucleus caudalis in the medulla and activate trigeminothalamic wide dynamic range neurons. Nociceptive-specific trigeminothalamic neurons receive input only from small Aδ and C afferents. Noxious information is transmitted directly to the thalamus, and ultimately to the cerebral cortex, and bypasses rostral trigeminal nuclei (main sensory nucleus and nucleus oralis). Input from the dorsal raphe nucleus and input from the nucleus raphe magnus are part of descending pathways that suppress the activity of nociceptive neurons in nucleus caudalis. (Adapted from Dubner, ref. 6.)

to involve rostral as well as caudal levels of the trigeminal nucleus [see (11) for review].

The remainder of this chapter is concerned with three major aspects of pain mechanisms in trigeminal nucleus caudalis: (a) incoming nociceptive signals; (b) the properties of trigeminothalamic or projection neurons in nucleus caudalis; and (c) modulation of the output of this projection system.

OBSERVATIONS AND DISCUSSION

Incoming Nociceptive Signals

Similar to findings with spinal cord afferents (3), there are three major types (Table 1) of primary trigeminal afferents that appear to be uniquely involved

TABLE 1. *Major types of nociceptive afferents innervating the monkey's face*

Afferent fiber type	Conduction velocity $\overline{X} \pm SD$ (m/sec)	Mechanical thresholds (von Frey filaments, grams of force)		Thermal thresholds (°C)	
		Median	Range	Median	Range
AHN	15.2 ± 9.9 $N=15$	0.4	0.2–15.0 $N=9$	43[a]	37–47[a] $N=15$
CPN	0.8 ± 0.2 $N=20$	1.2	0.07–8.5 $N=39$	46[a]	38–49[a] $N=37$
HTM	10.2 ± 7.2 $N=54$	1.3	0.2–125.0 $N=45$	47[b]	43–53[b] $N=9$

[a] Before sensitization.
[b] After sensitization.

in the transduction of tissue-damaging or noxious stimulation into discrete nerve impulses that are transmitted to the central nervous system (2, 8–10). In contrast to primary afferents activated by weak or innocuous mechanical and thermal stimuli (3,6), these nociceptive afferents respond exclusively or differentially to noxious stimuli. Two of these nociceptive afferents innervating the monkey's face, Aδ heat nociceptive (AHN) and C polymodal nociceptive (CPN) afferents, have similar general properties (Table 1 and Fig. 2A). They respond to intense thermal and mechanical stimuli and usually have small (1 to 2 mm) single

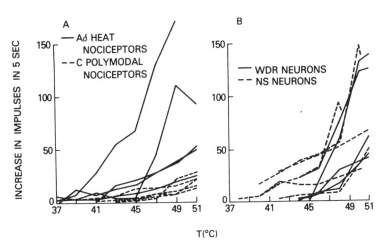

FIG. 2. A: Responses of five Aδ heat and five C polymodal nociceptive afferents to increases in receptive field temperature. The magnitude of the response expressed as the increase in impulses above spontaneous levels in the 5-sec period following the onset of the stimulus (temperature shift from 35°C to final temperatures of 37 to 51°C) is plotted against the final temperatures of individual trials. B: Responses of five wide dynamic range (WDR) and five nociceptive-specific (NS) neurons to receptive field skin temperature increases applied as described above. Both groups respond with the highest frequencies to skin temperatures in the noxious range (45 to 51°C). (Adapted from Price and Dubner, ref. 25.)

spot receptive fields. Thresholds to heat usually are below noxious levels (< 45°C), but almost all of these afferents are active at 45°C. Increases in stimulus intensity into the noxious range produce higher magnitude responses, with the greatest sensitivity occurring in the 45 to 51°C range. These afferents also respond to noxious mechanical stimuli (Table 1). Both AHNs and CPNs exhibit the property of sensitization and have lower thresholds and enhanced sensitivity to thermal stimuli after repeated exposure to noxious stimuli (2,9). The release of chemicals such as bradykinin and prostaglandin after skin injury may account for long-lasting sensitization (18) and may contribute, in part, to hyperalgesic areas of skin following tissue damage.

Although it is clear that AHNs and CPNs can provide information about noxious stimuli, they differ in some respects. As shown in Fig. 2A, both have stimulus-response functions that are monotonic in the 45 to 51°C range, but AHNs exhibit higher discharge rates. They also differ in their conduction velocities and fiber diameters; AHNs are finely myelinated Aδ afferents and CPNs are unmyelinated C afferents (Table 1). There is also additional evidence that AHNs contribute input essential to fast escape behavior in monkeys in response to noxious heat stimuli applied to the face (10). Monkeys trained in a reaction time task exhibit faster escape latencies to 51°C than to 49°C stimuli. Although CPNs probably contribute input to this behavior, only AHNs respond early enough in time to provide signals related to the fastest escape responses of these monkeys.

The third major type of nociceptor, high-threshold mechanoreceptive (HTM) afferents, has conduction velocities in the Aδ range and normally responds only to intense mechanical stimuli (Table 1). Thresholds are often below noxious levels but all are maximally sensitive in the noxious range. Receptive fields usually are single spots of 1 to 2 mm in diameter. Approximately 20 to 25% of HTMs respond to thermal stimuli after repeated exposure to noxious heat greater than 50°C. These heat-sensitive HTMs can be differentiated from AHNs by their higher thresholds, reduced sensitivity, and longer first spike latencies to noxious heat (9,10).

To summarize, small myelinated and unmyelinated afferents innervating the face exhibit specific responses to noxious thermal and mechanical stimuli. Their activity presumably is essential for the detection and discrimination of tissue-damaging or potentially tissue-damaging stimuli in the environment. These nociceptive afferents terminate at the level of trigeminal nucleus caudalis in the medulla. Recent studies (15) of afferent terminal degeneration after tooth pulp removal in cat indicate that unmyelinated axon terminals distribute in layer I (marginal zone) and small myelinated axons terminate in layers II and III (substantia gelatinosa). A similar restriction of small myelinated and unmyelinated axon terminals to the upper three layers also appears to exist in the spinal cord dorsal horn (22,23). The convergence of the different types of nociceptive and nonnociceptive afferents on trigeminothalamic caudalis neurons in the superficial and deep layers is discussed below.

Trigeminothalamic Neurons of Nucleus Caudalis

Similar to findings in the spinal cord dorsal horn [see (25) for review], there are two general categories of trigeminothalamic neurons in nucleus caudalis (Table 2) that receive direct or indirect input from small myelinated and unmyelinated afferents (8,11,26). The first class, referred to as *nociceptive-specific* neurons, responds only to intense mechanical or thermal stimuli, or both. Many are activated by nonnoxious intense pressure but respond maximally to noxious pinch. This class of neuron appears to receive direct or indirect input from HTMs and often from AHNs and/or CPNs. The second class, called *wide dynamic range* neurons, is activated by hair movement and weak mechanical stimuli (less than 5 g/mm^2) but responds maximally to noxious pinch. Many of these neurons respond to noxious heat. These neurons also appear to receive direct or indirect input from HTMs, and often from AHNs and CPNs. Their responses to low-threshold, tactile input and their brief latency responses to electrical stimulation of facial skin indicate that they also receive input from fast-conducting, large myelinated (Aβ) afferents. Large myelinated afferents innervating the skin of the face or limbs respond maximally to different types of innocuous mechanical stimuli such as hair movement, vibration, pressure, etc. (3,11,12,20). Their responses to noxious mechanical stimuli often are irregular or suppressed, and never of higher magnitude than those to innocuous mechanical stimuli.

There is a third general category of trigeminothalamic neurons[1] in nucleus caudalis that responds to light touch, pressure, or hair movement and appears to receive input exclusively from large myelinated Aβ afferents. Those *low-threshold mechanoreceptive* neurons do not respond to noxious heat or exhibit higher frequencies of discharge to noxious than to innocuous stimuli.

The locations of the three classes of trigeminothalamic neurons are shown in Figure 3. Nociceptive-specific neurons are located mainly in layer I (marginal

TABLE 2. *General categories of nucleus caudalis trigeminothalamic neurons*

Neuron type	Mean antidromic conduction velocity (m/sec)	Primary afferent convergence	Responses to heat	
			Warming	Noxious heat
Nociceptive specific	6.3	Aδ and sometimes C	+[a]	+
Wide dynamic range	11.6	Aβ + Aδ and/or C	+[a]	++
Low threshold	14.3	Aβ	—	—

++, Many neurons (> 50%); +, some neurons (< 50%); — no neurons.
[a] Above 38°C.

[1] Neurons activated exclusively by innocuous thermal stimuli have been reported, but whether they project directly to the thalamus is not yet known [see (11) for review].

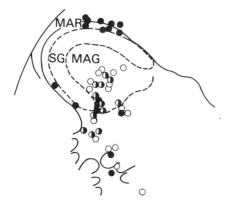

FIG. 3. Locations of wide dynamic range (◗) and nociceptive-specific (●) neurons in nucleus caudalis of the rhesus monkey; low-threshold mechanoreceptive neurons (○). These nucleus caudalis trigeminothalamic neurons projected to the ventroposterior nucleus of the thalamus. (Adapted from Price and Dubner, ref. 25.)

zone). Wide dynamic range neurons usually are found deep in layer IV (magnocellular zone) and in deeper layers. Low-threshold mechanoreceptive neurons usually are located in the superficial part of layer IV. All these neurons project directly to the thalamus in and near the ventroposterior medial nucleus. Note the absence of projection neurons from the substantia gelatinosa, an area presumed to contain excitatory and inhibitory interneurons involved in the modulation of input to the thalamic projection pathway (14).

The nociceptive input to the marginal zone is organized in a somatotopic fashion, as described previously for low-threshold mechanoreceptive input to the magnocellular layer (11). The mandibular division is located dorsomedially and the ophthalmic division, ventrolaterally (26,30). Furthermore, a somatotopic pattern is present in the rostrocaudal axis of nucleus caudalis. The nose and mouth are represented near the level of the obex, whereas scalp, preauricular skin, and lateral face are found most caudally (30). There is a gradual concentric shift of receptive field representation between these levels. These findings support the "onion skin" arrangement of facial dermatomes first described by Déjerine (4) and later supported by observations in patients undergoing trigeminal spinal tractotomy operations (21).

Both nociceptive-specific and wide dynamic range neurons have similar responses to noxious thermal stimuli (Fig. 2B). Thermal thresholds range from 38 to 50°C and stimulus-response functions are monotonic to final temperatures of 48 to 51°C. These stimulus-response functions are similar in form to those previously described for AHNs and CPNs (Fig. 2A). It appears that the information relayed by these primary afferents has converged on the same central neurons and has been transmitted in a highly secure fashion. However, these studies in nucleus caudalis were performed on anesthetized monkeys, and one might suspect that the response properties of such neurons would be different in awake, behaving monkeys since it is known that anesthetics alter ongoing and evoked central neuronal activity. In addition, there is considerable evidence that the output of these caudalis nociceptive neurons can be modified by descending influences from the cerebral cortex and other sites (6,24).

Modulation of the Output of Nucleus Caudalis

The most powerful inhibition of nociceptive neurons in trigeminal nucleus caudalis and the spinal cord dorsal horn is produced by stimulation of medullary midline raphe nuclei, midbrain periaqueductal gray, and diencephalic periventricular regions (24). Heat-induced responses of nociceptive-specific and wide dynamic range trigeminothalamic neurons can be suppressed for minutes by a 10- to 30-sec electrical stimulation of midbrain and diencephalic sites (19). A similar inhibitory effect on responses evoked by tooth pulp stimulation is observed in nucleus caudalis neurons (27). In the spinal cord, inhibition is produced by impulses traveling in a pathway from raphe magnus to spinal levels in the spinal cord dorsolateral quadrant (1,13,29). There are also direct projections from raphe magnus to trigeminal nucleus caudalis (1).

Recently, we have examined the dynamic properties of nociceptive-specific, wide dynamic range, and low-threshold mechanoreceptive neurons in nucleus caudalis in awake monkeys trained to discriminate and escape noxious heat stimuli. We have found that these neurons have more complex properties and a wider range of response capabilities in the awake monkey. Neuronal activity is strongly influenced by behavioral contingencies, supporting the concept that this region is subject to considerable descending modulatory control. The behavioral situation is similar to one we have described previously (7,10). The monkey initiates a trial by depressing a lighted panel button. At the same time, the temperature of a spring-loaded contact thermode applied to the upper hairy lip changes from 35°C to final temperatures varying from 37 to 49°C. Liquid reinforcement is available if the final temperature is less than 45°C and the monkey releases the panel within 2.0 sec of termination of the temperature increase. In one-sixth of the trials, the temperature increase is 45°C or greater and no reinforcement is available. Early releases on these trials terminate the temperature increase, thereby allowing the monkey to escape noxious heat stimuli. Thus, in order to receive liquid reinforcement, a monkey must in sequence (a) discriminate that a temperature increase at panel press is less than 45°C, (b) detect that the temperature increase has terminated, and (c) release the panel within 2.0 sec of termination of the temperature increase. Neuronal activity has been correlated with:

(a) light onset indicating the start of a trial;
(b) panel press and simultaneous temperature increase;
(c) temperature termination; and
(d) panel release to escape unrewarded and noxious heat trials ($\geq$ 45°C) or to secure reinforcement on innocuous temperature trials ($<$ 45°C).

Figure 4 shows some of the properties of one class of neuron that responds differentially to noxious heat and is capable of providing sensory signals related to the monkey's ability to discriminate temperature changes of 45° or greater from those less than 45°C. Peristimulus histograms have been plotted relative to panel press and simultaneous temperature increase for 47 and 49°C final

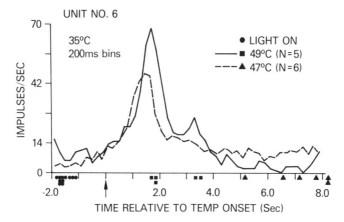

FIG. 4. Responses of a nucleus caudalis neuron in an awake monkey trained to discriminate and escape noxious heat stimuli applied to the face. Histograms are plotted relative to panel press and simultaneous temperature increase *(arrow)*. ———, average of five trials (49°C final temperature); – – – –, average of six trials (47°C final temperature). Time of occurrence of panel release (to escape or discriminate noxious stimuli) is shown on the abscissa: ■, 49°C; ▲, 47°C; ●, trial light onset. Base-line temperature is 35°C. The neuron was characterized with behaviorally unrelated, passive stimulation as nociceptive specific, and was located in layer V.

temperature trials. Escape or discrimination latencies to 49°C were all less than 4 sec, whereas latencies on 47°C trials were all greater than 4.0 sec. The greater increase in discharge of the neuron to 49°C temperatures than to 47°C occurred early enough to provide signals related to the shorter escape latencies at 49°C. No other class of neuron studied exhibited this early differential discharge.

These neurons usually are found in layer I or layer IV/V of nucleus caudalis, and receptive fields are limited to one or two ipsilateral trigeminal dermatomes. They are maximally sensitive to heat stimuli in the 45 to 49°C range with thresholds of 43 to 45°C. With behaviorally unrelated, passive stimulation, we determined that these neurons include both nociceptive-specific and wide dynamic range neurons previously studied in anesthetized monkeys. Thus, nociceptive-specific and wide dynamic range neurons provide discriminatory information about noxious heat stimuli in awake, behaving monkeys.

Figure 5 shows that the activity of this class of neuron can be modulated by the behavioral situation. On some trials, a signal is given to the monkey at the time of panel press, indicating that it will be a noxious trial of 49°C. This signal provides earlier information to the monkey than the temperature change to 49°C. The peristimulus histograms shown are plotted relative to panel press and simultaneous temperature increase for the unsignaled and signaled conditions. Note the earlier onset of the increase in discharge in the signaled condition. However, the magnitude of the response was reduced when the signal was present. The longer duration response in the signaled condition was due to a fixed stimulus duration of 4.0 sec and shows that there was a response to the tempera-

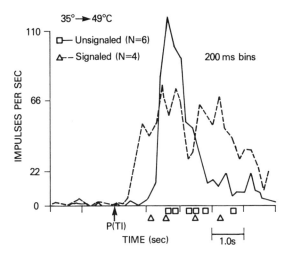

FIG. 5. Modulation of activity of a nucleus caudalis neuron to noxious heat (49°C) stimuli. Histograms are plotted relative to panel press and temperature increase [P(T1)]. ———, Response in the unsignaled condition averaged from six trials; — — —, response in the signaled condition averaged from four trials. The signal, a bright light mounted above the panel, was presented at panel press. Time of occurrence of panel release is shown on the abscissa: □, unsignaled condition; △, signaled condition. Base-line temperature is 35°C. The neuron was characterized with passive stimulation as a wide dynamic range neuron and was located in layer IV. See text for further details.

ture increase throughout the stimulus period. Thus, a signal predicting the occurrence of a noxious thermal stimulus can result in modulation of neural activity that includes a reduction in latency and magnitude of the response.

A second class of neuron observed in these studies shows another type of modulation. These neurons, as determined by behaviorally unrelated, passive stimulation, are very similar to some of the low-threshold mechanoreceptive neurons previously studied in anesthetized monkey. They are located in layer IV, exhibit maintained discharges to light tactile stimulation, and presumably receive input from slowly adapting mechanoreceptive afferents innervating the face (12). However, the maintained activity of some of these neurons is almost totally suppressed during the panel press period of the behaving monkeys. A typical response of one of these neurons is shown in Figure 6. The thermode was placed in the receptive field of the neuron and the histogram shows that there was maintained steady discharge of the neuron preceding panel press. At panel press and simultaneous temperature increase, activity almost ceased but returned to previous or higher levels at panel release. This suppression of activity is independent of temperature since it occurred in the absence of any temperature change (Fig. 6). In other experiments, we have demonstrated that this suppression of activity occurs during the animal's goal-directed behavior when (a) the probe is removed from the face, (b) it is placed outside the receptive field of the neuron, or (c) the experimenter initiates trials and provides reinforce-

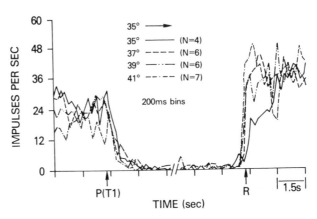

FIG. 6. Suppression of activity of a low-threshold mechanoreceptive neuron in nucleus caudalis during the panel press period. The histograms are plotted relative to panel press and simultaneous temperature increase [P(T1)] on the left, and panel release (R) on the right. Each pair of histograms is the response to a temperature shift from 35°C base line to a final temperature of 35 (no temperature change), 37, 39, or 41°C. N refers to the number of trials averaged in each pair of histograms. The neuron was located in layer IV.

ment at the appropriate time. The inhibition is absent on unreinforced, experimenter-initiated trials or during nonperformance-related stimulation. Thus, this suppression of activity takes place independent of peripheral somatosensory feedback from the face or hand. It appears to occur only in trials in which the monkey is attending to and preparing for the appropriate sensory cue and may function to suppress low-threshold mechanosensitive input irrelevant to the goal-directed behavior of the monkey.

The above behavioral and physiological findings in the awake monkey indicate that information about noxious stimuli probably is coded by the combined output of nociceptive-specific and wide dynamic range trigeminothalamic neurons and interneurons located in nucleus caudalis. These neurons receive input from nociceptive and nonnociceptive afferents, and mechanisms of convergence, central summation, inhibition, and descending control determine what sensory messages are relayed to more rostral brain centers. Descending modulation of these neurons appears to be a critical determinant of their output in the awake, behaving animal and probably is related to the multiple descending projections to nucleus caudalis from the cerebral cortex, brainstem midline raphe nuclei, and other reticular formation areas. The dynamic response capabilities of these neurons during goal-directed behaviors exceed those demonstrated in anesthetized animals.

SUMMARY

Trigeminal nucleus caudalis in the brainstem is a major component of the trigeminal nucleus concerned with orofacial nociception. It receives signals related to tissue-damaging (noxious) or potentially tissue-damaging environmental stimuli and conveys this information to higher brain centers via a central pathway that does not include the more rostral subdivisions of the trigeminal brainstem nucleus. Nucleus caudalis also sends projections to more rostral trigeminal subnuclei where it exerts a modulating influence on the output of trigeminothalamic neurons and interneurons. There are three major types of small myelinated and unmyelinated primary trigeminal afferents that respond exclusively or maximally to noxious stimuli and exhibit receptor-specific characteristics similar to those observed for primary afferents activated by weak or innocuous stimuli. The marginal and substantia gelatinosa layers of nucleus caudalis receive an exclusive projection of small myelinated and unmyelinated axons, including those activated primarily by noxious and thermal stimuli.

There are two categories of trigeminothalamic neurons in nucleus caudalis that receive nociceptive input. One type, nociceptive-specific neurons, responds only to near noxious and noxious stimuli. A second type, wide dynamic range neurons, is activated by hair movement and pressure but responds maximally to noxious stimuli. These neurons, studied in anesthetized monkey, are located in the marginal and deeper layers of nucleus caudalis. The earlier concepts of nucleus caudalis as only a relay station in the trigeminal pathway must be revised in light of the considerable modification of nociceptive information that can take place at this level. The output of these neurons is subject to considerable modulation from more rostral brain centers such as the cerebral cortex, midline brainstem raphe nuclei, and other reticular formation sites. This clearly is demonstrated in studies of neural activity in awake, behaving animals. In awake monkeys trained to discriminate and escape noxious thermal stimuli, nociceptive-specific and wide dynamic range neurons are observed and both are capable of providing discriminatory information related to the monkey's escape behavior. The activity of these neurons and other neurons is modulated by behavioral contingencies, indicating their wide response capabilities.

ACKNOWLEDGMENT

We appreciate the help of Sherry Berg who participated in the initial neural recording experiments in the awake monkey. We also wish to thank Patricia Wolskee, Robin Harris, and Henry Burris for their technical assistance in the same project.

REFERENCES

1. Basbaum, A. I., Clanton, C. H., and Fields, H. L. (1978): Three bulbospinal pathways from the rostral medulla of the cat: An autoradiographic study of pain modulating systems. *J. Comp. Neurol.,* 178:209–224.
2. Beitel, R. E., and Dubner, R. (1976): The response of unmyelinated (C) polymodal nociceptors to thermal stimuli applied to the monkey's face. *J. Neurophysiol.,* 39:1160–1175.
3. Burgess, P. R., and Perl, E. R. (1973): Cutaneous mechanoreceptors and nociceptors. In: *Hand-*

book of Sensory Physiology, Vol. II: Somatosensory System, edited by A. Iggo, pp. 29–78. Springer-Verlag, New York.

4. Déjerine, J. J. (1914): *Sémiologie des Affections du Système Nerveux.* Massion and Cie, Paris.
5. Denny-Brown, D., and Yanagisawa, N. (1973): The function of the descending root of the fifth nerve. *Brain,* 96:783–814.
6. Dubner, R. (1978): Neurophysiology of pain. *Dent. Clin. North Am.,* 22:11–30.
7. Dubner, R., Beitel, R. E., and Brown, F. J., (1976): A behavioral animal model for the study of pain mechanisms in primates. In: *Pain: New Perspectives in Therapy and Research,* edited by M. Weisenberg and B. Tursky, pp. 155–170. Plenum Press, New York.
8. Dubner, R., Gobel, S., and Price, D. D. (1976): Peripheral and central trigeminal "pain" pathways. In: *Advances in Pain Research and Therapy, Vol. 1: Proceedings of the First World Congress on Pain,* edited by J. J. Bonica and D. Albe-Fessard, pp. 137–148. Raven Press, New York.
9. Dubner, R., and Hu, J. W. (1977): Myelinated (Aδ) nociceptive afferents innervating the monkey's face. *J. Dent. Res.,* 56:A167.
10. Dubner, R., Price, D. D., Beitel, R. E., and Hu, J. W. (1977): Peripheral neural correlates of behavior in monkey and human related to sensory-discriminative aspects of pain. In: *Pain in the Trigeminal Region,* edited by D. J. Anderson and B. Matthews, pp. 57–66. Elsevier/North Holland Biomedical Press, Amsterdam.
11. Dubner, R., Sessle, B. J., and Storey, A. T. (1978): *The Neural Basis of Oral and Facial Function.* Plenum Press, New York.
12. Dubner, R., Sumino, R., and Starkman, S. (1974): Responses of facial cutaneous thermosensitive and mechanosensitive afferent fibers in the monkey to noxious heat stimulation. In: *Advances in Neurology, Vol. 4: Proceedings of the International Symposium on Pain,* edited by J. J. Bonica, pp. 61–71, Raven Press, New York.
13. Fields, H. L., Basbaum, A. I., Clanton, C. H., and Anderson, S. D. (1977): Nucleus raphe magnus inhibition of spinal cord dorsal horn neurons. *Brain Res.,* 126:441–453.
14. Gobel, S. (1978): Golgi studies of the neurons in layer II of trigeminal nucleus caudalis. *J. Comp Neurol.,* 180:395–414.
15. Gobel, S., and Binck, J. M. (1977): Degenerative changes in primary trigeminal axons and in neurons in nucleus caudalis following tooth pulp extirpations in the cat. *Brain Res.,* 132:347–354.
16. Gobel, S., Falls, W. M., and Hockfield, S. (1977): The division of the dorsal and ventral horns of the mammalian caudal medulla into eight layers using anatomical criteria. In: *Pain in the Trigeminal Region,* edited by D. J. Anderson and B. Matthews, pp. 443–453. Elsevier/North Holland Biomedical Press, Amsterdam.
17. Gobel, S., and Purvis, M. B. (1972): Anatomical studies of the organization of the spinal V nucleus: The deep bundles and the spinal V tract. *Brain Res.,* 48:27–44.
18. Handwerker, H. O. (1976): Influences of algogenic substances and prostaglandins on the discharges of unmyelinated cutaneous nerve fibers identified as nociceptors. In: *Advances in Pain Research and Therapy, Vol. 1: Proceedings of the First World Congress on Pain,* edited by J. J. Bonica and D. Albe-Fessard, pp. 41–45. Raven Press, New York.
19. Hayes, R. L., Price, D. D., Ruda, M. A., and Dubner, R. (1979): Suppression of nociceptive responses in the primate by electrical stimulation of the brain or morphine administration: Behavioral and electrophysiological comparisons. *Brain Res. (in press).*
20. Horch, K. W., Tuckett, R. P., and Burgess, P. R. (1977): A key to the classification of cutaneous mechanoreceptors. *J. Invest. Dermatol.,* 69:75–82.
21. Kunc, Z. (1970): Significant factors pertaining to the results of trigeminal tractotomy. In: *Trigeminal Neuralgia,* edited by R. Hassler and A. E. Walker, pp. 90–100. Georg Thieme Verlag, Stuttgart.
22. LaMotte, C. (1977): Distribution of the tract of Lissauer and the dorsal root fibers in the primate spinal cord. *J. Comp.Neurol.,* 172:529–561.
23. Light, A. R., and Perl, E. R. (1977): Differential termination of large-diameter and small-diameter primary afferent fibers in the spinal dorsal gray matter as indicated by labelling with horseradish peroxidase. *Neurosci. Lett.,* 6:59–63.
24. Mayer, D. J., and Price, D. D. (1976): Central nervous system mechanisms of analgesia. *Pain,* 2:379–404.
25. Price, D. D., and Dubner, R. (1977): Neurons that subserve the sensory-discriminative aspects of pain. *Pain,* 3:307–338.

26. Price, D. D., Dubner, R., and Hu, J. W. (1976): Trigeminothalamic neurons in nucleus caudalis responsive to tactile, thermal and nociceptive stimulation of monkey's face. *J. Neurophysiol.*, 39:936–953.
27. Sessle, B. J., Dubner, R., Hu, J. W., and Lucier, G. E. (1977): Modulation of trigeminothalamic relay and non-relay neurones by noxious, tactile and periaqueductal gray stimuli: Implications in perceptual and reflex aspects of nociception. In: *Pain in the Trigeminal Region,* edited by D. J. Anderson and B. Matthews, pp. 285–294. Elsevier/North Holland Biomedical Press, Amsterdam.
28. Sessle, B. J., and Greenwood, L. F. (1974): Influences of trigeminal nucleus caudalis on the responses of cat trigeminal brain stem neurons with orofacial mechanoreceptive fields. *Brain Res.,* 67:330–333.
29. Willis, W. D., Haber, L. H., and Martin, R. F. (1977): Inhibition of spinothalamic tract cells and interneurons by brain stem stimulation in the monkey. *J. Neurophysiol.,* 40:968–981.
30. Yokota, T., and Nishikawa, N. (1977): Somatotopic organization of trigeminal neurons within caudal medulla oblongata. In: *Pain in the Trigeminal Region,* edited by D. J. Anderson and B. Matthews, pp. 243–257. Elsevier/North Holland Biomedical Press, Amsterdam.

Mechanisms of Pain and Analgesic Compounds,
edited by R. F. Beers, Jr., and E. G. Bassett.
Raven Press, New York © 1979.

14. Descending Control Systems

J. Timothy Cannon and John C. Liebeskind

*Department of Psychology, University of California, Los Angeles,
Los Angeles, California 90024*

INTRODUCTION

The existence of brainstem controls on spinal reflexes and on ascending somatosensory pathways has been known for many years. In the past few years, much evidence has been provided that such controls can be exerted selectively on pain mechanisms. Several reviews have recently been published covering various aspects of this topic in detail (26,37,68,79,87,128,140). In the present chapter, we provide a brief overview of the major findings and conceptual issues in this area.

OBSERVATIONS AND DISCUSSION

Electrical stimulation of the midbrain periaqueductal gray matter in the rat induces powerful inhibition of pain responses across a wide variety of tests (44,89,109,125). This inhibition compares in potency to that achieved by high doses of morphine (85). Importantly, like morphine analgesia, this stimulation-produced analgesia (SPA) blocks even spinally mediated nociceptive reflexes (89), those known to be resistant to pharmacological inhibition except by narcotic analgesic drugs (50). Analgesic effects of similar magnitude have been seen in cat and monkey following periaqueductal electrical stimulation (47,91,98); in fact, several neurosurgical groups have successfully applied this technique to the alleviation of chronic pain states in man (1,23,54,61,111,112).

The anatomical locus of this pain inhibitory system is now known to include medial brainstem regions both rostral and caudal to the periaqueductal gray matter. A variety of medial, caudal diencephalic areas have proven to be effective SPA sites in rats (10,85,110) and monkeys (47) and to date have been the target of choice in neurosurgical trials (61,112). Other studies have revealed that the nucleus raphe magnus of the caudal brainstem is not only itself a site from which powerful pain inhibitory effects can be obtained (97,99,100,108), but is also an important relay conveying the centrifugal inhibitory message deriving from more rostral brainstem structures to the final site of pain inhibition in the spinal cord (37,114). Microinjections of morphine and other narcotic analgesic drugs into specific brain regions show that many of the same structures are involved in mediating opiate analgesia as well as SPA (33,65,66,87,103, 118,131,140,141,143). For example, even minute quantities of opiates injected into the periaqueductal gray induce analgesia as completely and powerfully as vastly larger systemic injections.

Some of the most salient features of SPA are:

(a) In a given animal, the analgesic effect may be seen in one body region, but at the same time not elsewhere (10,85,89,98).

(b) The analgesia can outlast the required brief period of brain stimulation, sometimes by many minutes or even several hours (61,85,89,112).

(c) For certain electrode placements in the brain, an animal will learn to press a bar to turn on the central stimulation only when he is also receiving a noxious peripheral stimulus, suggesting that under such circumstances brain stimulation is reinforcing because it reduces the perception of pain (89).

(d) Other deficits in sensory, motor, or emotional mechanisms are frequently not in evidence at the time pain inhibition is seen (26,87,89,101).

Such observations support the conclusion that this effect is specifically antinociceptive and cannot be explained by any other stimulation-produced disability. It seems, as we have previously suggested (78,89), that a natural or endogenous pain inhibitory system exists which is activated by direct electrical stimulation or by the administration of opiates and which then energizes descending controls serving to block the transmission of the pain message through the earliest synapses in the central pain path.

In the past few years, a great deal of new and exciting information has become available that has served to confirm and enrich this concept of an endogenous pain-suppressive system operating by the activation of centrifugal controls. Some of the most interesting of these findings are described below.

ATTENUATION OF NEURAL RESPONSES TO NOXIOUS STIMULI

Electrical stimulation of the periaqueductal gray matter and the nucleus raphe magnus, as well as morphine administration systemically or into the periaqueductal gray, have all been shown to exert a powerful and, in many instances, preferential inhibition on dorsal horn interneurons involved in pain mechanisms (15, 18,19,38,69,74,98,135). Similar observations have been made at the level of interneurons in the trigeminal complex (117). Neurons most affected appeared to be those responding specifically (marginal zone) or preferentially (lamina V) to noxious inputs. Some of the interneurons receiving this descending inhibitory control were identified by the antidromic activation technique as projecting to the thalamus (15,135). These studies have all been conducted in the anesthetized or decerebrate animal. Although the brainstem sites causing this inhibition have in some animals been previously studied behaviorally and confirmed to be analgesia producing, in other animals behaviorally ineffective sites nonetheless later proved to inhibit spinal nociceptive interneurons under anesthesia (98). It will be important in future studies of this genre to confirm the neurophysiological inhibition in awake animals with concurrent analgesia testing in order to assess the degree of correlation between the behavioral and the electrophysiological phenomena.

In other work, single or multiple unit recording techniques have been applied to studying both the responses in different brain areas evoked by noxious and nonnoxious stimuli and the effect on such responses of analgesic brain stimulation or morphine administration (94,97). Here again, these analgesic manipulations have been shown to exert good specificity in blocking preferentially the nociceptively driven cellular activity, whether lightly anesthetized or unanesthetized animals were employed.

DESCENDING PATHWAYS

Selective lesions of the spinal cord dorsolateral funiculus have been reported to abolish the analgesic effect of medial brainstem stimulation in the rat (14). They similarly block the inhibitory effect of such stimulation on spinal cord interneurons in the cat and monkey (38,135). Even more dramatically, the same lesions block the analgesic effect of morphine, whether administered locally into the periaqueductal gray matter (95) or even systemically in doses up to moderate levels (14,57). These lesions are known to interrupt serotonin-containing fibers descending to the cord from nucleus raphe magnus; and, in fact, recent autoradiographic data show that fibers from this nucleus terminate especially in those regions of the dorsal horn (marginal zone, substantia gelatinosa, and lamina V) where pain modulation is thought to occur (13). Analogous projections exist to the trigeminal nucleus caudalis (13).

These findings as well as those described in the preceding section illustrate the importance of descending or centrifugal systems underlying the analgesic effect of medial brainstem stimulation and opiate administration.

ROLE OF SEROTONIN

Drugs affecting serotonin, but also those affecting norepinephrine and dopamine, have been shown to alter SPA (2,4) much as they alter opiate analgesia (31,92,107,115). Particular interest has focused on serotonin since the cell bodies of the nucleus raphe magnus and the dorsal raphe nucleus (located within the periaqueductal gray matter) are known to be integral parts of the analgesia system and also serotonin containing. Drugs that interfere with serotinin's action have been found to reduce the potency of SPA (2,4) and morphine analgesia (126,137) as well as to block the efficacy of such procedures in inhibiting spinal cord nociceptive interneurons (51). Just as lesions of the serotonin-containing fibers in the dorsolateral funiculus interrupt SPA and opiate analgesia, destruction of the nucleus raphe magnus, whether accomplished pharmacologically (134) or electrolytically (108,138), has been shown to reduce or block morphine analgesia. That serotonin plays an important but not unique role in these antinociceptive systems is illustrated by the following observations. Stimulation in or near the dorsal raphe nucleus, as well as stimulation distant from these cells, can both inhibit spinal cord interneurons (51) and produce analgesia (4). However, antiserotoninergic drugs were seen to block the inhibitory effects of raphe stimulation without blocking the inhibitory effects caused by stimulation elsewhere (4,51). Clearly, nonserotoninergic pathways exist for mediating SPA.

OPIATE AND NONOPIATE ANALGESIC MECHANISMS

Considerable import has been attached to the finding that naloxone, a specific opiate antagonist drug, can at least partially block SPA (5,6,99,100). Of special interest is the recent observation that this drug can interrupt completely the pain-attenuating effect of medial brainstem stimulation in chronic pain patients (1,61,112). In a conceptually related set of experiments, it has been shown both in laboratory animals (84,86) and in man (61) that SPA manifests tolerance and, in fact, cross-tolerance with morphine. Such findings reinforce the idea that SPA and opiate analgesia share a common underlying mechanism of action, a common neurochemistry, just as SPA and morphine microinjection mapping studies suggest that these two phenomena share common sites of action. On the other hand, Akil et al. (5,6) found that naloxone only partially blocks SPA, and some investigators have completely failed to demonstrate this effect (96, 102,142). Similarly, tolerance to SPA and cross-tolerance between SPA and opiate analgesia have also been seen to be incomplete (84). It seems apparent from such observations that nonopiate mechanisms of analgesia also exist in the brain. Several additional findings strongly support this idea:

(a) Naloxone has been shown to diminish or block the analgesic effect of acupuncture and transcutaneous electrical stimulation in man (29,88,123) and in laboratory animals (105,106,136). Some of these same investigators, however, have failed to demonstrate any effect of naloxone on hypnotic analgesia in human subjects [(11,88); also see (45)].

(b) Subjecting rats to certain highly stressful procedures has been seen to induce analgesia which is according to some authors (3,22,30), and not to others (56), antagonized by naloxone.

In one study, although complete spinal transection blocked such stress-produced analgesia, dorsolateral funiculus lesions did not (57). Again, it seems evident that multiple descending analgesia systems exist, some possessing and some not a serotoninergic and/or opiate link. Much more work is required to sort out the apparently separate anatomy, physiology, and neurochemistry underlying these different forms of pain modulation.

EXCITATION OF THE MEDIAL BRAINSTEM BY OPIATES

Several recent investigations (97,132,133) appear to provide direct evidence that morphine administration and SPA selectively activate those medial brainstem areas (periaqueductal gray and nucleus raphe magnus) that are involved in mediating descending pain inhibition. These studies have employed multiple unit recording techniques in chronically prepared, awake animals and report uniformly large and reliable increases in spontaneous multiple unit activity after SPA (97), or after systemic (97,132) or intraventricular (133) morphine administration. By contrast, other investigations using single neuron recording methods and systemic or iontophoretic injections of opiates have generally reported inhibition of spontaneous firing rates (40,43,55,58). The reasons for this disparity are not known. It may be that multiple and single unit techniques exert different biases in the cell types from which they preferentially record. It is also true that the microelectrode studies have been conducted in the anesthetized or decerebrate animal, whereas the multiple unit studies were conducted in awake, intact preparations. In fact, it has recently been shown (132) that systemic morphine injections decrease multiple unit activity in the periaqueductal gray matter of urethane-anesthetized rats, but increase this same activity in awake animals. More evidence will be necessary to resolve this question, especially microelectrode data in unanesthetized, intact preparations. Until such evidence is forthcoming, the immediate effect of opiate drugs on cells involved in the mediation of pain inhibition cannot be determined. On the other hand, whether opiates directly excite such neurons or, by inhibiting them, release from tonic inhibition other neurons farther along in the modulation path, it seems abundantly clear that an essential excitation occurs somewhere in the descending path which permits pain modulation to be conveyed from the brainstem to the cord.

OPIATE RECEPTORS AND THE ENDORPHINS

One of the most dramatic series of studies in the recent history of neuroscience research has been the discovery of stereospecific opiate binding sites in the central nervous system (104,122,127), and the subsequent discovery and chemical identification of endogenous peptides that are apparently the natural ligands of these opiate receptors (32,52,62,63,121,129,130). As was immediately recognized, these findings are enormously significant in relation to the emerging picture of pain modulation described above. The first endogenous opioids found in the brain and sequenced by Hughes and colleagues (62,63) were the pentapeptides methionine- and leucine-enkephalin. Subsequently, other longer chain peptides were found in brain and pituitary (32,52,130), and the entire class of opiate-like peptides was given the more generic name "endorphins." The relationship between these discoveries and those described in earlier portions of this chapter appears solidified by the following observations:

(a) Opiate binding sites (9,71), as well as cell bodies and/or terminals containing the enkephalins (7,20,35,60,120) and another of the endorphins, β-endorphin (7,20), have been found to be distributed in the brain in close proximity to each other and to medial brainstem sites known to support SPA and morphine analgesia following microinjections.

(b) β-Endorphin and the enkephalins have been shown to induce analgesia following intraventricular injection (16,21,25,48,90,133) or administration directly into the peri-aqueductal gray matter (28,41,67,82,116). Some researchers, however, have reported negative findings with the enkephalins (21,67,77). Although the definitive explanation for this disparity is not known, it seems likely that negative results are related to the fact that the enkephalins (unlike β-endorphin) are enzymatically destroyed extremely rapidly in the brain, and that they will only be effective, therefore, if they are administered with sufficient accuracy, in sufficient quantity, and within a sufficiently compressed time period to allow them to exert a mass action on their appropriate receptor sites.

(c) Akil et al. (7) have reported that, in pilot work, continuous electrical stimulation at SPA sites in the periaqueductal gray of rats altered the amount of enkephalin-like material that could be detected in this region of the brain. Either an increase or decrease in such material could be produced depending on the duration of prior stimulation. These same investigators also found increases in enkephalin-like material in the cerebrospinal fluid (CSF) of chronic pain patients after the delivery of analgesic central stimulation (7).

(d) Several groups have reported that base-line CSF endorphin levels are lower than normal in chronic pain patients (7,119,124,129), and that these levels can be increased by analgesic electrical stimulation at acupuncture points (124). Notably, this increase did not occur in those patients successfully treated for pain localized above the lumbar dermatomes. Since the CSF was withdrawn from a lumbar puncture, these findings were taken to indicate that the endorphin level changes are not a general response to percutaneous electrical stimulation, but rather an effect specifically associated with the region of the nervous system in which the analgesia is being produced (124).

CONCLUDING REMARKS

It is difficult not to be impressed by the close apparent interrelationships among the various recent findings summarized in this review and the resulting homogeneity, almost monolithic quality, of the conceptual image that emerges from considering these data. Indeed, one must conclude that there is now a great deal of evidence suggesting the existence of a natural or endogenous pain inhibitory system having (a) a specialized anatomy involving descending paths from the medial brainstem to the spinal cord dorsal horn and trigeminal complex and (b) a specialized neurochemistry involving endogenous opioid peptides. Yet, reason and historical perspective compel caution. Much of the evidence just described suffers from recency and a consequent lack of sufficient opportunity to be replicated and extended. Simple ideas often become simplistic in the light of new information. We have already seen that multiple paths of modulation exist, some apparently opiate related, some not. Similarly, a causal link between dorsal horn neuronal inhibition and behaviorally defined analgesia is far from established, and a great deal of the circuitry and synaptic neurochemistry of the modulation paths has yet to be disclosed.

Three other major complexities can be briefly noted that will ultimately require integration into the descending endorphinergic pain inhibition story.

First, there is excellent evidence that opiate drugs and endorphins can exert a direct pain inhibitory action on the spinal cord. Opiate binding sites (8,72) and endorphins (60) are found in great density in those exact regions of the dorsal horn where pain inhibition is thought to take place. In fact, it has been reported that a significant proportion of the opiate binding sites in the dorsal horn disappear following dorsal rhizotomy, suggesting a presynaptic locus for such sites and, hence, a presynaptic site of action for opiate drugs (72). It has also been known for some time that nociceptive responding in dorsal horn interneurons is readily blocked by systemically administered opiates in the spinalized preparation (19,69,73,74). Similarly, more recent evidence shows that small quantities of opiates delivered into the subarachnoid space over the lumbar cord can produce analgesia in rats (139). Of even greater interest was the finding that naloxone injected into the same space could antagonize the analgesic action of systemically administered morphine (139). For a thorough and provocative discussion of the implications of these data, the reader is referred to the recent review by Yaksh and Rudy (140).

Second, very little is known about the natural mechanisms that access the supposed endogenous pain inhibitory system. When or by what circumstances is this system called into play? As mentioned above, stress can induce analgesia that, according to some investigations at least, is naloxone reversible (3,22,30). Consistent with these studies, it has been shown that stress causes increased endorphin release in the brain [(81); however, see (113)] and from the pituitary (53,113). Some studies have found that naloxone administered to drug-free experimental animals or human subjects exacerbates pain (24,39,64,70,76), but others have reported no effects (36,46,49). That this disparity may be attributable to intra- or interindividual differences is suggested by several recent investigations. For example, it has been shown that naloxone increases pain reactivity in rats to a greater or lesser degree as a function of a diurnal rhythm (39), presumably indicating that sensitivity to this drug co-varies with endorphin release. Similarly, it has also recently been reported that naloxone blocks placebo analgesia in placebo-responsive human subjects but does not change pain sensitivity in those unresponsive to placebo [(75); however, see (93)]. Whether or not any relationship exists between this observation and the reports of naloxone blocking acupuncture analgesia in man remains to be determined. In yet another demonstration related to this point, it has been reported (27) that pain sensitivity (tail-flick latency) in normal rats predicts the degree to which binding of labeled enkephalin later occurs; that is, the brains of animals who were more sensitive to pain exhibited higher binding of labeled enkephalin, suggesting lower occupation of receptor sites by endogenous ligand. Clearly, much more work of this sort needs to be done to establish the circumstances and pathways that access the endorphin systems of the brain and pituitary. That pain inhibition is the normal, physiological role of such systems can, until then, only be considered an intriguing hypothesis.

Finally, it is firmly established that opiate binding sites (8,9,59,71) and endorphins (7,20,60) are located in brain areas apparently unrelated to pain inhibition. It is generally considered that such sites must be involved in mediating other classic opiate effects, including respiratory, pupillary, and thermoregulatory changes (euphoria and dysphoria), and perhaps the motorial and pathological electrographic signs of opiate abstinence. Some data are available to suggest this is so. For example, it has been shown that rats will self-administer the enkephalins into the lateral ventricle (17), suggesting these peptides may play a role in natural mechanisms of reward. Moreover, other studies have implicated the endorphins in such diverse pathological syndromes as psychosis, epilepsy, and dyskinesia or rigidity (12,20,21,42,67,116,133). It seems evident that endorphins cannot be assigned a role exclusively in antinociception. In fact, there is evidence to suggest that the opiate binding sites mediating different endorphin effects not only are anatomically separate but also differ from each other in their pharmacological properties (34,41,80,83). The development of new pharmacological and histochemical tools will be required to dissect out these no doubt subtle differences.

REFERENCES

1. Adams, J. E. (1976): Naloxone reversal of analgesia produced by brain stimulation in the human. *Pain,* 2:161–166.
2. Akil, H., and Liebeskind, J. C. (1975): Monoaminergic mechanisms of stimulation-produced analgesia. *Brain Res.,* 94:279–296.
3. Akil, H., Madden, J., IV, Patrick, R. L., and Barchas, J. D. (1976): Stress-induced increase in endogenous opiate peptides: Concurrent analgesia and its partial reversal by naloxone. In: *Opiates and Endogenous Opioid Peptides,* edited by H. W. Kosterlitz, pp. 63–70. Elsevier, Amsterdam.
4. Akil, H., and Mayer, D. J. (1972): Antagonism of stimulation-produced analgesia by *p*-CPA, a serotonin synthesis inhibitor. *Brain Res.,* 44:692–697.
5. Akil, H., Mayer, D. J., and Liebeskind, J. C. (1972): Comparaison chez le rat entre l'analgésie induite par stimulation de la substance grise péri-aqueducale et l'analgésie morphinique. *CR Acad. Sci. [D] (Paris),* 274:3603–3605.
6. Akil, H., Mayer, D. J., and Liebeskind, J. C. (1976): Antagonism of stimulation-produced analgesia by naloxone, a narcotic antagonist. *Science,*191:961–962.
7. Akil, H., Watson, S. J., Berger, P. A., and Barchas J. D. (1978): Endorphins, β-LPH, and ACTH: Biochemical, pharmacological, and anatomical studies. In: *The Endorphins,* edited by E. Costa and M. Trabucchi, pp. 125–140. Raven Press, New York.
8. Atweh, S. F., and Kuhar, M. J. (1977): Autoradiographic localization of opiate receptors in rat brain. I. Spinal cord and lower medulla. *Brain Res.,* 124:53–67.
9. Atweh, S. F., and Kuhar, M. J. (1977): Autoradiographic localization of opiate receptors in rat brain. II. The brain stem. *Brain Res.,* 129:1–12.
10. Balagura, S., and Ralph, T. (1973): The analgesic effect of electrical stimulation of the diencephalon and mesencephalon. *Brain Res.,* 60:369–379.
11. Barber, J., and Mayer, D. (1978): Evaluation of the efficacy and neural mechanism of a hypnotic analgesia procedure in experimental and clinical dental pain. *Pain,* 4:41–48.
12. Barchas, J. D., Akil, H., Elliott, G. R., Holman, R. B., and Watson, S. J. (1978): Behavioral neurochemistry: Neuroregulators and behavioral states. *Science,* 200:964–973.
13. Basbaum, A. I., Clanton, C. H., and Fields, H. L. (1978): Three bulbospinal pathways from the rostral medulla of the cat: An autoradiographic study. *J. Comp. Neurol.,* 178:209–224.
14. Basbaum, A. I., Marley, N., O'Keefe, J., and Clanton, C. H. (1977): Reversal of morphine and stimulus-produced analgesia by subtotal spinal cord lesions. *Pain,* 3:43–56.
15. Beall, J. E., Martin, R. F., Applebaum, A. E., and Willis, W. D. (1976): Inhibition of primate spinothalamic tract neurons by stimulation in the region of the nucleus raphe magnus. *Brain Res.,* 114:328–333.
16. Belluzzi, J. D., Grant, N., Garsky, V., Sarantakis, D., Wise, C. D., and Stein, L. (1976): Analgesia induced in vivo by central administration of enkephalin in rat. *Nature,* 260:625–626.

17. Belluzzi, J. D., and Stein, L. (1977): Enkephalin may mediate euphoria and drive-reduction reward. *Nature*, 266:556–558.
18. Bennett, G. J., and Mayer, D. J. (1976): Effects of microinjected narcotic analgesics into the periaqueductal gray (PAG) on the response of rat spinal cord dorsal horn interneurons. *Soc. Neurosci. Abstr.*, II:928.
19. Besson, J. M., Wyon-Maillard, M. C., Benoist, J. M., Conseiller, C., and Hamann, K. F. (1973): Effects of phenoperidine on lamina V cells in the cat dorsal horn. *J. Pharmacol. Exp. Ther.*, 187:239–245.
20. Bloom, F. E., Rossier, J., Battenberg, E. L. F., Bayon, A., French, E., Henriksen, S. J., Siggins, G. R., Segal, D., Browne, R., Ling, N., and Guillemin, R. (1978): β-Endorphin: Cellular localization, electrophysiological and behavioral effects. In: *The Endorphins,* edited by E. Costa and M. Trabucchi, pp. 89–109. Raven Press, New York.
21. Bloom, F., Segal, D., Ling, N., and Guillemin, R. (1976): Endorphins: Profound behavioral effects in rats suggest new etiological factors in mental illness. *Science,* 194:630–632.
22. Bodnar, R. J., Kelly, D. D., Spiaggia, A., Ehrenberg, C., and Glusman, M. (1978): Dose-dependent reductions by naloxone of analgesia induced by cold-water stress. *Pharmacol. Biochem. Behav.,* 8:667–672.
23. Boëthius, J., Lindblom, U., Meyerson, B. A., and Widen, L. (1976): Effects of multifocal brain stimulation on pain and somatosensory functions. In: *Sensory Functions of the Skin in Primates,* edited by Y. Zotterman, pp. 531–548. Pergamon Press, Oxford.
24. Buchsbaum, M. E., Davis, G. C., and Bunney, W. E., Jr. (1977): Naloxone alters pain perception and somatosensory evoked potentials in normal subjects. *Nature,* 270:620–622.
25. Büscher, H. H., Hill, R. C., Römer, D., Cardinaux, F., Closse, A., Hauser, D., and Pless, J. (1976): Evidence for analgesic activity of enkephalin in the mouse. *Nature,* 261:423–425.
26. Cannon, J. T., Liebeskind, J. C., and Frenk, H. (1978): Neural and neurochemical mechanisms of pain inhibition. In: *The Psychology of Pain,* edited by R. A. Sternbach, pp. 27–47. Raven Press, New York.
27. Chance, W. T., White, A. C., Krynock, G. M., and Rosecrans, J. A. (1978): Conditional fear-induced antinociception and decreased binding of [^{3}H] N-Leu-enkephalin to the rat brain. *Brain Res.,* 141:371–374.
28. Chang, J. K., Fong, B. T. W., Pert, A., and Pert, C. B. (1976): Opiate receptor affinities and behavioral effects of enkephalin: Structure-activity relationship of ten synthetic peptide analogues. *Life Sci,* 18:1473–1482.
29. Chapman, C. R., and Benedetti, C. (1977): Analgesia following transcutaneous electrical stimulation and its partial reversal by a narcotic antagonist. *Life Sci.,* 21:1645–1648.
30. Chesher, G. B., and Chan, B. (1977): Footshock induced analgesia in mice: Its reversal by naloxone and cross-tolerance with morphine. *Life Sci.,* 21:1569–1574.
31. Cicero, T. J., Meyer, E. R., and Smithloff, B. R. (1974): Alpha-adrenergic blocking agents: Antinociceptive activity and enhancement of morphine-induced analgesia. *J. Pharmacol. Exp. Ther.,* 189:72–82.
32. Cox, B. M., Goldstein, A., and Li, C. H. (1976): Opioid activity of a peptide, β-lipotropin-(61–91), derived from β-lipotropin. *Proc. Natl. Acad. Sci. USA,* 73:1821–1823.
33. Criswell, H. E. (1976): Analgesia and hyperreactivity following morphine microinjection into mouse brain. *Pharmacol. Biochem. Behav.,* 4:23–26.
34. Della Bella, D., Casacci, F., and Sassi, A. (1978): Opiate receptors: Different ligand affinity in various brain regions. In: *The Endorphins,* edited by E. Costa and M. Trabucchi, pp. 271–277. Raven Press, New York.
35. Elde, R., Hökfelt, T., Johansson, O., and Terenius, L. (1976): Immunohistochemical studies using antibodies to leucine-enkephalin: Initial observations on the nervous system of the rat. *Neuroscience,* 1:349–351.
36. El-Sobky, A., Dostrovsky, J. O., and Wall, P. D. (1976): Lack of effect of naloxone on pain perception in humans. *Nature,* 263:783–784.
37. Fields, H. L., and Basbaum, A. I. (1978): Brainstem control of spinal pain-transmission neurons. *Annu. Rev. Physiol.,* 40:217–248.
38. Fields, H. L., Basbaum, A. I., Clanton, C. H., and Anderson, S. D. (1977): Nucleus raphe magnus inhibition of spinal cord dorsal horn neurons. *Brain Res.,* 126:441–453.
39. Frederickson, R. C. A., Burgis, V., and Edwards, J. D. (1977): Hyperalgesia induced by naloxone follows diurnal rhythm in responsivity to painful stimuli. *Science,* 198:756–758.

40. Frederickson, R. C. A., and Norris, F. H. (1976): Enkephalin-induced depression of single neurons in brain areas with opiate receptors—antagonism by naloxone. *Science,* 194:440–442.
41. Frenk, H., McCarty, B. C., and Liebeskind, J. C. (1978): Different brain areas mediate the analgesic and epileptic properties of enkephalin. *Science,* 200:335–337.
42. Frenk, H., Urca, G., and Liebeskind, J. C. (1978): Epileptic properties of leucine- and methionine-enkephalin: Comparison with morphine and reversibility by naloxone. *Brain Res.,* 147:327–337.
43. Gent, J. P., and Wolstencroft, J. H. (1976): Actions of morphine, enkephalin and endorphin on single neurons in the brain stem, including the raphe and periaqueductal gray, of the cat. In: *Opiates and Endogenous Opioid Peptides,* edited by H. W. Kosterlitz, pp. 217–224. Elsevier, Amsterdam.
44. Giesler, G. J., Jr., and Liebeskind, J. C. (1976): Inhibition of visceral pain by electrical stimulation of the periaqueductal gray matter. *Pain,* 2:43–48.
45. Goldstein, A., and Hilgard, E. R. (1975): Failure of the opiate antagonist naloxone to modify hypnotic analgesia. *Proc. Natl. Acad. Sci. USA,* 72:2041–2043.
46. Goldstein, A., Pryor, G. T., Otis, L., and Larsen, F. (1976): On the role of endogenous opioid peptides: Failure of naloxone to influence shock escape threshold in the rat. *Life Sci.,* 18:599–604.
47. Goodman, S. J., and Holcombe, V. (1976): Selective and prolonged analgesia in monkey resulting from brain stimulation. In: *Advances in Pain Research and Therapy, Vol. 1: Proceedings of the First World Congress on Pain,* edited by J. J. Bonica and D. Albe-Fessard, pp. 495–502. Raven Press, New York.
48. Graf, L., Szekely, J. I., Ronai, A. Z., Dunai-Kovacs, Z., and Bajusz, S. (1976): Comparative study on analgesic effect of Met^5-enkephalin and related lipotropin fragments. *Nature,* 263:240–242.
49. Grevert, P., and Goldstein, A. (1978): Endorphins: Naloxone fails to alter experimental pain or mood in humans. *Science,* 199:1093–1095.
50. Grumbach, L. (1966): The prediction of analgesic activity in man by animal testing. In: *Pain,* edited by R. S. Knighton and P. R. Dumke, pp. 163–182. Little, Brown, Boston.
51. Guilbaud, G., Besson, J. M., Oliveras, J. L., and Liebeskind, J. C. (1973): Suppression by LSD of the inhibitory effect exerted by dorsal raphe stimulation on certain spinal cord interneurons in the cat. *Brain Res.,* 61:417–422.
52. Guillemin, R., Ling, N., and Burgus, R. (1976): Endorphines, peptides d'origine hypothalamique et neurohypophysaire à activité morphinomimétique. Isolement et structure moléculaire de l'alpha-endorphine. *CR Acad. Sci. [D] (Paris),* 282:783–785.
53. Guillemin, R., Vargo, T., Rossier, J., Minick, S., Ling, N., Rivier, C., Vale, W., and Bloom, F. (1977): β-Endorphin and adrenocorticotropin are secreted concomitantly by the pituitary gland. *Science,* 197:1367–1369.
54. Gybels, J., and Cosyns, P. (1978): Modulation of clinical and experimental pain in man by electrical stimulation of thalamic periventricular gray. In: *Sensory Functions of the Skin in Primates,* edited by Y. Zotterman, pp. 521–530. Pergamon Press, Oxford.
55. Haigler, H. J. (1976): Morphine: Ability to block neuronal activity evoked by a nociceptive stimulus. *Life Sci.,* 19:841–858.
56. Hayes, R. L., Bennett, G. J., Newlon, P. G., and Mayer, D. J. (1978): Behavioral and physiological studies of non-narcotic analgesia in the rat elicited by certain environmental stimuli. *Brain Res.,* 155:69–90.
57. Hayes, R. L., Price, D. D., Bennett, G. J., Wilcox, G. L., and Mayer, D. J. (1978): Differential effects of spinal cord lesions on narcotic and non-narcotic suppression of nociceptive reflexes: Further evidence for the physiologic multiplicity of pain modulation, *Brain Res.,* 155:91–102.
58. Henry, J. L. (1976): Microiontophoresis of morphine and meperidine in the brain stem of the cat. In: *Advances in Pain Research and Therapy, Vol. 1: Proceedings of the First World Congress on Pain,* edited by J. J. Bonica and D. Albe-Fessard, pp. 615–620. Raven Press, New York.
59. Hiller, J., Pearson, J., and Simon, E. J. (1973): Distribution of stereospecific binding of the potent narcotic analgesic etorphine in the human brain: Predominance in the limbic system. *Res. Commun. Chem. Pathol. Pharmacol.,* 6:1052–1062.
60. Hökfelt, T., Ljungdahl, A., Terenius, L., Elde, R., and Nilsson, G. (1977): Immunohistochemi-

cal analysis of peptide pathways possibly related to pain and analgesia: Enkephalin and substance P. *Proc. Natl. Acad. Sci. USA,* 74:3081–3085.
61. Hosobuchi, Y., Adams, J. E., and Linchitz, R. (1977): Pain relief by electrical stimulation of the central gray matter in humans and its reversal by naloxone. *Science,* 197:183–185.
62. Hughes, J. (1975): Isolation of an endogenous compound from the brain with pharmacological properties similar to morphine. *Brain Res.,* 88:295–308.
63. Hughes, J., Smith, T. W., Kosterlitz, H. W., Fothergill, L. A., Morgan, B. A., and Morris, H. R. (1975): Identification of two related pentapeptides from the brain with potent opiate agonist activity. *Nature,* 258:577–579.
64. Jacob, J. J., Tremblay, E. C., and Columbel, M. (1974): Facilitation de réactions nociceptives par la naloxone chez la souris et chez le rat. *Psychopharmacologia (Berl.),* 37:217–223.
65. Jacquet, Y. F., and Lajtha, A. (1973): Morphine action at central nervous system sites in rat: Analgesia or hyperalgesia depending on site and dose. *Science,* 182:490–492.
66. Jacquet, Y. F., and Lajtha, A. (1976): The periaqueductal gray: Site of morphine analgesia and tolerance as shown by 2-way cross-tolerance between systemic and intracerebral injections. *Brain Res.,* 103:501–513.
67. Jacquet, Y. F., and Marks, N. (1976): The C-fragment of β-lipotropin: An endogenous neuroleptic or antipsychotogen? *Science,* 194:632–635.
68. Kerr, F. W. L., and Wilson, P. R. (1978): Pain. *Annu. Rev. Neurosci.,* 1:83–102.
69. Kitahata, L. M., Kosaka, Y., Taub, A., Bonikos, K., and Hoffert, M. (1974): Lamina-specific suppression of dorsal-horn unit activity by morphine sulfate. *Anesthesiology,* 41:39–48.
70. Kokka, N., and Fairhurst, A. S. (1977): Naloxone enhancement of acetic acid-induced writhing in rats. *Life Sci.,* 21:975–980.
71. Kuhar, M. S., Pert, C. B., and Snyder, S. H. (1973): Regional distribution of opiate receptor binding in monkey and human brain. *Nature,* 245:447–450.
72. LaMotte, C., Pert, C. B., and Snyder, S. H. (1976): Opiate receptor binding in primate spinal cord: Distribution and changes after dorsal root section. *Brain Res.,* 112:407–412.
73. LeBars, D., Menétrey, D., and Besson, J. M. (1976): Effects of morphine upon the lamina V type cells activities in the dorsal horn of the decerebrate cat. *Brain Res.,* 113:293–310.
74. LeBars, D., Menétrey, D., Conseiller, C., and Besson, J. M. (1975): Depressive effects of morphine upon lamina V cell activities in the dorsal horn of the spinal cat. *Brain Res.,* 98:261–277.
75. Levine, J. D., Gordon, N. C., and Fields, H. L. (1978): Evidence that the analgesic effect of placebo is mediated by endorphins. *Pain Abstr.,* 1:18.
76. Levine, J. D., Gordon, N. C., Jones, R. T., and Fields, H. L. (1978): The narcotic antagonist naloxone enhances clinical pain. *Nature,* 272:826–827.
77. Leybin, L., Pinsky, C., LaBella, F. S., Havlicek, V., and Rezek, M. (1976): Intraventricular Met⁵-enkephalin causes unexpected lowering of pain threshold and narcotic withdrawal signs in rats. *Nature,* 264:458–459.
78. Liebeskind, J. C., Mayer, D. J., and Akil, H. (1974): Central mechanisms of pain inhibition: Studies of analgesia from focal brain stimulation. In: *Advances in Neurology, Vol. 4: Proceedings of the International Symposium on Pain,* edited by J. J. Bonica, pp. 261–268. Raven Press, New York.
79. Liebeskind, J. C., and Paul, L. A. (1977): Psychological and physiological mechanisms of pain. *Annu. Rev. Psychol.,* 28:41–60.
80. Lord, J. A. H., Waterfield, A. A., Hughes, J., and Kosterlitz. H. W. (1977): Endogenous opioid peptides: Multiple agonists and receptors. *Nature,* 267:495–499.
81. Madden, J., IV, Akil, H., Patrick, R. L., and Barchas, J. D. (1976): Stress-included parallel changes in central opioid levels and pain responsiveness in the rat. *Nature,* 265:358–360.
82. Malick, J. B., and Goldstein, J. M. (1977): Analgesic activity of enkephalins following intracerebral administration in the rat. *Life Sci.,* 20:827–832.
83. Martin, W. R., Eades, C. G., Thompson, J. A., Huppler, R. E., and Gilbert, P. E. (1976): The effects of morphine and nalorphine-like drugs in the nondependent and morphine dependent chronic spinal dog. *J. Pharmacol. Exp. Ther.,* 197:517–532.
84. Mayer, D. J., and Hayes, R. (1975): Stimulation-produced analgesia: Development of tolerance and cross-tolerance to morphine. *Science,* 188:941–943.
85. Mayer, D. J., and Liebeskind, J. C. (1974): Pain reduction by focal electrical stimulation of the brain: An anatomical and behavioral analysis. *Brain Res.,* 68:73–93.

86. Mayer, D. J., and Murphin, R. (1976): Stimulation-produced analgesia (SPA) and morphine analgesia (MA): Cross-tolerance from application at the same brain site. *Fed. Proc.,* 35:385.
87. Mayer, D. J., and Price, D. D. (1976): Central nervous system mechanisms of analgesia. *Pain,* 2:379–404.
88. Mayer, D. J., Price, D. D., Rafii, A., and Barber, J. (1976): Acupuncture hypalgesia: Evidence for activation of a central control system as a mechanism of action. In: *Advances in Pain Research and Therapy, Vol. 1: Proceedings of the First World Congress on Pain,* edited by J. J. Bonica and D. Albe-Fessard, pp. 751–754. Raven Press, New York.
89. Mayer, D. J., Wolfle, T. L., Akil, H., Carder, B., and Liebeskind, J. C. (1971): Analgesia from electrical stimulation in the brainstem of the rat. *Science,* 174:1351–1354.
90. Meglio, M., Hosobuchi, Y., Loh, H. H., Adams, J. E., and Li, C. H. (1977): β-endorphin: Behavioral and analgesic activity in cats. *Proc. Natl. Acad. Sci. USA,* 74:774–776.
91. Melzack, R., and Melinkoff, D. F. (1974): Analgesia produced by brain stimulation: Evidence of a prolonged onset period. *Exp. Neurol.,* 43:369–374.
92. Messing, R. B., and Lytle, L. D. (1978): Serotonin-containing neurons: Their possible role in pain and analgesia. *Pain,* 4:1–21.
93. Mihic, D., and Binkert, E. (1978): Is placebo analgesia mediated by endorphin? *Pain Abstr.,* 1:19.
94. Morrow, T. J., and Casey, K. L. (1976): Analgesia produced by mesencephalic stimulation: Effect on bulboreticular neurons. In: *Advances in Pain Research and Therapy, Vol. 1: Proceedings of the First World Congress on Pain,* edited by J. J. Bonica and D. Albe-Fessard, pp. 503–510. Raven Press, New York.
95. Murfin, R., Bennett, G. J., and Mayer, D. J. (1976): The effect of dorsolateral spinal cord (DLF) lesions on analgesia from morphine microinjected into the periaqueductal gray matter (PAG) of the rat. *Soc. Neurosci. Abstr.,* II:946.
96. Oleson, T. D., and Liebeskind, J. C. (1976): Modification of midbrain and thalamic evoked responses by analgesic brain stimulation in the rat. In: *Advances in Pain Research and Therapy, Vol. 1: Proceedings of the First World Congress on Pain,* edited by J. J. Bonica and D. Albe-Fessard, pp. 487–494. Raven Press, New York.
97. Oleson, T. D., Twombly, D. A., and Liebeskind, J. C. (1978): Effects of pain attenuating brain stimulation and morphine on electrical activity in the raphe nuclei of the awake rat. *Pain,* 4:211–230.
98. Oliveras, J. L., Besson, J. M., Guilbaud, G., and Liebeskind, J. C. (1974): Behavioral and electrophysiological evidence of pain inhibition from midbrain stimulation in the cat. *Exp. Brain Res.,* 20:32–44.
99. Oliveras, J. L., Hosobuchi, Y., Redjemi, F., Guilbaud, G., and Besson, J. M. (1977): Opiate antagonist, naloxone, strongly reduces analgesia induced by stimulation of a raphe nucleus (centralis inferior). *Brain Res.,* 120:221–229.
100. Oliveras, J. L., Redjemi, F., Guilbaud, G., and Besson, J. M. (1975): Analgesia induced by electrical stimulation of the inferior centralis nucleus of the raphe in the cat. *Pain,* 1:139–145.
101. Oliveras, J. L., Woda, A., Guilbaud, G., and Besson, J. M. (1974): Inhibition of the jaw opening reflex by electrical stimulation of the periaqueductal gray matter in the awake, unrestrained cat. *Brain Res.,* 72:328–331.
102. Pert, A., and Walter, M. (1976): Comparison between naloxone reversal of morphine and electrical stimulation induced analgesia in the rat mesencephalon. *Life Sci.,* 19:1023–1032.
103. Pert, A., and Yaksh, T. (1974): Sites of morphine induced analgesia in the primate brain: Relation to pain pathways. *Brain Res.,* 80:135–140.
104. Pert, C. B., and Snyder, S. H. (1973): Opiate receptor: Demonstration in nervous tissue. *Science,* 179:1011–1014.
105. Pomeranz, B. (1978): Do endorphins mediate acupuncture analgesia? In: *The Endorphins,* edited by E. Costa and M. Trabucchi, pp. 351–360. Raven Press, New York.
106. Pomeranz, B., and Chiu, D. (1976): Naloxone blockade of acupuncture analgesia: Endorphin implicated. *Life Sci.,* 19:1757–1762.
107. Price, M. T. C., Fibiger, H. C. (1975): Ascending catecholamine systems and morphine analgesia. *Brain Res.,* 99:189–193.
108. Proudfit, H. K., and Anderson, E. G. (1975): Morphine analgesia: Blockade by raphe magnus lesions. *Brain Res.,* 98:612–618.

109. Reynolds, D. V. (1969): Surgery in the rat during electrical analgesia induced by focal brain stimulation. *Science,* 164:444–445.
110. Rhodes, D. L., and Liebeskind, J. C. (1978): Analgesia from rostral brain stem stimulation in the rat. *Brain Res.,* 143:521–532.
111. Richardson, D. E., and Akil, H. (1977): Pain reduction by electrical brain stimulation in man. I. Acute administration in periaqueductal and periventricular sites. *J. Neurosurg.,* 47:178–183.
112. Richardson, D. E., and Akil, H. (1977): Pain reduction by electrical brain stimulation in man. II. Chronic self-administration in the periventricular gray matter. *J. Neurosurg.,* 47:184–194.
113. Rossier, J., French, E. D., Rivier, C., Ling, N., Guillemin, R., and Bloom, F. E. (1977): Foot-shock induced stress increases β-endorphin levels in blood but not brain. *Nature,* 270:618–620.
114. Ruda, M. (1975): *Autoradiographic Study of the Efferent Projections of the Midbrain Central Gray of the Cat.* Ph.D. Dissertation, University of Pennyslvania, Philadelphia.
115. Saarnivaara, L. (1969): Effect of 5-hydroxytryptamine on morphine analgesia in rabbits. *Ann. Med. Exp. Biol. Fenn.,* 47:113–123.
116. Segal, D. S., Browne, R. G., Bloom, F., Ling, N., and Guillemin, R. (1977): β-Endorphin: Endogenous opiate or neuroleptic? *Science,* 198:411–414.
117. Sessle, B. J., Dubner, R., Greenwood, L. F., and Lucier, G. E. (1975): Descending influences of periaqueductal gray matter and somatosensory cerebral cortex on neurones in trigeminal brain stem nuclei. *Can. J. Physiol. Pharmacol.,* 54:66–69.
118. Sharpe, L. G., Garnett, J. E., and Cicero, T. J. (1974): Analgesia and hyperreactivity produced by intracranial microinjections of morphine into the periaqueductal gray matter of the rat. *Behav. Biol.,* 11:303–314.
119. Sicuteri, F., Anselmi, B., Curradi, C., Michelacci, S., and Sassi, A. (1978): Morphine-like factors in CSF of headache patients. In: *The Endorphins,* edited by E. Costa and M. Trabucchi, pp. 363–366. Raven Press, New York.
120. Simantov, R., Kuhar, M. J., Uhl, G. R., and Snyder, S. H. (1977): Opioid peptide enkephalin: Immunohistochemical mapping in rat central nervous system. *Proc. Natl. Acad. Sci. USA,* 74:2167–2171.
121. Simantov, R., and Snyder, S. H. (1976): Isolation and structure identification of a morphine-like peptide "enkephalin" in bovine brain. *Life Sci.,* 18:781–787.
122. Simon, E. J., Hiller, J. M., and Edelman, I. (1973): Stereospecific binding of the potent narcotic analgesic [^{3}H] etorphine to rat brain homogenate. *Proc. Natl. Acad. Sci. USA,* 70:1947–1949.
123. Sjölund, B., and Eriksson, M. (1976): Electro-acupuncture and endogenous morphine. *Lancet,* 2:1085.
124. Sjölund, B., Terenius, L., and Eriksson, M. (1977): Increased cerebrospinal fluid levels of endorphins after electro-acupuncture. *Acta Physiol. Scand.,* 100:382–384.
125. Soper, W. Y. (1976): Effects of analgesic midbrain stimulation on reflex withdrawal and thermal escape in the rat. *J. Comp. Physiol. Psychol.,* 90:91–101.
126. Tenen, S. S. (1968): Antagonism of the analgesic effect of morphine and other drugs by *p*-chlorophenylalanine, a serotonin depletor. *Psychopharmacologia (Berl.),* 12:278–285.
127. Terenius, L. (1972): Specific uptake of narcotic analgesics by subcellular fractions of the guinea-pig ileum. *Acta Pharmacol.,* 31:(Suppl. I):50.
128. Terenius, L. (1978): Endogenous peptides and analgesia. *Annu. Rev. Pharmacol. Toxicol.,* 18:189–204.
129. Terenius, L., and Wahlström, A. (1975): Morphine-like ligand for opiate receptors in human CSF. *Life Sci.,* 16:1759–1764.
130. Teschemacher, H., Opheim, K. E., Cox, B. M., and Goldstein, A. (1975): A peptide-like substance from pituitary that acts like morphine. I. Isolation. *Life Sci.,* 16:1771–1776.
131. Tsou, K., and Jang, C. S. (1964): Studies on the site of analgesic action of morphine by intracerebral micro-injection. *Sci. Sin.,* 13:1099–1109.
132. Urca, G. (1978): *Electrophysiological Correlates of Opiate Action in the Central Nervous System of the Rat.* Ph.D. Dissertation, University of California, Los Angeles.
133. Urca, G., Frenk, H., Liebeskind, J. C., and Taylor, A. N. (1977): Morphine and enkephalin: Analgesic and epileptic properties. *Science,* 197:83–86.
134. Vogt, M. (1974): The effect of lowering the 5-hydroxytryptamine content of the rat spinal cord on analgesia produced by morphine. *J. Physiol. (Lond.),* 236:483–498.

135. Willis, W. D., Haber, L. H., and Martin, R. F. (1977): Inhibition of spinothalamic tract cells and interneurons by brain stem stimulation in the monkey. *J. Neurophysiol.,* 40:968–981.
136. Woolf, C. J., Barrett, G. D., Mitchell, D., and Myers, R. A. (1977): Naloxone-reversible peripheral electroanalgesia in intact and spinal rats. *Eur. J. Pharmacol.,* 45:311–314.
137. Yaksh, T. L., DuChateau, J. C., and Rudy, T. A. (1976): Antagonism by methysergide and cinanserin of the antinociceptive action of morphine administered into the periaqueductal gray. *Brain Res.,* 104:367–372.
138. Yaksh, T. L., Plant, R., and Rudy, T. A. (1976): Incomplete blockade by raphe lesions of the antinociceptive actions of systemic morphine. *Eur. J. Pharmacol.,* 41:399–408.
139. Yaksh, T. L., and Rudy, T. A. (1977): Studies on the direct spinal action of narcotics in the production of analgesia in the rat. *J. Pharmacol. Exp. Ther.,* 202:411–428.
140. Yaksh, T. L., and Rudy, T. A. (1978): Narcotic analgesics: CNS sites and mechanisms of action as revealed by intracerebral injection techniques. *Pain,* 4:299–359.
141. Yaksh, T. L., Yeung, J. C., and Rudy, T. A. (1976): Systematic examination in the rat of brain sites sensitive to the direct application of morphine: Observation of differential effects within the periaqueductal gray. *Brain Res.,* 114:83–103.
142. Yaksh, T. L., Yeung, J. C., and Rudy, T. A. (1976): An inability to antagonize with naloxone the elevated thresholds resulting from electrical stimulation of the mesencephalic central gray. *Life Sci.,* 18:1193–1198.
143. Yeung, J. C., Yaksh, T. L., and Rudy, T. A. (1977): Concurrent mapping of brain sites for sensitivity to the direct application of morphine and focal electrical stimulation in the production of antinociception in the rat. *Pain,* 4:23–40.

Mechanisms of Pain and Analgesic Compounds,
edited by R. F. Beers, Jr., and E. G. Bassett.
Raven Press, New York © 1979.

15. Pain Mechanisms: Theoretical Approaches

Ronald Melzack and Stephen G. Dennis

Department of Psychology, McGill University, Montreal, Quebec, Canada

INTRODUCTION

The traditional specificity theory of pain, which is still widely taught in most medical schools, proposes that pain is a specific sensation and is subserved by a straight-through transmission system from somatic pain receptors to a pain center in the brain. The natural outcome of this concept of pain has been the development of neurosurgical techniques to cut the so-called pain pathway. When failures occur, they are attributed to an escape of "pain fibers," so that operations are carried out at successively higher levels of the nervous system. Generally, the results have been disappointing, particularly for low back pain, the neuralgias, and the myofascial pain syndromes. Not only does the pain tend to return in a substantial proportion of patients, but new pains may be "unmasked" and other iatrogenic complications, such as dysesthesias, "girdle pains," and various sensory–motor losses, may occur (17).

THE GATE CONTROL THEORY OF PAIN

During the past decade, the Gate Control Theory (16) has opened the way for a search for techniques to modulate the sensory input. The theory suggests that pain control may be achieved by the enhancement of normal physiological activities rather than their disruption by destructive, irreversible lesions. In particular, it has led to attempts to control pain by activation of inhibitory mechanisms.

Basically, the Gate Control Theory proposes that neural mechanisms in the dorsal horns of the spinal cord act like a gate that can increase or decrease the flow of nerve impulses from peripheral fibers to the central nervous system. Somatic input, therefore, is subjected to the modulating influence of the gate *before* it evokes pain perception and response. Melzack and Wall (16) proposed that large-fiber inputs tend to close the gate whereas small-fiber inputs generally open it, and that the gate is also profoundly influenced by descending inhibition from the brain. (These gating effects are assumed to be mediated by the substantia gelatinosa in the dorsal horns.) They further suggested that the sensory input is modulated at successive synapses from the spinal cord to the neural areas responsible for pain experience and response. Pain, they proposed, occurs when the number of nerve impulses that arrive at these areas exceeds a critical level.

Wall (24) has recently assessed the present-day status of the Gate Control Theory in light of new physiological research. It is apparent that the theory is alive and well despite considerable controversy and conflicting evidence. Although some of the physiological details may need revision, the concept of gating (or input modulation) is stronger than ever.

In an extension of the Gate Control Theory (Fig. 1), Melzack and Casey (12) have noted that the output of the dorsal horns is projected to the brain along three major ascending systems that contribute to the quality and pattern of pain experience and response. First, there is evidence (5,12) that several rapidly conducting pathways that project to the somatosensory thalamus and cortex contribute to the sensory–discriminative dimension of pain. In addition, the slowly conducting pathways, which project to the medial reticular areas of the brainstem and to the limbic system, are assumed to contribute to the motivational–affective dimension of pain. Finally, the most rapidly conducting systems are proposed (12,16) to comprise a "central control trigger" that activates neocortical or "higher central nervous system" processes, such as evaluation of the input in terms of past experience, which exert control over activity in both the discriminative and motivational systems. It is assumed that these three categories of activity interact with one another to provide perceptual information regarding the location, magnitude, and spatiotemporal properties of the noxious stimulus, motivational tendency toward escape or attack, and cognitive informa-

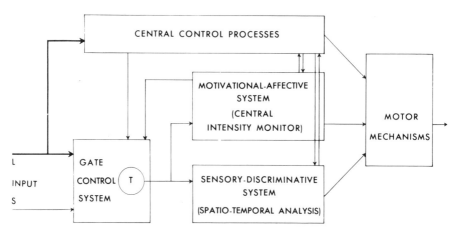

FIG. 1. Conceptual model of the sensory, motivational, and central control determinants of pain. The output of the transmission (T) cells of the gate control system projects to the sensory–discriminative system and the motivational–affective system. The central control trigger is represented by a line running from the large-fiber system to central control processes; these, in turn, project back to the gate control system and to the sensory–discriminative and motivational–affective systems. All three systems interact with one another and project to the motor system. (From Melzack and Casey, ref. 12.)

tion based on analysis of multimodal information, past experience, and probability of outcome of different response strategies. All three forms of activity, then, could influence motor mechanisms responsible for the complex patterns of overt responses that characterize pain.

Within the framework of the model, the word "pain" refers to a category of complex experiences, not to a kind of stimulation. Clearly, there are many varieties and qualities of experience that are simply categorized under the broad heading of pain because they defy more subtle verbal description. There are the pains of a stomach ulcer and a sprained ankle; there are headaches and toothaches. The pain of a coronary occlusion is uniquely different from the pain of a scalded hand. Pain is not a single, specific experience but a category of experiences, signifying a multitude of different, unique events having different causes and characterized by different qualities varying along sensory and affective dimensions (15).

TRANSCUTANEOUS ELECTRICAL NERVE STIMULATION

One of the major results of the Gate Control Theory was the discovery by Wall and Sweet (25) that selective activation of large fibers in peripheral nerves by direct or transcutaneous electrical stimulation produces striking relief of several forms of chronic pain associated with nerve lesions. After publication of that paper, many studies (8) have demonstrated the effectiveness of transcutaneous electrical nerve stimulation for a variety of pain states, including low back pain, pain related to reflex sympathetic dystrophy, and myofascial pains. The procedure, generally, is to allow the patient to wear the stimulating device so that electrical stimulation can be applied at low levels for long periods of time. The pain is rarely abolished but is often diminished to bearable levels so that patients who were previously immobilized are now able to work and lead more normal lives. To be sure, not all patients are helped, and some forms of chronic pain are relieved more than others; furthermore, some patients who are helped at first report decreasing effectiveness after several months. Nevertheless, the procedure is sufficiently effective and simple that it has become a major form of treatment of chronic pain.

The rationale underlying the procedure is the selective activation of large fibers to "close the gate" at spinal or higher levels. However, there is another way to inhibit pain signals. Major advances in neurophysiology during the past 10 years have shown that the descending control over the gate is extremely powerful. It is now known that areas in the brainstem exert a tonic descending inhibitory control over transmission through the dorsal horns (18). These areas are activated preferentially by small-fiber inputs usually produced by intense stimulation. It is apparent, then, that intense stimulation is potentially capable of inhibiting pain signals and may represent an important clinical approach to the modulation of pain (10).

HYPERSTIMULATION ANALGESIA

It is well known in Western medical practice that brief, intense stimulation of trigger points by dry needling (23), intense cold (23), or injection of normal saline (22) often produces prolonged relief of some forms of myofascial or visceral pain. This type of pain relief, which may be generally labeled as *hyperstimulation analgesia,* is one of the oldest methods used for the control of pain. It is sometimes known as "counter-irritation," and includes such methods of folk medicine as application of mustard plasters, ice packs, hot cups, or blistering agents to parts of the body. Some of these methods are still frequently used although there has not been (until recently) any theoretical or physiological explanation for their effectiveness. Suggestion and distraction of attention are the usual mechanisms invoked, but neither seems capable of explaining the power of the methods or the long duration of the relief they may afford.

This interest in folk medicine gained enormous impetus in recent years by the rediscovery of the ancient Chinese practice of acupuncture—inserting needles into specific body sites and twirling them manually. More recently, the Chinese have practiced electroacupuncture, in which electrical pulses are passed through the needles (19). We now know that the original claims that acupuncture can produce surgical analgesia (or anesthesia) have not been borne out by later investigation. However, acupuncture stimulation has recently been shown in several well-controlled clinical and experimental investigations (4) to provide substantial relief of pain. This is not surprising because it is now evident that there is nothing mysterious or magical about acupuncture; it is a form of *hyperstimulation analgesia* comparable to cupping or blistering the skin.

On the basis of these considerations, Melzack (11) developed the hypothesis that transcutaneous electrical stimulation could be administered the same way as acupuncture—for brief periods of time at moderate-to-high stimulation intensities. Consequently, he and his colleagues carried out three studies to determine whether acupuncture and transcutaneous electrical stimulation are comparable procedures.

The first study (11) examined the effects of brief, intense transcutaneous electrical stimulation at trigger points or acupuncture points on severe clinical pain. The data indicated that the procedure provides a powerful method for the control of several forms of pathological pain. The duration of relief frequently outlasted the 20-min period of stimulation by several hours, occasionally for days or weeks. Different patterns of the amount and duration of pain relief were observed. Daily stimulation carried out at home by the patient sometimes provided gradually increasing relief over periods of weeks or months.

The second study (6) compared the relative effectiveness of transcutaneous stimulation and acupuncture on low back pain. The results showed that both forms of stimulation at the same points produce substantial decreases in pain intensity but neither procedure is statistically more effective than the other. Most patients were relieved of pain for several hours, and some for one or more days. Statistical analysis also failed to reveal any differences in the duration of pain relief between the two procedures.

The third study (14) examined the correlation between trigger points and acupuncture points for pain. The results of the analysis showed that every trigger point reported in the Western medical literature has a corresponding acupuncture point. Furthermore, there is a close correspondence (71%) between the pain syndromes associated with the two kinds of points. This close correlation suggests that trigger points and acupuncture points for pain, although discovered independently and labeled differently, represent the same phenomenon and can be explained in terms of the same underlying neural mechanisms.

The relative advantages of transcutaneous electrical stimulation and acupuncture merit consideration. The chief advantage of acupuncture is that the procedure is of short duration—at intense levels, stimulation may sometimes last only a few minutes. The method, however, is invasive and requires licensed practitioners with specialized training. Transcutaneous electrical stimulation, on the other hand, is noninvasive, and once the appropriate points are located, it can be administered by paramedical personnel. Furthermore, once the procedure is found to be effective for a given patient, it can be self-administered by the patient with supervision by the physician.

CONCEPT OF A CENTRAL BIASING MECHANISM

There are three major properties of hyperstimulation analgesia:

(a) A moderate-to-intense sensory input is applied to the body to alleviate pain.
(b) The sensory input is sometimes applied to a site distant from the site of pain.
(c) The sensory input, which is usually of brief duration (ranging from a few seconds to 20 or 30 min) may relieve chronic pain for days, weeks, and sometimes permanently.

The relief of pain by brief, intense stimulation of distant trigger points (or acupuncture points) can be explained in terms of the Gate Control Theory. The most plausible explanation (10) seems to be that the brainstem areas which are known to exert a powerful inhibitory control over transmission in the pain signaling system may be involved. These areas, which may be considered to be a "central biasing mechanism" (10), receive inputs from widespread parts of the body and, in turn, project to widespread parts of the spinal cord and brain (Fig. 2). The stimulation of particular nerves or tissues by transcutaneous electrical stimulation or any other form of stimulation that activates small fibers could bring about an increased input to the central biasing mechanism, which would close the gates to inputs from selected body areas. The cells of the midbrain reticular formation are known to have large receptive fields, and the electrical stimulation of points within the reticular formation can produce analgesia in discrete areas of the body (2). It is possible, then, that particular body areas may project especially strongly to some reticular areas, and these, in turn, could "close the gate" to inputs from particular parts of the body.

There has been exciting recent support for this hypothesis. Direct electrical

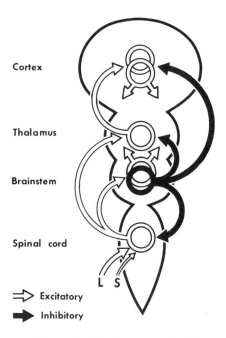

FIG. 2. Schematic diagram of the central biasing mechanism. Large and small fibers from a limb activate a neuron pool in the spinal cord, which excites neuron pools at successively higher levels. The central biasing mechanism, represented by the inhibitory projection system that originates in the brainstem reticular formation, modulates activity at all levels. When sensory fibers are destroyed after amputation or peripheral nerve lesion, the inhibitory influence decreases. This results in sustained activity at all levels that can be triggered repeatedly by the remaining fibers. L, large fibers; S, small fibers. (From Melzack, ref. 10.)

stimulation of the brainstem areas that produce analgesia inhibits the transmission of nerve impulses in dorsal horn cells that have been implicated in gate control mechanisms (18). Bilateral lesions of the dorsolateral spinal cord abolish these inhibitory effects and also abolish or reduce the analgesia produced by brainstem stimulation and morphine (3). Furthermore, the analgesia-producing brainstem areas are known to be highly sensitive to morphine, and their action is blocked by administration of naloxone (1). The demonstration that naloxone also blocks the analgesic effects of transcutaneous electrical stimulation (20) and acupuncture (9) thus provides powerful support for the hypothesis that intense stimulation activates a neural feedback loop through the brainstem analgesia-producing areas. There is still further exciting evidence to support the hypothesis: The analgesia-producing areas have been found to contain endogenous morphine-like compounds (endorphins), and electroacupuncture has been found to produce an increase in endorphins in cerebrospinal fluid in patients treated for chronic pain (21).

The prolonged relief of pain after only brief stimulation requires the additional postulation of prolonged, reverberatory activity in neural circuits that may underlie "memories" of earlier injury (7). These reverberatory circuits may be facilitated by low-level inputs, such as those from the pathological structures or processes that subserve trigger points or acupuncture points, and is disrupted for long periods of time (perhaps permanently) by a massive input produced by electrical or other intense stimulation. Furthermore, when pain is blocked, even briefly, the patient tends to become physically active and carry out normal motor activities such as walking and working. The normal, patterned proprioceptive inputs that result from these activities may prevent the resumption of the abnormal reverberatory neural activity that underlies prolonged pain.

THE CONCEPT OF A "PATTERN-GENERATING MECHANISM"

So far, we have dealt only with ways to increase the sensory input. However, doing the opposite is also a form of sensory modulation and, indeed, anesthetic blocks of sensory input often produce pain relief that outlasts the duration of the block (7). Successive blocks may relieve pain for increasingly long periods of time. Anesthetic blocks of trigger points, tender skin areas, peripheral nerves, or sympathetic ganglia would have the effect of diminishing the input through the gate and, thereby, would bring about a cessation of activity in reverberatory neural circuits. Thus, increasing or decreasing the input would have the same effect of disrupting abnormal neural activity. Moreover, in both cases, the relief of pain would permit normal motor activities that would tend to prevent the recurrence of abnormal central neural activity.

Recently, Melzack and Loeser (13) reviewed physiological evidence to show that deafferentation (such as root sections) produces abnormal physiological activity in spinal and brain cells deprived of input. The cells fire spontaneously in high-frequency bursts and may be triggered by inputs from adjacent structures; the abnormal firing may persist for hours after a single, brief triggering stimulus, and abnormal activity has been observed to persist for months.

On the basis of these data, as well as observations that paraplegics with total section of the spinal cord sometimes suffer severe pain below the level of the lesion, Melzack and Loeser suggested that denervated areas in the transmission pathways from dorsal horns to cortex may become "pattern-generating mechanisms." Their abnormal activity, they proposed, is capable of producing patterns of nerve impulses that give rise to pain. The cells that comprise these pattern-generating mechanisms receive inputs from multiple sources: the peripheral nervous system, the visceral and autonomic systems, the brain, as well as abnormal activity within the central nervous system based on prior injury (Fig. 3).

The implication of the model for therapy is that we should seek to modulate several of these sources at once. For example, analgesic drugs given in combination with transcutaneous electrical stimulation may permit a greater degree of control over pain than either one alone. The model suggests that cutting peripheral or central pathways is a deafferenting process that could increase the abnor-

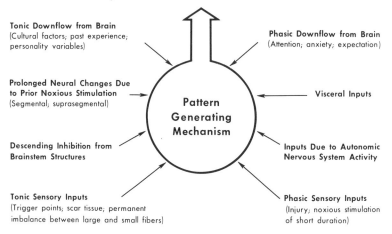

FIG. 3. Concept of a pattern-generating mechanism controlled by multiple inputs. (From Melzack and Loeser, ref. 13.)

mal firing. Instead, the emphasis of therapy should be to modulate the input by using all the techniques available to us, one at a time or in combination.

REFERENCES

1. Akil, H., Mayer, D. J., and Liebeskind, J. C. (1976): Antagonism of stimulation-produced analgesia by naloxone, a narcotic antagonist. *Science,* 191:961–962.
2. Balagura, S., and Ralph, T. (1973): The analgesic effect of electrical stimulation of the diencephalon and mesencephalon. *Brain Res.,* 60:369–379.
3. Basbaum, A. I., Marley, N. E. J., O'Keefe, J., and Clanton, C. H. (1977): Reversal of morphine and stimulus-produced analgesia by subtotal spinal cord lesions. *Pain,* 3:43–56.
4. Chapman, C. R., Chen, A. C., and Bonica, J. J. (1977): Effects of intrasegmental electrical acupuncture on dental pain: Evaluation by threshold estimation and sensory decision theory. *Pain,* 3:213–227.
5. Dennis, S. G., and Melzack, R. (1977): Pain-signalling systems in the dorsal and ventral spinal cord. *Pain,* 4:97–132.
6. Fox, E. J., and Melzack, R. (1976): Transcutaneous electrical stimulation and acupuncture: Comparison of treatment for low back pain. *Pain,* 2:141–148.
7. Livingston, W. K. (1943): *Pain Mechanisms.* Macmillan, New York.
8. Long, D. M. (1976): Use of peripheral and spinal cord stimulation in the relief of chronic pain. In: *Advances in Pain Research and Therapy, Vol. 1: Proceedings of the First World Congress on Pain,* edited by J. J. Bonica and D. Albe-Fessard, pp. 395–403. Raven Press, New York.
9. Mayer, D. J., Price, D. D., Barber, J., and Rafii, A. (1976): Acupuncture analgesia: Evidence for activation of a pain inhibitory system as a mechanism of action. In: *Advances in Pain Research and Therapy, Vol. 1: Proceedings of the First World Congress on Pain,* edited by J. J. Bonica and D. Albe-Fessard, pp. 751–754. Raven Press, New York.
10. Melzack, R. (1973): *The Puzzle of Pain.* Basic Books, New York.
11. Melzack, R. (1975): Prolonged relief of pain by brief, intense transcutaneous electrical stimulation. *Pain,* 1:357–373.
12. Melzack, R. and Casey, K. L. (1968): Sensory, motivational, and central control determinants

of pain: A new conceptual model. In: *The Skin Senses,* edited by D. Kenshalo, pp. 423–439. Charles C Thomas, Springfield, Ill.
13. Melzack, R., and Loeser, J. D. (1978): Phantom body pain in paraplegics: Evidence for a central "pattern generating mechanism" for pain. *Pain,* 4:195–210.
14. Melzack, R., Stillwell, D. M., and Fox, E. J. (1977): Trigger points and acupuncture points for pain: Correlations and implications. *Pain,* 3:3–23.
15. Melzack, R., and Torgerson, W. S. (1971): On the language of pain. *Anesthesiology,* 34:50–59.
16. Melzack, R., and Wall, P. D. (1965): Pain mechanisms: A new theory. *Science,* 150:971–979.
17. Noordenbos, W. (1959): *Pain.* Elsevier, Amsterdam.
18. Oliveras, J. L., Besson, J. M., Guilbaud, G., and Liebeskind, J. C. (1974): Behavioral and electrophysiological evidence of pain inhibition from midbrain stimulation in the cat. *Exp. Brain Res.,* 20:32–44.
19. Omura, Y. (1975): Electro-acupuncture: Its electrophysiological basis and criteria for effectiveness and safety. *Acupuncture and Electro-Therapeut. Res.,* 1:157–181.
20. Sjölund, B., and Eriksson, M. (1976): Electro-acupuncture and endogenous morphines. *Lancet,* 2:1085.
21. Sjölund, B., Terenius, L., and Eriksson, M. (1977): Increased cerebrospinal fluid levels of endorphins after electro-acupuncture. *Acta Physiol. Scand.,* 100:382–384.
22. Sola, A. E., and Williams, R. L. (1956): Myofascial pain syndromes. *Neurology,* 6:91–95.
23. Travell, J., and Rinzler, S. H. (1952): The myofascial genesis of pain. *Postgrad. Med.,* 11:425–434.
24. Wall, P. D. (1976): The modulation of pain by non-painful events. In: *Advances in Pain Research and Therapy, Vol. 1: Proceedings of the First World Congress on Pain,* edited by J. J. Bonica and D. Albe-Fessard, pp. 1–16. Raven Press, New York.
25. Wall, P. D., and Sweet, W. H. (1967): Temporary abolition of pain in man. *Science,* 155:108–109.

Mechanisms of Pain and Analgesic Compounds,
edited by R. F. Beers, Jr., and E. G. Bassett.
Raven Press, New York © 1979.

16. Discussion

Moderator: Kenneth L. Casey

Department of Physiology, University of Michigan, Ann Arbor, Michigan 48109

K. L. Casey: I think the sequence of these presentations has been very fortuitous. It started with a cellular approach to the hardware and ended with Ron Melzack's presentation, which brings up the issue of chronic pain and clinical pain problems. I will now raise the issue of the distinction between acute and chronic pain.

John Bonica, his colleagues, and other clinicians have been impressed with the difference between chronic and acute pain. The difference is very important, certainly as regards to the management of patients who come to see us with pain problems.

In the process of making that distinction, the issue is raised as to whether chronic and acute pain are physiologically distinct. To what extent is acute pain clearly different from chronic pain? We have been talking about neural mechanisms of pain, and except for the talk by Ron and the issues that he raised, the speakers have dealt with acute pain as produced in the laboratory. Do these studies of acute pain, which reveal pathways for pain perception, pathways for control of pain, and endogenous control mechanisms, bear upon the physiology and the chemistry of chronic pain? Do they have anything to say to the clinician who deals with chronic pain patients? Or, as the clinicians, are we left with speculation as to whether these studies have anything at all to do with clinical pain problems?

This raises the related question as to whether we should develop models of chronic pain in animals. Are we obliged to do that because of fundamental biological differences in the mechanisms of chronic and acute pain? This is a very serious question because there are strong arguments against developing chronic pain models. This is an issue that I think is important to clinicians and to those who are working on neural mechanisms of pain.

I would like to address this question to our speakers. Let me state it a little more specifically: to what extent, if any, do you feel that the neural mechanisms of acute pain differ from those of chronic pain?

F. W. L. Kerr: I shall start by saying that you can look at it this way: let us suppose for a moment that chronic pain is different from acute pain. In that case you have to presuppose a different circuitry for chronic pain. There is no evidence at all that there is a different circuitry. I believe that the same neurons that one activates with high threshold input, in the acute situation, are the same neurons that are going to be activated in the chronic situation.

Now, there is no question, as John Bonica has pointed out, that there is a striking difference between acute pain and chronic pain. We all agree with that. So, what is the difference? Let us say when we consider acute pain, you can jack up the stimulus intensity to whatever level you want until it is totally intolerable. If you had chronic pain with that type of intensity, every patient with chronic pain would commit suicide—there is little question about that. So I would propose that chronic pain has a low level of constant input and the majority of chronic pain is of that sort. The few patients who have high level of chronic pain input are liable to commit suicide, as you see with central pain and other pains that cannot be relieved.

I believe that with chronic pain as a result of constant input, you facilitate certain central nuclear activities in the same nuclei that are the receptor and relay nuclei for pain. So in effect you are dealing with the same pathways, the same nuclei, and then the question is: how about the affective motivational aspect that Ron Melzack and Ken Casey have brought to our attention? You have excited cells to which attention is directed because they are causing discomfort and because they are alerting the patient that something is wrong, and the more you concentrate on that, the more it comes to your attention. This may be the way that the mood modifying drugs may help considerably to relieve pain.

Then you get the things that John Liebeskind talked about with regard to the levels of enkephalins and normal endogenous systems that may run out of gas after a period of time. He mentioned that in the spinal fluid of patients with chronic pain, they may have low levels of endorphins; maybe they are running out of gas and therefore you have something else to add to it. So we are in, let us say, the primitive level of understanding of it, but a tremendously superior level to what we were 10, 15, or 20 years ago. We are beginning to get some scientific hints as to how these things are working. Chronic pain and acute pain follow the same pathways, but they have different central mechanisms that are facilitated by chronic input and by modifications and biochemicals and inhibitory systems that are inbuilt. That would be my tentative answer to that.

W. D. Willis: I would guess that in some chronic pain situations, where the affective overlay side of it is less in proportion to the responsive side of it, you could demonstrate some sort of interference with pain transmission in much the same way you do acute pain patients. But I could imagine that in a case of central pain that you couldn't do this. This must produce a good deal of discrepancy in different sorts of pains.

Not being a practicing clinician, I can't talk from experience, but I gather that the treatment of many forms of cancer pain, particularly from the lower part of the body, is managed very effectively by cordotomy; yet these patients may have chronic pain state. So it seems to me there is evidence for similar pathway for the responsive side of the pain stage.

R. Melzack: I think you have reached an extremely important question here. First of all, I think we should distinguish between phasic pain and tonic pain, phasic simply being the onset of the pain and then the tonic aspect being that which continues. Then, if it continues and continues, we have chronic pain. Now, chronic pain can be of two sorts: there is chronic pain that is due to metastasis, some obvious lesion. The pain just doesn't go away. But then in other cases, those unfortunate souls where nobody can find anything wrong— let's say the patient with low back pain where there doesn't seem to be any evidence of pathology. Nevertheless, the person feels pain.

Stephen Dennis, a member of our team, has been doing much of the same sort of work that John Liebeskind, David Mayer, and others have done but using a different sort of test. In the last 5 or 10 years, part of our work has been to get away from phasic pain, from brief pain, and try to approach tonic or chronic pain in the animal.

As Ken points out, there is a real ethical issue involved here. In the case of people, we have no problem because everybody in the hospital with chronic pain is someone that one can study. What I did then is to devise a test in which one can quite effectively measure pain in these people, can measure the sensory dimension of their pain, can measure the affective dimension of pain, and so forth. I think we should look at these kinds of pain instead of producing laboratory pains in people. Here are people in pain and we can do things with these people. They are happy to volunteer for experimentation and we can measure their pain.

In animals we have used what we call the formalin test that originated in my laboratory many years ago. One injects a little bit of turpentine or formalin to produce a pain—not excruciating—that lasts about an hour. We have all done it to ourselves. On a five-point scale, it would rate a number three for about 5 min. It is unpleasant and you may shake your hand for approximately 5 min but the hurt is quite bearable.

Applying this test to the cat, it immediately puts a paw to the mouth and licks vigorously, which is what we do if we get our skin pinched. Then after about 5 min of licking, the paw is simply favored, so the licking is given a rating of three. Holding the paw up is given a rating of two. Then the cat, after about 30 min, gingerly puts the paw on the floor. That is recorded as a rating of one. After 45 to 60 min, the cat walks normally and that is rated zero. So you can observe the number of each of these kinds of behavior every minute, get an average of these values over a 5-min period, and a beautiful curve can be plotted. One can then test a drug against the curve, so it brings us closer to chronic pain.

But I think one of the most important things that is happening in the field is our recognizing that chronic pain is very different from something like the tail flick, or the hot plate test, or any of these sorts of tests. Steven Dennis found that the biochemistry of the systems really are different. Serotonin seems to be extremely important in cases of phasic pain, but it is not all that important in types of more chronic or tonic pain that I have been talking about. I think we will have revealed some of the finer details of the biochemistry involved in these systems.

J. C. Liebeskind: I don't know how much can be added to what has already been said. I have been long impressed by the fact that pain can be measured in a lot of different ways, from the lowly spinal reflex all the way to much more complicated behaviors involving the highest centers in the nervous systems.

I think both acute and chronic pain can, under the appropriate circumstances, involve aspects of personality and higher nervous functions. Dr. Dubner provided an example in his talk today. Even in the most straightforward kind of acute pain situation, if you set up a situation appropriately and you have your eyes open to look at complicated aspects of the response permitted in the situation, you are going to see that these higher functions are going to express themselves and modulate pain.

It may just be in many chronic pain situations, as Drs. Fordyce and Bonica were stressing this morning, that pain behavior becomes functionally autonomous from its original stimulus source; it is all located in the frontal lobes, and has nothing more to do with the spinal cord, interneurons, and so on. When all is said and done, I believe that all levels of the nervous systems can be involved in any kind of pain, chronic or acute, and that therefore the anatomy is the same and it is only a question of which circumstances permit the expression of certain types of behavior involving different neural circuitry.

R. Dubner: I agree with what John Liebeskind has said. We do have examples of acute pain mimicking some aspects of chronic pain syndromes. An example was provided by Dave Mayer this morning in citing the work done by Don Price and his colleagues. As Norton Bush showed, there are three aspects of certain neuralgic pains such as postherpetic neuralgia, or causalgia, that are very characteristic. One is that the pain produced by stimulation summates with repeated stimulation; another aspect is that the pain outlasts the period of stimulation; the third aspect is that the pain very often radiates from the point of stimulation. These three characteristics can also be shown with acute pain models, such as the one that Don Price has developed. That is, with heat pain, or with electrical stimulation, you can show that second pain produced by this type of stimulation shows the same three characteristics: the pain summates with repeated stimulation; the pain outlasts the period of stimulation; and the pain radiates to another part of the limb outside the point of stimulation. So we can see in this instance that there are very close parallels between the acute pain situation and some of the processes involved in certain chronic pain syndromes.

J. J. Bonica: If I have done nothing during the past 30 years, what I have done today is probably as important as anything else. That is, I have stimulated some basic scientists to think about this matter. The fact is that you posed a question, Ken, as a neurophysiologist. You mentioned the neural mechanisms. The fact is that pain, both acute and chronic pain, involve not only neural mechanisms but, as you have so well described, higher centers.

I am not proposing that chronic pain involves different neural mechanisms, but I am saying that, in some instances, peripheral noxious stimulation over a period of time does something to the neuraxis that produces abnormal responses. After a period of time, this abnormal constant input, noxious input, produces some changes and perhaps the primary pathway is involved, but other pathways become involved and they develop this sustaining, closed loop neurons that have been described. It is very important to see there is a difference. There is not pain at the lowest segmental level. That is a reflex response to noxious stimulation. Pain is felt up here. I think that one could look at chronic pain as an abnormal function of any part of the system.

In some instances, I think this abnormal input produces an abnormal activity in the neuraxis. Even if you eliminate the peripheral input, the patient doesn't get complete, but partial relief or no relief at all. You can see this in chronic phases of reflexive dystrophies, causalgia, where many kinds of things can be done to relieve the patient permanently, but you don't do it in chronic pain cases. Then of course, there may be abnormal activity in the central nervous system without peripheral input.

I think you have to recognize that for many chronic pain patients, their problem is in the mind. I don't think that this is seen in the acute phase. If someone gets burned or someone hurts himself, you don't see this abnormal response that is seen in affective responses.

Finally, I wish to point out that if you take the blood pressure of somebody who has been stimulated actively, you will find he has an increase of heart rate, hyperventilation, and an endocrine response, but you don't see this in a chronic patient; the response is different. The autonomic and perhaps the psychophysiological response differs.

R. M. Kanner: Perhaps I couldn't see the forest for the trees. I would like to ask a couple of questions about some branches. Dr. Liebeskind said the level of enkephalins in CSF are down in patients with chronic pain and that with correct analgesia, they rise. One question that could be asked: is this simply a matter of finding that after continuing pain stimulation we are not seeing the enkephalins because they are bound to the receptor sites?

The second question is about serotonin levels in chronic pain. We know that serotonin levels have tremendous fluxes in migraine which may simply be a vascular response. Have serotonin levels in the CSF been measured in chronic pain patients?

F. W. L. Kerr: As far as the endorphin levels go, I don't think it would be a question of their sitting around so stably waiting to be bound. I think that what is seen is the influx into the ventricular system and into the spinal subarachnoid space, that this influx can be picked up and may be a sign of the amount of release that is tonically going on at that particular time. These are very exciting studies. They need further confirmation, but I think they are highly suggestive that indeed spontaneous fluctuations are evoked; fluctuations in this system may be mirroring very real differences in responsiveness to pain.

S. Hockfield: Dr. Kerr, you postulated inhibitory synapses to occur on the soma of the marginal neuron and excitatory synapses to occur on the dendrites. Have you seen any morphological differences between those synapses, differences in vesicle size, or anything else that would indicate they have the functions you postulated?

F. W. L. Kerr: We did an extensive study on this. I can't give you the figures because it was very complex by the time we had analyzed all the different types of synaptic vesicles. It would be very nice to say that the axosomatics on marginal neurons were flat vesicle synapses, and all the dendritic ones were round vesicle synapses, and so on. Unfortunately, that sort of thing doesn't happen. You have a mixture of synaptic endings.

The primary afferents that end on the dendrites tend to be mostly round vesicle synapses as one would anticipate, but when you get into the soma there is a mixture of some round vesicles, some mixed round and flat vesicles, and some that have dense core vesicles in them, too, occasionally. I can't give you the figures but will refer you to the paper by Narotzky and myself that was published in *Brain Research* (1978) and all the figures are there.

S. Hockfield: My second question concerns your mention of the lesions of Lissauer's tract. You said there is ample evidence that neurons of the substantia gelatinosa send their axons into Lissauer's tract and participate in propriospinal connections.

I am not sure that the evidence is that good for a couple of reasons. One point is that in Iggo's studies of substantia gelatinosa neurons, he could only antidromically activate less than 10% when he stimulated Lissauer's tract. Another point is that from Cajal's work, and I think you referred to LaMotte's work also, there is substantial evidence that primary afferents, especially the small myelinated and unmyelinated fibers, travel in Lissauer's tract; so when you leave Lissauer's tract, you are cutting primary afferents, and are the primary afferents endosomic neurilists, that you have illustrated? Are those inhibitory synapses?

F. W. L. Kerr: The majority of axons of lamina II gelatinosa cells that have been traced do in fact go into Lissauer's tract or into the pathways around the dorsal horn. That was the original observation of Cajal, which has been confirmed by Szentagothai, by Suguira, and by others.

In answer to the question about primary afferents in Lissauer's tract, you are quite correct. I didn't have time to go into the technical details. The majority of the primary afferents that ascend and descend in Lissauer's tract are in the medial part of that tract and if you do the tractotomy in the lateral half of the C_1 area or in the lumbar area, you can spare virtually all the primary afferents.

With regard to the antidromic activation studies by Iggo, that is true; he only got about 10% activation. But on the other hand, antidromic studies by Wall and Yaksh [*Exp. Neurol.*, 60:570–583 (1978)] resulted in the activation of the great majority of the neurons in gelatinosa. I recognize that there are conflicts such as you have pointed out, but I think they can be answered to this extent. We don't have the methods to do it perfectly.

S. Hockfield: I think there are two additional pieces of evidence, anatomical evidence, that both studies of Field and co-workers have shown that the majority, if not all, of the neurons in the substantia gelatinosa don't send their axons into Lissauer's tract, at least in their studies of the Golgi complex; I think that is a question that is still open.

F. W. L. Kerr: In answer to that, the neurons that lie deeper in the substantia gelatinosa—that is to say lamina III neurons—look very much like the short axon types, Golgi type II. The evidence for that comes particularly from the 1975 or 1976 paper by Mannen and Sugiura that shows this beautifully: axons coming out and breaking up in an enormous number of terminals, in laminae II, III, and IV, and that none of those go into the gelatinosa. So one has to specify what part of the gelatinosa the cells are from.

Furthermore, it is a fallacy to consider that all gelatinosa neurons are the same; the majority project into Lissauer's tract while a small number of them project into the spinothalamic tract; these are a different type of gelatinosa cells whose functions we know nothing about at the present.

L. S. Harris: I want to interject a word of caution about the interpretation of endorphin levels in this one experiment of the spinal cord and chronic pain. Specifically, the method of determining the endorphin levels, particularly as they exist in the spinal fluid, are not very specific or quantitative. So before we make a sweeping generalization from this one study, I think there is going to have to be a good deal more work done.

H. Lal: Dr. Melzack, acute pain in animals, when measured by the tail flick or tail withdrawal, is not affected no matter what you do to this animal in terms of producing another pain.

I have measured tail withdrawal by injecting formalin or histamine, or putting surgical clips on it but his tail stays constant. Any comment on this?

If you are measuring one pain and you produce another pain, it should alter the propensity. If one is measuring acute pain generated in an animal and subsequently cause another pain in this animal, the measurement does not change.

J. C. Liebeskind: Drs. Hayes and Mayer have done work that I think very much relates to that point. Certain kinds of pain or stressful procedures much like those that Ron Melzack was talking about are capable of altering pain responsiveness in the tail flick and hot plate tests. The story is not very neat and clear yet. One does tend to think of certain spinal reflexes as being immutable or not; they can be influenced. We don't know all the circumstances which do influence it, but certainly rotation, stress, and electric shock are capable of altering—very prominantly and for rather extensive periods of time—the rat tail flick response.

C. A. Winter: Several years ago, we showed that intraperitoneal injection of certain pain-producing substances would alter pain responses of animals. I think there are at least two different techniques that would probably be a little more of the chronic type than the injection he mentioned. One is in rats with adjuvant arthritis, in which pain persists for weeks. And if you think these rats are not experiencing pain, try putting a few of them together in a cage and see how they fight.

Another pain producing method, which can last a little longer than the acute pain usually measured in animals, is the response to the injection of urate crystals in the knee joint of a dog, for example. The degree to which that animal is willing to voluntarily use that limb has been very nicely measured by Dr. Van Arman. The thing that these two methods have in common is that they are both very sensitive to analgesic drugs in doses lower than those usually used in the more acute tests.

F. Sicuteri: I ask if Dr. Liebeskind has any experience about the activity of antiserotonin as an analgesic in animal that might match the efficiency of serotonin in the antinociceptor system.

J. C. Liebeskind: I think you have raised a very interesting question and I am not able to comment on it from the standpoint of direct experience. There have been some excellent reviews that have come out recently, particularly the one by Messing and Lytle that attempted to review the serotonin story; not a very straightforward situation but that there is evidence accumulating in many directions. The special case of migraine headache may have had more to do with the local or peripheral action of serotonin in blood levels. This is your specialty; I won't attempt to comment on it.

There are fragmentary bits of evidence here and there that are altering the serotonin picture. Serotonin can have a profound effect in laboratory animals involved in certain kinds of pain tests. I am reasonably persuaded that the serotonin is an important mediator in the antinociceptive effects of morphine. The evidence is reasonably strong there, as well as that in the antinociceptive effects of stimulation-produced analgesia and brain stimulation when that stimulation is applied to serotonin-containing cells.

But as you pointed out, mechanisms of analgesia that do not involve serotonin are also present. The system is certainly very complex and I would not call serotonin synapses an essential link in the antinociceptive effect of these various manipulations.

F. Sicuteri: Dr. Melzack, I am wondering if the improvement following the operation you discussed is totally due to psychological mechanisms, because it can also be due to the hemorrhagic shock.

R. Melzack: It could well be; there are probably many mechanisms involved in the relief of pain in such cases. What interested me was that this procedure represented an intense sensory input—but you are quite right. With such a loss of blood during one of those operations, who wants to admit he has a headache? You know the story of a patient who goes to the doctor for a cure for a chronic cough. He is told to drink a bottle of castor oil—then you will be afraid to cough.

F. W. L. Kerr: I have a comment or two on Professor Sicuteri's comment. First, that there was no evidence of the patient being in hemorrhagic shock whatsoever; a big man like that can lose three or four times that amount of blood before signs of shock develop.

Second, the follow-up was inadequate because it was stated that they came back to see this man 1 month later; many of the pain patients one sees who have had something spectacular done to them will come back in a month stating that they are pain-free. This may be simply a placebo effect together with the emotional and psychological effects that go with it. If you follow this patient for a year or two, the result may be much less impressive. Long-term follow-up is indispensable in pain patients; those marvelous operations came and went, because everybody was enthusiastic about them for 3 to 6 months but after a few years, the results are much less satisfactory.

R. Melzack: I fully agree with your comment about the follow-up. McNett, who made the film, has been in touch with the patient and apparently the pain really has gone. As I said before, who would admit to having pain?

Mechanisms of Pain and Analgesic Compounds,
edited by R. F. Beers, Jr., and E. G. Bassett.
Raven Press, New York © 1979.

17. Introduction to Section C: Endogenous Substances Having Analgesic Action

Hans W. Kosterlitz

*Unit for Research on Addictive Drugs, University of Aberdeen,
Aberdeen AB9 1AS, Scotland*

The title of this section has been deliberately called "Endogenous Substances Having Analgesic Action." We did not entitle it the "Endogenous Analgesic System," which would raise controversial questions. In my opinion it is rather doubtful that there is any evidence for the view that analgesia is a physiological phenomenon. There may be exceptional situations in which analgesic mechanisms may become activated as, for instance, in soldiers who have been severely injured and yet do not appear to experience pain, or possibly in childbirth: however, we do not know enough about these situations.

Therefore, I would like to ask that the term "endogenous analgesic system" not be used. There is another good reason for this request because, quite clearly, analgesia, even when produced pharmacologically, is only one function of the opioid peptides and it may not be the most important one. We probably should call it the "opioid peptidergic system." It may also reduce confusion if we were to avoid "endorphin system" as a general term and confine it to designate neurones containing β-endorphin. We now know that there are three opioid peptides of importance: β-endorphin, methionine-, and leucine-enkephalins.

Since this section is in memory of Dr. Seevers, I would like to relate an experience I had. In 1962 we first decided to look into the mode of action of narcotic analgesics at a molecular level and it was by that time that we had developed certain of our models. In those days, we used the so-called peristaltic reflex of the guinea pig ileum, which is elicited by distending the lumen of the ileum suspended in an organ bath. Another model was based on contractions of the cat nictitating membrane, elicited by stimulation of its postganglionic nerves. At that time, I visited the United States because I wanted to meet the people who were leaders in the field of narcotic analgesic drugs and I was a newcomer to this area of research. I visited Dr. Seevers' laboratory and he very kindly invited me to present a seminar on our work. At the end he said (those who knew Dr. Seevers will appreciate it), "Dr. Kosterlitz, what you have said is all very interesting but I don't think that I can believe a word of it." During the discussion that followed, I asked, "How can I make you believe it?" He replied, "Well, there is one condition: we'll send you coded samples of various narcotic and nonnarcotic drugs and if you get the majority of them right, we will start to believe in your models." Well, we were very lucky. We got correct answers for five of the six samples. We thought Dr. Seevers was rather shrewd because he gave us what we thought were two samples of morphine and it turned out that the sixth sample was nalorphine. At that time we really did not know enough about the action of compounds with dual agonist and antagonist actions which will be discussed later this week.

I wanted to tell this story because in the early days of the use of the guinea pig ileum as a model, people used to ask me, "What on earth has the intestine to do with the brain?" After we had convinced Dr. Seevers that we could predict, in fact, the potency of drugs and also their agonist and antagonist components, both he and Dr. Nathan Eddy gave us their support. Without it we may not have had the good fortune of finding the opioid peptides. The guinea pig ileum and, particularly, the mouse vas deferens proved to be very good monitoring systems in the search for the opioid peptides.

Recalling the origin of the studies on the enkephalins, I would like to mention three other authors in this section who helped John Hughes and myself in deciding to look for an endogenous compound. In their paper published in 1972, Akil, Mayer, and Liebeskind showed that stimulation of the pericentral gray had an antinociceptive effect. The key result, as far as we were concerned, was the observation that this effect was reversed by naloxone.

Mechanisms of Pain and Analgesic Compounds,
edited by R. F. Beers, Jr., and E. G. Bassett.
Raven Press, New York © 1979.

18. Possible Physiological Significance of Multiple Endogenous Opioid Agonists

Hans W. Kosterlitz

*Unit for Research on Addictive Drugs, University of Aberdeen,
Aberdeen AB9 1AS, Scotland*

INTRODUCTION

On present evidence it would appear that there are in the central nervous system two independent peptidergic systems. The first is represented by the short chain peptides, methionine-enkephalin (β-lipotropin$_{61-65}$) and the leucine^{65} analog or leucine-enkephalin (15) and is spread unevenly throughout the brain, spinal cord, and peripheral autonomic nervous system (9,14,26). The second system contains the long chain peptide, β-endorphin (β-lipotropin$_{61-91}$) and is centered around the hypothalamus-pituitary axis with extensions into the midline regions of the diencephalon and anterior pons (3,25,30).

OBSERVATIONS AND DISCUSSION

Interactions of the Opioid Peptides with Opiate Receptors

The question arises of whether the short and long chain opioid peptides interact with one and the same receptor or whether there are several receptors subserving different physiological functions. Already before the discovery of the endogenous opioid peptides, Martin and his colleagues (20,21), from experiments on the chronic spinal dog, had adduced evidence for the view that the action of certain semisynthetic and synthetic surrogates cannot be explained on the basis of a single opiate receptor. This view was supported by investigations on the *in vitro* models of the guinea pig ileum and mouse vas deferens (16); the results led to the same conclusions as those obtained by Martin and his colleagues, namely that, apart from the μ-receptors mediating the action of classical morphine-like compounds, receptors of a different type (κ-receptors) were present in the central and peripheral nervous systems.

The findings obtained with the opioid peptides could not be fitted into this concept (19). Methionine-enkephalin (β-lipotropin$_{61-65}$), the Leu^{65} analog leucine-enkephalin, β-endorphin (β-lipotropin$_{61-91}$), and its putative metabolic breakdown product, γ-endorphin (β-lipotropin$_{61-77}$) behaved differently from μ-agonists and κ-agonists in the four assay models used by Lord et al. (19).

TABLE 1. *Assessment of the relative potencies of opioid peptides and morphine by four parallel assays*[a]

Compound	Inhibition of contractions of			Inhibition of binding of		
	Mouse vas deferens	Guinea pig ileum	Gpi/Mvd	^{3}H-Leucine-enkephalin	^{3}H-Naltrexone	Naltrexone/ Leu-enkephalin
Methionine-enkephalin	1	0.11	0.11	1	0.18	0.18
Leucine-enkephalin	1.6	0.04	0.025	0.76	0.05	0.066
Morphine	0.03	0.19	6.3	0.01	0.07	7.0
Tyr-D-Ala²-Gly-MePhe-Met(0)-ol	1.1	2.0	1.8	0.03	0.40	13.3
β-endorphin	0.32	0.38	1.2	1.31	0.66	0.5
γ-endorphin	0.46	0.05	0.11	0.02	0.01	0.5

[a] The binding tests were performed at 0 to 4°C for 150 min to reduce enzymatic degradation (19; Waterfield et al., *unpublished observations*).

When the relative potencies are referred to those of methionine-enkephalin in the mouse vas deferens and in the binding test with ^{3}H-leucine-enkephalin as standard units, values are obtained which allow a direct comparison between the four assay systems (Table 1). In the guinea pig ileum, the potency of methionine-enkephalin has only 11% of that in the mouse vas deferens; similarly its potency to inhibit ^{3}H-naltrexone binding is only 18% of that to inhibit ^{3}H-leucine-enkephalin binding. Compared with methionine-enkephalin, the potency of leucine-enkephalin is increased in the mouse vas deferens and lowered in the guinea pig ileum; its affinity to the ^{3}H-leucine-enkephalin binding site is lowered only a little, with a concomitant decrease of 70% in affinity to the ^{3}H-naltrexone binding site. When morphine is compared with the two enkephalins, it is found that it is more potent in the guinea pig ileum but has a very much reduced activity in the mouse vas deferens. This finding is mirrored by the very low affinity of morphine to the ^{3}H-leucine-enkephalin binding site, whereas the affinity to the ^{3}H-naltrexone binding site is of the same order of magnitude as that of the enkephalins.

β-Endorphin behaves very differently in these parallel assays although the first five amino acids are identical with the sequence of methionine-enkephalin (15). It is resistant to the action of exopeptidases but is cleaved by an endopeptidase present in the pituitary at residues 77 to 78 to give γ-endorphin or β-lipotropin$_{61-77}$ (13). β-Endorphin is unique amongst the opioid peptides in that it is equipotent or nearly so in the two pharmacological models and in the binding tests. This characteristic property may, at least in part, explain its high antinociceptive and other activities (10,11,18). On the other hand, the putative catabolic product γ-endorphin has only 1.5% of the binding affinity of β-endorphin although, for as yet unexplained reasons, it still shows considerable activity in the mouse vas deferens and, to a lesser extent, in the guinea pig ileum. In this context, it should be remembered that the binding assays were performed at 0 to 4°C while the two tissue models were maintained at 36 to 37°C; little is known about the differences in the temperature coefficients of binding of the various opioids.

Pharmacological Pattern of Enkephalin Analogs

Since the biological half-life of the two naturally occurring enkephalins is very short, many attempts have been made to design stable analogs with strong antinociceptive activity. It is therefore important to know which alterations in the molecule are permissible without concomitant changes in the pattern of pharmacological activity. If, in position 2 of leucine-enkephalin, glycine was replaced by the unnatural D-alanine, the potencies in both guinea pig ileum and mouse vas deferens were increased by factors of 14 and 7, respectively, without altering significantly the affinities to the ^{3}H-naltrexone and ^{3}H-leucine-enkephalin binding sites (Table 2). This effect was most likely due to a decrease in the enzymatic degradation of the peptide in the pharmacological models

TABLE 2. *Assessment of the relative potencies of analogs of leucine-enkephalin by four parallel assays*[a]

Compound	Inhibition of contractions of		Inhibition of binding of	
	Mouse vas deferens	Guinea pig ileum	³H-Leucine-enkephalin	³H-Naltrexone
Tyr-*Gly*-Gly-Phe-*L-Leu*	1.6	0.04	0.76	0.05
Tyr-*D-Ala*-Gly-Phe-*L-Leu*	9.4	0.61	0.56	0.06
Tyr-*D-Ala*-Gly-Phe-*D-Leu*	29	0.37	0.34	0.04

[a] The binding tests were performed at 0 to 4°C for 150 min to reduce enzymatic degradation (19). The units of reference were the same as in Table 1: the inhibitory effects of methionine-enkephalin in the mouse vas deferens and in the ³H-leucine-enkephalin assay (Waterfield et al., *unpublished observations*).

maintained at 36 to 37°C, while the binding assays were carried out at 0 to 4°C. Replacement of L-Leu by D-Leu increased activity in the mouse vas deferens (2) without a major change in the affinity to the binding sites; on the other hand, the activity in the guinea pig ileum was reduced somewhat. The pharmacological pattern was, therefore, still of the type characteristic of leucine-enkephalin, perhaps even to an exaggerated extent since the peptide was much more potent in the mouse vas deferens than in the guinea pig ileum and the affinity for the ³H-leucine-enkephalin binding site was much higher than that for the ³H-naloxone binding site (Waterfield, et al., *unpublished observations*). This peptide has been shown (1) to have antinociceptive activity after injection into the cerebral ventricles. When the C-terminal amino acid residue of the enkephalins was replaced by amides of proline (27), the most important change was an increase in the activity in the guinea pig ileum; there was also an increase in the affinity for the ³H-naltrexone binding site with a simultaneous loss in affinity for the ³H-leucine-enkephalin binding site. Székely et al. (27) found that such compounds have antinociceptive activity after intravenous and subcutaneous injection. In this context, it is of particular interest to compare the methionine-enkephalin analog, Tyr-D-Ala-Gly-MePhe-Met(O)-ol (FK 33–824, Sandoz) introduced by Roemer et al. (24), with the enkephalins and morphine (Table 1). It is about as potent as the enkephalins in the mouse vas deferens but 20 times more potent in the guinea pig ileum. It has a very low affinity for the ³H-leucine-enkephalin binding site but is more potent than methionine-enkephalin at the ³H-naltrexone binding site. It therefore follows that this potent analog has lost at least some of the characteristics of methionine-enkephalin and has become rather more similar to morphine. In a trial on human volunteers, non-morphine-like side effects were observed after intramuscular injections of 0.025 to 1.2 mg, which gave peak plasma concentrations of 25 to 80 nM (29).

Alterations at the two terminal amino acid residues of the enkephalins have considerable effects on their pharmacological pattern. When the C-terminal leucine of D-Ala²-leucine-enkephalin is decarboxylated, the relative potency is increased in the guinea pig ileum and markedly decreased in the mouse vas deferens, while the affinity for the naltrexone binding site is improved and that for the enkephalin binding site diminished. When the leucine residue is removed, the resulting tetrapeptide is less active than the parent compound; the loss in activity is more pronounced in the mouse vas deferens and in its affinity to the leucine-enkephalin binding site, showing the importance of Leu[5] or Met[5] for the enkephalin-like properties of the pentapeptides. This shift in potencies is aggravated when the C-terminal phenylalanine of the tetrapeptide is decarboxylated and the N-terminal primary amino group made secondary by the introduction of a methyl group (Waterfield et al., *unpublished observation*).

It has been stressed (19) that the low effectiveness of naloxone against the action of the naturally occurring opioid peptides in the mouse vas deferens is strong supporting evidence for the view that the δ-receptors of the mouse vas deferens are different from the μ-receptors with which the classical opiates interact. However, from the fact that the opioid peptides are active in the guinea pig ileum and that their action is antagonized by naloxone as readily as that of morphine, it follows that they can interact also with μ-receptors. If the view is correct that in the mouse vas deferens the enkephalins and endorphins interact preferentially with δ-receptors less sensitive to the antagonist effect of naloxone than the μ-receptors, then naloxone should be a weaker antagonist against enkephalin analogs which retain their enkephalin-like pharmacological pattern, as for instance Tyr-D-Ala-Gly-Phe-D-Leu, than against enkephalin analogs which are more morphine-like, as for instance Tyr-D-Ala-Gly-NH(CH$_2$)$_2$Ph or Tyr-D-Ala-Gly-MePhe-Met(O)-ol. The results obtained with several analogs are compatible with this concept. It has been found that, in the mouse vas deferens, the equilibrium dissociation constant (K_e) of naloxone against normorphine is about 2; the corresponding values against methionine-enkephalin or β-endorphin are about 22 (19). Whereas the K_e value against Tyr-D-Ala-Gly-Phe-D-Leu is 32, the corresponding value against Tyr-D-Ala-Gly-NH(CH$_2$)$_2$Ph is only 5.7 and that against Tyr-D-Ala-Gly-MePhe-Met(O)-ol, 4.1 (Waterfield, et al., *unpublished observation*).

Possible Physiological Significance

The analysis of the possible physiological functions of the opioid peptides is even now, in 1978, in its early stages. Therefore, great care has to be taken to avoid speculation for which the experimental basis is insecure. It is likely that the peptides will mimic the actions of morphine, such as limitation of experience of pain, euphoric changes of mood, depression of respiration, changes in the extrapyramidal motor system, and constipation. Although it is not possible at present to allocate different physiological functions to the different peptides and to the receptors represented by the enkephalin and naltrexone binding sites, it is likely that the various peptides, the long chain endorphins and short chain enkephalins, may subserve different physiological functions. This concept may have its structural basis on the apparent independence of the enkephalin and endorphin systems (3).

The naturally occurring methionine- and leucine-enkephalins are poor antinociceptive agents, even after injection into the cerebral ventricles or directly into the brain substance, because they are rapidly inactivated by peptidases. Enzyme-resistant analogs such as D-Ala^2-methionine-enkephalin amide, N-CH$_3$-Tyr^1-methionine-enkephalin amide, and particularly the Pro^5 analogs and FK 33–824, are potent antinociceptive peptides (10,11,22,24,27). It is not clear yet how far the antinociceptive effect is correlated with affinity to the naltrexone or enkephalin binding sites.

Although the longer chain peptides are resistant to the action of exopeptidases, their antinociceptive potencies vary greatly. β-Endorphin or C-fragment is the most potent of these peptides; its antinociceptive effect after injection into the cerebral ventricles has been found to be at least equal to, and by most observers, greater than that of morphine (5,6,10,11,18,22). The effect of β-endorphin is long lasting as is that of the enzyme-resistant pentapeptides in contrast to the transient effects of the naturally occurring enkephalins. Since the onset of action of the natural enkephalins is rapid and the action is readily terminated enzymatically, they are good candidates for a possible role of inhibitory neurotransmitters or neuromodulators, particularly for rapid transients.

Other important actions of the opioid peptides affect the control of motor activity. For instance, microinjection of morphine or D-Ala^2-methionine-enkephalin amide into the nucleus accumbens of the limbic forebrain of the rat causes hypermotility which is reversed by naloxone (23). On the other hand, injection of β-endorphin into the periaqueductal grey, the cisterna magna, or the lateral ventricles leads to catatonia (4,17,28). Methionine-enkephalin is ineffective but N-CH$_3$-Tyr^1-methionine-enkephalin amide produces catatonia (6).

It is well known that morphine stimulates the release of prolactin and growth hormone from the pituitary. It has been shown that these effects are mimicked by methionine-enkephalin and β-endorphin when injected intraventricularly (7,8,12). Two facts make β-endorphin particularly suitable for such an endocrine control function: it is present in high concentration in the hypothalamus-pituitary axis and it is more resistant to enzymatic inactivation than the enkephalins.

CONCLUSIONS

The evidence presented in this paper indicates that the opioid peptidergic system is complex. The three agonists, methionine-enkephalin, leucine-enkephalin, and β-endorphin have different pharmacological patterns in the four assay systems used in this investigation. It may be of particular importance that they vary in their relative affinities to the enkephalin and naloxone binding sites. There is so far insufficient evidence to allocate different physiological functions to the different peptides.

ACKNOWLEDGMENTS

These investigations were supported by grants from the Medical Research Council, the National Institute on Drug Abuse (DA 00662), and the Committee on Problems of Drug Dependence.

REFERENCES

1. Baxter, M. G., Goff, D., Miller, A. A., and Saunders, I. A. (1977): Effect of a potent synthetic opioid pentapeptide in some antinociceptive and behavioural tests in mice and rats. *Br. J. Pharmacol.,* 59:455–456P.
2. Beddell, C. R., Clark, R. B., Hardy, G. W., Lowe, L. A., Ubatuba, F. B., Vane, J. R., Wilkinson, S., Chang, K.-J., Cuatrecasas, P., and Miller, R. J. (1977): Structural requirements for opioid activity of analogues of the enkephalins. *Proc. R. Soc. Lond. [Biol],* 198:249–265.
3. Bloom, F., Battenberg, E., Rossier, J., Ling, N., and Guillemin, R. (1978): Neurons containing β-endorphin in rat brain exist separately from those containing enkephalin: Immunocytochemical studies. *Proc. Natl. Acad. Sci. USA,* 75:1591–1595.
4. Bloom, F., Segal, D., Ling, N., and Guillemin, R. (1976): Endorphins: Profound behavioral effects in rats suggest new etiological factors in mental illness. *Science,* 194:630–632.
5. Bradbury, A. F., Feldberg, W., Smyth, D. G., and Snell, C. R. (1976): Lipotropin C-fragment: An endogenous peptide with potent analgesic activity. In:*Opiates and Endogenous Opioid Peptides,* edited by H. W. Kosterlitz, pp. 9–17. North-Holland, Amsterdam.
6. Bradbury, A. F., Smyth, D. G., Snell, C. R., Deakin, J. F. W., and Wendlandt, S. (1977): Comparison of the analgesic properties of lipotropin C-fragment and stabilized enkephalins in the rat. *Biochem. Biophys. Res. Commun.,* 74:748–754.
7. Dupont, A., Cusan, L., Garon, M., Labrie, F., and Li, C. H. (1977): β-Endorphin: Stimulation of growth hormone release in vivo. *Proc. Natl. Acad. Sci. USA,* 74:358–359.
8. Dupont, A., Cusan, L., Labrie, F., Coy, D. H., and Li, C. H. (1977): Stimulation of prolactin release in the rat by intraventricular injection of β-endorphin and methionine-enkephalin. *Biochem. Biophys. Res. Commun.,* 75:76–82.
9. Elde, R., Hökfelt, T., Johansson, O., and Terenius, L. (1976): Immunohistochemical studies using antibodies to leucine-enkephalin: Initial observations on the nervous system of the rat. *Neuroscience,* 1:349–351.
10. Feldberg, W., and Smyth, D. G. (1977): Analgesia produced in cats by the C-fragment of lipotropin and by a synthetic pentapeptide. *J. Physiol. (Lond.),* 265:25–27P.
11. Feldberg, W., and Smyth, D. G. (1977): C-fragment of lipotropin—an endogenous potent analgesic peptide. *Br. J. Pharmacol.,* 60:445–453.
12. Ferland, L., Fuxe, K., Eneforth, P., Gustafsson, J.-A., and Skett, P. (1977): Effects of methionine-enkephalin on prolactin release and catecholamine levels and turnover in the median eminence. *Eur. J. Pharmacol.,* 43:89–90.
13. Gráf, L., and Kenessey, A. (1976): Specific cleavage of a single peptide bond (residues 77–78) in β-lipotropin by a pituitary endopeptidase. *FEBS Lett.,* 69:255–260.
14. Hughes, J., Kosterlitz, H. W., and Smith, T. W. (1977): The distribution of methionine-enkephalin and leucine-enkephalin in the brain and peripheral tissues. *Br. J. Pharmacol.,* 61:639–647.
15. Hughes, J., Smith, T. W., Kosterlitz, H. W., Fothergill, L. A., Morgan, B. A., and Morris, H. R. (1975): Identification of two related pentapeptides from the brain with potent opiate agonist activity. *Nature,* 258:577–579.
16. Hutchinson, M., Kosterlitz, H. W., Leslie, F. M., Waterfield, A. A., and Terenius, L. (1975): Assessment in the guinea-pig ileum and mouse vas deferens of benzomorphans which have strong antinociceptive activity but do not substitute for morphine in the dependent monkey. *Br. J. Pharmacol.,* 55:541–546.
17. Jacquet, Y. F., and Marks, N. (1976): The C-fragment of β-lipotropin: An endogenous neuroleptic or antipsychotogen. *Science,* 194:632–635.
18. Loh, H. H., Tseng, L. F., Wei, E., and Li, C. H. (1976): β-Endorphin as a potent analgesic agent. *Proc. Natl. Acad. Sci. USA,* 73:2895–2898.

19. Lord, J. A. H., Waterfield, A. A., Hughes, J., and Kosterlitz, H. W. (1977): Endogenous opioid peptides: Multiple agonists and receptors. *Nature,* 267:495–499.
20. Martin, W. R. (1967): Opioid antagonists. *Pharmacol. Rev.,* 19:463–521.
21. Martin, W. R., Eades, C. G., Thompson, J. A., Huppler, R. E., and Gilbert, P. E. (1976): The effects of morphine- and nalorphine-like drugs in the nondependent and morphine-dependent chronic spinal dog. *J. Pharmacol. Exp. Ther.,* 197:517–532.
22. Pert, A. (1976): Behavioural pharmacology of D-alanine^2-methionine-enkephalin amide and other long-lasting opiate peptides. In: *Opiates and Endogenous Opioid Peptides,* edited by H. W. Kosterlitz, pp. 87–94. North-Holland, Amsterdam.
23. Pert, A., and Sivit, C. (1977): Neuroanatomical focus for morphine and enkephalin-induced hypermotility. *Nature,* 265:645–647.
24. Roemer, D., Buescher, H. H., Hill, R. C., Pless, J., Bauer, W., Cardinaux, F., Closse, A., Hauser, D., and Huguenin, R. (1977): A synthetic enkephalin with prolonged parenteral and oral analgesic activity. *Nature,* 268:547–549.
25. Rossier, J., Vargo, T. M., Minick, S., Ling, N., Bloom, F. E., and Guillemin, R. (1977): Regional dissociation of β-endorphin and enkephalin contents in rat brain and pituitary. *Proc. Natl. Acad. Sci. USA,* 74:5162–5165.
26. Simantov, R., Kuhar, M. J., Uhl, G. R., and Snyder, S. H. (1977): Opioid peptide enkephalins: Immunohistochemical mapping in the rat central nervous system. *Proc. Natl. Acad. Sci. USA,* 74:2167–2171.
27. Székely, J. I., Rónai, A. Z., Dunai-Kovács, Z., Miglécz, E., Berzétri, I., Bajusz, S., and Gráf, L. (1977): (D-Met^2,Pro^5)-Enkephalin amide: A potent morphine-like analgesic. *Eur. J. Pharmacol.,* 43:293–294.
28. Tseng, L. F., Loh, H. H., and Li, C. H. (1977): Human β-endorphin: Development of tolerance and behavioral activity in rats. *Biochem. Biophys. Res. Commun.,* 74:390–396.
29. Von Graffenried, B., del Pozo, E., Roubicek, J., Krebs, E., Pöldinger, W., Burmeister, P., and Kerp, L. (1978): Effects of the synthetic enkephalin analogue FK 33–824 in man. *Nature,* 272:729–730.
30. Watson, S. J. (1978): Immunocytochemical studies of the endogenous opiate peptides and related substances (*this volume*).

Mechanisms of Pain and Analgesic Compounds,
edited by R. F. Beers, Jr., and E. G. Bassett.
Raven Press, New York © 1979.

19. Release, Biosynthesis, and Metabolism of the Enkephalins

John Hughes

*Department of Biochemistry, Imperial College of Science and Technology,
London SW7 2AZ, England*

INTRODUCTION

The mechanisms involved in catecholamine synthesis, release, and inactivation are perhaps the most clearly understood of all neurotransmitter systems. It was therefore somewhat of a shock to realize that the principles learned as a "catecholaminologist" were perhaps of little avail when applied to putative peptide neurotransmitters. The elucidation of the principles underlying the control of catecholamine synthesis and the discovery of the importance of the catecholamine uptake systems made it possible to advise strategems for determining the physiological activity and importance of the catecholamine systems *in vivo.* However, it is now apparent that a somewhat different approach may be needed for studying a new class of putative neurotransmitters that appear to rival and even exceed the catecholamines in terms of their distribution and possible physiological and pathological importance. These new putative neurotransmitters are the opioid pentapeptides leucine[5]-enkephalin (Leu-enk) and methionine[5]-enkephalin (Met-enk). These were the first opioid peptides to be identified (22) and there is now general agreement that these peptides constitute a major proportion of the opioid-like activity to be found in the brain and spinal cord (21,29,40).

Kosterlitz and Hughes (25) originally proposed that the enkephalins might function as neurotransmitters or neuromodulators. At first there was doubt in some people's minds that the enkephalins were true endogenous ligands for the opiate receptor(s). It was suggested that the pentapeptides might be just proteolytic degradation products of the larger endorphins (12,39); however, the experimental results of several groups do not support this view (21,40,51). Thus, fixation of proteolytic enzymes by microwave irradiation or by formaldehyde perfusion results in an increased yield of brain enkephalins—not a decrease which would be expected if the peptides were artifacts resulting from postmortem proteolysis. It is perhaps of interest, however, that it now seems likely that the two pituitary endorphins, lipotropin$_{61-76}$ and $_{61-77}$ (α- and δ-endorphin) are artifacts arising from limited proteolysis of β-endorphin during the extraction of pituitary tissue (39).

Biochemical and histochemical studies have provided support for the proposed neurotransmitter role of the enkephalins. Subcellular fractionation studies have shown that the peptides are concentrated in the synaptosomal fraction of brain homogenates (19,29,37). Immunofluorescent studies (7,16,36,50) have revealed a widespread system of enkephalin-containing nerves in the brain, spinal cord, and gastrointestinal tract; and colchicine has been employed to demonstrate the existence of numerous groups of enkephalin-containing cells bodies (15). Many of these neurons appear to be interneuron such as in the spinal cord (40) where rhizotomy or cord section does not affect the number of enkephalin-positive fibers. One possible, long Leu-enk-containing pathway has been described however, running from the caudoputamen to the globus pallidus (6). These findings do not, of course, constitute proof for a neurotransmitter role but it is encouraging and of some significance that the antibodies used in the above studies do not lead to a cross-reaction with pituitary endorphins and that recently a quite separate system of β-endorphin-containing neurons has been described in the brain (4). In absolute amounts there appears to be approximately ten times more enkephalin (300 to 400 pmoles/g) than β-endorphin (30 pmoles/ g) in whole brain.

In the following sections the evidence relating to a transmitter function for the enkephalins, particularly in terms of measuring their release and turnover under various physiological and pathological conditions, is discussed. By analogy with the catecholamines, we need to know far more about the biogenesis and metabolism of the enkephalins before we can reliably attempt to study enkephalin turnover *in vivo*.

OBSERVATIONS AND DISCUSSION

Pharmacological Evidence for Enkephalin Neurotransmission

It is not surprising that many attempts to demonstrate a physiological role for the enkephalins have centered round studies on pain perception in man and antinociception in animals. In general, the results have been variable and somewhat difficult to interpret. If endogenous opioids play a role in the modulation of pain processes then it would appear reasonable to assume that opioid antagonists should increase the perception of, or the reaction to, painful stimuli. However, several factors may complicate this experimental strategem. First, the complex nature of pain perception and, in particular, the psychological nature of an individual's response, makes it difficult to devise suitable experimental conditions for obtaining an objective assessment of any change. In this respect it is perhaps easier to measure avoidance or nociceptive reactions but here one is faced with the problem that a major effect of morphine, and by implication the enkephalins, is on the psychological reaction to pain and not on pain thresholds.

Second, there may be alternative pain modulatory systems distinct from the endogenous opioids. The existence of alternate or parallel systems might well nullify the effects of blocking the endogenous opioid system. Despite these provisos, sufficient evidence has been obtained to indicate a role for the endogenous opioids in pain modulation. In a series of carefully designed experiments, Jacob and his co-workers (24,46) have shown that naloxone decreases the pain threshold in mice. These experiments demonstrated that it is important to use naive animals and to carefully adjust for optimal conditions in the hot plate antinociception test. Jacob also found that the effect of naloxone decreased at high dosages, thus making it necessary to observe the effects of a range of doses in order to obtain an optimal effect. Finally, and most importantly, these same workers have shown that the lowering of the pain threshold by opioid antagonists is a stereoselective effect (46).

Our search for the endogenous opiate ligand was considerably stimulated by the observation of Akil and Liebeskind, who showed that stimulation-evoked antinociception in the rat was partially reversed by naloxone. These results have been confirmed and extended (1), and this remains among the most compelling evidence for a sensory modulation role for the endogenous opioids. It has now been reported that naloxone can reverse the analgesic response of brain stimulation in patients (28) and these results correlate with the increase in enkephalin/endorphin levels in the cerebrospinal fluid of such patients (see later section).

There have been very few other studies on the *in vivo* effects of naloxone in systems not concerned with sensory perception/analgesia. However, naloxone has been reported to enhance spinal reflexes in cats (3,11) and to inhibit the release of prolactin and growth hormone from rat pituitary gland (8).

The results of *in vitro* studies with naloxone have been more consistent than the *in vivo* studies. This is possibly due to the fact that in the former, experimental conditions are more easily controlled and that a considerable range of stimuli may be employed for obtaining optimal conditions. The high concentration of enkephalins in the guinea pig ileum (21) and their localization in nerve fibers (7) has made this a very suitable model for studying enkephalin neurotransmission. Van Neuten et al. (47) originally showed that the fatigue induced by repetitive peristalsis in the guinea pig ileum could be reversed on addition of naloxone. These are possibly the most physiological conditions yet employed for demonstrating an effect of naloxone. Normally, electrically evoked single twitches of the guinea pig ileum are not affected by naloxone, provided the tissue is in good condition and supramaximal stimuli are employed. However, Waterfield and Kosterlitz (49) were able to show that naloxone increases both the spontaneous and electrically evoked output of acetylcholine from this tissue. Presumably, naloxone does not normally increase the size of the mechanical response because the output of acetylcholine is already sufficient to evoke a maximal response. These same workers also showed that the enhancement of acetylcholine release was a stereospecific effect.

It is possible to demonstrate an effect of naloxone on the mechanical response to nerve stimulation in the guinea pig ileum. Puig et al. (32) showed that single evoked twitches of this tissue were inhibited by a period of high-frequency stimulation. Naloxone and stereoselective opiate antagonists could partially prevent this inhibition of the single twitches. We have confirmed this effect (19) and provided evidence that the inhibition is probably not due to a large release of enkephalin into the bathing medium, but possibly involves the repetitive firing of enkephalin nerve units.

Naloxone has also been shown to increase the potassium-evoked release of norepinephrine from isolated slices of rat occipital cortex (44) and it is likely that other isolated brain preparations will prove useful for studying this type of effect, since the enkephalins have been shown to inhibit the release of acetylcholine and dopamine (43), as well as norepinephrine.

STUDIES ON ENKEPHALIN RELEASE

In Vivo Studies

A number of investigations have been carried out on human patients in an attempt to correlate cerebrospinal fluid levels of opioid peptides with various physiological or pathological states. Terenius and his co-workers (45) have made the most extensive studies to date. They have used the opiate receptor binding assay to show that opioid peptide levels in the lumbar cerebrospinal fluid increase during intracerebral electrical stimulation or during electroacupuncture. Unfortunately, the chemical nature of the opioid material detected in these studies is not known. Terenius considers that the opioid material has a MW of approximately 1,200 and is not identical to any known sequence of β-lipotropin. This material may, in fact, be similar to the ϵ-endorphin described by Hughes et al. (21).

Our studies (2) are in general agreement with those of Terenius' group. Thus, there are barely detectable levels of opioid material in normal cerebrospinal fluid (0.5 to 2 pmoles/ml of Met-enk equivalents) but this increases significantly some 0.5 to 1 hr after electrial stimulation with electrodes implanted at a site near the posterior aspect of the third ventricle medial to the nucleus parafascicularis. However, our studies indicate that the opioid in question is Met-enk or a very closely allied peptide since there was good correlation between three independent methods of assay: bioassay on the mouse vas deferens, opiate receptor assay, and radioimmunoassay with Met-enk antibodies. Interestingly, both our results and those of Terenius yield very similar quantitative values although it is quite possible that this is fortuitous and that Terenius is studying a quite different peptide that is also released into the cerebrospinal fluid during electroanalgesia.

In collaboration with Dr. J. Miles of Liverpool, we have also assayed cerebrospinal fluid samples from patients receiving alcohol injections into the pituitary. This procedure gives very good pain relief (partially destroying the pituitary and ventral hypothalamus in the process) but, unlike brain stimulation, there is no corresponding rise in opioid levels. Obviously further work is required to identify the nature of the opioid material in the cerebrospinal fluid. The existence of other unidentified endorphins will, if confirmed, complicate the interpretation of the relationship between stimulation-produced analgesia and the enkephalins.

Changes in Content of Brain Enkephalins

In general one would not expect to obtain much information from studies on tissue content of enkephalins unless it was possible to specifically block synthesis or metabolism so as to obtain an estimate of turnover (see later section). Total brain content of enkephalin does show a diurnal rhythm (8). Chronic or acute treatment with morphine, naloxone, or physostigmine does not significantly alter brain enkephalin levels (19). However, Hong et al. (17) have found that chronic treatment with cataleptogenic antipsychotics such as haloperidol causes a significant (up to twofold) increase in the Met-enk content of the neostriatum, globus pallidus, and nucleus accumbens of rats. A similar effect was noted after chronic treatment with lithium (10). Enkephalin levels in the hypothalamus and hindbrain were not altered by these drugs. This drug-induced effect of tissue content may prove to be a useful tool for probing enkephalinergic mechanisms but it is not known at present whether the effect reflects a change in the biogenesis or release of enkephalin.

In Vitro Release of Enkephalins

One of the major criteria for establishing a neurotransmitter role for the enkephalins has now been met, namely, the direct demonstration of a calcium-dependent release of enkephalin from neuronal stores in response to depolarizing stimuli. Most of the experiments to date have employed isolated preparations of the striatum or globus pallidus, tissues that are extremely rich in enkephalin. We initially showed that synaptosomal preparations of striatum (38) release enkephalin into the superfusate when exposed to 50 mM potassium. In these experiments, the basal release of enkephalin, measured by bioassay, was between 0.1% to 0.2% of the total tissue content per 15 min period. In the presence of 50 mM potassium and 2.54 mM calcium there was a release of some 1.9% of the total tissue content in 15 min. This potassium-evoked release increased to 4.4% in the presence of 5.08 mM calcium and lessened to 0.6% in the absence of calcium. No attempt was made to prevent metabolism of enkephalin in these experiments and it is likely that the release was, in fact, much greater.

The potassium-evoked release of enkephalin has also been shown with perfused slices of rat striatum (30) or rat globus pallidus (23). Both of these studies showed that the potassium-induced release was calcium dependent. Iversen et al. (23) used bacitracin to block the proteolytic breakdown of enkephalin and found that $9.6 \pm 1.8\%$ of the total tissue content was released during a 6-min exposure to potassium, but release was significantly less in the absence of bacitracin.

We selected veratridine as a depolarizing stimulus in our studies on isolated, superfused slices of guinea pig striatum (14), since this is a more specific agent than potassium. However, in the absence of enzyme inhibitors, the release of enkephalin was small and variable. It was found that less than 50% of added exogenous enkephalin could be recovered from the superfusion system. Addition of the dipeptides Tyr-Tyr, Leu-Leu and Leu-Gly (0.1 mM each) to the medium increased the recovery of added enkephalin from 47 to 97%. Under these conditions we could demonstrate a reproducible, tetrodoxin-sensitive release of Met-enk and Leu-enk (Fig. 1); the chemical identity of the enkephalins was confirmed by chromatography. It was found that veratridine released Met-enk and Leu-enk in the same proportions as that found in the tissue stories. Osborne et al.

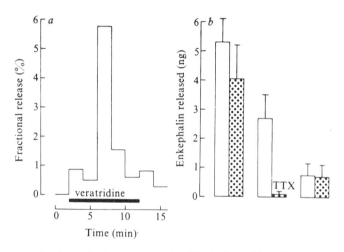

FIG. 1. Release of enkephalin from guinea pig striatal slices. The slices were superfused (1.1 ml/min) for 45 min with Krebs solution at 36°C and gassed with 95% O_2 and 5% CO_2. **a:** 600-μm thick sagittal sections from two striata weighing approximately 300 mg were exposed to veratridine (50 μM) for 10 min. The superfusate was collected at 2-min intervals. Fractional release refers to the total enkephalin activity (assayed as Met-enkephalin) released into the superfusate expressed as a percentage of the tissue content. **b:** 450-μm thick sagittal sections from one striatum weighing approximately 150 mg were exposed to veratridine (50 μm) for 3 min every 30 min. The superfusate was collected for 12 min from the start of veratridine exposure. The open columns represent the output of enkephalin on three successive exposures to veratridine. The stippled columns represent the output of enkephalin from tissues in which the second exposure to veratridine was made in the presence of 1.6 μM tetrodotoxin (TTX). All outputs were assayed as Met-enkephalin. Each column represents the means from three experiments, the vertical bar indicating SEM. In both **a** and **b**, Leu-Leu, Tyr-Tyr, and Leu-Gly (each 1 mM) were present in the superfusing fluid for 5 min before exposure to veratridine and throughout the collection periods. All samples (superfusate and tissues) were chromatographed on only Amberlite CG-400 and XAD-2 columns with a recovery of 90 to 100%. No attempt was made to separate Leu-enkephalin from Met-enkephalin. (From Henderson et al., ref. 14.)

(30), using specific antisera for detecting the two peptides, also concluded that both Leu-enk and Met-enk were released by potassium.

We have also performed experiments to check that the source of the enkephalin released from brain slices is not due to the extracellular cleavage of a larger endorphin. We found no evidence for a significant conversion of α- or β-endorphin to Met-enk when the endorphins were added to the superfusion system.

Iversen et al. (23) noted a marked loss (up to 60%) of the enkephalin content of the globus pallidus during a 40-min superfusion. This was not observed in experiments on striatal slices (14,30). The reason for this is unclear but it may be that the globus pallidus is not such a suitable preparation as the striatum for long-term release studies. We have also noted that transverse slices of striatum were distinctly inferior to sagittal sections for enkephalin release studies. It may be that it is important to maintain an intact cell body-axonal unit in these studies; at present, there is little information as to the anatomy of enkephalin pathways, although one caudatoputamen-globus pallidus pathway has been described.

Biogenesis of Enkephalins

Studies with insulin, parathyroid hormone (42), and the neurohypophyseal hormones (9) have shown that peptide hormones and neurohormones are derived from the proteolytic cleavage of larger prohormones that are formed by RNA-directed ribosomal synthesis. The most detailed studies on neuronal peptides have been carried out with oxytoxin and vasopressin (9). It has been shown that after injection of labeled amino acids into the supraoptic nucleus, there is an initial synthesis of large precursors in the cell bodies, followed by the gradual conversion (within 1 to 2 hr) to vasopressin and oxytoxin. This conversion proceeds by way of intermediate size precursors as the secretory granules are transported along the magnocellular neuron.

The presence of the Met-enk sequence at residues 61 to 65 of β-lipotropin was originally adduced as evidence for a similar process for the elaboration of the enkephalins. Indeed, it has now been shown that a large molecular weight (31,000) protein is present in the pituitary (27) and brain (35) and which contains the sequences of both lipotropin and adrenocorticotropic hormone. However, if lipotropin or β-endorphin are intermediates in the biogenesis of Met-enk, then it is likely that they are short-lived since the immunochemical localization of these larger peptides does not correspond to that of the enkephalin-containing neurons (4,51). Unidentified opioid peptides larger than enkephalin have been detected in extracts of striatum (38) or globus pallidus (53) and these may well be intermediates in the formation of enkephalin.

In general, it appears that the production of very large precursor proteins allows the rapid and efficient transfer of ribosomal products to the Golgi apparatus for packaging. The life of the initial translation products is quite short (30 to 60 min) and further conversion to the final product may require a similar period of time. An interesting point is that a peptidergic neuron may well contain, within the secretory granules, several cleavage products from the original precursor (9). Some, like neurophysin, may have a role in the storage of the biologically active neurohormone, but survival of these cleavage products means that they too may be released from nerve terminals with the other granule contents.

We have obtained direct evidence that Leu-enk and Met-enk are derived from the products of ribosomal protein synthesis (18,41). Incorporation of ^{3}H-tyrosine into the enkephalins was studied in isolated preparations of the guinea pig myenteric plexus and slices of guinea pig striatum. The peptides were purified to radiochemical homogeneity by high pressure liquid chromatography and thin layer chromatography. The results from the two tissues were very similar. A linear incorporation of ^{3}H-tyrosine into both enkephalins was only observed after an initial lag period of 1 to 2 hr following incubation with the labeled amino acid. The incorporation of ^{3}H-tyrosine could be prevented when protein synthesis inhibitors such as cycloheximide or puromycin were included in the incubation medium during the labeling period. Cycloheximide or puromycin had little or no effect when added after the initial lag period, indicating a specific effect on ribosomal synthesis. The rate of incorporation of ^{3}H-tyrosine into Met-enk was much more rapid than that of Leu-enk. In both tissues, the incorporation of ^{3}H-tyrosine was linear with time between 2 to 6 hr after the initial labeling period and, indeed, it continued linearly with time up to 12 hr in the myenteric plexus.

In our experiments the lag period of 1 to 2 hr must represent the time taken for the labeled amino acid to be chased through the intermediate precursor stage. Whether this also represents the time taken for transport from the cell body to the nerve terminal cannot yet be determined, since the biochemical analysis includes all the components of the neuron.

There is still no information regarding the identity of the precursor for Leu-enk, although our experiments suggest that there must be one, since both Leu-enk and Met-enk are products of protein synthesis. The lower rate of Leu-enk synthesis presumably reflects the generally lower concentration of this peptide compared to Met-enk in tissue stores. Biochemical studies have shown (21,40) that the proportions of Leu-enk and Met-enk vary considerably in different brain areas, but it has not been possible to demonstrate separate Met-enk- and Leu-enk-containing neurons by histochemical techniques. It seems most unlikely that Leu-enk is an error of gene expression and, indeed, this peptide is the major enkephalin present in cow brain (40). It is possible that Leu-enk derives from a vestigial mechanism not entirely discarded when evolutionary processes selected one of two possible enkephalin peptides. This could occur if there was a common precursor to both enkephalins and the cleavage enzymes were not entirely specific for the Met-enk precursor. Nevertheless, Leu-enk has a different pharmacological profile than that of Met-enk and I consider it more likely that Leu-enk has a separate and specific biological role of its own.

A consequence of the mechanisms underlying enkephalin biogenesis is that cell body synthesis is the only source for replenishment of nerve ending stores. It is most unlikely that neuronal reuptake or local nerve ending synthesis exist as for the biogenic amines. At present, we have no information as to whether the enkephalin neuron can respond rapidly to an increased turnover of peripheral stores. Further, since opiate activity is retained, although to a lesser degree, on extension of the C-terminal sequence of enkephalin, then it is possible that under extreme physiological activity or pathological conditions larger and biologically active precursors of the enkephalins could be released from immature or metabolically deficient secretory granules. This may have implications in the etiology of certain behavioral dysfunctions; Terenius (45) has discussed the evidence for the involvement of endorphins in certain psychiatric disease states.

CONCLUDING REMARKS

The weight of evidence at present supports the view that the enkephalins function as neurotransmitters in the central and peripheral nervous system. Further advances in our knowledge of the physiology of these peptides will no doubt be obtained from studies on enkephalin turnover and release. It seems unlikely that really specific inhibitors of enkephalin biosynthesis or breakdown will become available in the near future. For example, metabolism of the enkephalins proceeds primarily through N-terminal cleavage of tyrosine by an aminopeptidase(s) that appears to have a wide regional and subcellular distribution (13). Also, an efficient inactivation can occur via C-terminal hydrolysis. The development of specific inhibitors for these processes is a daunting prospect.

It is possible to inhibit enkephalin biosynthesis with cycloheximide or puromycin, and we have used this effect to estimate enkephalin turnover in the guinea pig myenteric plexus (20). Intracerebral injection of puromycin also markedly reduces the endogenous brain content of the enkephalins. However, this approach cannot be used to estimate turnover *in vivo* because of the many side effects associated with the use of protein synthesis inhibitors. We are presently developing methods for following enkephalin turnover *in vivo* by following the incorporation of labeled amino acids into the peptides. However, an accurate assessment of enkephalin turnover will depend on a full knowledge of the precursor product relationship.

ACKNOWLEDGMENTS

I wish to thank my colleagues H. W. Kosterlitz, A. T. McKnight, and R. P. Sosa for their collaboration and advice. The experiments described in this paper were carried out with the aid of grants from the National Institute on Drug Abuse (to H. W. Kosterlitz) and from the Medical Research Council (to J. Hughes and H. W. Kosterlitz).

REFERENCES

1. Akil, H., Mayer, D. J., and Liebeskind, J. C. (1976): Antagonism of stimulation produced analgesia by naloxone, a narcotic antagonist. *Science,* 191:961–962.
2. Akil, H., Richardson, D. E., Hughes, J., and Barchas, J. D. (1978): Enkephalin-like material in ventricular cerebrospinal fluid of pain patients after analgetic focal stimulation. *Science,* 201:463–465.
3. Bell, J. A., and Martin, W. R. (1977): The effects of narcotic antagonists, naloxone, naltrexone and nalorphine on spinal cord C-fibre reflexes evoked by electrical stimulation of radiant heat. *Eur. J. Pharmacol.,* 42:147–154.
4. Bloom, F., Battenberg, E., Rossier, J., Ling, N., and Guillemin, R. (1978): Neurons containing β-endorphin in rat brain exist separately from those containing enkephalin: Immunocytochemical studies. *Proc. Natl. Acad. Sci. USA,* 75:1591–1595.
5. Cocchi, D., Santagostino, A., Gil-Ad, I., Ferri, S., and Müller, E. E. (1977): Leu-enkephalin-stimulated growth hormone and prolactin release in the rat: comparison with the effect of morphine. *Life Sci.,* 20:2041–2045.
6. Cuello, A. C., and Paximos, G. (1978): Evidence for long Leu-enkephalin striopallidal pathway in rat brain. *Nature,* 271:178–180.
7. Elde, R., Hökfelt, T., Johansson, O., and Terenius, L. (1976): Immunohistochemical studies using antibodies to leucine-enkephalin: Initial observations on the nervous system of the rat. *Neuroscience,* 1:349–351.
8. Frederickson, R. C. A. (1977): Enkephalin pentapeptides: A review of current evidence for a physiological role in vertebrate neurotransmission. *Life Sci.,* 21:23–42.
9. Gainer, H., Sarne, Y., and Brownstein, M. J. (1977): Biosynthesis and axonal transport of rat neurohypophysial proteins and peptides. *J. Cell Biol.,* 73:366–381.
10. Gillin, J. C., Hong, J. S., Yang, H-Y. T., and Costa, E. (1978): Met^5-enkephalin content in brain regions of rat treated with lithium. *Proc. Natl. Acad. Sci. USA,* 75:2991–2993.
11. Goldfarb, J., and Hu, J. W. (1976): Enhancement of reflexes by naloxone in spinal cats. *Neuropharmacology,* 15:785–792.
12. Goldstein, A. G., (1976): Opioid peptides (endorphins) in pituitary and brain. *Science,* 193:1081–1086.
13. Hambrook, J. M., Morgan, B. A., Rance, M. J., and Smith, C. F. C. (1976): Mode of deactivation of the enkephalins by rat and human plasma and rat brain homogenates. *Nature,* 262:782–784.
14. Henderson, G., Hughes, J., and Kosterlitz, H. W. (1978): *In vitro* release of Leu- and Met-enkephalin from the corpus striatum. *Nature,* 271:677–679.
15. Hökfelt, T., Elde, R., Johansson, O., Terenius, L., and Stein, L. (1977): The distribution of enkephalin-immunoreactive cell bodies in the rat central nervous system. *Neuroscience Lett.,* 5:25–31.
16. Hökfelt, T., Ljungdahl, A., Terenius, L., Elde, R., and Nilsson, G. (1977): Immunohistochemical analysis of peptide pathways possibly related to pain and analgesia: enkephalin and substance P. *Proc. Natl. Acad. Sci. USA,* 74:3081–3085.
17. Hong, J. S., Yang, H-Y. T., Fratta, W., and Costa, E. (1978): Rat striatal methionine-enkephalin content after chronic treatment with cataleptogenic and non-cataleptogenic anti-schizophrenic drugs. *J. Pharmacol. Exp. Ther. (in press).*
18. Hughes, J., Kosterlitz, H. W., and McKnight, A. T. (1978): The incorporation of ^{3}H-tyrosine into the enkephalins of striatal slices of guinea-pig brain. *Br. J. Pharmacol.,* 63:396P.
19. Hughes, J., Kosterlitz, H. W., McKnight, A. T., Sosa, R. P., Lord, J. A. H., and Waterfield, A. A. (1978): Pharmacological and biochemical aspects of the enkephalins. In: *Centrally Acting Peptides,* edited by J. Hughes, pp. 179–193. Macmillan Press, London.
20. Hughes, J., Kosterlitz, H. W., and Sosa, R. P. (1978): Enkephalin release from the myenteric plexus of the guinea-pig small intestine in the presence of cycloheximide. *Br. J. Pharmacol.,* 63:397P.
21. Hughes, J., Kosterlitz, H. W., and Smith, T. W. (1977): The distribution of methionine-enkephalin and leucine-enkephalin in the brain and peripheral tissues. *Br. J. Pharmacol.,* 61:639–647.
22. Hughes, J., Smith, T. W., Kosterlitz, H. W., Fothergill, L. A., Morgan, B. A., and Morris, H. R. (1975): Identification of two related pentapeptides from the brain with potent opiate agonist activity. *Nature,* 258:577–579.

23. Iversen, L. L., Iversen, S. D., Bloom, F. E., Vargo, T., and Guillemin, R. (1978): Release of enkephalin from rat globus pallidus *in vitro. Nature,* 271:679–681.
24. Jacob, J. J., Tremblay, E. C., and Colombel, M. C. (1974): Facilitation de réactions nociceptive par la naloxone chez la souris et chez le rat. *Psychopharmacologia,* 37:217–223.
25. Kosterlitz, H. W., and Hughes, J. (1975): Some thoughts on the significance of enkephalin, the endogenous ligand. *Life Sci.,* 17:91–96.
26. Levine, J. D., Gordon, N. C., Jones, R. T., and Fields, H. L. (1978): The narcotic antagonist naloxone enhances clinical pain. *Nature,* 272:826–827.
27. Mains, R. E., Eipper, B. A., and Ling, N. (1977): Common precursor to corticotropins and endorphins. *Proc. Natl. Acad. Sci. USA,* 74:3014–3018.
28. Mayer, D. J., Price, D. D., and Rafii, A. (1977): Antagonism of acupuncture analgesia in man by the narcotic antagonist naloxone. *Brain Res.,* 121:368–372.
29. Osborne, H., Höllt, V., and Herz, A. (1978): Subcellular distribution of enkephalins and endogenous opioid activity in rat brain. *Life Sci.,* 22:611–618.
30. Osborne, H., Höllt, V., and Herz, A. (1978): Potassium-induced release of enkephalins from rat striatal slices. *Eur. J. Pharmacol.,* 48:219–221.
31. Pomeranz, B., and Chiu, D. (1976): Naloxone blockade of acupuncture analgesia: endorphin implicated. *Life Sci.,* 19:1757–1762.
32. Puig, M. M., Gascon, P., Craviso, G. L., and Musacchio, J. M. (1977): Endogenous opiate receptor ligand: electrically induced release in the guinea pig ileum. *Science,* 195:419–420.
33. Rossier, J., Vargo, T. M., Minick, S., Ling, N., Bloom, F. E., and Guillemin, R. (1977): Regional dissociation of β-endorphin and enkephalin contents in rat brain and pituitary. *Proc. Natl. Acad. Sci. USA,* 74:5162–5165.
34. Rubinstein, M., Stein, S., and Udenfriend, S. (1977): Isolation and characterisation of the opioid peptides from rat pituitary: β-endorphin. *Proc. Natl. Acad. Sci. USA,* 74:4969–4972.
35. Rubinstein, M., Stein, S., and Udenfriend, S. (1978): Characterization of pro-opiocortin, a precursor to opioid peptides and corticotropin. *Proc. Natl. Acad. Sci. USA,* 75:669–671.
36. Simantov, R., Kuhar, M. J., Uhl, G. R., and Snyder, S. H. (1977): Opioid peptide enkephalin: immunohistochemical mapping in rat central nervous system. *Proc. Natl. Acad. Sci. USA,* 74:2167–2171.
37. Simantov, R., Snowman, A. M., and Snyder, S. H. (1976): A morphine like factor 'enkephalin' in rat brain: subcellular location. *Brain Res.,* 107:650–657.
38. Smith, T. W., Hughes, J., Kosterlitz, H. W., and Sosa, R. P. (1976): Enkephalins: isolation, distribution and function. In: *Opiates and Endogenous Opioid Peptides,* edited by H. W. Kosterlitz, pp. 57–62. Elsevier/North Holland, Amsterdam.
39. Smyth, D. G., and Snell, C. R. (1977): Metabolism of the analgesic peptide lipotropin C-fragment in rat striatal slices. *FEBS Lett.,* 78:225–228.
40. Snyder, S. H., Uhl, G. R., and Kuhar, M. J. (1978): Comparative features of enkephalin and neurotensin in the mammalian central nervous system. In: *Centrally Acting Peptides,* edited by J. Hughes, pp. 85–97. Macmillan, London.
41. Sosa, R. P., McKnight, A. T., Hughes, J., and Kosterlitz, H. W. (1977): Incorporation of labelled amino acids into the enkephalins. *FEBS Lett.,* 84:195–198.
42. Steiner, D. F., (1976): Peptide hormone precursors: Biosynthesis processing and significance. In: *Peptide Hormones,* edited by J. A. Parsons, pp. 49–64. Macmillan, London.
43. Subramanian, N., Mitznegg, P., Sprügel, W., Domschke, W., Domschke, S., Wünsch, E., and Demling, L. (1977): Influence of enkephalin on K⁺-evoked efflux of putative neurotransmitters in rat brain. Selective inhibition of acetylcholine and dopamine release. *Naunyn-Schmiedebergs Arch. Pharmacol.,* 299:163–165.
44. Taube, H. D., Borowski, E., Endo, T., and Starke, K. (1976): Enkephalin, a potential modulator of noradrenaline release in rat brain. *Eur. J. Pharmacol.,* 38:377–380.
45. Terenius, L., and Wahlström, A. (1978): Physiological and clinical relevance of endorphins. In: *Centrally Acting Peptides,* edited by J. Hughes, pp. 161–178. Macmillan, London.
46. Tremblay, E., Colombel, M. C., and Jacob, J. J. (1976): Précipitation et prévention de l'abstinence chez le rat et chez la souris en etat de dépendance aiguë. Comparison de la naloxone, de la naltrexone et de la diprenorphine. *Psychopharm. Bull.,* 49:41–48.
47. Van Neuten, J. M., Janssen, P. A. J., and Fontaine, J. (1976): Unexpected reversal effects of naloxone on the guinea pig ileum. *Life Sci.,* 18:803–808.
48. Van Vugt, D. A., Bruni, J. F., and Meites, J. (1978): Naloxone inhibition of stress-induced increase in prolactin secretion. *Life Sci.,* 22:85–90.

49. Waterfield, A. A. and Kosterlitz, H. W. (1975): Stereospecific increase by narcotic agonists of evoked acetylcholine output in the guinea-pig ileum. *Life Sci.,* 16:1787–1792.
50. Watson, S. J., Akil, H., Sullivan, S. and Barchas, J. D. (1977): Immunocytochemical localization of methionine enkephalin: preliminary observation. *Life Sci.,* 21:733–738.
51. Watson, S. J., Barchas, J. C. and Li, C. H. (1977): β-Lipotropin: Localization of cells and axons in rat brain by immunocytochemistry. *Proc. Natl. Acad. Sci. USA,* 74:5155–5158.
52. Yang, H-Y. T., Hong, J. S. and Costa, E. (1977): Regional distribution of Leu- and Met-enkephalin in rat brain. *Neuropharmacology,* 16:303–307.
53. Yang, H-Y. T., Fratta, W., Hong, J. S., DiGiulio, A. M. and Costa, E. (1978): Detection of two endorphin like peptides in nucleus caudatus. *Neuropharmacology,* 17:433–438.

Mechanisms of Pain and Analgesic Compounds,
edited by R. F. Beers, Jr., and E. G. Bassett.
Raven Press, New York © 1979.

20. Anatomy of the Endogenous Opioid Peptides and Related Substances: The Enkephalins, β-Endorphin, β-Lipotropin, and ACTH

Stanley J. Watson* and Jack D. Barchas

Department of Psychiatry and Behavioral Sciences, Stanford University School of Medicine, Stanford, California 94305

INTRODUCTION

Specific information on the endogenous opiate peptides has come rapidly over the last few years. Soon after Hughes et al. (14) described the structure of the enkephalins (the methionine and leucine forms), there were several reports of the existence of other opiate peptides derived from the C-terminus of β-lipotropin (β-LPH) (5,7,19,32). Both the enkephalins and the C-fragment of β-LPH [also known as β-endorphin (β-end)] have been shown to exhibit many of the pharmacological properties of opiates (2,6,10,40–42). In this report we shall summarize our current anatomical knowledge of the two brain opioid systems: the enkephalins and β-end. We shall attempt to emphasize primarily those anatomical features which appear critical for a better understanding of pain transmission and modulation.

OBSERVATIONS AND DISCUSSION

Enkephalins

Concurrent with the demonstration of opiate activity for enkephalins and β-LPH fragments, there arose a major question about the relationship between methionine-enkephalin (Met-enk) and β-end. Since the full structure of Met-enk was present at the N-terminus of β-end, it was suggested that they both derived from the same system in the brain or in the pituitary. As the active form in the brain had not been determined, it was hypothesized that Met-enk was a breakdown product of β-end, or alternatively that β-end was the precursor of Met-enk. Soon after these questions were raised, Elde et al. (8) demonstrated enkephalin-positive neurons in rat brain. Other enkephalin immunocytochemical studies were carried out by several laboratories (11,12,15,16,28,29,33,37). The

---

* Present address: Mental Health Research Institute, University of Michigan School of Medicine, Ann Arbor, Michigan 48109.

results of these studies were in remarkable agreement, showing that enkephalin was found in small faint cells and beaded fibers throughout the brainstem (Figs. 1 and 2). More thorough visualization of enkephalin cells required the use of colchicine (11,12,16,28,33) or vinblastine (15). From a structural point of view, it was apparent that these enkephalin cells and fibers in the brain exhibited the synthesis and storage characteristics of neuromodulators. There seemed little anatomical support for enkephalin as exclusively the breakdown product of β-end. Rather, a role of enkephalin as a putative neurotransmitter appeared more likely. The general outline of the enkephalin system can be seen in Fig. 3. In general, enkephalin cells are seen in many nuclei ranging from the spinal cord throughout the medulla, pons, and midbrain to limbic structures and striatum.

Of particular interest are the areas with enkephalin fibers and cells potentially associated with the action of plant opiates. For example, the cells in laminae I, II, and V and in the trigeminal system are well positioned for modulating some of the morphine analgesia seen in these structures. Other pain-related enkephalin sites would seem to be the lateral reticular n., raphe pontis, and magnus, and periaqueductal central gray area. The n. parabrachilis is reported to be involved in respiration and has many enkephalin cells and fibers. More rostrally, in the dorsal medial aspect of the thalamus (periventricular n.), there is a heavy concentration of enkephalin fibers. This general region has been associated with analgesia and opiate addiction and withdrawal (30,34).

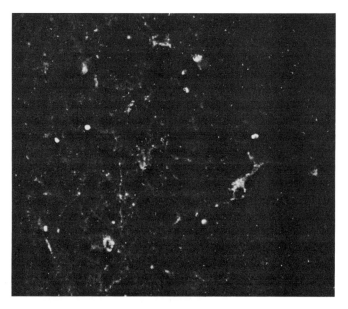

FIG. 1. Leu-enk-positive cell in the anterior hypothalamus. Note unstained nucleus and beaded enkephalin fibers. Section from a colchicine pretreated (50 μg i.c.v., 48 hr prior to sacrifice) adult rat. Dark field fluorescein preparation, ×120.

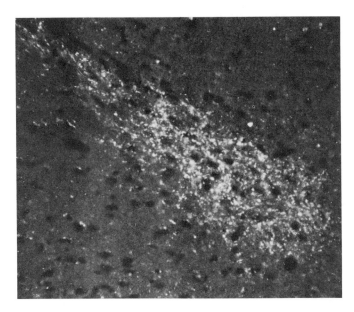

FIG. 2. Met-enk-positive fiber bundle extending from the midthalamus toward the lateral thalamic n. Section from a normal rat. Dark field fluorescein preparation, ×100.

IMMUNOCYTOCHEMISTRY OF ENKEPHALIN CELLS

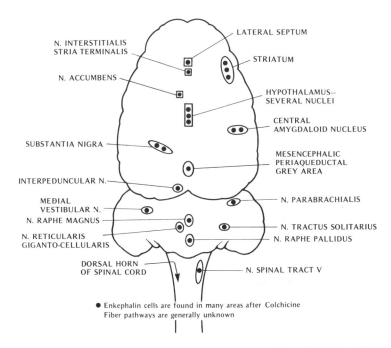

N. INTERSTITIALIS STRIA TERMINALIS

N. ACCUMBENS

SUBSTANTIA NIGRA

INTERPEDUNCULAR N.

MEDIAL VESTIBULAR N.

N. RAPHE MAGNUS

N. RETICULARIS GIGANTO-CELLULARIS

DORSAL HORN OF SPINAL CORD

LATERAL SEPTUM

STRIATUM

HYPOTHALAMUS— SEVERAL NUCLEI

CENTRAL AMYGDALOID NUCLEUS

MESENCEPHALIC PERIAQUEDUCTAL GREY AREA

N. PARABRACHIALIS

N. TRACTUS SOLITARIUS

N. RAPHE PALLIDUS

N. SPINAL TRACT V

● Enkephalin cells are found in many areas after Colchicine
Fiber pathways are generally unknown

FIG. 3. Horizontal schematic illustration of enkephalin-positive cells in the rat brain.

The many enkephalin-positive structures in the hypothalamus are correlated with certain endocrine control areas. Motor systems are also heavily invested with enkephalin neurons. The caudate seems to contain enkephalin cells, whereas the globus pallidus has extremely dense terminal fields. Finally, the enkephalins are well situated in limbic structures for possible control of affective state and mood. There are large enkephalin cells in the septum with fibers near the lateral ventricle. The n. accumbens and amygdala are also heavily invested with enkephalin cells and fibers. Thus, the distribution of the enkephalins appears to correlate well with many of the effects associated with plant opiates: analgesia, respiratory depression, tolerance, endocrine changes, motor effects, and modification of affect.

β-LPH and β-end

While the hypothesis of Met-enk as a breakdown product had become less tenable, the possibility that β-end merely served as its precursor in brain remained viable. Simultaneously, several groups were able to demonstrate the presence of β-end-like immunoreactivity (3,35) and β-LPH-like immunoreactivity (18, 38,43) in rat brain, utilizing β-LPH and antiserum provided by Dr. C. H. Li.

Surprisingly, these studies refuted the second hypothesis, by showing that β-end had a unique distribution, quite distinct from Met-enk, and was therefore

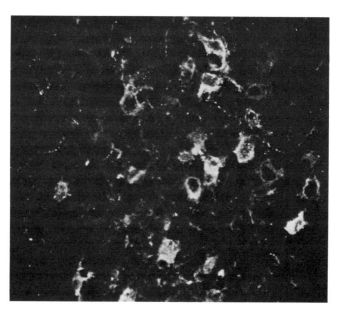

FIG. 4. β-End-positive cells in the periarcuate region of the rat hypothalamus; note the unstained nuclei. Colchicine pretreated as in Fig. 1. Dark field fluorescein preparation, ×120.

not just a precursor of enkephalin. The anatomical studies of β-LPH and β-end were in agreement in describing a system with a single major cell group in the periarcuate region of the hypothalamus (Fig. 4) with a very widespread fiber system. These β-LPH/β-end fibers were visualized mainly in the medial hypothalamus (Fig. 5), amygdala, basal septal nuclei, n. accumbens, periventricular thalamus, periaqueductal central gray area (Fig. 6), and locus coeruleus (Fig. 7). There were major differences between this system and the enkephalins. For example, very sparse β-LPH/β-end activity was seen in the central amygdala, striatum, and lateral septum, whereas enkephalin was abundant in these areas. On the other hand, the β-LPH/β-end cells were in the arcuate region of the hypothalamus where there were relatively few enkephalin fibers and no major enkephalin cell concentrations. Yet the possibility remained that the β-LPH/β-end system was somehow a part of the enkephalin system. Rossier et al. (27) carried out a study demonstrating that enkephalin and β-end were found in different ratios across brain regions. In further support of the differences between the enkephalin and β-end systems, we have carried out several lesions demonstrating differential effects on β-LPH and Met-enk in two brain areas (36). A unilateral hypothalamic lesion (aimed at β-LPH cells) produced a significant decrease in β-LPH but not in Met-enk in both the hypothalamus and midbrain. On the other hand, a lesion in the periaqueductal central gray produced

FIG. 5. β-End-positive fibers in the paraventricular n. of the hypothalamus. Colchicine pretreated as in Fig. 1. These fibers are easily visible without such pretreatment. Dark field fluorescein preparation, ×120.

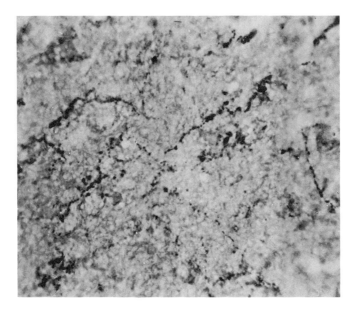

FIG. 6. β-LPH-positive fibers in the periaqueductal central gray area of normal rat; note the fine beaded appearance. Light field peroxidase preparation, ×200.

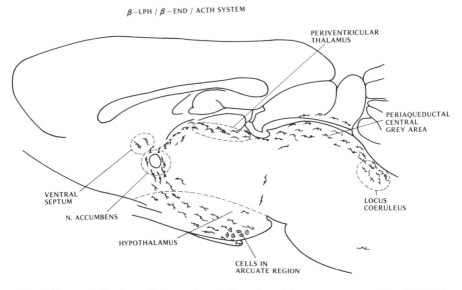

FIG. 7. Parasagittal schematic illustration of the cell and fiber system containing β-LPH/β-end/ACTH in rat brain. Cells are found near the arcuate n. with fibers distributed widely in the brainstem.

a modest decrease in midbrain β-LPH and a major decrease in Met-enk; in the hypothalamus Met-enk was also decreased but β-LPH was unchanged. Thus, in anatomical, biochemical, and lesion studies the enkephalins and β-LPH/β-end seem to be located in separate neuronal pools. To date there is no example of cellular overlap between the two systems. It is quite possible, however, that Met-enk is synthesized from β-LPH and β-end, but that these two longer peptides are rapidly cleared and are only present in enkephalin neurons briefly and in small quantities.

ACTH, β-LPH, and β-end

In pituitary studies of β-LPH, Moon et al. (23) demonstrated that β-LPH was located in the corticotrophs of the anterior lobe and all the cells of the intermediate lobe. Bloom et al. (4) subsequently visualized β-end in the same two cell groups. In an electron microscopic study of the pituitary, Pelletier (24) showed that β-LPH and ACTH were located in the same cells and granules. This, along with evidence suggesting the covariation in pituitary β-LPH, MSH, and ACTH, led to the elegant studies of Mains et al. (21) and Roberts and Herbert (26), who demonstrated that pituitary ACTH and β-LPH (and therefore β-end) share a common 31,000-dalton precursor. The same biosynthetic pattern for β-LPH, β-end, and ACTH has not yet been demonstrated in the brain. However, there is evidence supporting the hypothesis of a common 31,000-dalton precursor in the brain as well as in the pituitary. At about the same time that β-end (3,35) and β-LPH (38,43) were visualized in brain, Krieger et al. (17) demonstrated ACTH-like immunoreactivity in brain extracts. It was not clear how ACTH was stored or whether it had any relationship to the β-LPH/β-end system. In an immunocytochemical study using an ACTH 11–24 antibody (provided by R. E. Mains and B. A. Eipper), we have been able to demonstrate ACTH-positive cells and fibers in rat brain (Fig. 8) (39). Again, only one major cell group was seen with a widespread fiber pattern. The ACTH distribution was very similar to that seen with β-end and β-LPH, in that all three immunoreactivities were located in cells in the arcuate region of the hypothalamus and had very similar fiber distributions.

In a recent study, we have demonstrated that the antibodies toward ACTH, β-LPH, and β-end bind to the same hypothalamic cells (36). The ACTH antibody does not cross-react with β-LPH or β-end, while the β-LPH antibody is < 1% cross-reactive with β-end and not detectably cross-reactive with ACTH. The β-end antibody recognized totally the C-terminus of β-LPH, but it does not react with ACTH. All antisera were blocked only by the appropriate peptides. After each antiserum treatment, the same cells and fibers were visible. It was concluded that these three antisera were either binding their respective peptides or portions of the 31,000-dalton precursor. This study strongly supports the hypothesis that ACTH, β-end, and β-LPH share a common cellular origin and biochemical precursor in pituitary and brain.

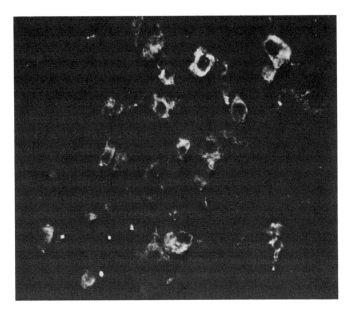

FIG. 8. ACTH-positive cells in the periarcuate n. of the hypothalamus; note the unstained nuclei. Colchicine pretreated as in Fig. 1. Dark field fluorescein preparation, ×120.

OVERVIEW

Immunocytochemical studies of the brain enkephalins, β-LPH, β-end, and ACTH have led to an interesting set of conclusions and hypotheses. From studies of Met-enk and Leu-enk, it seems clear that these substances are stored as though they are neuromodulators. Their general distribution argues for relatively short pathways, local circuit, and interneuronal functions. They appear ideally situated for modulation of many of the pharmacological effects of plant opiates. As yet no difference between Met-enk and Leu-enk distribution has been detected in spite of several such efforts. It has been hypothesized that they are, in fact, located in the same neurons. If that is the case, then they may be synthesized and released together. In studies of multiple opiate receptors, Akil et al. (1) have been able to demonstrate differing ratios of Met-enk to Leu-enk binding across brain regions. It may be that both enkephalins are released from the same neurons but act on somewhat different subpopulations of receptor sites. If that is the case, then the issues of biosynthesis, transmitter feedback control, and receptor specificity, to mention a few, become much more complex than in one transmitter system.

The anatomical studies of β-end, β-LPH, and ACTH reveal that all three are stored in a fashion consonant with a neuromodulator or neuromodulator precursor role. Again, two potentially active peptides (β-end and ACTH) appear to be contained within a single neuronal pool, raising important theoretical questions about their interactions, their biosynthetic regulation, and receptor controls. It is known that β-end has opiate-like properties (as do Met-enk and Leu-enk) and probably acts through an opiate receptor. However, ACTH has only minimal action on opiate receptors in the nanomolar range (31). ACTH has biological activity in the brain (9) but no specific receptor has been demonstrated for it. Two of the major questions in the "opiate" field are the nature of the ACTH-β-end interaction and whether ACTH acts on a unique receptor.

As was mentioned earlier, the β-end/ACTH system appears quite separate from enkephalin systems. Yet there are several major areas of overlap between the neuronal distributions of these two brain opiate systems. The hypothalamus, n. accumbens, periventricular n. of thalamus, periaqueductal central gray area and locus coeruleus—to name a few—exhibit both types of immunoreactivities. In these areas it would seem difficult to separate the role of enkephalin from that of β-end. For example, electrical stimulation of several of these core gray regions is known to be especially effective in producing analgesia in rat (22), cat (20), and humans (13,25). Currently, it is not possible to determine whether enkephalin or β-end (or both) is involved in the production of this electrically-induced analgesia (see Akil et al., *this volume*). Careful work will be required in order to tease apart the role of the two opioid systems in this mode of pain control.

From a speculative point of view, many of the higher structures that appear to be involved in the actions of the plant opiates could be under the control of both enkephalin and β-end systems. For example, the role of the noradrenergic systems, the sensory integration in the periaqueductal gray area, transmission through the thalamus, and affective-limbic changes could all be modulated by either opiate peptide system. Below the level of the locus coeruleus there are few β-end/ACTH fibers, whereas the enkephalin system continues to be quite heavy with them. Thus, analgesic effects in the cord and medulla are more likely to be enkephalinergic.

It is clear that the investigator of pain systems needs to focus a great deal more on specific opiate anatomy as it subsumes physiology. The problem is likely to be very complex as there are many points where enkephalin and endorphin systems could influence a pain signal as it travels from the earliest spinal level through midbrain to its final limbic perceptual expression.

ACKNOWLEDGMENTS

Stanley J. Watson is supported by a training fellowship No. MH-11028 of the National Institute of Mental Health and a Bank of America-Giannini Foundation Postdoctoral Fellowship. Jack D. Barchas is recipient of Research Scientist Development Award No. MH-24161. This work was supported in part by Program-Project Grant No. MH-23861, National Institute of Mental Health.

REFERENCES

1. Akil, H., Watson, S., and Barchas, J. D. (1979): Distribution and kinetic properties of methionine and leucine enkephalin binding sites in rat brain *(in preparation)*.
2. Belluzzi, J. D., Grant, N., Garsky, V., Sarantakis, D., Wise, C. D., and Stein, L. (1976): Analgesia induced *in vivo* by central administration of enkephalin in rat. *Nature*, 260:625–626.
3. Bloom, F., Battenberg, E., Rossier, J., Ling, N., and Guillemin, R. (1978): Neurons containing β-endorphin in rat brain exist separately from those containing enkephalin: immunocytochemical studies. *Proc. Natl. Acad. Sci. USA*, 75:1591–1595.
4. Bloom F., Battenberg, E., Rossier, J., Ling, N., Leppaluoto, J., Vargo, T. M., and Guillemin, R. (1977): Endorphins are located in the intermediate and anterior lobes of the pituitary gland, not in the neurohypophysis. *Life Sci.*, 20:43–48.
5. Bradbury, A. F., Feldberg, W. F., Smyth, D. G., and Snell, C. R. (1976): Lipotropin C-fragment: an endogenous peptide with potent analgesic activity. In: *Opiates and Endogenous Opioid Peptides*, edited by H. W. Kosterlitz, pp. 9–17. North-Holland, Amsterdam.
6. Büscher, H. H., Hill, R. C., Römer, D., Cardinaux, F., Closse, A., Hauser, D., and Pless, J. (1976): Evidence for analgesic activity of enkephalin in the mouse. *Nature*, 261:423–425.
7. Cox, B. M., Opheim, K. E., Teschemacher, H., and Goldstein, A. (1975): A peptide-like substance from pituitary that acts like morphine. 2. Purification and properties. *Life Sci.*, 16:1777–1782.
8. Elde, R., Hökfelt, T., Johansson, O., and Terenius, L. (1976): Immunohistochemical studies using antibodies to leucine-enkephalin: initial observations on the nervous system of the rat. *Neuroscience*, 1:349–351.
9. Gispen, W. H., Van Ree, J. M., and deWied, D. (1977): Lipotropin and the central nervous system. In: *International Review of Neurobiology, Vol. 20*, edited by T. R. Smythies and R. J. Bradley, pp. 209–249. Academic Press, New York.
10. Gráf, L., Szekely, J. I., Ronai, A. Z., Dunai-Kovacs, Z., and Bajusz, S. (1976): Comparative study on analgesic effect of Met^5-enkephalin and related lipotropin fragments. *Nature*, 263:240–242.
11. Hökfelt, T., Elde, R., Johansson, O., Terenius, L., and Stein, L. (1977): The distribution of enkephalin-immunoreactive cell bodies in the rat central nervous system. *Neurosci. Lett.*, 5:25–31.
12. Hökfelt, T., Ljungdahl, A., Terenius, L., Elde, R., and Nilsson, G. (1977): Immunohistochemical analysis of peptide pathways possibly related to pain and analgesia: Enkephalin and substance P. *Proc. Natl. Acad. Sci. USA*, 74:3081–3085.
13. Hosobuchi, Y., Adams, J. E., and Linchitz, R. (1977): Pain relief by electrical stimulation of the central grey matter in humans and its reversal by naloxone. *Science*, 197:183–186.
14. Hughes, J., Smith, T. W., Kosterlitz, H. W., Fothergill, L. A., Morgan, B. A., and Morris, H. R. (1975): Identification of two related pentapeptides from the brain with potent opiate agonist activity. *Nature*, 258:577–579.
15. Jacobowitz, D. M., Silver, M. A., and Soden, W. (1979): Mapping of the localization of leucine-enkephalin containing axons and cell bodies of the rat forebrain. In: *Endorphins in Mental Health Research*, edited by E. Usdin and W. Bunney. Macmillan, New York *(in press)*.
16. Johansson, O., Hökfelt, T., Elde, R. P., Schultzberg, M., and Terenius, L. (1978): Immunohistochemical distribution of enkephalin neurons. In: *Advances in Biochemical Psychopharmacology, Vol. 18*, edited by E. Costa and M. Trabucchi, pp. 51–70. Raven Press, New York.
17. Krieger, D. T., Liotta, A., and Brownstein, M. J. (1977): Presence of corticotropin in brain of normal and hypophysectomized rats. *Proc. Natl. Acad. Sci. USA*, 74:648–652.
18. Krieger, D. T., Liotta, A., Suda, T., Palkovits, M., and Brownstein, M. J. (1977): Presence of immunoassayable, β-lipotropin in bovine brain and spinal cord: lack of concordance with ACTH concentrations. *Biochem. Biophys. Res. Commun.*, 73:930–936.
19. Li, C. H., and Chung, D. (1976): Isolation and structure of an untriakontapeptide with opiate activity from camel pituitary glands. *Proc. Natl. Acad. Sci. USA*, 73:1145–1148.
20. Liebeskind, J. C., Guilbaud, G., Besson, J.-M., and Oliveras, J.-L. (1973): Analgesia from electrical stimulation of the periaqueductal gray matter in the cat: behavioral observations and inhibitory effects on spinal cord interneurons. *Brain Res.*, 50:441–446.
21. Mains, R. E., Eipper, B. A., and Ling, N. (1977): Common precursor to corticotropins and endorphins. *Proc. Natl. Acad. Sci. USA*, 74:3014–3018.

22. Mayer, D. J., Wolfle, T. L., Akil, H., Carder, B., and Liebeskind, J. C. (1971): Analgesia from electrical stimulation in the brainstem of the rat. *Science,* 174:1351–1354.
23. Moon, H. D., Li, C. H., and Jennings, B. M. (1973): Immunohistochemical and histochemical studies of pituitary β-lipotrophs. *Anat. Rec.,* 175:524–538.
24. Pelletier, G., Leclerc, R., Labrie, F., Cote, J., Chretien, M., and Les, M. (1977): Immunohisto-chemical localization of β-lipotropic hormone in the pituitary gland. *Endocrinology,* 100:770–776.
25. Richardson, D. E., and Akil, H. (1977): Pain reduction by electrical brain stimulation in man. I. Acute administration in periaqueductal and periventricular sites. *J. Neurosurg.,* 47:178–183.
26. Roberts, J. L., and Herbert, E. (1977): Characterization of a common precursor to corticotropin and β-lipotropin: Identification of β-lipotropin peptides and their arrangement relative to cortico-tropin in the precursor synthesized in a cell-free system. *Proc. Natl. Acad. Sci. USA,* 74:5300–5304.
27. Rossier, J., Vargo, T. M., Minick, S., Ling, N., Bloom, F. E., and Guillemin, R. (1977): Regional dissociation of β-endorphin and enkephalin contents in rat brain and pituitary. *Proc. Natl. Acad. Sci. USA,* 74:5162–5165.
28. Sar, M., Stumpf, W. E., Miller, R. J., Chang, K.-J., and Cuatrecasas, P. (1978): Immunohisto-chemical localization of enkephalin in rat brain and spinal cord. *J. Comp. Neurol.,* 182:17–39.
29. Simantov, R., Kuhar, M. J., Uhl, G. R., and Snyder, S. H. (1977): Opioid peptide enkephalin: immunohistochemical mapping in rat central nervous system. *Proc. Natl. Acad. Sci. USA,* 74:2167–2171.
30. Teitelbaum, H., Catravas, G. N., and McFarland, W. L. (1974): Reversal of morphine tolerance after medial thalamic lesions in rat. *Science,* 185:449–451.
31. Terenius, L., Gispen, W. H., and deWied, D. (1975): ACTH-like peptides and opiate receptors in the rat brain: Structure-activity studies. *Eur. J. Pharmacol.,* 33:395–399.
32. Teschemacher, H., Opheim, K. E., Cox, B. M., and Goldstein, A. (1975): A peptide-like substance from pituitary that acts like morphine. I. Isolation. *Life Sci.,* 16:1771–1776.
33. Uhl, G. R., Goodman, R. R., Kuhar, M. J., and Snyder, S. H. (1978): Enkephalin and neuroten-sin: immunohistochemical localization and identification of an amygdala-fugal pathway. In: *Advances in Biochemical Psychopharmacology, Vol. 18,* edited by E. Costa and M. Trabucchi, pp. 71–87. Raven Press, New York.
34. Watson, S., Akil, H., and Barchas, J. D. (1977): A possible role for the dorsal periventricular catecholamine bundle in stimulation produced analgesia: A behavioral and histochemical study. *Brain Res.,* 130:335–342.
35. Watson, S. J., Akil, H., and Barchas, J. D. (1979): Immunohistochemical and biochemical studies of the enkephalins, β-endorphin, and related peptides. In: *Endorphins in Mental Health Research,* edited by E. Usdin, W. E. Bunney, and N. S. Kline. Macmillan, New York *(in press).*
36. Watson, S. J., Akil, H., Richard, C. W., and Barchas, J. D.: (1978): Evidence for two separate opiate peptide neuronal systems and the coexistence of β-lipotropin, β-endorphin, and ACTH immunoreactivities in the same hypothalamic neurons. *Nature,* 275:226–228.
37. Watson, S. J., Akil, H., Sullivan, S. O., and Barchas, J. D. (1977): Immunocytochemical localiza-tion of methionine enkephalin: Preliminary observations. *Life Sci.,* 21:733–738.
38. Watson, S. J., Barchas, J. D., and Li, C. H. (1977): β-Lipotropin: Localization of cells and axons in rat brain by immunocytochemistry. *Proc. Natl. Acad. Sci. USA,* 74:5155–5158.
39. Watson, S. J., Richard, C. W., and Barchas, J. D. (1978): Corticotropin in rat brain: immunocyto-chemical localization in cells and axons. *Science,* 200:1180–1182.
40. Wei, E., and Loh, H. (1976): Chronic intracerebral infusion of opiates and peptides with osmotic minipumps and the development of physical dependence. In: *Opiates and Endogenous Opioid Peptides,* edited by H. W. Kosterlitz, pp. 303–310. North-Holland, Amsterdam.
41. Wei, E., and Loh, H. (1976): Physical dependence on opiate-like peptides. *Science,* 190:1262–1263.
42. Wei, E. T., Tseng, L. F., Loh, H. H., and Li, C. H. (1977): Comparison of the behavioral effects of β-endorphin and enkephalin analogs. *Life Sci.,* 21:321–327.
43. Zimmerman, E. A., Liotta, A., and Krieger, D. T. (1978): β-Lipotropin in brain: Localization in hypothalamic neurons by immunoperoxidase technique. *Cell Tissue Res.,* 186:393–398.

Mechanisms of Pain and Analgesic Compounds,
edited by R. F. Beers, Jr., and E. G. Bassett.
Raven Press, New York © 1979.

21. Pain Control by Focal Brain Stimulation in Man: Relationship to Enkephalins and Endorphins

Huda Akil,* D. E. Richardson,** and Jack D. Barchas

Department of Psychiatry and Behavioral Sciences, Stanford University School of Medicine, Stanford, California 94305

INTRODUCTION

The use of focal electrical stimulation of specific brain loci to relieve intractable pain in human subjects has pointed to a number of theoretical and clinical issues. These range from evaluating the efficacy and practicality of such stimulation as a tool for pain relief, to questions of multiple mechanisms of pain control and relationships between stimulation-produced analgesia (SPA) and the opioids endogenous to brain and pituitary. In this chapter, we shall attempt to summarize our results with SPA in man, pointing out both the advantages and the limitations of this approach. We shall also present data linking this analgesia to activation of endogenous opioids (endorphins) along with some observations that suggest involvement of further pain-modulating mechanisms. Finally, we shall outline some future research direction, based on our recently acquired knowledge of brain and pituitary enkephalins and endorphins.

We undertook the work in human patients based on information about stimulation-produced analgesia gathered in animals (3,18,20). This animal work suggested that electrical activation of specific periaqueductal and periventricular loci produced a decrease in pain responsiveness comparable to the effect of a large dose of morphine. Further, this reduction in withdrawal reflexes to noxious input—termed SPA—was shown to be partially blocked by the opiate antagonist naloxone (3,4) and to be dependent on monoaminergic integrity (5). The anatomical distribution of SPA-producing sites, the effect of naloxone, and the demonstration of "tolerance" and cross-tolerance with morphine (19) led to the suggestion that SPA activates an endogenous pain inhibitory system that is also sensitive to opiates (3,5,18,20). Early reports of an endogenous opiate-like factor (14) and the subsequent discovery of enkephalin (15) and β-endorphin (16) led to the more specific hypothesis that SPA works, at least in part, by releasing

---

* Present address: Mental Health Research Institute, University of Michigan School of Medicine, Ann Arbor, Michigan 48109; ** Department of Neurosurgery, Louisiana State University, New Orleans, Louisiana 70024.

endogenous opioids, whereas morphine produces its effects by directly activating opiate receptors (4,19,21). Some of the work described below was designed to test this latter hypothesis.

OBSERVATIONS AND DISCUSSION

Summary of Clinical Results

While the investigation of brain stimulation as a tool for pain relief in man predates the discovery of endogenous opioids, its theoretical underpinnings were clearly based on the notion of activating an endogenous pain inhibitory system. This was to play an important role in our approach because we did not attempt to "mask" the pain by activating sensory pathways in brain (cf. 12), nor did we set out to "jam" transmission along pain pathways by producing a functional lesion with electrical stimulation. Rather, we searched for sites where electrical stimulation would lead to a diminution of pain responsiveness with minimal sensory, motor, or autonomic concomitants.

The first set of studies (23) involved an examination of anatomical loci that might produce analgesia on stimulation in man. Previously, Heath and Mickle (10) had reported pain relief by septal stimulation in one patient, but Gol (9) reported very mixed results from this same site in a study with more subjects. Since most of the work in rat and cat had been carried out in the central gray area, we set out to study this area. However, Nashold et al. (22) reported noxious side effects from stimulation of the central gray area in human subjects. Further, some early reports suggested the involvement of the medial thalamic and periventricular sites in opiate analgesia (cf. 21). Therefore, a number of medial thalamic and periventricular sites en route to the central gray target were examined. The studies were carried out acutely, in the operating room, on intractable pain patients scheduled for thalamotomy for pain relief. We received informed consent to stimulate along periventricular and periaqueductal sites prior to the thalamotomy. The patients were, as usual, under local anesthesia, and could therefore describe any stimulation-induced changes in pain or other sensations. The experimental details of these studies have been described elsewhere (23). The results in five subjects led to the conclusion that central gray stimulation caused substantial decreases in pain, but was marred by a number of unpleasant side effects. On the other hand, stimulation of a periventricular site adjacent to the posterior commissure (Schatelbrand and Bailey ATLAS, coordinates: $Fp = 10$; $Ht = 0$; $Lat = 2$ to 5 mm) produced analgesia with minimal side effects.

Chronic implants in the periventricular area were initiated in May 1973. Candidates were screened carefully to determine the cause of pain, and to avoid selection of subjects with severe psychological problems. The two stages of the surgical procedure involved implanting the electrode under local anesthesia and securing the electrode-receiver assembly (Medtronics Corporation) under general anesthesia. Typically, a period of a few days separates the two stages during which the effectiveness of the stimulator is determined. After the receiver is implanted, the patient is instructed in the use of the pocketsize Medtronics stimulator, and followed up on an outpatient basis. We have reported the surgical details and the first eight case studies (24). The effectiveness of the procedure is assessed by using the patient's reports of changes in chronic pain and by testing acute pain with pinprick, radiant heat applied to the finger tip, ischemic pain, and acute exacerbation of the chronic pain. Criteria for evaluating efficiency of the stimulation were established around four factors: (a) completeness of pain relief during and after stimulation; (b) duration of analgesia after the termination of stimulation; (c) accompanying side effects; and (d) long-term effectiveness. This last factor was of particular interest because of our concern about the development of opiate-like tolerance. The results of this first group of subjects demonstrated the potential usefulness of this technique as a clinical tool. Six of the eight patients obtained significant pain relief with minimal side effects for long duration (up to several hours) for periods lasting from several months to several years.

We have since summarized our results from a subsequent group of 22 patients, yielding a total population of 30 subjects. The cases were followed up for 1 to 48 months with a mean period of 18½ months. Of the 30 patients, 3 were "tested out"—i.e., the electrode was not permanently internalized because early percutaneous testing did not yield significant pain relief. The remainder were evaluated along the scales described above. The patients suffered from a wide range of illnesses ranging from low back pain (33% of all cases) to cancer, paraplegia, spinal arachnoiditis, spinal cord injury, thalamic pain, scoliosis, postherpetic neuralgia, phantom limb pain, arthritis, and atypical face pain. As a result of the procedure, 18 of the 30 subjects reported "marked" to "complete" pain relief, i.e., a decrease of over 50% in their pain ratings. The mean duration of analgesia after cessation of the stimulation was 3.8 hr, ranging from a few minutes to 24 hr. The most common side effect observed was temperature paresthesia (16/30), i.e., a mild change in temperature perceived at a localized site, most commonly in the contralateral face, neck, and arm or in the back. Other side effects involved "tingling" paresthesias (11/30), visual blurring or nystagmus (8/30), emotional responses such as "startle or nervousness" (4/30), and vertigo (2/30). The most serious complication seen was postoperative meningitis (3/30). Other complications were primarily mechanical, involving broken wiring (3/30), electrode migration (2/30), or failure of the device (1/30). Subjectively, the patients described their pain as "floating away" on stimulation. Others reported a "tightening up" in the painful area, followed by disappearance of the pain. Although four subjects reported tension associated with the stimulation, most of the patients emphasized the feeling of relief and relaxation that accompanied or followed the stimulation. Typically, the treatment resulted in improved sleep patterns, increased physical activity, and enhanced social and personal interactions.

The cases that were considered "failures" are of interest since they shed light on some of the limitations of the treatment. Eight of the 30 subjects have made little or no use of their stimulators. Only one of these subjects exhibited no relief at all from the outset. The remaining patients exhibited a reticence to withdraw from narcotics, or resumed the use of narcotics when their pain was exacerbated at a later time. Finally, in four cases, the stimulation produced good but extremely short-lived analgesia, outlasting the stimulation by only a few minutes. This required almost continuous stimulation, leading to short-term habituation and loss of effectiveness. This habituation is unlike "tolerance" in that it occurs over a period of a few hours. However, abstaining from use of stimulation for a few days leads to a complete return of effectiveness.

Continuous use can lead to a decrease in usefulness. However, long-term effectiveness has exceeded our expectations, since 60% of our patients still obtain good to excellent relief with over 18 months of use. Few of the patients have exhibited a steady increase in the current intensity necessary for analgesia. It is our impression that this is due to the judicious use of the device to prevent "overstimulation." We have emphasized to our patients the necessity to minimize the use of the stimulator and to employ the lowest effective current parameters. We have hypothesized that if the patient waits until the pain returns prior to restimulation, this might allow the levels of neurotransmitters involved to recover between stimulation, thus minimizing longer-term adaption. Further, if receptor occupancy is critical for analgesia, and if continued occupancy leads to tolerance, then the intermittent stimulation may allow the receptors to return to a "normal" state of occupancy between uses. This hypothesis requires systematic testing in animals. Nonetheless, we have adopted this course because it appears safe and potentially critical for clinical usefulness.

It is apparent that focal stimulation in these subjects produces differential effects on acute versus chronic pain. Lower currents are necessary for effective control of clinical pain. Further, analgesia for acute pain outlasts stimulation for only a few minutes, whereas chronic pain can remain attenuated for several hours after the termination of current. It is unclear whether this is merely due to different intensities of the two classes of discomfort or to a difference in the specific mechanisms that are activated by the stimulation and that modulate the two types of sensations.

Relationship Between SPA in Man and Endogenous Opioids

We have three lines of evidence linking the effects of stimulation of the periventricular gray area in man to the activation of endogenous opioids.

Anatomical Evidence

The first is merely circumstantial and is based on the anatomy of opioids. We have reported that in man (23), as in rat (25), analgesia can be obtained from a number of sites surrounding the aqueduct of Sylvius and the third ventricle. These areas are rich in both enkephalins and β-endorphin. The medial thalamic region in particular is, at least in the rat, one of the richest areas in β-endorphin activity arising from the cell bodies of the hypothalamic periarcuate region (6,8,26). If human anatomy is similar, then it is not inconceivable that we would be activating both opioid systems—enkephalin and β-endorphin—when stimulating this region.

Naloxone Effects

The second line of evidence derives from a preliminary study of the effect of naloxone on SPA in four of our patients. This study was conducted in a double-blind, cross-over design. It involved two sessions, two days apart: a saline control session and a naloxone session. Three indices of analgesia were employed:

(a) the patient's rating of his chronic pain (on a scale of 0 to 10, from nonexistent to excruciating);
(b) the latency of the withdrawal response to radiant heat applied to the index finger;
(c) the duration of pain relief after the termination of stimulation.

The patients were asked not to self-administer any stimulation for 24 hr prior to testing. At the beginning of each session, base-line pain responsiveness was determined. The patient's rating of his own pain was obtained, and the latency of the withdrawal reflex to heat was measured. Electrical stimulation was then administered for 10 min at the parameters usually employed by the patient. The effect of this stimulation on pain was assessed by radiant heat testing and subjective rating. With the stimulation still in progress, the patient received an intravenous injection of either naloxone (1 mg) or saline. Testing of pain was conducted at 2-min intervals for 20 min after drug administration. The stimulation was then terminated, and the patient asked to note the time at which his pain returned, and to rate its level. Each patient served as his own control, with half the patients undergoing the naloxone session first, and the other half the saline session first. Tables 1 and 2 summarize the effect of naloxone on SPA-induced changes in latency to radiant heat. The estimated latency for each subject is based on the mean of three trials.

TABLE 1. *Effect of stimulation and naloxone (1 mg) or saline on latency of withdrawal from radiant heat*

	Latency of withdrawal (min)	
	Saline session	Naloxone session
Base-line latency	4.5 ± 0.5	4.5 ± 0.4
Effect of 10 min of stimulation	4.9 ± 0.6	5.0 ± 0.6
Infusion effect, 10-min post-injection, continued stimulation	4.8 ± 0.6	4.5 ± 0.5

TABLE 2. *Difference scores between latency prior to infusion with 10 min of stimulation and latency after infusion with continued stimulation*[a]

Patient	Latency (min)	
	Saline session	Naloxone session
1	0.4	0.6
2	0.1	0.2
3	0.1	0.6
4	−0.3	0.6
x	0.08	0.5

[a]Paired *t*-test: $t = 2.365$—not significant ($p < 0.1$).

As can be seen, the patients were quite variable amongst themselves with respect to the withdrawal latencies. However, the within-subject variability was very small (on the order of 0.05 min). Two of the four subjects who exhibited marked increases in response time on stimulation (0.8 and 1-min increase), clearly responded with a drop in latency of 0.6 min on the naloxone day, but exhibited no change on the saline day.

The effect of naloxone in reversing SPAs effect on clinical pain was more difficult to assess. In one case, the base-line score was so different between the 2 days that a valid comparison could not be made. One patient exhibited no clear effect of naloxone either during the stimulation or after cessation of the current. The two remaining patients showed some effects of naloxone. One subject required twice the duration of stimulation on the naloxone day as compared to the saline day before he achieved complete relief of pain. His base-line score was identical prior to stimulation on both sessions. The other patient experienced a complete reversal of the stimulation effect 10 min after naloxone infusion, and complained that his pain had returned to prestimulation intensity in spite of continued stimulation. The saline infusion, on the other hand, was followed by continued pain relief for a period of 90 min. It should be noted that, in this study, we attempted a reversal of the stimulation effect after it was in progress for 10 min. This may be more difficult to achieve than the prevention of stimulation effects by prior administration of naloxone. Still, this work suggests some effects of naloxone on SPA in man—and is consonant with the results of Hosobuchi et al. (13), demonstrating a similar effect in their pain patients.

Release of Endogenous Opioids by SPA in Man

We have recently described the existence of an enkephalin-like material in the cerebrospinal fluid (CSF) of human subjects (7). This material resembles enkephalin in its interactions with opiate receptor assays and radioimmunoassay, as well as its behavior on several chromatographic systems. Whalström and

Terenius (27) have described the existence of two fractions in CSF with opiate-like activity: a high molecular weight substance, and an enkephalin-like, lower molecular weight factor. We have therefore studied the effect of analgesic electrical stimulation on the levels of this enkephalin-like material in ventricular CSF. Samples were obtained from eight subjects during the first stage of surgery. The first was a base-line sample collected from an intraventricular catheter prior to stimulation. Three or four other samples were collected over a 20-min period after electrical stimulation. The samples were immediately frozen on dry ice to halt possible degradation. Three sets were shipped to John Hughes for bioassay. The remainder were chromatographed and measured using the binding of labeled opiates to brain membrane homogenates. The details of the procedures have been described elsewhere (1). The results indicated that 20 min of analgetic electrical stimulation led to a significant rise in the levels of this opioid material in CSF.

Taken together, the above results suggest a role of endogenous opioids in the analgesia obtained by pain patients when they self-administer current in the periventricular region. However, this does not preclude the role of other mechanisms of pain modulation in this analgesia. The complexity of the responses to chronic and acute pain, the interactions with affective state of the subjects, the variable effect of naloxone points to the interactions of multiple systems of pain appreciation and inhibition. This notion is supported by findings in animals demonstrating different types of analgesia with opioid and non-opioid components (2,21).

Future Directions

The recently accumulated information on endogenous opioid systems points to a number of issues that requires study in our investigation of SPA in man. It is now clear that β-endorphin is a separate system, distinct from enkephalin systems within the brain (8,26, also Watson and Barchas, *this volume*). This brain β-endorphin system arises from a single group of cell bodies localized in the periarcuate hypothalamic region, projecting to structures throughout the brainstem. The enkephalin system, on the other hand, involves multiple cell groups with shorter processes. As mentioned previously, both opioids are localized in loci known to produce analgesia when stimulated. Yet, the specific role of each of the opioids in pain control is unknown. We are currently carrying out studies in which the β-endorphin cell group is stimulated in rat and changes in pain responsiveness assessed. The naloxone reversibility of any analgesia seen at this site will be examined. Since β-endorphin is degraded more slowly than enkephalin, it is tempting to speculate that stimulation of β-endorphin pathways might lead to longer-lasting analgesia. Examination of the potential role of the two peptides in modulating the short-lived control of acute pain versus the longer-lasting inhibition of chronic pain is, obviously, the next step.

Clearly, the endogenous opioids serve functions outside of pain modulation.

Thus, the role of their activation in observed changes in mood, affect, or sleep patterns warrants closer attention. Further, the interaction between the brain and pituitary opioids deserves investigation. We are currently examining changes in blood levels of opioids and related peptides in stimulated patients.

Finally, opioids do not exist in isolation. They exhibit close anatomical relationships with catecholamines (6,26, also Watson and Barchas, *this volume*). This is supported by our finding of interactions between SPA and monoamine altering drugs in rat (5) and by the potentiation of SPA by amitriptyline in man (24). There are further indications of interactions with substance P (11). We have suggested that medial thalamic stimulation may be particularly useful because it activates a nexus of interacting neuromodulators at a site critical for biasing pain transmission and appreciation (25). The role of these various substances in SPA remains to be elucidated.

Electrical stimulation in man has proven to be both an exciting source of insight into pain modulation and a useful clinical tool. We have only begun to uncover its complexities—a great deal remains to be learned.

ACKNOWLEDGMENTS

Huda Akil is the recipient of Sloan Foundation Fellowship in Neurophysiology, BR 16091. Jack D. Barchas holds Research Scientist Development Award MH 24161. This work was supported by NIMH Program-Project Grant MH 23861, NIDA grant DA 01522, and a grant from the Office of Naval Research.

REFERENCES

1. Akil, H., Richardson, D. E., Hughes, J., and Barchas, J. D. (1978): Enkephalin-like material in ventricular cerebrospinal fluid of pain patients after analgetic focal stimulation. *Science,* 201:463–465.
2. Akil, H., Madden, J., IV, Patrick, R., and Barchas, J. D. (1976): Stress-induced increase in endogenous opiate peptides: Concurrent analgesia and its partial reversal by naloxone. In: *Opiates and Endogenous Opioid Peptides,* edited by H. W. Kosterlitz, pp. 63–70. Elsevier/North-Holland, Amsterdam.
3. Akil, H., Mayer, D. J., and Liebeskind, J. C. (1972): Comparison chez le rat entre l'analgesie induite par stimulation de la substance grise periaqueducale et l'analgesie morphinique. *C. R. Acad. Sci. [D] (Paris),* 274:3603–3605.
4. Akil, H., Mayer, D. J., and Liebeskind, J. C. (1976): Antagonism of stimulation-produced analgesia by naloxone, a narcotic antagonist. *Science,* 191:961–962.
5. Akil, H., and Liebeskind, J. C. (1975): Monoaminergic mechanisms of stimulation-produced analgesia. *Brain Res.,* 94:279–296.
6. Akil, H., Watson, S. J., Berger, P. A., and Barchas, J. D. (1978): Endorphins, β-LPH, and ACTH: biochemical, pharmacological and anatomical studies. In: *The Endorphins: Advances in Biochemical Psychopharmacology, Vol. 18,* edited by E. Costa and E. M. Trabucchi, pp. 125–140. Raven Press, New York.
7. Akil, H., Watson, S., Sullivan, S., and Barchas, J. D. (1978): Enkephalin-like material in normal human cerebrospinal fluid: measurement and levels. *Life Sci.,* 23:121–125.
8. Bloom, F. E., Battenberg, E., Rossier, J., Ling, N., and Guillemin, R. (1978): Neurons containing β-endorphin in rat brain exist separately from those containing enkephalin: Immunocytochemical studies. *Proc. Natl. Acad. Sci. USA,* 75:1591–1595.

9. Gol, A. (1967): Relief of pain by electrical stimulation of the septal area. *J. Neurol. Sci.,* 5:115–120.
10. Heath, R. G., and Mickle, W. A. (1960): Evaluation of seven years' experience with depth electrode studies in human patients. In: *Electrical Studies on the Unanesthesized Brain,* edited by E. R. Ramey and D. S. O'Doherty, pp. 214–247. Hoeber, New York.
11. Hökfelt, T., Kellerth, J. O., Ljungdahl, A., Nilsson, G., Nygards, A., and Pernow, B. (1977): Immunohistochemical localization of substance P in the central and peripheral nervous system. In: *Neuroregulators and Psychiatric Disorders,* edited by E. Usdin, D. Hamburg, and J. Barchas, pp. 299–311. Oxford University Press, New York.
12. Hosobuchi, Y., Adams, J. E., and Fields, H. L. (1974): Chronic thalamic and internal capsular stimulation for the control of facial anesthesia dolorosa and dysesthesia of thalamic syndrome. In: *Advances in Neurology, Vol. 4: Proceedings of the International Symposium on Pain,* edited by J. J. Bonica, pp. 783–787. Raven Press, New York.
13. Hosobuchi, Y., Adams, J. E., and Linchitz, R. (1977): Pain relief by electrical stimulation of the central gray matter in humans and its reversal by naloxone. *Science,* 197:183–186.
14. Hughes, J. (1975): Isolation of an endogenous compound from the brain with pharmacological properties similar to morphine. *Brain Res.,* 88:295–308.
15. Hughes, J., Smith, T. W., Kosterlitz, H. W., Fothergill, L. A., Morgan, B. A., and Morris, H. R. (1975): Identification of two related pentapeptides from the brain with potent opiate agonist activity. *Nature,* 258:577–579.
16. Li, C. H., and Chung, D. (1976): Isolation and structure of an untriakontapeptide with opiate activity from camel pituitary glands. *Proc. Natl. Acad. Sci. USA,* 73:1145–1148.
17. Liebeskind, J. C., Guilbaud, G., Besson, J.-M., and Oliveras, J.-L. (1973): Analgesia from electrical stimulation of the periaqueductal gray matter in the cat: Behavioral observations and inhibitory effects on spinal cord interneurons. *Brain Res.,* 50:441–446.
18. Liebeskind, J. C., Mayer, D. J., and Akil, H. (1974): Central mechanisms of pain inhibition: Studies of analgesia from focal brain stimulation. In: *Advances in Neurology, Vol. 4: Proceedings of the International Symposium on Pain,* edited by J. J. Bonica, pp. 261–268. Raven Press, New York.
19. Mayer, D. J., and Hayes, R. (1975): Stimulation-produced analgesia: Development of tolerance and cross-tolerance to morphine. *Science,* 188:941–943.
20. Mayer, D. J., Wolfle, T. L., Akil, H., Carder, B., and Liebeskind, J. C. (1971): Analgesia from electrical stimulation in the brainstem of the rat. *Science,* 174:1351–1354.
21. Mayer, D. J., and Price, D. D. (1976): Central nervous system mechanisms of analgesia. *Pain,* 2:379–404.
22. Nashold, B. S., Jr., Wilson, W. P., and Slaughter, D. G. (1969): Sensations evoked by stimulation in the midbrain of man. *J. Neurosurg.,* 30:14–24.
23. Richardson, D. E., and Akil, H. (1977): Pain reduction by electrical brain stimulation in man. I. Acute administration in periaqueductal and periventricular sites. *J. Neurosurg.,* 47:178–183.
24. Richardson, D. E., and Akil, H. (1977): Pain reduction by electrical brain stimulation in man. II. Chronic self-administration in the periventricular gray matter. *J. Neurosurg.,* 47:184–194.
25. Watson, S., Akil, H., and Barchas, J. D. (1977): A possible role for the dorsal periventricular catecholamine bundle in stimulation produced analgesia: A behavioral and histochemical study. *Brain Res.,* 130:335–342.
26. Watson, S. J., Akil, H., and Barchas, J. D. (1979): Immunohistochemical and biochemical studies of the enkephalins, β-endorphin, and related peptides. In: *Endorphins in Mental Health Research,* edited by E. Usdin, W. E. Bunney, and N. S. Kline. Macmillan, New York *(in press).*
27. Whalström, A., Johansson, L., and Terenius, L. (1976): Characterization of endorphins (endogenous morphine-like factors) in human CSF and brain extracts. In: *Opiates and Endogenous Opioid Peptides,* edited by H. W. Kosterlitz, pp. 49–56. Elsevier/North Holland, Amsterdam.

Mechanisms of Pain and Analgesic Compounds,
edited by R. F. Beers, Jr., and E. G. Bassett.
Raven Press, New York © 1979.

22. Endorphins and Pain: A Critical Review

Avram Goldstein

Addiction Research Foundation, Palo Alto, California 94304

INTRODUCTION

Circumstantial Evidence for a Role of Endorphins in Pain Modulation

The discovery of opioid peptides in the brain (53) and pituitary (20,84) led to the natural assumption that they represented an endogenous system for producing analgesia (40). Three years later, matters appear not to be quite so straightforward (83). The evidence implicating these peptides in analgesia, however indirectly, may be summarized as follows:

(a) Since opiates are known to act at the specific opiate receptors at various levels of the spinal axis to produce analgesia (5,6,80,92,93), and since the opioid peptides clearly interact with these same receptors, one has to suppose that *if and when* the peptides are released at the receptor sites, analgesia should result.

(b) The distribution of enkephalinergic neurons at various levels of the cerebrospinal axis, in close association with pain pathways, especially in substantia gelatinosa, seems to implicate them in some way in the modulation of pain. Enkephalins are in terminals of short neurons and in close relationship to the opiate receptors (34,49,50,67,87). β-endorphin is in terminals of a different system of long neurons (78,88).

(c) Administration of enkephalins (at high doses) or of β-endorphin into the cerebroventricular system or at certain sites in brain or spinal cord results in analgesia, as does administration of morphine by the same route (24,25,32, 36,47,61,89,93). A mechanism that secreted endorphins (especially β-endorphin) into the ventricles would probably result in analgesia. The rapid breakdown of enkephalin probably accounts for its evanescent activity and poor apparent potency, because these pentapeptides are highly potent in neuroblastoma x glioma cells that contain opiate receptors (58), and because enkephalin congeners stabilized against enzymic attack are also highly potent *in vivo* (28,29,73,77, 82,86,95).

(d) Stimulation-produced analgesia first suggested the possibility of endogenous opiate-like substances, because this analgesia is at least partially blocked and reversed by the specific opiate antagonist naloxone (3,4). Electrical stimulation in brain regions known to be rich in enkephalins or β-endorphin apparently releases the opioid peptides and thus causes analgesia. The mechanism is uncertain, however, and it could be complex (65). For example, local release of enkephalins at the stimulation site could inhibit release of an inhibitory neurotransmitter, thus causing excitation of a downflowing pathway, which in turn stimulates enkephalin release in the substantia gelatinosa.

(e) Acupuncture analgesia, both in animals (74,75) and in man (66), is blocked by naloxone. In the animal experiments, electroacupuncture suppressed the response of spinal cord dorsal horn cells to noxious stimuli at the limb. Naloxone blockade was dramatic and complete, implying that somehow the electrical needle stimulation caused enkephalin release in the substantia gelatinosa. The time course of the effects and the dependence upon an intact pituitary suggest the release, perhaps by secretion back into the cerebroventricular system, of a long-acting peptide like β-endorphin. It should be noted, however, that this experiment was done in mice, where hypophysectomy frequently results in damage to the median eminence; it cannot be concluded, therefore, whether it is the pituitary or the hypothalamus that must be intact for acupuncture to work.

(f) Opioid peptides have been shown to inhibit the potassium-stimulated release of substance P from terminals of dorsal root ganglion cells (57,63), just as opiates and opioid peptides inhibit release of acetylcholine from myenteric plexus neurons and of norepinephrine from sympathetic terminals in vas deferens (52). This finding is consistent with the view that the short enkephalin interneurons could be stimulated to inhibit release of substance P from terminals of the bipolar sensory neurons known to conduct pain stimuli and to contain substance P (50).

Thus, there is ample circumstantial evidence linking the opioid peptides to some kind of pain-modulatory role. It is important to distinguish, however, between artificially stimulated release of these substances and physiological mechanisms for their release. The central question about the opioid peptides is: What natural circumstances cause their release, and under those circumstances, do they modify pain?

The administration of opioid peptides directly into the brain or spinal cord carries no weight in this argument; of course, they do what morphine is known to do, including causing analgesia. What we need to know is when and where the endogenous stores are released in sufficient quantity to produce analgesia. Nor can measurement of the content of opioid peptides in whole brain or brain regions after various treatments yield unambiguous results [cf. (18) for the same argument applied to other neurotransmitters]. If the content increases, for example, after footshock stress (64), does this mean that synthesis was increased, or that release was decreased, or that degradation was inhibited, or that a reuptake mechanism became more efficient, or what? And if the same stress causes some type of analgesia, how can any conclusion be drawn about the relationship of that analgesia to the change in brain content of opioid peptides?

OBSERVATIONS AND DISCUSSION

Rationale for the Use of Naloxone as an Experimental Tool

It follows that until better methods are developed for reliably measuring the release (turnover) of neurotransmitters *in vivo* at the specific sites of action, we are limited to the use of receptor antagonists. If we know that a receptor is blocked by a given antagonist, we have a right to use that antagonist as a probe to see what those receptors are doing. If they are quiescent (i.e., not occupied by any endogenous agonist), the antagonist will be without effect. If they are active (i.e., occupied by an endogenous agonist), the antagonist will turn them off, and the consequence must be an altered physiological state. If the active state of the receptors causes a measurable physiological effect, as indeed it should, it follows that the antagonist (at sufficient dosage to occupy the receptors) should cause a measurable reduction or abolition of that effect.

With respect to pain modulation, if enkephalinergic neurons are tonically active and suppressing pain input in the spinal cord, the specific antagonist naloxone should intensify pain. If enkephalinergic neurons are not tonically active but are activated by painful stimuli under certain conditions, naloxone should intensify pain under those conditions.

Naloxone Effects on Nociceptive Responses

Surprisingly, the preponderance of evidence on the effect of naloxone on pain, both in laboratory animals and in humans, has been negative, ambiguous, or conflicting, and even the positive results have been less than dramatic. Tables 1 and 2, taken from a review by B. M. Cox and E. R. Baizman (19), summarize the studies to date.

One of the earliest animal experiments was a test of naloxone in an automated quantitative system for determining the footshock threshold for pole jump escape in trained rats (41). Up to dosages just short of those causing gross behavioral deficits, (e.g., 100 mg/kg), naloxone was absolutely without effect on the escape threshold. A positive control was that naloxone, at low dosage, completely antagonized the threshold-raising effect of morphine. Similar negative effects were observed in a shock-titration paradigm in squirrel monkeys at 0.3 to 10 mg/kg (30).

The latency to squeak following a thermal stimulus to the nose in mice was shortened slightly by naloxone (0.9 mg/kg) (75), but formic acid or PGE_1-induced writhing in mice was unaffected at a similar dose (16).

Conflicting results have been reported with the tail flick response to a thermal stimulus in rats—both reduction of response latency by naloxone (2 mg/kg) (10) and no effect at various doses (72,94). Increased writhing in response to acetic acid was noted at 4 mg/kg (59), but in another experiment naloxone (10 mg/kg) had no effect on forepaw pain due to formalin injection (70).

TABLE 1. *Effects of naloxone on pain thresholds*[a]

Method of measure of pain sensitivity	Specie	Effect of naloxone	Dose of naloxone	Ref.
Hot plate test	Mouse	Reduction of response latency	0.01–30 mg/kg	55
Hot plate test	Mouse	Reduction of response latency	0.5–4 mg/kg	34,37
Hot plate test	Mouse	Reduction of response latency	0.03–10 mg/kg	46
Heat on nose: squeak response	Mouse	Reduction of response latency	0.9 mg/kg	75
Formic acid or PGE₁-induced writhing	Mouse	No effect	1 mg/kg	16
Shock escape threshold	Rat	No effect	12.5–100 mg/kg	41
Tail flick test (thermal stimulus)	Rat	Reduction of response latency	2 mg/kg	10
Tail flick test (thermal stimulus)	Rat	No effect	1, 10, or 20 mg/kg	72,90,94
Acetic acid-induced writhing	Rat	Increased frequency of writhing	4 mg/kg	59
Shock titration	Squirrel monkey	No effect	0.3–10 mg/kg	30
Electrical stimulation of arm: verbal report	Man	No effect	0.4 or 0.8 mg i.v.	31
Ischemic muscle pain: verbal report	Man	No effect	2 or 10 mg i.v.	44
Electrical stimulation of arm: verbal report, and measurement of evoked potential from scalp	Man	Threshold lowered in insensitive subjects, but raised in pain sensitive subjects	2 mg i.v.	13
Cold water pain: verbal report	Man	No effect	1 or 10 mg i.v.	45
Nociceptive reflex of lower limb	Man	Reduced threshold in subject cogenitally insensitive to pain	Not stated	23
Clinical pain following oral surgery: subjective judgement	Man	Increase in pain severity	9 mg i.v.	60

[a] From Cox and Baizman, ref. 19.

TABLE 2. *Effects of naloxone on analgesia produced by various experimental procedures*[a]

Method of production of analgesia	Method of measurement of pain sensitivity	Specie	Effect of naloxone	Dose of naloxone	Ref.
Stimulation of specific brain regions	Tail flick test	Rat	Partial antagonism	1 mg/kg	3,4
	Tail flick test	Rat	Inconsistent antagonism	1 or 10 mg/kg	72
	Tail flick test	Rat	No antagonism	20 mg/kg	94
	Response to forceps pinch, or electrical tooth stimulation	Cat	Antagonism	0.3 mg/kg	71
	Pathological pain: verbal report	Man	Antagonism	0.05–0.2 mg i.v.	1
	Pathological pain: verbal report	Man	Antagonism	0.1–1.0 mg i.v.	51
Acupunctural analgesia	Heat on nose: squeak response	Mouse	Antagonism	0.9 mg/kg	75
	Electrical tooth stimulation: verbal report	Man	Antagonism	0.8 mg i.v.	66
Transcutaneous electrical stimulation	Electrical tooth stimulation: verbal report	Man	Partial antagonism	0.4 mg i.v.	15
	Acute trauma pain (fractured ribs)	Man	No antagonism	0.8 mg i.v.	91
	Tail flick test	Rat	Antagonism	1 mg/kg	90
Hypnosis	Ischemic muscle pain: verbal report	Man	No antagonism	10 mg i.v.	39
	Electrical tooth stimulation: verbal report	Man	No antagonism	0.8 mg i.v.	7
Vaginal stimulation	Electrical stimulation of tail: squeak response	Rat	No antagonism	1 or 10 mg/kg	21
Cold water stress	Flinch jump test	Rat	Partial antagonism	10 mg/kg	11
Footshock stress	Tail flick test	Rat	Partial antagonism	10 mg/kg	2
	PGE₁-induced writhing frequency	Mouse	Antagonism	1 mg/kg	16
Nonopiate drugs: Nitrous oxide	Phenylbenzoquinone	Mouse	Antagonism	5 mg/kg	9
	Acetic acid-induced writhing	Mouse	Antagonism	5 mg/kg	8
Aspirin and ethanol	Acetic acid-induced writhing	Mouse	No antagonism	5–100 mg/kg	8
Substance P	Hot plate test	Mouse	Partial antagonism	60 ng/mouse i.c.v.	81
Substance P	Hot plate test	Mouse	Partial antagonism	0.2 mg/kg	35

[a]From Cox and Baizman, ref. 19.

Other evidence implicating endogenous opioids in a physiological response to noxious stimuli comes from the experiments of Akil et al. (2,64) with severe footshock stress in rats. After 30 or 60 min of continuous unavoidable footshock, tail flick latency was for a brief period prolonged (typically by 2 to 3 sec), and this effect was only partially antagonized by naloxone. Massive stress of this kind produces obvious gross derangements of behavior, in the presence of which the tail flick response could be delayed for a few seconds by nonspecific depression of alertness, attention, or motor control. However, Hayes et al. (48), in a preliminary report, claim to have ruled out such nonspecific factors, and to have confirmed the analgesic effect of footshock by the tail flick, hot plate, and noxious pressure methods.

In a rather similar study, Chance et al. (14) produced analgesia in conditioned rats by merely placing them on the grid without administering shock. This was associated with certain changes in opiate-binding capacity of brain membranes, possibly reflecting increased occupancy by endogenous ligands. Unfortunately, it was not reported if this analgesia could be blocked by naloxone.

Footshock stress (10 min) produced a very slight but significant reduction in the number of abdominal constrictions in mice after injection of formic acid or PGE_1, and the slight effect after formic acid (but not after PGE_1) was blocked by naloxone (1 mg/kg). In the same experiment, the analgesic effects of morphine (1 mg/kg) were very much greater than those attributed to footshock (16).

Reinterpretation of Naloxone Hyperalgesia in Mice

The strongest evidence suggesting that nociceptive inputs in experimental animals can be suppressed by endogenous opioids comes from the Jacob experiment (55), replicated in our laboratory (45), and by Frederickson (35–37). Mice on a hot plate give two different responses. After a few seconds a paw lick reaction is seen. Much later, at about 120 sec, the animals jump. Naloxone has no effect on the paw lick response, but greatly reduces the jump latency (as though intensifying the nociceptive input) at very low doses. This phenomenon has been interpreted to mean "that thermo-nociceptive stimulation releases endogenous ligands which temper the reaction and are antagonized by naloxone and related drugs" (54). Thus, the jump latency observed in normal mice is supposed to be prolonged relative to what it would have been in the absence of endorphins, and the latency reducing effect of naloxone is attributed to abolition of the postulated prolongation by endorphins.

Experiments by Priscilla Grevert in my laboratory (43) cast serious doubt upon this interpretation. The Jacob experiment was repeated with hypophysectomized mice (many of which also had median eminence damage). The purpose of the experiment was to ascertain if the pituitary was the source of the putative endogenous opioid supposed to be responsible for the "prolonged" (i.e., normal) jump latency. If it were, hypophysectomized animals should have shorter jump latencies, comparable to those seen in normal mice after naloxone treatment, and furthermore, naloxone should have no further latency reducing action. On the other hand, if the putative endogenous opioid were independent of the pituitary (e.g., enkephalin in substantia gelatinosa), hypophysectomized mice should have the same latencies as normal mice, and naloxone should have its usual latency reducing effect. Neither outcome was seen. The results (Fig. 1), repeated in many animals and in several independent experiments, were unambiguous. The jump latencies of hypophysectomized mice were not significantly different from normal, but naloxone was now entirely without effect.

These results are incompatible with the previous interpretation. They show that the latency reducing effect of naloxone requires the presence of the pituitary (or median eminence). Since we also showed that the antagonism of morphine analgesia by naloxone was unaffected by hypophysectomy, it cannot be argued that the pituitary is required for naloxone blockade of opiate receptors. The most parsimonious explanation is that secretion of a *pituitary hyperalgesic factor* is stimulated by naloxone. Such a factor could be under tonic inhibitory control by enkephalin or another endorphin, and its release by naloxone would be analo-

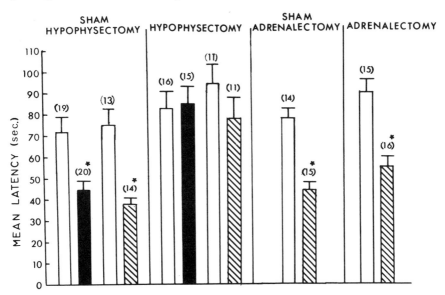

FIG. 1. Jump latencies. Mean (+ SEM) latency (seconds) of sham hypophysectomized, hypophysectomized, sham adrenalectomized, and adrenalectomized mice to jump off a $55 \pm 1°C$ hot plate 10 min after s.c. injections of saline *(clear bar)*, 1 mg/kg naloxone *(dark bar)*, or 3 mg/kg naloxone *(hatched bar)*. The appropriate saline control group is to the left of each experimental group. All mice, except the hypophysectomized and sham hypophysectomized mice that received 3 mg/kg of naloxone and their saline controls, were tested during the normal dark period. The number of mice in each group is in parentheses. The following day, the 3 mg/kg naloxone groups with hypophysectomy or sham hypophysectomy were placed on a hot plate at 62°C. All the mice had jump latencies of 10 sec or less. Thus, the failure of naloxone to reduce latency in hypophysectomized animals were not due to an impaired ability to jump faster. Asterisks denote values significantly less than the saline controls ($p < 0.001$). (From Grevert et al., ref. 43.)

gous to the naloxone stimulation of luteinizing hormone (LH) release. In any case, the jump latency of normal mice would not be under a tempering influence of endogenous opioids. Possibly relevant here is the dramatic and permanent analgesic effect that hypophysectomy can sometimes produce, in intractable cancer pain (69), an action that is not antagonized by naloxone (68).

This reinterpretation of the hyperalgesic action of naloxone on hot plate behavior calls into question all experiments with various kinds of noxious stimuli, in which naloxone had a hyperalgesic effect. To sustain the conclusion that endorphins exert direct analgesic actions on opiate receptors in the pain pathways in those experiments, it would seem necessary to show that the same results are obtained after hypophysectomy.

Naloxone on Pain in Humans

In human volunteers, in our laboratory, using both ischemic exercise forearm pain and cold water immersion pain, intravenous naloxone up to 10 mg was absolutely without effect on subjective pain ratings, and there was also no effect on mood (an early finding of slightly increased anxiety could not be replicated) (44,46). Similar negative findings, usually at lower doses, have been reported by others (31). In one study using electric shock to the arm, the pain threshold of pain-insensitive subjects was lowered slightly by naloxone (2 mg i.v.), but the threshold was raised in pain-sensitive subjects (13). Dental pain after tooth extraction was somewhat increased in severity after naloxone (9 mg i.v.) (60).

Was Enough Naloxone Used in the Negative Experiments?

It is reasonable to ask if, in the experiments with negative outcome, naloxone was used at sufficient dosage to occupy the opiate receptors. Here it is relevant to recall that less than 1 mg of the antagonist suffices to produce dramatic resuscitation of victims of heroin overdosage and also to abolish profound analgesia caused by opiates (56). It has been argued, however, that a much higher naloxone concentration is required to compete with the opioid peptides than with exogenous opiates at receptor sites (52,62).

We now know that the hormonal effects of endogenous opioids are blocked by very low naloxone (or naltrexone) doses. Thus, as little as 0.2 mg/kg in laboratory animals is sufficient to cause a substantial increase in release of LH (12) and a decrease in release of growth hormone (GH) and prolactin from pituitary (17,22,27,33,38,42,76,79,85). These effects are exactly what would be expected if endogenous opioids were acting like morphine—to inhibit LH release and to stimulate GH and prolactin release. It may be concluded that release of these hormones is under tonic inhibitory or excitatory regulation through opiate receptors. And most important, these results provide concrete evidence that low doses of naloxone effectively block a certain class of endorphin action.

It could be argued that opiate receptors in the pain pathways differ from those controlling hormone release. It is noteworthy, however, that stimulation-produced analgesia can be blocked by very low doses of naloxone in the cat (71), and by as little as 0.2 mg in man (1,51). Acupuncture analgesia, in animals (74,75) and in man (66), is also blocked by low doses of naloxone, although hypnosis analgesia is not (7,39). There is both positive and negative evidence on the ability of naloxone to block analgesia produced by transcutaneous stimulation (15,90,91).

A case of congenital insensitivity to pain responded dramatically to naloxone (1.2 mg i.v.) (23). The greatly elevated pain threshold was temporarily brought into the normal range, whereas the same dose of naloxone had no effect on the pain thresholds of normal subjects. This experiment suggests that strong tonic activation of analgesia receptors by endogenous opioids is a pathological rather than a physiological condition.

Thus, although *in vitro* opiate receptor binding studies indicate that naloxone is somewhat less effective in competing with enkephalin than with opiate alkaloids, there seems to be no doubt that *in vivo*, low-to-moderate doses of naloxone do block certain endorphin-mediated effects. These include not only hormonal effects, but analgesia produced by artificial stimulation (directly in the brain or by electroacupuncture) or in congenital insensitivity to pain. I conclude that the negative experiments cannot be blamed on insufficient naloxone dosage.

SUMMARY

That the enkephalin-containing neurons and their receptors are optimally placed to inhibit noxious inputs is evident, and it is also true that neuronal terminals containing β-endorphin could secrete into the cerebroventricular system, where administration of exogenous β-endorphin is known to produce analgesia. Artificial stimulation by electrodes in the brain or by acupuncture apparently releases endorphins to cause analgesia. Moreover, evolutionary considerations suggest important survival value for the endorphins and their receptors.

How, then, can we rationalize the paucity of evidence for a physiological, naloxone-blocked modulatory influence on pain? I suggest that with respect to analgesia, in contrast to control of pituitary hormone release, the endorphin system is not tonically active, except in pathological states. This view is supported by the finding of Duggan et al. (26) that naloxone did not increase the firing of cat dorsal horn cells in response to noxious stimuli. Moreover, the opioid antinociceptive system is not activated readily or quickly by acute noxious stimuli of moderate intensity. Possibly chronic pathological pain is required, or pain in association with overwhelming stress.

The complex mechanisms of nociception were themselves perfected over millions of years of evolution, and for obvious reasons. A counter-mechanism would seem to have survival value only in facilitating escape from a predator, as part of a fight or flight response to a life-threatening situation, or to reduce the intensity of chronic pain. Animal experiments with naloxone should therefore simulate more closely the association of pain with life-or-death encounters, and should also employ chronic pathological pain. Human studies should focus upon naloxone in chronic clinical pain. Differential diagnosis between chronic pain of organic and psychological origin is notoriously difficult. It would be interesting to study whether naloxone exacerbates the former preferentially, with a view to improved diagnosis. Sufficiently stressful experiments in which very severe acute or chronic pain is produced in human volunteers are certainly ruled out by ethical considerations.

ACKNOWLEDGMENT

The experimental studies were supported by grant DA–1199 from the National Institute on Drug Abuse.

REFERENCES

1. Adams, J. E. (1976): Naloxone reversal of analgesia produced by brain stimulation in the human. *Pain,* 2:161–166.
2. Akil, H., Madden, J., IV, Patrick, R. L., and Barchas, J. D. (1976): Stress-induced increase in endogenous opiate peptides: Concurrent analgesia and its partial reversal by naloxone. In: *Opiates and Endogenous Opioid Peptides,* edited by H. W. Kosterlitz, pp. 63–70. Elsevier/North-Holland, Amsterdam.
3. Akil, H., Mayer, D. J., and Liebeskind, J. C. (1972): Comparaison chez le rat entre l'analgesie induite par stimulation de la substance grise péri-aqueducale et l'analgésie morphinique. *C. R. Acad. Sci. [D] (Paris),* 274:3603–3605.
4. Akil, H., Mayer, D. J., and Liebeskind, J. C. (1976): Antagonism of stimulation-produced analgesia by naloxone, a narcotic antagonist. *Science,* 191:961–962.
5. Atweh, S. F., and Kuhar, M. J. (1977): Autoradiographic localization of opiate receptors in rat brain. II. The brain stem. *Brain Res.,* 129:1–12.
6. Atweh, S. F., and Kuhar, M. J. (1977): Autoradiographic localization of opiate receptors in rat brain. III. The telencephalon. *Brain Res.,* 134:393–405.
7. Barber, J., and Mayer, D. (1977): Evaluation of the efficacy and neural mechanism of a hypnotic analgesia procedure in experimental and clinical dental pain. *Pain,* 4:41–48.
8. Berkowitz, B. A., Finck, A. D., and Ngai, S. H. (1977): Nitrous oxide analgesia: Reversal by naloxone and development of tolerance. *J. Pharmacol. Exp. Ther.,* 203:539–547.
9. Berkowitz, B. A., Ngai, S. H., and Finck, A. D. (1976): Nitrous oxide "analgesia": Resemblance to opiate action. *Science,* 194:967–968.
10. Berntson, G. G., and Walker, J. M. (1977): Effect of opiate receptor blockade on pain sensitivity in the rat. *Brain Res. Bull.,* 2:157–159.
11. Bodnar, R. J., Kelly, D. D., Spiaggia, A., and Glusman, M. (1977): Analgesia produced by cold water stress: Effect of naloxone. *Fed. Proc.,* 36:1010.
12. Bruni, J. F., Van Vugt, D., Marshall, S., and Meites, J. (1977): Effects of naloxone, morphine and methionine enkephalin on serum prolactin, luteinizing hormone, follicle stimulating hormone, thyroid stimulating hormone and growth hormone. *Life Sci.,* 21:461–466.
13. Buchsbaum, M. E., Davis, G. C., and Bunney, W. E., Jr. (1977): Naloxone alters pain perception and somatosensory evoked potentials in normal subjects. *Nature,* 270:620–622.
14. Chance, W. T., White, A. C., Krynock, G. M., and Rosecrans, J. A. (1978): Conditional fear-induced antinociception and decreased binding of [^{3}H]N-Leu-enkephalin to rat brain. *Brain Res.,* 141:371–374.
15. Chapman, C. R., and Benedetti, C. (1977): Analgesia following transcutaneous electrical stimulation and its partial reversal by a narcotic antagonist. *Life Sci.,* 21:1645–1648.
16. Chesher, G. B., and Chan, B. (1977): Footshock induced analgesia in mice: Its reversal by naloxone and cross tolerance with morphine. *Life Sci.,* 21:1569–1574.

17. Cocchi, D., Santagostino, A., Gil-Ad, I., Ferri, S., and Muller, E. E. (1977): Leu-enkephalin-stimulated growth hormone and prolactin release in rat: Comparison with effect of morphine. *Life Sci.,* 20:2041–2045.

18. Cooper, J. R., Bloom, F. E., and Roth, R. H., editors (1974): *The Biochemical Basis of Neuropharmacology, 2nd edition.* Oxford University Press, New York.

19. Cox, B. M., and Baizman, E. R. (1979): Physiological functions of endorphins. In: *Endorphins,* edited by R. M. S. Bell and J. B. Malick. Marcel Dekker, New York *(in press).*

20. Cox, B. M., Opheim, K. E., Teschemacher, H., and Goldstein, A. (1975): A peptide-like substance from pituitary that acts like morphine. 2. Purification and properties. *Life Sci.,* 16:1777–1782.

21. Crowley, W. R., Rodriguez-Sierra, J. F., Komisaruk, B. R. (1977): Analgesia induced by vaginal stimulation in rats is apparently independent of a morphine-sensitive process. *Psychopharmacology,* 54:223–225.

22. Cusan, L., Dupont, A., Kledzik, G. S., Labrie, F., Coy, D. H., and Schally, A. V. (1977): Potent prolactin and growth hormone releasing activity of more analogs of Met-enkephalin. *Nature,* 268:544–547.

23. Dehen, H., Willer, J. C., Boureau, F., and Cambier, J. (1977): Congenital insensitivity to pain and endogenous morphine-like substances. *Lancet,* 2:293–294.

24. Duggan, A. W., Hall, J. G., and Headley, P. M. (1977): Enkephalins and dorsal horn neurones of the cat: Effects on responses to noxious and innocuous skin stimuli. *Br. J. Pharmacol.,* 61:399–408.

25. Duggan, A. W., Hall, J. G., and Headley, P. M. (1977): Suppression of transmission of nociceptive impulses by morphine: Selective effects of morphine administered in the region of the substantia gelatinosa. *Br. J. Pharmacol.,* 61:65–76.

26. Duggan, A. W., Hall, J. G., Headley, P. M., and Griersmith, B. T. (1977): The effect of naloxone on the excitation of dorsal horn neurones of the cat by noxious and non-noxious cutaneous stimuli. *Brain Res.,* 138:185–189.

27. Dupont, A., Cusan, L., Garon, M., Labrie, F., and Li, C. H. (1977): β-Endorphin: Stimulation of growth hormone release *in vivo. Proc. Natl. Acad. Sci. USA,* 74:358–359.

28. Dutta, A. S., Gormley, J. J., Hayward, C. F., Morley, J. S., Shaw, J. S., Stacey, G. J., and Turnbull, M. J. (1977): Analgesia following intravenous administration of enkephalin analogues. *Br. J. Pharmacol.,* 61:P481–P482.

29. Dutta, A. S., Gormley, J. J., Hayward, C. F., Morley, J. S., Shaw, J. S., Stacey, G. J., and Turnbull, M. J. (1977): Enkephalin analogues eliciting analgesia after intravenous injection. *Life Sci.,* 21:559–562.

30. Dykstra, L. A., and McMillan, D. E. (1977): Electric shock titration: Effects of morphine, methadone, pentazocine, nalorphine, naloxone, diazepam and amphetamine. *J. Pharmacol. Exp. Ther.,* 202:660–669.

31. El-Sobky, A., Dostrovsky, J. O., and Wall, P. D. (1976): Lack of effect of naloxone on pain perception in humans. *Nature,* 263:783–784.

32. Feldberg, W., and Smyth, D. G. (1977): C-fragment of lipotropin—an endogenous potent analgesic peptide. *Br. J. Pharmacol.,* 60:445–453.

33. Ferland, L., Fuxe, K., Enefoth, P., Gustafsson, J. A., and Skett, P. (1977): Effects of methionine-enkephalin on prolactin release and catecholamine levels and turnover in the median eminence. *Eur. J. Pharmacol.,* 43:89–90.

34. Frederickson, R. C. A. (1977): Enkephalin pentapeptides—a review of current evidence for a physiological role in vertebrate neurotransmission. *Life Sci.,* 21:23–42.

35. Frederickson, R. C. A., Burgis, V., and Edwards, J. D. (1977): Hyperalgesia induced by naloxone follows diurnal rhythm in responsivity to painful stimuli. *Science,* 198:756–758.

36. Frederickson, R. C. A., Burgis, V., Harrell, C. E., and Edwards, J. D. (1978): Dual actions of substance P on nociception: Possible role of endogenous opioids. *Science,* 199:1359–1362.

37. Frederickson, R. C. A., Nickander, R., Smithwick, E. L., Shuman, R., and Norris, F. H. (1976): Pharmacological activity of met-enkephalin and analogues *in vitro* and *in vivo:* Depression of single neuronal activity in specified brain regions. In: *Opiates and Endogenous Opioid Peptides,* edited by H. W. Kosterlitz, pp. 239–246. Elsevier/North-Holland, Amsterdam.

38. Gold, M. S., Redmond, D. E. Jr., and Donabedian, R. K. (1978): Prolactin secretion, a measurable central effect of opiate-receptor antagonists. *Lancet,* 1:323–324.

39. Goldstein, A., and Hilgard, E. R. (1975): Failure of the opiate antagonist naloxone to modify hypnotic analgesia. *Proc. Natl. Acad. Sci., USA,* 72:2041–2043.

40. Goldstein, A. (1976): Opioid peptides (endorphins) in pituitary and brain. *Science,* 193:1081–1086.
41. Goldstein, A., Pryor, G. T., Otis, L. S., and Larsen, F. (1976): On the role of endogenous opioid peptides: Failure of naloxone to influence shock escape threshold in the rat. *Life Sci.,* 18:599–604.
42. Grandison, L., and Guidotti, A. (1977): Regulation of prolactin release by endogenous opiates. *Nature,* 270:357–359.
43. Grevert, P., Baizman, E. R., and Goldstein, A. (1978): Naloxone effects on a nociceptive response of hypophysectomized and adrenalectomized mice. *Life Sci.,* 23:723–728.
44. Grevert, P., and Goldstein, A. (1977): Effects of naloxone on experimentally induced ischemic pain and on mood in human subjects. *Proc. Natl. Acad. Sci., USA,* 74:1291–1294.
45. Grevert, P., and Goldstein, A. (1977): Some effects of naloxone on behavior in the mouse. *Psychopharmacology,* 53:111–113.
46. Grevert, P., and Goldstein, A. (1978): Endorphins: Naloxone fails to alter experimental pain or mood in humans. *Science,* 199:1093–1095.
47. Guillemin, R. (1977): Endorphins, brain peptides that act like opiates. *N. Engl. J. Med.,* 296:226–228.
48. Hayes, R. L., Bennett, G. J., Newlon, P., and Mayer, D. J. (1976): Analgesic effects of certain noxious and stressful manipulations in the rat. *Soc. Neurosci. Abstr.,* II:939.
49. Hökfelt, T., Elde, R., Johansson, O., Terenius, L., and Stein, L. (1977): The distribution of enkephalin-immunoreactive cell bodies in the rat central nervous system. *Neurosci. Lett.,* 5:25–31.
50. Hökfelt, T., Ljungdahl, A., Terenius, L., Elde, R., and Nilsson, G. (1977): Immunohistochemical analysis of peptide pathways possibly related to pain and analgesia: Enkephalin and substance P. *Proc. Natl. Acad. Sci. USA,* 74:3081–3085.
51. Hosobuchi, Y., Adams, J. E., and Linchitz, R. (1977): Pain relief by electrical stimulation of the central gray matter in humans and its reversal by naloxone. *Science,* 197:183–186.
52. Hughes, J., and Kosterlitz, H. W. (1977): Opioid peptides. *Br. Med. Bull.,* 33:157–161.
53. Hughes, J., Smith, T. W., Kosterlitz, H. W., Fothergill, L. A., Morgan, B. A., and Morris, H. R. (1975): Identification of two related pentapeptides from the brain with potent opiate agonist activity. *Nature,* 258:577–579.
54. Jacob, J. J. C., and Ramabadran, K. (1977): Opioid antagonists, endogenous ligands and nociception. *Eur. J. Pharmacol.,* 46:393–394.
55. Jacob, J. J., Tremblay, E. C., and Colombel, M. C. (1974): Facilitation de réactions nociceptives par la naloxone chez la souris et chez le rat. *Psychopharmacologia (Berl.),* 37:217–223.
56. Jaffe, J. F., and Martin, W. R. (1975): Narcotic analgesics and antagonists. In: *The Pharmacological Basis of Therapeutics, 5th edition,* edited by L. S. Goodman and A. Gilman, pp. 245–283, Macmillan, New York.
57. Jessell, T. M., and Iversen, L. L. (1977): Opiate analgesics inhibit substance P release from rat trigeminal nucleus. *Nature,* 268:549–551.
58. Klee, W. A., Lampert, A., and Nirenberg, M. (1976): Dual regulation of adenylate cyclase by endogenous opiate peptides. In: *Opiates and Endogenous Opioid Peptides,* edited by H. W. Kosterlitz, pp. 153–159. Elsevier/North-Holland, Amsterdam.
59. Kokka, N., and Fairhurst, A. S. (1977): Naloxone enhancement of acetic acid-induced writhing in rats. *Life Sci.,* 21:975–980.
60. Levine, J. D., Gordon, N. C., Jones, R. T., and Fields, H. L. (1978): The narcotic antagonist naloxone enhances clinical pain. *Nature,* 272:826–827.
61. Li, C. H. (1977): β-endorphin: A pituitary peptide with potent morphine-like activity. *Arch. Biochem. Biophys.,* 183:592–604.
62. Lord, J. A. H., Waterfield, A. A., Hughes, J., and Kosterlitz, H. W. (1977): Endogenous opioid peptides: Multiple agonists and receptors. *Nature,* 267:495–499.
63. Macdonald, R. L., and Nelson, P. G. (1978): Specific opiate-induced depression of transmitter release from dorsal root ganglion cells in culture. *Science,* 199:1449–1451.
64. Madden, J., IV, Akil, H., Patrick, R. L., Barchas, J. D. (1977): Stress-induced parallel changes in central opioid levels and pain responsiveness in the rat. *Nature,* 265:358–360.
65. Mayer, D. J., and Price, D. D. (1976): Central nervous system mechanisms of analgesia. *Pain,* 2:379–404.
66. Mayer, D. J., Price, D. D., and Rafii, A. (1977): Antagonism of acupuncture analgesia in man by the narcotic antagonist naloxone. *Brain Res.,* 121:368–372.

67. Miller, R. J., Chang, K-J., Cooper, B., and Cuatrecasas, P. (1978): Radioimmunoassay and characterization of enkephalins in rat tissues. *J. Biol. Chem.,* 253:531–538.
68. Misfeldt, D. S., and Goldstein, A. (1977): Hypophysectomy relieves pain not via endorphins. *N. Engl. J. Med.,* 297:1236–1237.
69. Moricca, G. (1974): Chemical hypophysectomy for cancer pain. *Adv. Neurol.,* 4:707–714.
70. North, M. A. (1977): Naloxone reversal of morphine analgesia but failure to alter reactivity to pain in the formalin test. *Life Sci.,* 22:295–302.
71. Oliveras, J. L., Hosobuchi, Y., Redjemi, F., Guilbaud, G., and Besson, J. M. (1977): Opiate antagonist, naloxone, strongly reduces analgesia induced by stimulation of a raphe nucleus (centralis inferior). *Brain Res.,* 120:221–229.
72. Pert, A., and Walter, M. (1976): Comparison between naloxone reversal of morphine and electrical stimulation induced analgesia in the rat mesencephalon. *Life Sci.,* 19:1023–1032.
73. Pert, C. B., Bowie, D. L., Pert, A., Morell, J. L., and Gross, E. (1977): Agonist-antagonist properties of *N*-allyl-[D-Ala]²-Met-enkephalin. *Nature,* 269:73–75.
74. Pomeranz, B., Cheng, R., and Law, P. (1977): Acupuncture reduces electrophysiological and behavioral responses to noxious stimuli: Pituitary is implicated. *Exp. Neurol.,* 54:172–178.
75. Pomeranz, B., and Chiu, D. (1976): Naloxone blockade of acupuncture analgesia: Endorphin implicated. *Life Sci.,* 19:1757–1762.
76. Rivier, C., Vale, W., Ling, N., Brown, M., and Guillemin, R. (1977): Stimulation *in vivo* of secretion of prolactin and growth hormone by β-endorphin. *Endocrinology,* 100:238–241.
77. Roemer, D., Buescher, H. H., Hill, R. C., Pless, J., Bauer, W., Cardinaux, F., Closse, A., Hauser, D., and Huguenin, R. (1977): A synthetic enkephalin analogue with prolonged parenteral and oral analgesic activity. *Nature,* 268:547–549.
78. Rossier, J., Vargo, T. M., Minick, S., Ling, N., Bloom, F. E., and Guillemin, R. (1977): Regional dissociation of β-endorphin and enkephalin contents in rat brain and pituitary. *Proc. Natl. Acad. Sci. USA,* 74:5162–5165.
79. Shaar, C. J., Frederickson, R. C. A., Dininger, N. B., and Jackson, L. (1977): Enkephalin analogues and naloxone modulate the release of growth hormone and prolactin: Evidence for regulation by an endogenous opioid peptide in brain. *Life Sci.,* 21:853–860.
80. Simon, E. J. (1976): The opiate receptors. *Neurochem. Res.,* 1:3–28.
81. Stewart, J. M., Getto, C. J., Neldner, K., Reeve, E. B., Krivoy, W. A., and Zimmerman, E. (1976): Substance P and analgesia. *Nature,* 262:784–785.
82. Székely, J. I., Rónai, A. Z., Dunai-Kovács, Z., Miglécz, E., Berzétri, I., Bajusz, S., and Gráf, L. (1977): (D-Met², Pro⁵)-Enkephalinamide: A potent morphine-like analgesic. *Eur. J. Pharmacol.,* 43:293–294.
83. Terenius, L. (1978): Endogenous peptides and analgesia. *Annu. Rev. Pharmacol. Toxicol.,* 18:189–204.
84. Teschemacher, H., Opheim, K. E., Cox, B. M., and Goldstein, A. (1975): A peptide-like substance from pituitary that acts like morphine. 1. Isolation. *Life Sci.,* 16:1771–1776.
85. Van Vugt, D. A., Bruni, J. F., and Meites, J. (1978): Naloxone inhibition of stress-induced increase in prolactin secretion. *Life Sci.,* 22:85–90.
86. Walker, J. M., Sandman, C. A., Berntson, G. G., and McGivern, R. F. (1977): Endorphin analogs with potent and long-lasting analgesic effects. *Pharmacol. Biochem. Behav.,* 7:543–548.
87. Watson, S. J., Akil, H., Sullivan, S., and Barchas, J. D. (1977): Immunocytochemical localization of methionine enkephalin: Preliminary observations. *Life Sci.,* 21:733–738.
88. Watson, S. J., Barchas, J. D., and Li, C. H. (1977): β-lipotropin: Localization of cells and axons in rat brain by immunocytochemistry. *Proc. Natl. Acad. Sci. USA,* 74:5155–5158.
89. Wei, E. T., Tseng, L. F., Loh, H. H., and Li, C. H. (1977): Comparison of the behavioral effects of β-endorphin and enkephalin analogs. *Life Sci.,* 21:321–327.
90. Woolf, C. J., Barrett, G. D., Mitchell, D., and Myers, R. A. (1977): Naloxone-reversible peripheral electroanalgesia in intact and spinal rats. *Eur. J. Pharmacol.,* 45:311–314.
91. Woolf, C. J., Mitchell, D., Myers, R. A., and Barrett, G. D. (1978): Failure of naloxone to reverse peripheral transcutaneous electro-analgesia in patients suffering from acute trauma. *S. Afr. Med. J.,* 53:179–180.
92. Yaksh, T. L. (1978): Opiate receptors for behavioral analgesia resemble those related to the depression of spinal nociceptive neurons. *Science,* 199:1231–1233.
93. Yaksh, T. L., Huang, S. P., Rudy, T. A., and Frederickson, R. C. A. (1977): The direct and specific opiate-like effect of met⁵-enkephalin and analogues on the spinal cord. *Neuroscience,* 2:593–596.

94. Yaksh, T. L., Yeung, J. C., and Rudy, T. A. (1976): An inability to antagonize with naloxone the elevated nociceptive thresholds resulting from electrical stimulation of the mesencephalic central gray. *Life Sci.,* 18:1193–1198.
95. Yamashiro, D., Tseng, L-F., and Li, C. H. (1977): [D-Thr^2,Thz^5]- and [D-Met^2,Thz^5]-Enkephalinamides: Potent analgesics by intravenous injection. *Biochem. Biophys. Res. Commun.,* 78:1124–1129.

Mechanisms of Pain and Analgesic Compounds,
edited by R. F. Beers, Jr., and E. G. Bassett.
Raven Press, New York © 1979.

23. Discussion

Moderator: Hans W. Kosterlitz

A. Goldstein: I want to comment on the papers by Hans Kosterlitz and John Hughes. In working with peptides, there are two general things that may happen; then there is one special thing that may happen during investigations of enkephalins and endorphins. Enzymic or nonenzymic breakdowns of the peptides may occur during processing and work-up. There may also be a loss of peptides by adsorption to glass and plastic surfaces, which is particularly serious at low concentrations of the peptides. There is really no good solution to the problem.

Another difficulty is the tendency of methionine to become oxidized; in some assays this oxidation may render the results invalid. The degree of oxidation depends on the conditions of the processing of the materials.

I now want to comment on two matters: first, the question of the alleged difference of the relative distribution of methionine- and leucine-enkephalin. Since there is no published evidence that the possibility of differential loss, breakdown, or oxidation has been adequately assessed, variations in the ratio of the two enkephalins in different parts of the brain may be artifactual.

The same considerations apply to the arguments for multiple opiate receptors. I think one has to be very careful for the reason Hans Kosterlitz showed you in one of his slides, namely, the increase in potency that occurs when the enkephalins are protected against breakdown. Therefore, one has to demonstrate for each tissue, in which different opiate receptors are alleged to be present on the basis of different responses to peptides and alkaloids, that there is no differential breakdown or oxidation going on.

H. W. Kosterlitz: I think we are all in agreement with what Avram Goldstein said. As far as the receptors are concerned, it is quite clear that the present evidence is indirect and circumstantial. However, with regard to breakdown in the binding tests, this has been minimized by working at low temperatures.

J. Hughes: Avram, you are quite right that enkephalin is subject to oxidation in any of the assays. We have been aware of this possibility all along and have taken precautions as far as it is possible. As regards the differential distribution of the peptides, we have measured the recoveries of added methionine- and leucine-enkephalin and I am fairly certain that the differences we see are real differences and not due to degradation or oxidation. Moreover, the variations in the ratio of the two enkephalins have been seen in several laboratories which use different methods for assaying them. So I am convinced that there are differences in the distribution of the two enkephalins.

K. L. Casey: Among the papers that have been presented at this Symposium so far, the one by H. Akil in collaboration with D. E. Richardson and J. D. Barcha has potentially very pronounced implications as regards the function of these peptides and the organization of pain systems in the brain in relation to clinical medicine.

My first question relates to the selection of the patients. I notice, for example, that most of the people fell into the categories of low back pain and I would like to know a little more about the diagnosis. Further, what was the pathology of the patients with scoliosis?

My next question deals with the methods used for testing these patients for analgesia, both inside and outside the operating room. Looking at the organization of the central nervous system, I find it difficult to accept the idea that stimulation in the periventricular gray is going to produce such a localized and selective effect.

H. Akil: I was hoping for a chance to say something about patient selection. We used only patients with well characterized medical histories; we did not take just somebody who said he had low back pain unless we could pin it down to some sort of trauma or other specific problem that was the source of that pain. We purposely used a wide variety of pain patients because we wanted to make sure that the effect of our procedure was not due to the fortuitous selection of one subcategory.

As far as the drugs are concerned, I would say that 90% of our patients were withdrawn entirely from all drugs prior to starting any procedure. We always discussed with them possible alternatives for alleviating pain. The patients were subjected to a battery of tests, including the Minnesota Multiphasic Personality Inventory. So we tried as much as possible to select patients with identifiable pain, with an identifiable cause who had been withdrawn from medication and continued to have very specific pain. Probably the acid test for the procedure was the cancer patients who had multiple types of pain.

Pain testing was done in the operating room on patients who were only under local anesthesia. They might have had a small dose of diazepam prior to surgery. Afterward, a number of the patients were given amitriptyline along with the stimulation because we found it enhanced the duration of the analgesia beyond the cessation of stimulation. Before we tested the patients in the laboratory, we asked them not to stimulate for 24 hr prior to the test. The tests were radiant heat applied to the extremities, pin pricks, and ischemic pain; we asked them to assess their chronic pain on a rating scale. Moreover, we obtained information from their families.

F. Sicuteri: Dr. Akil, would you please give us more information about the visual syndrome due to stimulation?

H. Akil: There is mostly some visual blurring that can be altered by changing the frequency of stimulation, as can the other side effects. There is no doubt in my mind that if we went above, say, 20 Hz, we would see all kinds of other phenomena. We had to work very closely with the patient to select frequencies that minimized nystagmus and sensory side effects to produce the desired reduction in pain.

H. W. Kosterlitz: Dr. Akil, obviously electrical stimulation is very nonphysiological.

H. Akil: That's right.

H. W. Kosterlitz: The question is: Do we know anything at all about the physiological activation of this pathway?

H. Akil: No.

H. W. Kosterlitz: Would it be possible to train people to activate it without electrical stimulation?

H. Akil: I think the studies of Dave Meyer on hypnosis and acupuncture and those of A. Goldstein and E. Hilgard, in which they looked at hypnotic analgesia and its reversibility by naloxone, probably came the closest to the problem of whether one can activate the system in a less aggressive way than we did. Their results were negative for hypnosis and positive for acupuncture. We do not know if it is possible to activate the system in something by yoga or something like it. When I experienced labor and delivery recently, I was struck by the effectiveness of the Lamaze technique as a means of controlling pain. I don't think that has been studied enough.

H. W. Kosterlitz: The fact that we apparently find it very difficult to activate the pathways that modify pain in such a way that we can control excessive pain is of importance for their physiological functions.

H. Akil: But as you have pointed out repeatedly, analgesia is not a normal state as much as catalepsy is not a normal state. I am sure there are neurological situations where you can see tremor epilepsy but clearly you are swinging a system far away from its homeostatic situation. It is really a difficult question for a good reason.

H. W. Kosterlitz: I deliberately asked this question to bring up this particular difficulty.

W. A. Check: I have a question prompted by the suggestions about multiple receptors. I should like to suggest a very simple control which may have been done already, namely, to let enkephalins compete in binding assays against other neurotransmitters. Such a procedure would try to settle the question whether there is cross-reaction with other transmission systems.

H. W. Kosterlitz: As far as is known, there is no cross-reaction.

A. Taub: I am intrigued by the mention of three procedures that may be considered to act as substitutes for the electrical stimulation. One of them was the use of amitriptyline, the second was the combined use of amitriptyline and fluphenazine, and the third was the withdrawal of opiates. I wonder whether there is any evidence that withdrawal of opiates in some way activates the so-called morphinomimetic systems, and whether any of the psychotropic drugs have also an activating effect. What was the percentage of patients who might have dropped out because of morphine withdrawal and the associated relief of pain, and because of the administration of amitriptyline and fluphenazine?

H. Akil: I would say that a good 50% of the patients, when you withdraw them and try them on alternate therapies, can be handled with drugs without any further manipulations. I really don't know whether the opiate withdrawal and the lack of pain after opiate withdrawal is due to psychological or physiological reasons and I don't personally know of any evidence that shows any unequivocal changes after withdrawal.

H. O. J. Collier: About 3 years ago when you and John Hughes were speculating about the enkephalins, you thought that enkephalins might be liberated by one neuron to act on another, or they might possibly be liberated by one neuron to act on itself.

I wonder if you have gotten any evidence since then which would help decide this issue.

H. W. Kosterlitz: This is at the moment still an unanswerable question although the work of Tomas Hökfelt has demonstrated co-existence of enkephalins and catecholamines in the chromaffin cells of the adrenal medulla. Enkephalins are also present in the preganglionic cholinergic fibers innervating the adrenal medulla.

A. Herz: Dr. Kosterlitz, is there any evidence that central effects of opiates are mediated by different types of receptors? Further, what is their relationship to the different types of receptors described by W. R. Martin?

H. W. Kosterlitz: The answer to the first part is simple: we have at present no information.

The second question is difficult to answer because two different techniques have been employed. Dr. Martin used the results of behavioral and neurological tests as a basis for his hypothesis of μ-, κ-, and σ-receptors. On the other hand, our differentiation of receptors is based on pharmacological *in vitro* and binding tests.

As far as I know, Dr. Martin has so far not obtained any data on enkephalins and endorphins. With regard to the opiates themselves, there are first the μ-agonists, which are morphine-like drugs. However, certain compounds, for instance, the ketazocines of Sterling–Winthrop and the N-dimethylfurylbenzomorphans of Boehringer Ingelheim do not seem to interact with the μ-receptors but rather with another class, the κ-receptors. In this respect, our data agree with those of Martin who was the first to postulate that the ketazocines interacted with the κ-receptors and not with the μ-receptors.

J. C. Liebeskind: I have a brief comment on Dr. Herz' question. We feel we have some very sketchy evidence of different functions mediated by different opiate receptor types in the rat brain. As we suggested in a recent article in *Science,* it may be that epileptogenic properties of the enkephalins are more attributable to their action on the δ-receptors and the analgesic properties to that on the μ-receptors; however, the evidence is still very limited.

R. W. Houde: I offer a brief comment on Dr. Akil's paper. We have evidence that introduction of β-endorphin into the cerebral spinal fluid produces analgesia. We have administered doses as high as 7.5 mg β-endorphin through an intraventricular catheter attached to a subcutaneous Ommaya reservoir. This procedure led to prolonged morphine-like effects of analgesia associated with drowsiness and some disorientation. On intravenous administration, the volume of distribution was very small and there was no analgesia after 5 mg β-endorphin.

G. W. Pasternak: Would you speculate a little on the multiple site theory demonstrated several years ago, namely, that there are at least two binding sites with different affinities within the brain for agonists and antagonists. One can actually destroy, by chemical or enzymic means, one of the sites without affecting the other. Please comment on this possible relationship to your multiple site theory.

H. W. Kosterlitz: We have no information on this point.

L. A. Chahl: Dr. Goldstein, how significant do you think is the fact that the pituitary is outside the blood brain barrier for the assessment of analgesic tests?

A second question is, does adrenalectomy affect the latency in hot plate testing?

A. Goldstein: The second question I can answer first. The slide showed that the latencies in adrenalectomized animals were normal and that the reaction to naloxone was also normal.

My answer to the first question is that I don't know. It is clear that some former ideas about the pituitary are pretty much abandoned now. There is flow of substances between the anterior to posterior lobes and from the pituitary back up into the stalk and the median eminence. I therefore think it is likely that any effects of pituitary peptides on pain would be through that route rather than through the bloodstream.

I think it has to be recognized that no receptors for β-endorphin have been identified in the periphery. Moreover, the concentrations of β-endorphin that circulate in the blood are by two orders of magnitude below the affinities of any of the known opiate receptors.

So I think the notion of any kind of analgesic effect mediated by the secretion of pituitary opioid peptide into the blood is most unlikely.

F. W. L. Kerr: Dr. Goldstein, you referred to the case from France which had been well studied. I recollect that, like some people with congenital indifference to pain, the patient has severe mental deficit. I wonder whether we should put much store by one case even though it appears to be rather well studied.

A. Goldstein: We shouldn't put store by one case of anything. That is fairly obvious.

I mentioned it because naloxone had a striking result but I don't think my argument depended on that at all. I think I cited other ample evidence showing the effectiveness of low doses of naloxone.

K. L. Casey: I just want to be sure I understand the thrust of Dr. Goldstein's speculation. As I understand it, you are hypothesizing on all the evidence you cited, that an algogenic substance is normally present in the pituitary, the release being activated by naloxone. Is that correct?

A. Goldstein: That is the conclusion that we are forced to by the evidence.

K. L. Casey: Are there any circumstances under which you might imagine the algogenic substance would be released other than by naloxone? In other words, we now have another problem that is as difficult to deal with as the first one. Under what circumstances might you imagine that the algogenic substance is released—only in severe pain? Would you elaborate on that a little?

A. Goldstein: Obviously I don't know. One purpose of presenting material like this is to stimulate other people to think of other interpretations and experiments. This would suggest the value of experiments in which one looked deliberately for other ways of releasing pituitary hyperalgesic substances.

H. O. J. Collier: As I see it, the essence of Goldstein's hypothesis on the hypophysis is that a hyperalgesic substance is released from the pituitary of both animals and man. As Dr. Ferreira has stated, the prostaglandins are hyperalgesic both centrally and peripherally. Hence, it might be worth looking for prostaglandin release by a pituitary mechanism.

K. L. Casey: You would expect to see at the clinical level fairly major differences between the ways hypophysectomized people and people who have an intact pituitary gland respond to or react to metastic carcinoma. Perhaps I am misunderstanding this terribly.

A. Goldstein: I think the clinicians need to resolve this question of hypophysectomy for pain. What is described in the literature by those people who get this effect (and I am influenced by one such patient at Stanford whom I saw), is a dramatic, complete, immediate, and permanent alleviation of intractable deep cancer pain. This occurs in patients with tumors that are not necessarily hormone-dependent. Since these patients do not have any disturbance in the appreciation of epicritic pain, it has to be assumed that there is something very different about the kind of pain that is generated from metastatic cancer. It seems to involve the pituitary hyperalgesic substance in some way.

R. W. Houde: Dr. Goldstein, I would like to address the same question because the response to hypophysectomy that one sees is not that consistent. While it does occur and while it may be very dramatic, it most commonly occurs in breast cancer, or prostatic cancer, or metastic disease in the bone but even there not consistently. Therefore, I am not so sure that your hypothesis holds up. Moreover, these patients may have a return of pain later in the course of their disease. So I have real reservations about what you say.

A. Goldstein: The hypothesis that I advanced in no way depends on clinical results. I think that clinicians should settle what the problem is because dramatic cases have been reported and there are other cases in whom hypophysectomy does not work; there seems to be something out of control in this clinical procedure. But the proposed hypothesis, I repeat, is forced by on us the experimental data that I presented in mice. I suggest that if someone has an alternative interpretation of those data, he should advance a counterhypothesis.

R. W. Houde: The patients who have hypophysectomies in our hospital are checked by endocrine measures to decide whether the hypophysectomy is complete or not. I might point out that in Moricca's method of injecting alcohol or phenol in the hypophysis, it apparently has been shown that the injected material courses along the stalk into the hypothalamus and down along the base.

A Goldstein: It is very important and I should have mentioned it in my presentation. Hypophysectomized mice are very likely to have median eminence damage. It is very difficult to obtain commercially hypophysectomized mice without such damage. It is a good idea to check that out. Many of our mice did have median eminence damage and the effects that I described could therefore be due to that, rather than to the hypophysectomy itself.

A. Taub: Dr. Goldstein, you have found that the mice jump off the plate faster when they get naloxone and you postulate that perhaps they feel more pain. I understand that is what you mean by hyperalgesia. Would you postulate that the mice actually feel something?

I would suggest that your experiment is ambiguous because you have no idea why the mice jump off the plate and you haven't devised an experimental control to demonstrate that, if the mice can't feel anything, they will not jump off the plate.

I should add that your experiment is not only ambiguous but the material that you present is very ambiguous. For example, you quote without any question the data that suggest that the so-called acupunctural effect is affected by naloxone.

We really can't accept the idea that the effect of hypophysectomy in chronic pain is based upon data obtained from acupuncture, the effect of which is not very well established. We must have unambiguous experiments with unambiguous results before we worry about hypotheses. Then we clinicians will start to sharpen up our clinical data.

A. Goldstein: I certainly agree with you. No one could deny that unambiguous data are useful to have.

As to the two specific questions, one doesn't try to attribute feelings to mice. The effect that we are talking about is the effect that has been universally studied in all experiments on nociception and antinociception. We have chosen the hot plate technique to study this effect. What we have shown is that the effects of naloxone in shortening the latency disappears after hypophysectomy. That is an unambiguous fact and it has nothing to do with what the mice feel or don't feel. But it does have to do with the interpretation that others have placed on that same experiment. That is all that needs to be said. The problem does need some thinking about, because previously those studies fit into a comfortable framework in which one thought that the enkephalinergic systems are active here and that naloxone shuts them off and therefore everything was all right. What I am saying is that the problem needs rethinking.

As to the second part of your question, I really must reject the criticism. It wasn't my function here to review all the data that are in the literature on acupuncture or anything else. I was referring to what I consider the well-controlled and carefully done experiments of Pomeranz on cats and mice and of David Mayer on humans. Both are consistent in showing clearly measurable effects of acupuncture which are abolished by very low doses of naloxone. That was the purpose of mentioning it.

A. Taub: The point I wanted to make was the difficulty of extrapolating from animal to man and of talking about analgesia in this context. You really must at the same time do controlled experiments which account for all other possible effects that naloxone can exert other than on conscious experience. What I am appealing for is this: when we decide to extrapolate from the animal to human system, the first thing we must do is eliminate rigorously the possibility that what is happening is merely reflex.

F. W. L. Kerr: I would like to get back to the matter of the striking effect that you get in some cases of hypophysectomy and suggest another possibility that has not been considered and which struck me a long time ago on seeing pain disappear completely and immediately after hypophysectomy in cases of breast cancer. We still don't know what the pain mechanism is in cancer and whether it is generated by metastic tumors invading the plexuses, the periosteum, or for other reasons. However, the indications for the hypophysectomy was the attempt to cause involution of the tumors.

It is quite possible that, immediately after hypophysectomy, a marked change occurs at the tumor level itself and it may be unnecessary to postulate that an algogenic substance is released by the pituitary. There may be a rapid decrease in the vascular blood supply which may markedly modify mechanical and chemical factors at the tumor level. Dr. Goldstein, would you like to consider the possibility?

A. Goldstein: I would like not to consider that because I am not at all an expert clinician in relation to hypophysectomized patients. Had I omitted any reference to that phenomenon, it would have been correctly criticized since there is such strong evidence in our work that the pituitary may have a hyperalgesic effect in animals. I don't know what relationship that has to this phenomenon in man.

Mechanisms of Pain and Analgesic Compounds,
edited by R. F. Beers, Jr., and E. G. Bassett.
Raven Press, New York © 1979.

24. Introduction to Section D: Peripheral Mechanisms of Pain and Analgesia

S. H. Ferreira

Department of Pharmacology, Faculty of Medicine of Ribeirão Preto, São Paulo, Brazil

It is our intention to present some aspects from our work that may be of some practical and theoretical importance, and that have been selected in order to stimulate discussion. The speakers have in common the fact that, at some point during their career, they have studied the participation of an inflammatory mediator in some "painful situation," either trying to understand its relevance to the ongoing process or how drugs are capable of interfering in its synthesis, release, or action. I believe (and this is a point for discussion) that pain treatable with aspirin-like drugs or even opioids results from the participation of some mediator of inflammation and is not solely due to structual tissue changes that occur during inflammation.

I am sure you all understand that we are dealing with a very complex subject, pain, and that our experiments and theories may lead us to error. But, I believe in Francis Bacon's remark that "truth comes out of error more easily than out of confusion." We do not mind to be in error; in fact, we are struggling to get out of confusion.

Mechanisms of Pain and Analgesic Compounds,
edited by R. F. Beers, Jr., and E. G. Bassett.
Raven Press, New York © 1979.

25. Pain Induced by Inflammatory Mediators

Loris A. Chahl

Department of Physiology, University of Queensland, St. Lucia, Queensland, 4067 Australia

INTRODUCTION

Pain and Nociception

A large number of substances of diverse chemical nature are released during the inflammatory response. Several of these substances have been shown to induce pain, as well as some of the vascular changes characteristic of inflammatory states. Those which have been most fully investigated for their pain-inducing activity include histamine, 5-hydroxytryptamine, acetylcholine, bradykinin, prostaglandins, and potassium and hydrogen ions. Other substances are also known to be released from cellular elements such as platelets and leukocytes during the inflammatory response. Some of these are high-molecular weight proteins and enzymes, but little is known of their pain-inducing actions.

Pain in its most complete sense can only be studied in conscious man. Experiments in man must be of a very limited nature, and thus many investigations have been on nociception in animals. Studies in animals are made difficult by the necessity to find a reliable response to the stimulus under investigation. Since all experiments on conscious animals are fraught with ethical considerations, in many studies nociception has been investigated in anesthetized animals using indices such as autonomic reflexes which may be still present.

Experimental Techniques Used to Study Pain and Nociception

Pain

Pain induced by chemicals applied into or onto the skin of conscious human subjects has been widely investigated. The cantharidine blister base technique developed by Armstrong et al. (1) was an important advance in the study of substances inducing cutaneous pain in man, since it overcame some of the problems of other techniques such as pain induced by the pressure of injected solutions.

The blister base is an inflammatory site itself, and the technique could be criticized in light of recent evidence that there is potentiation among some mediators of inflammation (15). It should also be remembered that the top layer of the skin has been removed and the chemicals might be placed in contact with axons which do not have the usual receptive area present. So little is known of the mechanisms by which chemicals activate the nerves that this is not yet a valid reason for criticism of results using this technique. Despite these possible limitations, the technique has shown which substances are potentially painful to man. Keele and Armstrong (34) obtained evidence that the stimulation of "pain" nerve fibers by some chemicals was by action on specific receptors in the pharmacological sense, since they were antagonized by their appropriate blocking agents; i.e., acetylcholine could be blocked by nicotinic receptor blocking agents. There was also no crossed tachyphylaxis between many of the agents.

The pain-inducing action of chemicals on deeper tissues in man has been, of necessity, less studied, although pain induced on intramuscular or intravascular injection has been recorded for some substances.

Nociception

Nociception in conscious animals has been studied using responses such as writhing in mice, withdrawal of limbs in response to applied pressure, and vocalization in animals such as dogs. In anesthetized animals, "pseudoaffective" reactions such as reflex rise in blood pressure or changes in respiration have been commonly used as indices of nociception. The activities of pain-inducing substances on afferent nerves from skin, muscle, or viscera have been investigated employing electrophysiological techniques of recording from single or multiple afferent units dissected from whole nerves. In these studies, the substances have been administered by retrograde intraarterial injection into the blood supplying the region from which recordings were being made, or by injection or direct application to the tissue under investigation. The former technique was used by Fjällbrant and Iggo (17) to investigate the action of 5-hydroxytryptamine, histamine, acetylcholine, and crude bradykinin on cutaneous afferent nerves from the cat hind limb skin. The technique has been applied by several workers since to study the effect of pain-inducing substances on cutaneous (3,9), muscle (18,20,46,47), and visceral nerves [see reviews (37,50)]. The limitation of this type of technique is that the level of firing in the afferent units which would produce nociception in the animal if it were conscious is unknown, and it can only be assumed that doses of the substances which produce detectable firing in the nerves would result in pain. It could also be argued that the intraarterial method of application of the drugs is an unnatural one since, during inflammatory states, the mediators might not usually reach the afferent nerves and/or their terminals via the blood stream. However, other methods of administration such as injection into the tissues would be likely to cause local pressure and excitation of several types of afferent units.

NATURE OF THE NOCICEPTORS RESPONDING TO CHEMICALS

Cutaneous and Subcutaneous

Nociceptors are those which respond only to damaging or near-damaging stimuli. They are often referred to as "high-threshold" receptors. In mammalian skin, two major types of nociceptors have been identified (6):

(a) The mechanical nociceptors respond only to strong mechanical stimuli, but are not responsive to thermal or chemical stimuli. Many of these receptors have thinly myelinated afferent fibers conducting in the Aδ range, and appear to be involved in the sensation of sharp pain such as occurs with pinprick. Mechanical nociceptors with unmyelinated (C) fibers have been found in cutaneous nerves but these appear to originate in subcutaneous tissues and differ from those from skin in that they respond to irritant chemicals placed on broken skin (4).

(b) The mechanical and thermal nociceptors respond to both strong mechanical and thermal stimuli. A large subgroup of these are the polymodal nociceptors which have unmyelinated afferent fibers and represent from 40 to 90% of randomly sampled C-fiber afferent units in cat and monkey cutaneous nerves (6,43). These nociceptors respond to strong mechanical stimuli, noxious heat, and irritant chemicals applied to the skin and they have afferent fibers which are among the slowest conducting of all sensory units. One striking property of most polymodal nociceptors is their change in responsiveness and appearance of background activity, particularly after noxious heating (4). Following heating there is a decrease in threshold for subsequent heating, often accompanied by a decrease in threshold to mechanical stimulation, provided the initial heat stimulus was not strong enough to inactivate the receptors. These sensitizing effects occur rapidly and may last for several hours (6).

It is unlikely that any cutaneous sensation will be found to be related to excitation of only one sensory receptor type in the skin. Nevertheless, as has been suggested by Burgess and Perl (6), the properties of the polymodal nociceptors, especially their sensitization, would appear to be of great importance for the pain associated with inflammation. It is common experience that inflammatory sites are hyperalgesic and have a lowered threshold to mechanical and thermal stimuli. Smolin (56) has obtained electrophysiological evidence that, in inflamed skin of cats and dogs, sensitization to tactile stimulation of mechanoreceptors with C-fibers occurred, particularly of those with the slowest conducting C-fibers which were presumably the polymodal nociceptors.

Adequate information of the relationship between the qualities of known pain stimuli in man and activities evoked in cutaneous receptors by these same stimuli is not yet available. It is possible that the infinite variety in quality of pain sensation is provided by different patterns of activity produced by various stimuli, not only in nociceptors but also in other receptors. At the present time therefore, any conclusions about pain sensation based on the activity in the nociceptors must be drawn with caution.

Muscle and Visceral

Less information is available about nociceptors in muscle and viscera. Muscle afferent units with group IV fibers (unmyelinated) and group III fibers (thinly myelinated) have been found which have the characteristics of polymodal nociceptors (36). However, there is no known population of specific nociceptors in viscera although visceral pain is a well-known experience (37).

PAIN-INDUCING ACTIONS OF INFLAMMATORY MEDIATORS

Each of the frequently studied inflammatory mediators has been proposed at some time to be a final common mediator for chemically induced pain. However it is equally likely that the afferent nerve terminal, like other nerve terminals, is equipped with a variety of pharmacological receptors which are capable of being acted upon to initiate a chain of events leading to action potentials in the nerve. It would also seem likely that the receptor populations of afferent nerve terminals might vary, from one tissue to another, in their proportions or in their sensitivities to chemicals.

Comparison of the threshold doses and concentrations of mediators producing pain and nociception would be useful, although such comparison is difficult because of the varying experimental techniques which have been used and the lack of knowledge of the concentrations actually reaching the nerve terminals. Although the data is incomplete, it is apparent that pain and nociception occur at relatively high concentrations compared with those which produce other pharmacological responses (Table 1). This probably introduces a safety factor so that nociception is not produced until high local levels of these mediators are present, such as might occur in pathological inflammatory states.

Pain in Man

On the blister base, acetylcholine, potassium ions, acids (hydrochloric or lactic < pH 3), histamine, 5-hydroxytryptamine, and bradykinin were all found to produce pain (1,34). There was some tachyphylaxis or desensitization of the blister base following application of most of the agents, which was particularly marked following 5-hydroxytryptamine. Bradykinin and 5-hydroxytryptamine were the most potent substances tested (14,34). Pain induced by histamine was followed by itching.

On injection into the skin, histamine (41,55), potassium ions (41,55), acid (41), and 5-hydroxytryptamine (41) have been reported to produce pain of short duration, whereas acetylcholine produced no pain on injection alone (41,55) but induced pain in the presence of histamine (55). This interaction between

TABLE 1. Concentrations and doses of inflammatory mediators inducing pain, nociception, and activity in afferent nerves

Mediator	Pain in man			Nociception in animals	Activity in afferent nerves	
	Blister base	Skin injection	Parenteral injection		Cutaneous	Muscle
Acetylcholine	5×10^{-5} M[a] (34)[b]	nil (41,55)	5×10^{-5} moles[c] (25,60)	2–3×10^{-6} moles[c] (24,58); 5×10^{-5} M[c] (35)	10^{-7} moles[c] (17); 2.5×10^{-8} moles[c] (32)	
Hydrogen ions	pH < 3 (34)	pH < 6.2 (41)	pH < 6.5[d] (40)	pH < 6[c] (48)		
Potassium ions	3×10^{-2} M (34)	3–4×10^{-2} M (41,55)	7×10^{-2} M[d] (40); 4×10^{-4} moles/min[c] (23,42)	3×10^{-4} moles[c] (24); 3×10^{-2} M[c] (35)	8×10^{-6} moles[c] (32)	5×10^{-5} moles[c] (18)
Histamine	10^{-5} M (34) (itch 10^{-7} M)	10^{-3} M (55); 6×10^{-4} M (41)	nil[c] (53) (headache 5×10^{-7} moles)	5×10^{-7} moles[c] (24); 5×10^{-5} moles[c] (35)	3×10^{-8} moles[c] (17); 2.5×10^{-7} moles[c] (32)	2.5×10^{-7} moles[c] (18)
5-Hydroxytryptamine	10^{-7} M (34)	6×10^{-3} M (41)	nil[c,e] (54)	nil (58); 2×10^{-7} moles[c] (24); 2.5×10^{-6} M[c] (35)	10^{-8} moles[c] (3,17); 5×10^{-7} moles[c] (32)	3×10^{-8} moles[c] (18)
Bradykinin	10^{-7} M (28,34)	nil (33); 5×10^{-9} moles (28)	nil[e] (54); nil[d,f] (33); 1–2×10^{-9} moles[c] (5,54); 1×10^{-9} moles[g] (33)	2×10^{-9} moles[c] (24); 3×10^{-10} moles[c] (58); 5×10^{-7} M[c] (35)	nil[c] (9,17); 5×10^{-9} moles[c] (3); 5×10^{-11} moles[c] (32)	5×10^{-9} moles[c] (18)
Prostaglandins E₁	nil (27)	10^{-2} M (15)		nil[c] (16); 3×10^{-8} moles/kg[g] (12); nil[c] (16)	nil[c] (9)	
E₂			3×10^{-9} moles/min[e] (22); 3×10^{-10} moles/min[e] (11)	3×10^{-7} moles/kg[g] (12); 6×10^{-9} moles daily[f] (59)		

[a]Concentrations are expressed as molar concentrations (M) and doses in moles (moles). [b]Numbers in parentheses are references. [c]Intraarterial. [d]Intramuscular. [e]Intravenous. [f]Subcutaneous. [g]Intraperitoneal.

acetylcholine and histamine could not be demonstrated on the blister base (34). Many investigators have demonstrated that histamine pricked into the skin or injected into the superficial layers produces itch (34). Intraepidermal injections of bradykinin produced pain and a flare, both of which were absent in denervated skin (28). Kantor et al. (33), however, found that they could not evaluate the pain-inducing action of intradermal injections of bradykinin since the effect produced was not much greater than that produced by the vehicle.

Prostaglandin E_1 did not produce pain on the blister base (27) but in high doses produced pain on intradermal injection, which was more prolonged than that produced by agents such as acetylcholine, bradykinin, or histamine (15). The lower doses of various prostaglandins used by Crunkhorn and Willis (13) did not produce pain. On subdermal infusion for 2 hr, prostaglandin E_1 produced hyperalgesia and a potentiation of the responses to histamine and bradykinin (15). Ferreira (15) has suggested that a possible explanation for the lack of effect of prostaglandin E_1 on the blister base might be that it is an inflamed site already hyperalgesic and application of prostaglandin E_1 might be unable to elicit a further response.

Some mediators have been tested by parenteral injection for pain-inducing actions on deeper tissues in man. Potassium injected intramuscularly (40) or intravascularly (23,42) produced pain. Intramuscular injection of acids has also been reported to produce prolonged pain in muscles, similar to that resulting from exercise of muscles under ischemic conditions (40,45). Acetylcholine has been found to produce severe, short-lasting pain on intraarterial injection (25,60), whereas histamine and 5-hydroxytryptamine alone have not been found to be painful on intravascular administration (54); however, histamine is notable for producing headache (53), and intravenous 5-hydroxytryptamine potentiated the pain response to bradykinin (54). There have been conflicting observations on the pain-inducing action of parenteral injection of bradykinin. Intraarterial injection of bradykinin was found to produce pain by Burch and DePasquale (5) and Sicuteri (54), but it was not found to be more painful than other vasodilators in the subjects used in the experiments of Fox et al. (19). Bradykinin was not painful on intramuscular (33), subcutaneous (33) or intravenous injection (54), but pain was produced by low doses injected intraperitoneally (33). Intravenous injections of prostaglandins, including prostaglandin E_2, however, have been found to be painful (11,22).

Nociception in Animals

The effects of inflammatory mediators on the pseudoaffective responses of dogs and cats have been extensively studied by Guzman et al. (24). Intraarterial, but not intravenous injection, of potassium chloride, acetylcholine, histamine, 5-hydroxytryptamine, and bradykinin produced nociception when injected into somatic or visceral arteries. Bradykinin was the most potent of these algesic agents. The nociceptive response of dogs to intraarterial 5-hydroxytryptamine was not confirmed by Taira and Nakano (58) but these workers found that 5-hydroxytryptamine sensitized somatic nociceptors to the actions of acetylcholine and bradykinin (49). Intraarterial injections of acid solutions below pH 6 were found to elicit pseudoaffective reactions in dogs (48). Ferreira et al. (16) found that intraarterial injection of prostaglandins E_1 and E_2 produced little nociceptive action when injected into dog spleen but potentiated the response to bradykinin. Juan and Lembeck (32) also found that infusion of prostaglandin E_1 into rabbit ears potentiated the reflex fall in blood pressure to bradykinin. The E-type prostaglandins injected intraperitoneally have been found to be among the most powerful substances to evoke abdominal constrictions in mice (12). Daily subcutaneous injections of prostaglandin E_2 into rat paws have also been reported to produce marked hyperalgesia (59).

The observations of Khayutin et al. (35) should be considered when drawing conclusions from results using the reflex pressor response as an index of nociception. These workers showed that pressor responses in cats produced by injection of small doses of 5-hydroxytryptamine, histamine, potassium ions, acetylcholine, and bradykinin into the perfused small intestine with the nerve supply intact were the result of specific tissue receptor excitation, whereas the nociceptive reflex pressor responses occurred at higher concentrations.

Activity in Afferent Nerves

Fjällbrant and Iggo (17) showed that several types of cutaneous afferent units from cat skin were excited by inflammatory agents. Not only high-threshold units with C fibers were excited by 5-hydroxytryptamine, histamine, and acetylcholine, but also large myelinated units with the characteristics of slowly adapting mechanoreceptors type II. This has since been confirmed in several studies of inflammatory mediators on cutaneous nerves (3,9). However, studies on muscle afferents have shown that only unmyelinated units (group IV) and thinly myelinated units (group III) were excited by inflammatory mediators whereas larger myelinated fibers in muscle nerves were unresponsive (46). It is possible that firing in myelinated mechanoreceptors in the skin occurs in response to increased fluid pressure from the edema which is produced by inflammatory mediators. Units responding to this type of stimulus might not be present in muscle.

Electrophysiological experiments have demonstrated that acetylcholine, histamine, and 5-hydroxytryptamine excite cutaneous afferent units (17,32). There have been, however, conflicting reports on the action of bradykinin on cutaneous nerves. Fjällbrant and Iggo (17) using impure bradykinin in cats, and Chahl and Iggo (9) using pure bradykinin in rats, were unable to show any definite action of bradykinin, whereas Beck and Handwerker (3) found that bradykinin excited both myelinated and unmyelinated fibers in cat cutaneous nerve. The latter workers also found that bradykinin enhanced the response of unmyelinated nociceptors to noxious radiant heat. Chahl and Iggo (9) found that prostaglandin E_1 alone had little action on cutaneous afferent nerves but, following a 10-

min intraarterial infusion of a low dose of prostaglandin E_1, bradykinin excited afferent nerves.

Excitation of muscle afferent units has been shown to occur with acetylcholine, potassium ions, histamine, 5-hydroxytryptamine, and bradykinin (18,20,36, 46,47). Although the effects of chemicals and inflammatory mediators have been investigated on visceral afferent nerve units (37,50), it is uncertain whether the observations relate to nociception or to reflex control of the tissue.

From the available results it can be concluded that acetylcholine and hydrogen and potassium ions induce pain in all tissues if administered in sufficient concentration. It is likely that hydrogen and potassium ions produce nonspecific depolarization of nerve terminals. Histamine and 5-hydroxytryptamine, although potent on the blister base and in producing firing in afferent nerves, seem to produce short-lasting pain especially in somatic tissues. The role of 5-hydroxytryptamine is controversial. The response to 5-hydroxytryptamine is tachyphylactic and the results obtained on intravascular administration have been variable. It would appear that the action of 5-hydroxytryptamine in potentiating responses to other mediators might be more important than its direct pain-inducing action.

Not all studies are in agreement with bradykinin being a potent algesic agent. It is very potent on the blister base and on intraarterial injection, particularly into dog spleen. However, the lack of activity in afferent nerves found in some studies and the marked potentiation of its effect by low concentrations of prostaglandins make it necessary to consider whether bradykinin is an effective algesic agent in its own right or it requires the presence of a low concentration of a prostaglandin (or prostaglandin precursor) for its action to be manifest. Indeed, the blister base is an inflammatory site itself which might have prostaglandins present, and resting release of prostaglandins has been shown to occur in dog spleen (16). It is possible that experimental differences might explain the varying results obtained with bradykinin. Further experiments on the pain-inducing action of bradykinin are required to establish the dependence of its action on the presence of prostaglandins. Likewise, it would seem that prostaglandins themselves are not potent pain-inducers but act to potentiate other mediators.

PAIN AND INFLAMMATION

All pain-inducing substances produce some degree of inflammatory response. It is interesting that potentiation of edema responses also occurs between inflammatory mediators, e.g., the potentiation of bradykinin and histamine by prostaglandin E_1 and of bradykinin by 5-hydroxytryptamine (7). Some pain-inducing substances have marked direct effects on blood vessels to produce vascular changes leading to edema, but others appear to produce their inflammatory responses indirectly via stimulation of the sensory nerves (2,30). This type of response has been called "neurogenic" (30). Even mediators such as histamine and 5-hydroxytryptamine, which produce edema mainly via their direct actions on blood vessels, produce some component of neurogenic edema (2). It would therefore appear that any agent which induces pain and thus firing in nociceptive afferent units causes release of a substance(s) from the nerves which is itself capable of inducing or enhancing the edema response (2,29). This conclusion is supported by the finding that electrical stimulation of rat cutaneous nerves produces edema (10,21,30). A useful tool in the study of the role of the sensory nervous system in inflammation is capsaicin, the active principle in the fruits of various species of *Capsicum*. It was found by Jancsó (29) to have the ability to cause pain and inflammation in rats on first exposure but, after repeated exposure of local sites or after repeated subcutaneous injection, the animals became unresponsive to capsaicin and to certain other irritating chemicals although responses to physical stimuli were normal. It appeared, therefore, that a certain population of sensory nerves could be selectively destroyed by capsaicin. It is tempting to suggest that the polymodal nociceptors might be those which are rendered nonfunctional by capsaicin and that it is these nerve fibers which contain the neurogenic edema-producing agent.

The nature of the agent which is released from the sensory nerves is unknown but its existence has been postulated for many years (39). One strong candidate is the peptide, substance P, which has been found by Hökfelt et al. (26) to be localized in some primary sensory neurons. Substance P has been suggested to be the mediator of antidromic vasodilatation (38) and cutaneous hyperalgesia (44). In support of this, substance P has many properties which would qualify it for these roles: viz., it produces vasodilatation (52) and edema (8), it excites afferent units in low doses (32), and it potentiates other inflammatory mediators (8). Unexpectedly, the pure peptide did not produce pain on the blister base (57). Perl et al. (51) have recently found that the agent producing sensitization of polymodal nociceptors is unlikely to be 5-hydroxytryptamine, histamine, hydrogen or potassium ions, a prostaglandin, or kinin. It would be interesting to know whether substance P would sensitize polymodal nociceptors.

Recently Jancsó et al. (31) have found that treatment of neonatal rats with capsaicin produced permanent destruction of some of the afferent nerve fibers in the dorsal roots and spinal cord, a permanent loss of response to noxious chemicals, and loss of ability to produce neurogenic edema. Although agents such as 6-hydroxydopamine, which produce selective destruction of sympathetic nerves, have been known for several years, this is the first report of a substance which is capable of selective chemical destruction of portion of the afferent nervous system. Capsaicin promises to be a useful tool in the study of the mechanisms involved in pain induction by inflammatory mediators.

SUMMARY

There is still much to be learnt about the pain-inducing actions of inflammatory mediators. It seems that during the inflammatory response pain is induced by several mediators acting in concert. Therefore, study of the interactions between the mediators must be considered of paramount importance and will no doubt be the topic of many future investigations. It also seems likely that the sensory nerve terminal might prove to be an important link between pain induced by the mediators and the magnitude of the inflammatory response.

ACKNOWLEDGMENT

The original work of the author was supported by a research grant from the National Health and Medical Research Council of Australia.

REFERENCES

1. Armstrong, D., Dry, R. M. L., Keele, C. A., and Markham, J. W. (1953): Observations on chemical excitants of cutaneous pain in man. *J. Physiol. (Lond.)*, 120:326–351.
2. Arvier, P. T., Chahl, L. A., and Ladd, R. J. (1977): Modification by capsaicin and compound 48/80 of dye leakage induced by irritants in the rat. *Br. J. Pharmacol.*, 59:61–68.
3. Beck, P. W., and Handwerker, H. O. (1974): Bradykinin and serotonin effects on various types of cutaneous nerve fibers. *Pflügers Arch.*, 347:209–222.
4. Bessou, P., and Perl, E. R. (1969): Response of cutaneous sensory units with unmyelinated fibers to noxious stimuli. *J. Neurophysiol.*, 32:1025–1043.
5. Burch, G. E., and DePasquale, N. P. (1962): Bradykinin, digital blood flow, and the arteriovenous anastomoses. *Circ. Res.*, 10:105–115.
6. Burgess, P. R., and Perl, E. R. (1973): Cutaneous mechanoreceptors and nociceptors. In: *Handbook of Sensory Physiology, Vol. 2: Somatosensory System,* edited by A. Iggo, pp. 29–78. Springer-Verlag, Heidelberg.
7. Chahl, L. A. (1976): Interactions of bradykinin, prostaglandin E_1, 5-hydroxytryptamine, histamine and adenosine-5'-triphosphate on the dye leakage response in rat skin. *J. Pharm. Pharmacol.*, 28:753–757.
8. Chahl, L. A. (1977): Interactions of substance P with putative mediators of inflammation and ATP. *Eur. J. Pharmacol.*, 44:45–49.
9. Chahl, L. A., and Iggo, A. (1977): The effects of bradykinin and prostaglandin E_1 on rat cutaneous afferent nerve activity. *Br. J. Pharmacol.*, 59:343–347.
10. Chahl, L. A., and Ladd, R. J. (1976): Local oedema and general excitation of cutaneous sensory receptors produced by electrical stimulation of the saphenous nerve in the rat. *Pain*, 2:25–34.
11. Collier, J. G., Karim, S. M. M., Robinson, B., and Somers, K. (1972): Action of prostaglandins A_2, B_1, E_2 and $F_{2\alpha}$ on superficial hand veins of man. *Br. J. Pharmacol.*, 44:374P–375P.
12. Collier, H. O. J., and Schneider, C. (1972): Nociceptive response to prostaglandins and analgesic actions of aspirin and morphine. *Nature [New Biol.]*, 236:141–143.
13. Crunkhorn, P., and Willis, A. L. (1971): Cutaneous reactions to intradermal prostaglandins. *Br. J. Pharmacol.*, 41:49–56.
14. Elliott, D. F., Horton, E. W., and Lewis, G. P. (1960): Actions of pure bradykinin. *J. Physiol. (Lond.)*, 153:473–480.
15. Ferreira, S. H. (1972): Prostaglandins, aspirin-like drugs and analgesia. *Nature [New Biol.]*, 240:200–203.
16. Ferreira, S. H., Moncada, S., and Vane, J. R. (1973): Prostaglandins and the mechanism of analgesia produced by aspirin-like drugs. *Br. J. Pharmacol.*, 49:86–97.
17. Fjällbrant, N., and Iggo, A. (1961): The effect of histamine, 5-hydroxytryptamine and acetylcholine on cutaneous afferent fibers. *J. Physiol. (Lond.)*, 156:578–590.
18. Fock, S., and Mense, S. (1976): Excitatory effects of 5-hydroxytryptamine, histamine and potassium ions on muscular group IV afferent units: A comparison with bradykinin. *Brain Res.*, 105:459–469.
19. Fox, R. H., Goldsmith, R., Kidd, D. J., and Lewis, G. P. (1961): Bradykinin as a vasodilator in man. *J. Physiol. (Lond.)*, 157:589–602.
20. Franz, M., and Mense, S. (1975): Muscle receptors with group IV afferent fibres responding to application of bradykinin. *Brain Res.*, 92:369–383.
21. Garcia Leme, J., and Hamamura, L. (1974): Formation of a factor increasing vascular permeabil-

ity during electrical stimulation of the saphenous nerve in rats. *Br. J. Pharmacol.*, 51:383–389.

22. Gillespie, A. (1972): Prostaglandin-oxytocin enhancement and potentiation and their clinical applications. *Br. Med. J.*, 1:150–152.
23. Glover, W. E., Roddie, I. C., and Shanks, R. G. (1962): The effect of intra-arterial potassium chloride infusions on vascular reactivity in the human forearm. *J. Physiol. (Lond.)*, 163:22P–23P.
24. Guzman, F., Braun, C., and Lim, R. K. S. (1962): Visceral pain and the pseudaffective response to intra-arterial injection of bradykinin and other algesic agents. *Arch. Int. Pharmacodyn. Ther.*, 136:353–384.
25. Harvey, A. M., and Lilienthal, J. L. (1941): Observations on the nature of myasthenia gravis. *Bull. Johns Hopkins Hosp.*, 69:566–577.
26. Hökfelt, T., Kellerth, J-O., Nilsson, G., and Pernow, B. (1975): Experimental immuno-histochemical studies on the localization and distribution of substance P in cat primary sensory neurons. *Brain Res.*, 100:235–252.
27. Horton, E. W. (1963): Action of prostaglandin E_1 on tissues which respond to bradykinin. *Nature*, 200:892–893.
28. Horton, E. W. (1963): The role of bradykinin in the peripheral nervous system. *Ann. NY Acad. Sci.*, 104:250–257.
29. Jancsó, N. (1960): Role of the nerve terminals in the mechanism of inflammatory reactions. *Bull. Millard Fillmore Hosp.*, 7:53–77.
30. Jancsó, N., Jancsó-Gábor, A., and Szolcsányi, J. (1967): Direct evidence for neurogenic inflammation and its prevention by denervation and by pretreatment with capsaicin. *Br. J. Pharmacol.*, 31:138–151.
31. Jancsó, G., Kiraly, E., and Jancsó-Gábor, A. (1977): Pharmacologically induced selective degeneration of chemosensitive primary sensory neurones. *Nature*, 270:741–743.
32. Juan, H., and Lembeck, F. (1974): Action of peptides and other algesic agents on paravascular pain receptors of the isolated perfused rabbit ear. *Naunyn Schmiedebergs Arch. Pharmacol.*, 283:151–164.
33. Kantor, T. G., Jarvik, M. E., and Wolff, B. B. (1967): Bradykinin as a mediator of human pain. *Proc. Soc. Exp. Biol. Med.*, 126:505–507.
34. Keele, C. A., and Armstrong, D. (1964): *Substances Producing Pain and Itch.* Edward Arnold, London.
35. Khayutin, V. M., Baraz, L. A., Lukoshkova, E. V., Sonina, R. S., and Chernilovskaya, P. E. (1976): Chemosensitive spinal afferents: Thresholds of specific and nociceptive reflexes as compared with thresholds of excitation for receptors and axons. In: *Somatosensory and Visceral Receptor Mechanisms: Progress in Brain Research, Vol. 43*, edited by A. Iggo and O. B. Ilyensky, pp. 293–306. Elsevier, Amsterdam.
36. Kumazawa, T., and Mizumura, K. (1977): Thin-fiber receptors responding to mechanical, chemical, and thermal stimulation in the skeletal muscle of the dog. *J. Physiol. (Lond.)*, 273:179–194.
37. Leek, B. F. (1977): Abdominal and pelvic visceral receptors. *Br. Med. Bull.*, 33:163–168.
38. Lembeck, F. (1953): Zur Frage der zentralen Übertragung afferenter Impulse. III. Mitteilung. Das Vorkommen und die Bedeutung der Substanz P in den dorsalen Würzien des Rückenmarks. *Naunyn Schmiedebergs Arch. Pharmacol.*, 219:197–213.
39. Lewis, T. (1936): Experiments relating to cutaneous hyperalgesia and its spread through somatic nerves. *Clin. Sci.*, 2:373–423.
40. Lewis, T. (1938): Suggestions relating to the study of somatic pain. *Br. Med. J.*, 1:321–325.
41. Lindahl, O. (1961): Experimental skin pain induced by injection of water soluble substances in humans. *Acta Physiol. Scand.*, 51 (Suppl 179):1–89.
42. Lowe, R. D., and Thompson, J. W. (1962): The effect of intra-arterial potassium chloride infusion upon forearm blood flow in man. *J. Physiol. (Lond.)*, 162:69–70P.
43. Lynn, B. (1975): Somatosensory receptors and their CNS connections. *Annu. Rev. Physiol.*, 37:105–127.
44. Lynn, B. (1977): Cutaneous hyperalgesia. *Br. Med. Bull.*, 33:103–108.
45. Maison, G. L. (1939): Studies on the genesis of ischemic pain: the influence of the potassium, lactate and ammonium ions. *Am. J. Physiol.*, 127:315–321.
46. Mense, S. (1977): Nervous outflow from skeletal muscle following chemical noxious stimulation. *J. Physiol. (Lond.)*, 267:75–88.

47. Mense, S., and Schmidt, R. F. (1974): Activation of group IV afferent units from muscle by algesic agents. *Brain Res.,* 72:305–310.
48. Moore, R. M., Moore, R. E., and Singleton, A. O. (1934): Experiments on the chemical stimulation of pain-endings associated with small blood vessels. *Am. J. Physiol.,* 107:594–602.
49. Nakano, T., and Taira, N. (1976): 5-Hydroxytryptamine as a sensitizer of somatic nociceptors for pain-producing substances. *Eur. J. Pharmacol.,* 38:23–29.
50. Paintal, A. S. (1977): Thoracic receptors connected with sensation. *Br. Med. Bull.,* 33:169–174.
51. Perl, E. R., Kumazawa, T., Lynn, B., and Kenins, P. (1976): Sensitization of high threshold receptors with unmyelinated (C) afferent fibers. In: *Somatosensory and Visceral Receptor Mechanisms: Progress in Brain Research, Vol. 43,* edited by A. Iggo and O. B. Ilyensky, pp. 263–277. Elsevier, Amsterdam.
52. Pernow, B. (1953): Studies on substance P. Purification, occurrence and biological actions. *Acta Physiol. Scand.,* 29 (Suppl. 105):57–64.
53. Pickering, G. W., and Hess, W. (1933–34): Observations on the mechanism of the headache produced by histamine. *Clin. Sci.,* 1:77–101.
54. Sicuteri, F. (1968): Sensitization of nociceptors by 5-hydroxytryptamine in man. In: *Pharmacology of Pain: Proceedings of Third International Pharmacology Meeting, Vol. 9,* edited by R. K. S. Lim, D. Armstrong, and E. G. Pardo, pp. 57–86. Pergamon Press, Oxford.
55. Skouby, A. P. (1953): The influence of acetylcholine, curarine and related substances on the threshold for chemical pain stimuli. *Acta Physiol. Scand.,* 29:340–352.
56. Smolin, L. N. (1976): The peripheral mechanisms of sensitization of inflamed tissues. In: *Somatosensory and Visceral Receptor Mechanisms: Progress in Brain Research, Vol. 43,* edited by A. Iggo and O. B. Ilyensky, pp. 307–309. Elsevier, Amsterdam.
57. Stewart, J. M., Getto, C. J., Neldner, K., Reeve, E. B., Krivoy, W. A., and Zimmermann, E. (1976): Substance P and analgesia. *Nature,* 262:784–785.
58. Taira, N., and Nakano, T. (1974): Is intra-arterial 5-hydroxytryptamine a potent algogenic substance in the dog? *Eur. J. Pharmacol.,* 25:113–116.
59. Willis, A. L., and Cornelsen, M. (1973): Repeated injection of prostaglandin E_2 in rat paws induces chronic swelling and a marked decrease in pain threshold. *Prostaglandins,* 3:353–357.
60. Wilson, A., and Stoner, H. B. (1947): The effect of the injection of acetylcholine into the brachial artery of normal subjects and patients with myasthenia gravis. *Q. J. Med.,* 16:237–243.

Mechanisms of Pain and Analgesic Compounds,
edited by R. F. Beers, Jr., and E. G. Bassett.
Raven Press, New York © 1979.

26. Local Mechanisms in Dental Pain

Leif Olgart

Department of Pharmacology, Karolinska Institutet, S-104 01 Stockholm, Sweden

INTRODUCTION

One characteristic feature of the tooth is that it can give rise to pain in response to a variety of external stimuli. For many years this has stimulated dentists and physiologists to investigate the specific mechanisms by which intradental sensory nerves are activated, both in normal teeth and in teeth with pulpal inflammation. This chapter presents some of the general views about pain mechanisms in the tooth and some recent findings from our laboratory.

OBSERVATIONS AND DISCUSSION

Activation of Intradental Sensory Nerves by External Stimuli

The familiar sensitivity of the tooth to external stimuli was long difficult to understand, since the enamel and the peripheral parts of the dentin are devoid of nervous structures. Much interest has therefore been focused on the dentin, which is a mineralized tissue (70% inorganic material) with approximately 30,000 tubules/mm². The dentinal tubules having a diameter of about 1 μm, are filled mainly with extracellular fluid, and run continuously through the whole dentin layer from the pulp to the dentin-enamel junction. At their pulpal end, specialized cells (odontoblasts) are located with their processes running some 200 μm into the tubules. The main function of these cells is to elaborate dentin. However, the odontoblasts may also play a role in dental pain mechanisms (Fig. 1).

Experimental proof that sensory fibers are present in dentinal tubules in close contact with the odontoblasts has been provided by several recent independent studies. Our own piece of evidence was based on experiments in the cat in which resection of the mandibular nerve was shown to produce degeneration of myelinated fibers in the pulp and of their terminals within the dentinal tubules (2). The neurons penetrate into the tubules to a distance of 100 to 200 μm. In this section of the tubules, free nerve endings can be seen running along with the odontoblasts, forming tight junctions with their processes. In the coronal portion of human and animal teeth, such nerve structures can be seen in up to 40% of the dentinal tubules.

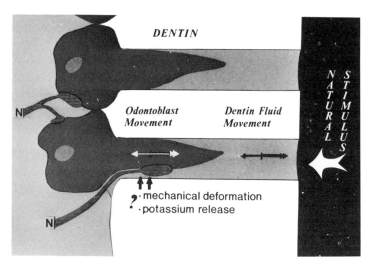

FIG. 1. Diagram showing odontoblasts and their relation to sensory nerve fibers (N) in the pulp and in dentinal tubules. Non-noxious pain stimuli applied to outer dentinal surface produce fluid movements which impinge on odontoblasts and nerve endings. Mechanical stimuli, evaporation, sugar solutions, and cold cause outward movements, while heat causes inward movements.

Thus, the inner dentin is innervated but the main part of the dentin and its tubules is devoid of sensory nerves. Pain evoked by surface stimulation of the tooth or of exposed dentin has therefore to be explained by some indirect mechanism. According to Brännström and Åström (4), pain stimuli are transmitted to the nerve structures by a hydrodynamic link. This conclusion has been reached by studying the effect of well-known clinical pain stimuli on dentinal fluid movements *in vitro*. It has thus been shown by Brännström and colleagues that painful stimuli (e.g., a stream of air, cold, and mechanical probing on exposed surface dentin) produce rapid outward movements of fluid in the dentinal tubules. Local application of a hypertonic solution (e.g., sugar) and heat, which are other "natural" dental pain stimuli, also produce displacement of the dentinal tubule content. Thus, a common property of the different stimuli that produce pain in teeth seems to be their ability to initiate fluid movements across dentin. This may cause some interaction between the nerve endings and the odontoblasts.

The mechanism by which an action potential is initiated is under debate and is still not known with certainty. According to one theory, mechanical disruption of the membrane of the nerve ending initiates the nerve response. An alternative explanation is that potassium may leak out of the odontoblast as a result of disruption of the cell, thus causing depolarization of the nerve ending. However, convincing evidence has still to be presented to establish the specific mechanism of excitation.

It is generally considered that nerve fibers involved in dental pain elicited by physical stimuli are mainly of the Aδ-type and that these fibers are likely to be mechanosensitive in nature. The pain response to natural stimuli is usually of short duration in teeth with uninflamed pulps and the stimulus does not seem to cause any damage to the tissue. The duration of the response thus seems to be mainly related to the short period of fluid movement in the dentinal tubules.

Recording of Intradental Sensory Nerve Activity

Impulses originating from intradental nerve fibers can be recorded within the teeth of animals and man. By preparing two dentinal cavities in the tooth, electrodes can be placed in contact with the exposed dentin and nerve impulses visualized and counted using standard electrophysiological equipment (Fig. 2). Such nerve impulses are, in all probability, related to activity in the myelinated nerves within the pulp, as previously described. A temporal correlation between nerve impulses and the sensation of pain elicited by relevant clinical stimuli has been established (5,14).

Measurements of Pulpal Blood Flow

Changes in pulpal blood flow can be measured indirectly using a radioactive depot of an easily diffusible solute (^{125}I) placed in a dentinal cavity (6). The tracer enters the pulp by diffusion and is transported in capillary blood at a

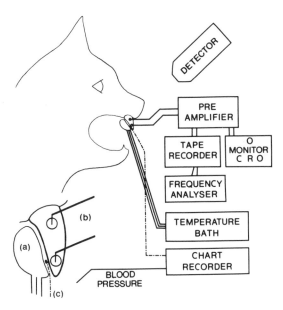

FIG. 2. Experimental set up for recording of intradental sensory nerve activity and blood flow. Inset represents enlargement of tooth, thermode (a), electrodes (b) in cavities, and thermocouple circuit (c). The incisal cavity is used as a depot for radioactive tracers.

rate which changes in parallel with the transport function of the blood flow. This rate is monitored by an external scintillation detector (Fig. 2).

Using the two methods in combination it is possible to study changes in both parameters in the same region in the pulp. It has been shown that this can be done without causing any appreciable damage to the pulp tissue.

Sympathetic Vasomotor Control of Sensory Neurones in the Pulp

In previous studies (6) it was demonstrated that reduction of blood flow in the cat pulp induced by activation of sympathetic nerves to the oral tissues causes a transient increase in sensory nerve excitability, followed by a period of depressed nerve activity. Application of thermal stimuli (which under normal conditions cause excitation) is without such effect under conditions of reduced pulpal blood flow. These results show that the excitability of intradental sensory neurons depends on the integrity of the pulpal circulation and indicate that the sympathetic vasomotor control of the teeth may modulate the resulting afferent flow of nerve impulses from this tissue.

Studies on Increased Sensory Nerve Activity

It has been clinically established that when the tooth and its dentin are subjected to carious decay and/or chemical and thermal insults, a state of exaggerated pain response to external stimuli or spontaneous pain may develop. It is also well known that such clinical insults will produce inflammatory changes in the pulp and that the tissue reactions develop as a result of the transport of stimuli (heat, toxic products) through the dentin and its tubules. There is, however, a poor correlation between morphological signs of pulp inflammation and reports of pain in human subjects (15). This indicates that increased excitability in intradental nerves may preferentially be related to functional disturbances, rather than to morphological alterations in the tissue.

One approach we have used to study the initial reactions in pulp inflammation and pain is the application of certain chemicals to exposed dentin or noxious heat to the tooth surface while recording nerve activity and blood flow in the tooth.

Compound 48/80 (Burroughs Wellcome) is one substance that has been used widely to study initial mechanisms in inflammation. The principal action of this agent is to release histamine by degranulating mast cells. Other biologically active agents, such as slow reacting substance (SRS) and prostaglandins, may also be released or formed. What stimulated our interest in compound 48/80 was the observation that it induced long-lasting nerve activity following local application to the cat and dog pulp. The activity starts after a delay of some minutes and persists for several hours after removal of compound 48/80. During this time, the neurons show enhanced susceptibility to cold stimulation applied to the tooth surface. It was also found that pulpal blood flow was influenced concomitantly with the increased nerve activity and that the expected reduction in blood flow in response to sympathetic nerve activation was absent for a period of several hours following the application of compound 48/80. Our curiosity was aroused further when we found that the effect of compound 48/80 could be blocked by pretreatment with disodium cromoglycate (local application and intraarterial infusion). This finding supported our previous theory that the action of compound 48/80 on the nerves is an indirect one, and suggested that mast cells take a part in sensory nerve excitation in the pulp. However, our previous studies have shown that substances known to be released or formed in association with mast cell degranulation in the cat are without excitatory effects on intradental nerves. Thus, histamine, SRS, prostaglandin E_2, and arachidonic acid fail to excite or influence the excitability of the neurons, even if the agents are applied in combination to exposed pulps in pharmacological doses. It is therefore tempting to assume that if these biologically active substances are involved in the nerve excitation their action is indirect, possibly mediated via vascular changes in the pulp since their vasoactive efficacy is well documented. Such a mechanism of excitation may be related to a local increase in intrapulpal pressure due to outward filtration of fluid from the vessels (16) and pressure effects on the mechanosensitive sensory receptors (8,13).

Among the biologically active substances we have tested in the tooth preparation so far, 5-hydroxytryptamine (5-HT) seems to be the only one which regularly causes nerve excitation. This finding led us to introduce 5-HT antagonists in combination with compound 48/80 in a series of experiments. It was found that systemic pretreatment with methysergide in a dose range of 10 to 15 μg/kg markedly reduced the nervous response to compound 48/80, while nerve activity induced by other means (e.g., application of hypertonic salt solutions and aconitine, which act directly on the nerves) was not influenced by methysergide. This may imply that 5-HT is involved in excitation of sensory nerves during the initial stages of pulp inflammation. However, validation of this hypothesis requires more substantial evidence than has been obtained in these experiments.

To our surprise, we found in further experiments that when methysergide (and also tetrodotoxin) was given systemically after compound 48/80 there was a complete absence of effect on the established nerve activity. The lack of effect in this situation may be ascribed to the local circulatory arrest induced by compound 48/80 and thus to a subsequent incomplete distribution of the blocking agents to the pulp. These observations demonstrate that circulatory alterations have to be considered when studying sensory functions in the pulp.

Nerve activity of an inflammatory nature can also be induced by repeated application of noxious heat to the tooth of the cat (1). In Fig. 3 the nervous response to three consecutive brief heat stimulations is shown. Each produced an immediate burst of impulses, presumably due to direct stimulation of the nerves by displacement of the dentinal fluid *(vide supra)*. Following the third stimulation, a phase of prolonged nerve activity developed. To analyze this

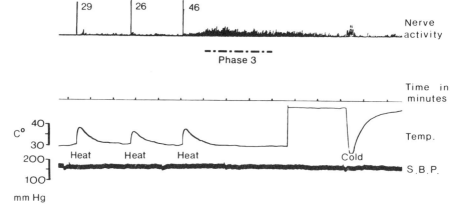

FIG. 3. Heat-induced sensory nerve activity in the cat tooth. Heat stimulus (80 to 90°C) was applied repeatedly on the incisal tooth surface for periods of 1 sec. Temperature is registered at the tooth surface at ½ crown length. Values of nerve activity, time, temperature, and systemic blood pressure are shown. Mean impulse frequency for period ⎯.⎯.⎯ was calculated and is given in Table 1. (From Ahlberg, ref. 1.)

response in some detail and to study if some algogenic agent is involved, nonsteroidal antiinflammatory drugs were administered. Special interest was focused on indomethacin, diclofenac sodium, and naproxen since they are potent inhibitors of prostaglandin synthesis. Table 1 shows the inhibitory effect of these drugs on heat-induced nerve activity as compared to the response obtained in contralateral teeth stimulated before drug administration. The blocking effect of indomethacin was dose-dependent (ID_{50} 0.04 to 0.2 mg/kg) in a dose range where no unspecific effects of the drug are to be expected. These results thus

TABLE 1. *Inhibitory effect of pretreatment with nonsteroidal antiinflammatory drugs on heat-induced nerve activity*[a]

	Control		Pretreatment		
Drug and dosage	No. of teeth	Mean phase 3 activity imp/sec $\bar{\chi} \pm SD$	No. of teeth	Mean phase 3 activity imp/sec $\bar{\chi} \pm SD$	Reduction percent of control, $\bar{\chi} \pm SD$
Indomethacin 5 mg/kg	5	15.7 ± 4.6	7	2.0 ± 0.9	86 ± 7.9 $p < 0.001$[b]
Diclofenac sodium 5 mg/kg	9	7.7 ± 2.9	13	2.0 ± 1.6	75 ± 12.3 $p < 0.001$[b]
Naproxen 15 mg/kg	2	19.2 ± 2.3	2	1.3 ± 0.3	93 ± 2.1

[a] From Ahlberg, ref. 1.
[b] Student's *t*-test.

indicate that prostaglandins are involved in certain stages of heat-induced pulp inflammation and that, in such situations, they act as mediators of increased sensory nerve activity. Whether this effect of prostaglandins or their intermediates is due to a direct action on the nerves remains to be determined. An interesting finding in this context is that when the antagonists were given after the heat stimuli, and during the established nerve activity, they had no effect. This again suggests that circulatory changes must be considered when attempting to explain inflammatory pain mechanisms in the dental pulp.

Effects of Sensory Nerve Stimulation on Blood Flow

The relationship between vascular and neural functions in the pulp may also be demonstrated by direct activation of sensory nerves. In the experiment illustrated in Fig. 4, changes in pulpal blood flow were induced by electrical stimula-

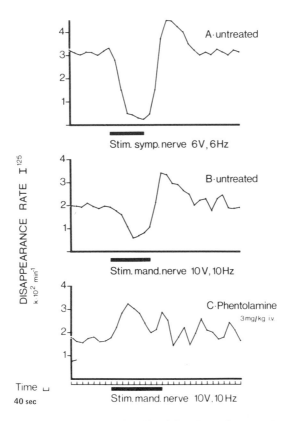

FIG. 4. Effect of nerve stimulation on pulpal blood flow in cat lower canine tooth. Ipsilateral stimulation of cervical sympathetic nerve trunk **(A)** and mandibular nerve **(B)** reduced disappearance rate. Mandibular nerve stimulation after α-receptor blockade (phentolamine, 3 mg/kg) increased disappearance rate **(C)**.

tion of the ipsilateral sympathetic and mandibular nerves in the cat. Figure 4A shows the expected reduction in blood flow upon sympathetic stimulation. In the same experiment, stimulation of the mandibular nerve resulted in a similar reduction in blood flow (Fig. 4B). This indicates that the mandibular nerve contains sympathetic fibers. After systemic administration of an α-adrenoceptor blocking drug (phentolamine), subsequent mandibular nerve stimulation induced an increase in pulpal blood flow (Fig. 4C). Such a vasodilatory response is not altered by previous intravenous injection of atropine, propranolol, or mepyramine and is therefore not likely to be mediated by acetylcholine, catecholamines, or histamine. The effect may instead be related to the well-known phenomenon of antidromic vasodilatation, which has been considered to be due to a neurohumor released from nerve endings of unmyelinated C-fibers (9). The authors cited showed that in the skin tissue reactions developed resembling those of an acute inflammatory reaction following sensory nerve stimulation. The nature of the mechanism is still unclear. Valuable information has, however, been obtained in recent immunohistochemical studies showing that sensory nerve endings contain a peptide with immunological characteristics similar to those of substance P (SP).

The presence of SP in the pulp has been demonstrated in cat, dog, and human teeth (11). In the cat pulp SP is localized to small, possibly unmyelinated fibers which are frequently observed close to blood vessels (Fig. 5). All SP fibers in the pulp disappear after transection of the inferior alveolar nerve but not following extirpation of the superior cervical ganglion (12). These observations imply that the SP-containing nerves in the pulp are of sensory origin since no convincing evidence of any other type of innervation to this tissue has been presented (3). The unmyelinated appearance of the SP-containing fibers is interesting, since it has long been assumed that dental pain is mediated by Aδ fibers. However, our observations are supported by some recent electron microscopic and electrophysiological studies reporting that, in all probability, afferent C-fibers are present in the dental pulp. Their role in dental pain will certainly be a matter of great interest in future research.

The question of whether SP plays a role in peripheral sensory nerves cannot be answered at present. The close relation of SP-positive nerves to blood vessels and the fact that SP causes vasodilatation when injected intraarterially to the cat pulp (7) supports the idea put forward by Lembeck (10) that it might produce the vascular effects induced by sensory nerve stimulation, commonly referred to as the axon reflex. If so, a release of SP would be expected upon sensory nerve stimulation. Results indicative of such release were recently obtained in our laboratory (11). Thus, it could be demonstrated that the amount of SP-like immunoreactivity is increased in exudate collected from the exposed cat pulp following electrical stimulation of the inferior alveolar nerve. Even if a definite conclusion cannot yet be drawn as to the role of SP in the dental pulp, it is tempting to assume that SP plays a role in the development of the inflammatory response associated with injury and pain in the tooth.

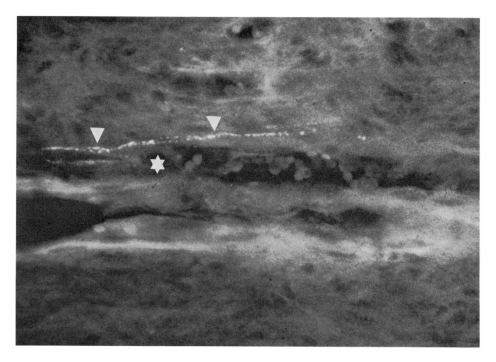

FIG. 5. Immunofluorescence micrograph of cat dental pulp after incubation with antiserum to substance P (SP). SP-positive fibers ▼, are seen running close to a blood vessel (★). ×340.

REFERENCES

1. Ahlberg, K. F. (1978): Dose-dependent inhibition of sensory nerve activity in the feline dental pulp by anti-inflammatory drugs. *Acta Physiol. Scand.*, 102:434–440.
2. Arwill, T., Edwall, L., Lilja, J., Olgart, L., and Svensson, S. E. (1973): Ultrastructure of nerves in the dentinal-pulp border zone after sensory and autonomic nerve transection in the cat. *Acta Odontol. Scand.*, 31:273–281.
3. Bender, I. B., and Seltzer, S. (1975): *The Dental Pulp.* J. B. Lippincott, Philadelphia.
4. Brännström, M., and Åström, A. (1972): The hydrodynamics of the dentine: its possible relationship to dentinal pain. *Int. Dent. J.*, 22:219–227.
5. Edwall, L., and Olgart, L. (1977): A new technique for recording of intradental sensory nerve activity in man. *Pain,* 3:121–125.
6. Edwall, L., and Scott, D., Jr. (1971): Influence of changes in microcirculation on the excitability of the sensory unit in the tooth of the cat. *Acta Physiol. Scand.*, 82:555–566.
7. Gazelius, B., Olgart, L., Edwall, L., and Trowbridge, H. O. (1977): Effects of Substance P on sensory nerves and blood flow in the feline dental pulp. In: *Pain in the Trigeminal Region,* edited by D. J. Anderson and B. Matthews, pp. 95–101. Elsevier/North-Holland, Amsterdam.
8. Halkumäki, M. O. K., and Nähri, M. V. O. (1973): Effect of intrapulpal pressure stimulation on the activity of sensory nerves of dental pulp. *Acta Physiol. Scand.*, 88:584–586.
9. Jancsó, N., Jancsó-Gábor, A., and Szolcsányi, J. (1967): Direct evidence for neurogenic inflammation and its prevention by denervation and by pretreatment with capsaicin. *Br. J. Pharmacol.*, 31:138–151.
10. Lembeck, F., Gamse, R., and Juan, H. H. (1977): Substance P and sensory nerve endings. In: *Substance P (Nobel Symposium 37),* edited by U. S. von Euler and B. Pernow, pp. 169–181. Raven Press, New York.

11. Olgart, L., Gazelius, B., Brodin, E., and Nilsson, G. (1977): Release of Substance P-like immuno-reactivity from the dental pulp. *Acta Physiol. Scand.,* 101:510–512.
12. Olgart, L., Hökfelt, T., Nilsson, G., and Pernow, B. (1977): Localization of Substance P-like immunoreactivity in nerves in the tooth pulp. *Pain,* 4:153–159.
13. Paintal, A. S. (1976): Natural and paranatural stimulation of sensory receptors. In: *Sensory Functions of the Skin,* edited by Y. Zotterman, pp. 3–12. Pergamon Press, New York.
14. Scott, D., Jr. (1972): The arousal and suppression of pain in the tooth. *Int. Dent. J.,* 22:20–32.
15. Seltzer, S. (1972): Classification of pulpal pathosis. *Oral Surg.,* 34:269–287.
16. Van Hassel, H. J. (1971): Physiology of the human dental pulp. *Oral Surg.,* 32:126–134.

Mechanisms of Pain and Analgesic Compounds,
edited by R. F. Beers, Jr., and E. G. Bassett.
Raven Press, New York © 1979.

27. The Nature of Pain in Headache and Central Panalgesia

Federigo Sicuteri

Department of Clinical Pharmacology, University of Florence, Florence, Italy

INTRODUCTION

Nociception is a function that results in pain and depends mainly on the activity of the antinociceptive system (ANS), a multiintegrated and flexible apparatus capable of modulating the inflow of pain sensations. Emotions from emergencies, such as anger, terror, sex, and pain itself, activate the ANS with a result of analgesia. The ANS is calibrated so that only stimuli, capable of damaging tissues, arrive at the consciousness. A weakening of the ANS provokes an amplification of nociception, which causes a lowering of pain threshold and an increase of pain. To distinguish it from that provoked by physiological or peripheral stimuli, this type is called pathological spontaneous, hallucinatory, or central pain. The qualitative and quantitative characteristics of physiological pain are overturned in central pain. Analogous to other dysfunctions, one can speak of "dysnociception," which focuses on the impairment of the nociceptive system. When the ANS is affected by gross lesions (e.g., tissue softness, tumors, inflammation), organic central pain occurs (12,20,34). Organic central pain is rather stable in regions, side, intensity, and quality. When the ANS is impaired by functional biochemical disorders, pain can be labeled as nonorganic central pain (56) and is characterized by instability of regions, side, intensity, and quality. The most common expression of nonorganic central pain is idiopathic headache, migraine included (42), whereas a less common one is central panalgesia (42, 52,56). Idiopathic headache is considered to be due to a weakening of the rostral section of the ANS (47,48), whereas in central panalgesia the entire ANS is thought to be impaired (48,52,56). According to the thesis of the central nature of pain, idiopathic headache requires a well-defined nosological collocation as the most common disease of the nociceptive system. Strong evidence supporting the thesis of the central, in contrast to that of the peripheral, nature of pain is discussed below.

WHY CENTRAL?

Clinical Aspects

Characteristics of Pain

If pain is postulated as central in nature, the following characteristics (12,20) are probable: (a) poor localization, (b) over-reaction to painful stimuli, (c) frequent association with paresthesias, and (d) exacerbation of emotional and sensory stimuli. These are well-known characteristics of pain in idiopathic headache. If failure of the ANS is considered biochemical in nature, one can expect the pain to be unstable in regions (left, right idiopathic headache) and in time (biorhythms of idiopathic headache pain).

Exacerbatory Mechanisms

Since the pain threshold is lowered, pain arises or is exacerbated from mechanical (head jolting) stimuli, or from emotional or pharmacological (alcohol, nitroglycerin) vasodilatation, pulsation, and prolonged muscular contraction of the scalp and neck (using the latter two types of headache according to the conventional definition). A violent and prolonged emotion, capable of activating the ANS (in spite of its weakening), can cancel a preexisting idiopathic headache. Physiopathological conditions such as sleep, catamenia, pregnancy, sexual intercourse, stress, and fever, subserved by the same ANS neurotransmitters, can influence idiopathic headache.

Extracephalic Pains

When a pain arises from peripheral stimulation, the pain threshold of nonaffected areas increases (30). As expected, in nonorganic central pain the deep pain threshold is not increased but lowered significantly in nonaffected areas (10). Idiopathic headache sufferers often complain of spontaneous pain in extracephalic regions such as the neck, shoulders, back, and legs. In a few patients, a systemic pain syndrome (central panalgesia) has been described and labeled according to its mechanism (42,54).

Biochemical Aspects

Although in animals it is possible to demonstrate a direct correlation between the ANS neurotransmitters, primarily 5-hydroxytryptamine (5-HT), dopamine, morphine-like factors, and nociception (1,21,25,31,59), in man only indirect evidence has been obtained (55). An involvement of serotonin in migraine was suggested many years ago by our group (17,40,58) (Fig. 1) and other investigators have endorsed this concept (3,11). The recent central theory of idiopathic headache (42,48) rests on a possible deficiency of 5-HT, thought to be the main transmitter of the ANS; in animals, its deficiency in periaquaductal gray matter has been shown to induce hyperalgesia (1,21). Maintenance of the ANS 5-HT patrimony is required for morphine to exhibit its analgesic effect in animals (32). This finding enables one to suggest a correlation between it and the observation that morphine addiction is practically unknown among idiopathic headache sufferers. This correlation depends mainly on the poor analgesic effect of morphine on migraine, supporting the hypothesis of an involvement of morphine-like factors in idiopathic headache (48,49). Morphine-like factors were lowered

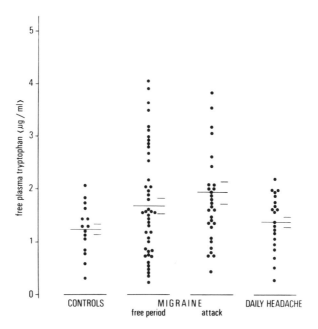

FIG. 1. The increase of free plasma tryptophan during migraine attack is significant when compared with controls.

in the cerebrospinal fluid of sufferers of trigeminal neuralgia (61) and in a pilot study of idiopathic headache sufferers (50).

Pharmacological Aspects

If the turnover of ANS neurotransmitters is defective in idiopathic headache, one must expect both an influence on pain by administration of drugs affecting the metabolism of the ANS transmitters and an increased sensibility (supersensitivity) of peripheral and central (brain) receptors to neurotransmitters or correlated agonists.

Drugs Affecting ANS Neurotransmitters

If ANS neurotransmitters (5-HT in particular) are deficient in the brainstem of idiopathic headache sufferers, drugs capable of depleting brain 5-HT are expected to aggravate pain. In fact, reserpine (27) and fenfluramine (13) in acute doses precipitate pain only in idiopathic headache sufferers. Parachlorophenylalanine (fenclonine), an inhibitor of 5-HT synthesis, chronically administered to idiopathic headache sufferers, provokes an impressive systemic pain syndrome that is reversible on discontinuation of the drug (42,51). In normal subjects, this compound does not induce pain (9). The pain-precipitating capacity of *p*-chlorophenylalanine is exclusive in idiopathic headache sufferers, providing further evidence of a precarious 5-HT turnover in their ANS. More recently, chronic treatment with *p*-chlorophenylalanine has been observed to provoke pain in parkinsonian patients (66). According to the 5-HT deficiency hypothesis, serotonin precursors such as tryptophan and 5-hydroxytryptophan would be expected to improve migraine (43). Drugs capable of enhancing the activity of 5-HT, such as methysergide, LSD-25, ergotamine, and GC-94 in man (2,57) and in animals (18,19,39), have a positive effect on idiopathic headache. The therapeutic effect of these drugs does not seem to involve a blockade of serotonin, as 5-HT antagonism is observed only at plasma concentrations of these drugs resulting from larger than clinical doses. The possibility that central serotoninergic neurons react to classic migraine drugs (e.g., methysergide) in a manner similar to that of 5-HT has been claimed recently in the elegant investigations of Higler and Aghajanan (23).

Peripheral Supersensitivity

Vascular Smooth Muscle (Computerized Venotest)

The cut of a nerve induces a loss of agonist in neuronal terminals, a specific increase of receptor sensitivity to agonists (denervation supersensitivity), and a local loss of monoamine oxidase activity (6,7,33,35). Decentralization provokes a similar phenomenon except that supersensitivity is concerned not only with one, but a multiplicity of agonists (64). Using an original technique (computerized venotest), we observed a strong increase (10- to 50-fold) of vein sensitivity to 5-HT and norepinephrine at the acme and end of a migraine attack, as depicted in Fig. 2 (54). This increase may be due to an increased receptor sensitivity, or a loss of local monoamine oxidase activity, or both. The postulated decrease in platelet monoamine oxidase activity (50%) in migraine was subsequently confirmed (38,53).

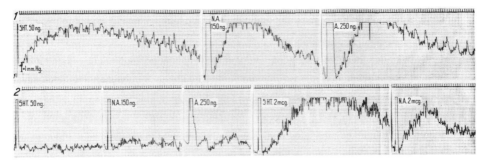

FIG. 2. Venotest recordings of dorsal veins. **Top panel:** An example of serotonin (5-HT), norepinephrine (NA), and epinephrine (A) supersensitivity at the end of a migraine attack. **Bottom panel:** During a migraine-free period.

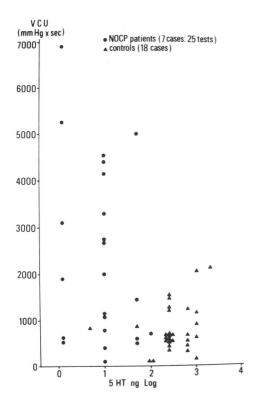

FIG. 3. Vein supersensitivity to 5-HT in sufferers of nonorganic central pain (NOCP) compared with control subjects. Venospasm is expressed in venoconstrictive units (1 U equals an increase of 1 mm Hg of local vein pressure per sec).

An impressive monoamine supersensitivity was observed, by employing the computerized venotest, in 40% of patients suffering from central panalgesia (CPA), a newly defined systemic pain syndrome (42,48,52,56). Supersensitivity in CPA involves dopamine, tyramine, and, to a dramatic extent (up to 2,000-fold), 5-HT (Fig. 3). In these CPA patients, no important changes in levels of free plasma and platelet 5-HT were found. The most typical case, a 35-year-old woman with debilitating CPA, was tested 21 times on different occasions and her supersensitivity to 5-HT varied between 100 and 2,000 times that of the control (Fig. 4). The pains of CPA patients were previously interpreted by other clinicians as manifestations of hysteria or masked depression. This striking monoamine supersensitivity is the first objective measure of these patients. Vein supersensitivity of CPA sufferers is suggestively analogous to that of the nictitating membrane in decentralized cats (33) where the sensitivity to norepinephrine and 5-HT is increased 10- and 70-fold, respectively.

Iris Smooth Muscle (Pupil-Test)

The iris of idiopathic headache sufferers dilates more and for longer time periods than in normal subjects after conjunctival administration of phenylephrine, a direct agonist of α-receptors (Fig. 5). However, after oral doses of fenflura-

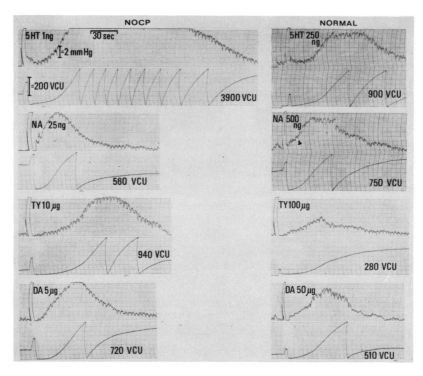

FIG. 4. Supersensitivity in a typical case of a systemic NOCP sufferer **(left panel)** compared with a control subject **(right panel)**. 5-HT, serotonin; NA, norepinephrine; TY, tyramine; and DA, dopamine. VCU described in Fig. 3 legend.

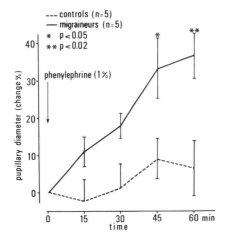

FIG. 5. Supersensitivity of the iris α-receptors in headache sufferers. The agonist (phenylephrine) was instilled in the conjunctival sac.

mine (a norepinephrine-releasing drug), the pupil of idiopathic headache sufferers dilates less and for a shorter period of time when compared to normal subjects (13,16). It is of significance that this supersensitivity is ipsilateral in cluster headaches and lasts many months after the cluster ends (14). Miosis following conjunctival application of guanethidine (an agent depleting the norepinephrine level) is more persistent and pronounced than in normal subjects (16). All of these observations are compatible with a supersensitivity of the iris α-adrenoceptors that is due to a local deficiency of norepinephrine.

Central Supersensitivity

The Chemotrigger Zone

Vomiting during migraine attack is one of the most frequent events and is clearly central in nature. Apomorphine and levodopa, when acutely administered in small doses, provokes nausea and vomiting, more so in idiopathic headache sufferers than in control subjects. This occurs because of a supersensitivity of dopamine receptors which subserve the chemotrigger zone (55). Idiopathic headache sufferers exhibit the same sensitivity when given L-5-hydroxytryptophan (55) because of a local release of dopamine and chemotrigger zone stimulation (32).

Vasopressor Centers

Collapse due to orthostatic hypotension frequently occurs during a migraine attack. Bromocriptine is a specific agonist for dopamine receptors subserving vasopressor centers by inhibiting this hypotension. Idiopathic headache sufferers, when tested with a small (2.5 mg) oral dose of α-bromocriptine, display a greater standing arterial hypotension than do the controls; in many cases a dramatic standing hypotension provokes an initial fainting that can be interrupted by the patient assuming a supine position.

Hallucinatory Structures

Elementary (white and colored scintillations) or more elaborate hallucinations, perceptive distortions (micropsia), together with a feeling of enlarged hands, feet, and eyes are experienced by a few migraineurs during their attacks (62). Idiopathic headache sufferers experience significantly more hallucinatory events than the control population following administration of a small dose of 5-HT analog drugs, such as psylocibin and LSD-25 (15). A correlation between hallucinations, serotoninergic neurons, LSD-25, psylocibin, and other 5-HT analog drugs has been demonstrated. σ-Receptors have an affinity for exogenous and endogenous opiates; when stimulated by such, they provoke hallucinations (29). Pentazocine exhibits a high affinity for σ-receptors (29) and administration of it to idiopathic headache sufferers induces dysphoria, depersonalization, and hallucinations, sometimes to a dramatic extent (48). During occasional attacks of migraine with visual aura, naloxone, if given promptly at the start of an aura, reduces the intensity and duration of scintillations (F. Sicuteri, *unpublished observations*). The hallucinations of idiopathic sufferers following pentazocine administration could be interpreted as a supersensitivity of sigma opiate receptors, due to a deficiency of morphine-like factors. The lowered levels of morphine-like factors in the cerebrospinal fluid of idiopathic headache sufferers can be of significance (49,50).

WHY NOT PERIPHERAL?

Pain from idiopathic headache is considered physiological and peripheral in nature since it can be provoked by mechanical stimuli (dilatation and pulsation of cranial vessels), or chemical stimuli (release of pain-producing substances in tissues of the head), or muscular stimuli (psychogenic sustained contraction of muscles of the scalp, face, nucha, and neck). In this section, the peripheral mechanism concept will be examined as we hypothesize that pain is, in nature, central.

Peripheral (Vascular and Muscular) Factors

Vascular Mechanisms

Only those biological agents (e.g., histamine, bradykinin, and prostaglandins) capable of stimulating pain receptors can provoke headache in normal subjects; in idiopathic headache sufferers, the pain is more intense (Fig. 6). These substances are also capable of inducing pain when injected into the carotid, digitally occluded to avoid vasodilatation (41). Nitroglycerin, papaverine, and similar drugs provoke intracranial vasodilatation but not pain; in fact, an impressive intracranial vasodilatation bordering on a slight collapse can be induced by inhaling amyl nitrate without which the normal subject complains of idiopathic headache. Spontaneous (from emotional stimuli) or pharmacological dilatation becomes painful when the pain threshold is lowered, as often happens in idiopathic headache sufferers. Vasodilatation, as other ancillary troubles (vomiting, depression, and fever) when present, must be considered as aggravating phenomena of idiopathic headache. Ergotamine constricts the vessels and breaks the idiopathic headache attacks, but other powerful vasoconstricting agents (such as vasopressin, norepinephrine and angiotension) usually do not stop the attack. Ergotamine, as well as other antimigrainous drugs, enhances the spasmogenic activity of 5-HT on the dorsal vein of the hand (2,57) and vessels of nasal mucosa of dogs (18,19,39). Similarly, ergotamine might enhance 5-HT at the ANS level, correcting the critical loss of physiological analgesia. In agreement with this interpretation, others have shown that ergot drugs are stimulating agents of 5-HT receptors (8,23,60).

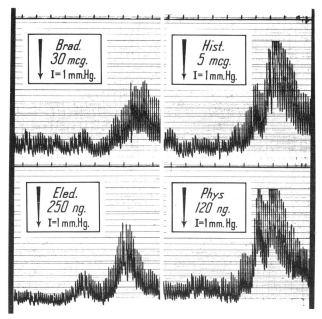

FIG. 6. Electromanometric registration of CSF during a diagnostic spinal puncture of a headache sufferer. An increase of CSF pressure indicates an increase of intracranial vasodilatation. Brad., bradykinin; Hist., histamine; Eled., eledoisin; and Phys., physalaemin.

Muscle Contraction

Muscular activity during ischemia provokes pain sooner in idiopathic headache sufferers than in normals (10) because the former have a lower deep pain threshold in comparison to controls. Pain, of whatever origin (including central), provokes a defensive muscle contraction. A psychogenic muscle contraction is usually not painful, but it becomes so if the pain threshold has been lowered. In such cases, muscle contraction is not the primary but accessory mechanism of tension headache. The electromyographic activity of the temporalis, trapezius, and forearm flexors of tension headache sufferers was the same as that of normal subjects; the EMG of the frontalis depicted a significant difference, but without any correlation to the area of pain (5). Some investigations confirmed an increased EMG activity of frontalis (65,67), whereas others disagree with this conclusion after observing no increase of frontalis or other muscular EMG activity during headache (22). The critical questions concerning the existence of muscle contraction headache are the following: Why is not tension muscle contraction painful in a number of subjects, and is the muscle contraction the cause or an aggravating consequence of pain?

DISCUSSION

All nervous or nonnervous functions are subject to disorders or diseases; nociception is not an exception to this rule. The most common expression of the central dysnociception is idiopathic headache, migraine included. A functional failure of the ANS could be the basis for idiopathic headache; this failure is credibly biochemical in nature. Some indirect evidence suggests a deficiency of the ANS neurotransmitters such as 5-HT, dopamine, and morphine-like factors. Dysnociception can be reversible or irreversible, depending on the therapeutic distinction of tractable and intractable idiopathic headache. The central theory, initially proposed following one of our studies in clinical pharmacology (42), has been supported by pharmacological (mostly conditions of supersensitivity) and biochemical (5-HT precursor, morphine-like factors, and monoamine oxidase activity) studies (36,40,44–46,49,51). However, some pharmacological mechanisms must be reconsidered: methysergide, first used in migraine therapy (40), must be now considered as a 5-HT enhancing agent (or a 5-HT agonist), rather than an antiserotoninic one (2,18,19,39,48,57). The idiopathic headache therapeutic armamentarium has been enriched by L-tryptophan and L-5-hydroxytryptophan both of which are able to pass the blood-brain barrier (43). An analogy can be proposed between Parkinson's disease (striatal dopamine deficiency, employing L-DOPA as treatment) and idiopathic headache (5-HT deficiency of the ANS system, treated with L-tryptophan). My own thesis concerning the central nature of pain has been affirmed by some authors (26,28,68), whereas another author (surprisingly) has not quoted the original paper (4).

According to the central theory, changes of vasomotility (constriction and dilatation), as well as psychogenic muscle contraction, are not primary mechanisms but accessory phenomena that occasionally aggravate the pain. The most convincing support for this novel theory is the infrequent evolution of serious idiopathic headache in CPA (42,52). In this syndrome, until now labeled as hysteria or masked depression, a striking supersensitivity to monoamines (and to a dramatic extent, to 5-HT), is found in 40% of patients. This stable supersensitivity is similar to the transitory one, even if to a minor extent, during migraine attack (54); the vein supersensitivity in idiopathic headache and CPA parallels the supersensitivity to multiple monoamines detected in the nictitating membrane of the decentralized cats (33,63). Perhaps the most convincing support for this theory emerges from the clinic: Many clinical aspects and influences of internal or external factors (biorhythms, emotion, sex, catamenias, pregnancy, sleep, and drugs), which are difficult to understand by applying the peripheral (vascular, muscular) theory, become more interpretable when the physician examines his patients by speculating, under the perspective of this theory, in terms of central dysnociception.

SUMMARY

A failure of the structures that centrally modulate the pain is proposed as the primary substrate of idiopathic headache, migraine included. Monoamines (5-HT and dopamine) and neuropeptides (morphine-like factors) are the neurotransmitters of the ANS; therefore, a deficiency of their turnover could be the biochemical background for the ANS dysfunction, of which the most common expression is idiopathic headache. Spontaneous vasoconstriction and vasodilatation are never painful in normals with physiological nociception; in these subjects, idiopathic headache can be provoked only by drugs (such as histamine, bradykinin, and prostaglandins) capable of stimulating nociceptors. Spontaneous or pharmacological dilatation is painful only in dysnociceptors because of a lowering of pain threshold. The same criticisms are valid for the interpretation of idiopathic headache, conventionally thought to be due to a contraction of the scalp musculature. A most convincing support for the present theory is CPA, a newly described syndrome representing an infrequent evolution of idiopathic headache. By using the computerized venotest, a high supersensitivity to dopamine, norepinephrine, and 5-HT can be found in some CPA patients. Such supersensitivity is credibly an expression of a neurotransmitter deficiency in the brainstem, according to the concept of supersensitivity resulting from decentralization. An analogy between vein supersensitivity in CPA and that of the nictitating membrane of decentralized cats is suggested.

ACKNOWLEDGMENT

These investigations were conducted under grants from the National Council of Research, Rome, Italy.

REFERENCES

1. Akil, H., and Liebeskind, J. C. (1975): Monoaminergic mechanisms of stimulation-produced analgesia. *Brain Res.,* 94:279–296.
2. Anselmi, B., Del Bianco, P. L., de Vos, C. J., Galli, P., Lamar, J. C., Schonbaum, E., Sicuteri, F., and van der Veen, F. (1976): Clinical and animal pharmacology of migraine: New perspectives. In: *Clinical Pharmacology of Serotonin,* edited by F. Sicuteri and E. Schonbaum, pp. 45–59. Karger, Basel.
3. Anthony, M., Hinterberger, H., and Lance, J. H. (1967): Plasma serotonin in migraine and stress. *Arch. Neurol.,* 16:544–552.
4. Appenzeller, O. (1975): Hypothesis: Pathogenesis of vascular headache of the migrainous type: The role of impaired central inhibition. *Headache,* 15:177–179.
5. Boxtel, van A., and Roozeveld, van der ven J. (1978): Differential EMG activity in subjects with muscle contraction headache related to mental effort. *Headache,* 17:233–237.
6. Burn, J. H., and Robinson, J. (1953): Hypersensitivity of the denervated nictitating membrane and amine oxidase. *J. Physiol. (Lond.),* 120:224–229.
7. Cannon, W. B. (1939): A law of denervation. *Am. J. Med. Sci.,* 198:737–750.
8. Corrodi, H., Farnebo, L. O., Fuxe, K., and Hamberger, B. (1975): Effect of ergot drugs on central 5-hydroxytryptamine neurons: Evidence for 5-hydroxytryptamine release or 5-hydroxytryptamine receptor stimulation. *Eur. J. Pharmacol.,* 30:172–181.
9. Cremata, V. Y., and Koe, B. K. (1966): Clinical pharmacological evaluation of *p*-chlorophenylalanine: A new serotonin depleting agent. *Clin. Pharmacol. Ther.,* 7:768–776.
10. Curradi, C., Giovanni, M. D., Caternolo, M., and Sicuteri, F. (1976): Esplorazione del dolore extracefalico indotto nelle cefalee essenziale. *Minerva Med.,* 67:1840–1844.
11. Curzon, C., Barrie, M., and Wilkinson, M. I. P. (1969): Relationship between headache and amine changes after administration of reserpine to migrainous patients. *Neurosurg. Psychiat.,* 32:555–561.
12. Dejerine, J., and Roussy, G. (1906): La syndrome thalamique. *Rev. Neurol. (Paris),* 14:521–531.
13. Del Bene, E., Anselmi, B., Del Bianco, P. L., Fanciullacci, M., Galli, P., Salmon, S., and Sicuteri, F. (1977): Fenfluramine headache: A biochemical and monoamine receptorial human study. In: *Headache: New Vistas,* edited by F. Sicuteri, pp. 101–109. Biomedical Press, Florence.

14. Fanciullacci, M. (1979): Iris adrenergic impairment in idiopathic headache. *Headache,* 19 *(in press).*
15. Fanciullacci, M., Franchi, G., and Sicuteri, F. (1974): Hypersensitivity to lysergic acid diethylamide (LSD-25 and psilocybin) in essential headache. *Experientia,* 30:1441–1442.
16. Fanciullacci, M., Galli, P., Pietrini, U., and Sicuteri, F. (1977): Adrenergic supersensitivity of the pupil in idiopathic headache. *Experientia,* 33:1082–1083.
17. Fanciullacci, M., Salmon, S., Bonciani, M., and Sicuteri, F. (1977): Free and total plasma tryptophan in idiopathic headache. In: *Headache: New Vistas,* edited by F. Sicuteri, pp. 83–91. Biomedical Press, Florence.
18. Fozard, J. R. (1975): Review: The animal pharmacology of drugs used in the treatment of migraine. *J. Pharm. Pharmacol.,* 27:297–321.
19. Fozard, J. R. (1977): The mechanism by which migraine prophylactic drugs modify vascular reactivity in vitro. In: *Headache: New Vistas,* edited by F. Sicuteri, pp. 259–278. Biomedical Press, Florence.
20. Garcin, R. (1968): Thalamic syndrome and pain of central origin. In: *Pain,* edited by A. Soulariac, J. Cahn, and J. Charpentier, pp. 521–541. Academic Press, New York.
21. Harvey, J. A., and Lints, C. E. (1971): Lesions in the medial forebrain bundle: Relationship between pain sensitivity and telencephalic content of serotonin. *J. Comp. Physiol. Psychol.,* 74:28–35.
22. Haynes, S. N., Griffin, P., Mooney, D., and Parise, M. (1975): Electromyographic biofeedback and relaxation instructions in the treatment of muscle contraction headaches. *Behav. Res. Ther.,* 6:672–678.
23. Higler, H. J., and Aghajanan, G. K. (1977): Serotonin receptors in the brain. *Fed. Proc.,* 36:2159–2164.
24. Hosobuchi, Y., and Wemmer, J. (1977): Disulfiram inhibition of development of tolerance to analgesia induced by central gray stimulation in humans. *Eur. J. Pharmacol.,* 43:385–387.
25. Hughes, J. (1975): Isolation of an endogenous compound from the brain with the pharmacological properties similar to morphine. *Brain Res.,* 88:295–308.
26. Hyyppa, M. T., and Kangasniemi, P. (1977): Variation of plasma-free tryptophan and CSF-5-HIAA during migraine. *Headache,* 17:25–27.
27. Kimball, R. W., and Friedman, A. P. (1961): Studies on pathogensis of migraine. *Recent Adv. Biol. Psych.,* 3:200–206.
28. Lance, J. W. (1969): *The Mechanism and Management of Headache.* Butterworths, London.
29. Martin, W. R. (1976): Naloxone. *Ann. Intern. Med.,* 85:765–768.
30. Merskey, H., and Evans, P. R. (1975): Variations in pain complaint threshold in psychiatric and neurological patients with pain. *Pain,* 1:73–79.
31. Messing, R. B., and Lytle, L. D. (1978): Serotonin-containing neurons: Their possible role in pain and analgesia. *Pain,* 4:1–21.
32. Peng, M. T. (1963): Locus of emetic action of epinephrine and dopa in dogs. *J. Pharmacol. Exp. Ther.,* 139:345–349.
33. Pluchino, S. (1972): Direct and indirect effects of 5-hydroxytryptamine and tyramine on cat smooth muscle. *Naunyn Schmiedebergs Arch. Pharmacol.,* 272:189–224.
34. Riddoch, G. (1938): Clinical features of central pain. *Lancet,* 1:1093.
35. Rosenthal, M. E., and Di Palma, J. R. (1962): Acute tolerance to nor-epinephrine in dogs. *J. Pharmacol. Exp. Ther.,* 136:336–343.
36. Salmon, S., Fanciullacci, M., Bonciani, M., and Sicuteri, F. (1978): Plasma tryptophan in migraine. *Headache,* 17:238–241.
37. Samanin, R., Gumulka, W., and Valzelli, L. (1970): Reduced effect of morphine in midbrain raphe lesioned rats. *Eur. J. Pharmacol.,* 10:339–343.
38. Sandler, M., Youdin, M. B. H., Southgate, J., and Hannington, E. (1970): The role of tyramine in migraine: Some possible biomedical mechanisms. In: *Background to Migraine,* edited by A. L. Cochrane, pp. 103–112. Heinemann Medical Books, London.
39. Schonbaum, E., Vargaftig, B. B., Lefort, K., Lamar, J. C., and Hasenack, T. (1975): An unexpected effect of serotonin antagonists on the canine nasal circulation. *Headache,* 15:180–187.
40. Sicuteri, F. (1959): Prophylactic and therapeutic properties of l-methyl-lysergic acid butanolamide in migraine. *Int. Arch. Allergy,* 15:300–307.
41. Sicuteri, F. (1970): Bradykinin and intracranial circulation in man. In: *Bradykinin, Kallidin and Kallikrein,* edited by E. Erdos, pp. 482–515. Springer-Verlag, Berlin.
42. Sicuteri, F. (1971): Pain syndrome in man following treatment with *p*-chlorophenylalanine. *Pharmacol. Res. Commun.,* 3:401–407.

43. Sicuteri, F. (1972): 5-Hydroxytryptophan in the prophylaxis of migraine. *Pharmacol. Res. Commun.,* 4:213–219.
44. Sicuteri, F. (1974): Headache biochemistry and pharmacology. *Arch. Neurobiol. (Madr.),* 37:27–65.
45. Sicuteri, F. (1976): Headache: Disruption of pain modulation. In: *Advances in Pain Research and Therapy, Vol 1,* edited by J. J. Bonica and D. Albe-Fessard, pp. 871–880. Raven Press, New York.
46. Sicuteri, F. (1976): Migraine pathophysiology: New vistas. *Clin. Neurol. (Jpn.),* 16:865–866.
47. Sicuteri, F. (1976): Migraine, a central biochemical dysnociception. *Headache,* 16:145–159.
48. Sicuteri, F. (1977): Headache as metonymy of non-organic central pain. In: *Headache: New Vistas,* edited by F. Sicuteri, pp. 18–67. Biomedical Press, Florence.
49. Sicuteri, F. (1978): Mini-review: Endorphins, opiate receptors and migraine headache. *Headache,* 17:253–257.
50. Sicuteri, F., Anselmi, B., Curradi, C., Michelacci, S., and Sassi, A. (1978): Morphine-like factors in CSF of headache patients. In: *The Endorphins,* edited by E. Costa and M. Trabucchi, pp. 363–366. Raven Press, New York.
51. Sicuteri, F., Anselmi, B., and Del Bianco, P. L. (1973): 5-Hydroxytryptamine supersensitivity as a new theory of headache and central pain: A clinical pharmacological approach with parachlorophenylalanine. *Psychopharmacologia (Berl.),* 29:347–356.
52. Sicuteri, F., Anselmi, B., and Del Bianco, P. L. (1978): Systemic non-organic central pain: a new syndrome with decentralization supersensitivity. *Headache,* 18:133–136.
53. Sicuteri, F., Buffoni, F., Anselmi, B., and Del Bianco, P. L. (1971): Monoamine oxidase activity in migraine and arterial hypertension. In: *Proceedings International Headache Symposium,* edited by D. Dalessio, T. Dalsgaard-Nielsen, and S. Diamond, pp. 195–200. Sandoz, Ltd., Basel.
54. Sicuteri, F., Del Bianco, P. L., and Fanciullacci, M. (1966): Variazioni di sensibilità alla 5-HT e alle catecolamine durante l'attacco emicranico. Test della venocostrizione. *Boll. Soc. Ital. Biol. Sper.,* 42:843–844.
55. Sicuteri, F., Fanciullacci, M., and Del Bene, E. (1977): Dopamine system and idiopathic headache. In: *Headache: New Vistas,* edited by F. Sicuteri, pp. 239–250. Biomedical Press, Florence.
56. Sicuteri, F., Fanciullacci, M., and Michelacci, S. (1978): Decentralizaion supersensitivity in headache and central panalgesia. In: *Research and Clinical Studies in Headache, Vol. 6,* edited by A. P. Friedman, M. E. Granger, and M. Critchley, pp. 19–33. Karger, Basel.
57. Sicuteri, F., Franchi, G., and Fanciullacci, M. (1974): New perspectives on analgesia from ergotamine and methysergide in migraine. *2nd Hung. Congr. Pharmacol. Soc. Abstracts,* Abstr. 1/28.
58. Sicuteri, F., Testi, A., and Anselmi, B. (1961): Biochemical investigations in headache: Increase in the hydroxyindoleacetic acid excretion during migraine attacks. *Int. Arch. Allergy,* 19:55–58.
59. Snyder, S. H., and Simantov, R. (1977): The opiate receptor and opioid peptides. *J. Neurochem.,* 26:13–20.
60. Sofia, R. D., and Vassar, H. B. (1975): The effect of ergotamine and methysergide on serotonin metabolism in the rat brain. *Arch. Int. Pharmacodyn. Ther.,* 216:40–50.
61. Terenius, L., and Wahlstrom, A. (1975): Morphine-like ligand for opiate receptors in human CSF. *Life Sci.,* 16:1759–1764.
62. Todd, J. (1955): The syndrome of Alice in wonderland. *Can. Med. Assoc. J.,* 73:701–704.
63. Trendelenburg, U. (1966): Mechanisms of supersensitivity and subsensitivity to sympathomimetic amines. *Pharmacol. Rev.,* 18: 629–640.
64. Trendelenburg, U., Maxwell, R. A., and Pluchino, S. (1970): Methoxamine as a tool to assess the importance of intraneuronal uptake of l-norepinephrine in the cat's nictitating membrane. *J. Pharmacol. Exp. Ther.,* 172:91–99.
65. Tunis, M. M., and Wolff, H. G. (1954): Studies on headache: Cranial artery vasoconstriction and muscle contraction headache. *Arch. Neurol. Psychiat.,* 71:425–434.
66. Van Woert, M. H., Ambani, L. M., and Levine, R. J. (1972): Clinical effects of parachlorophenylalanine in Parkinson's disease. *Dis. Nerv. Syst.,* 33:777–780.
67. Vaughn, R., Pall, M. L., and Haynes, S. N. (1977): Frontalis EMG response to stress in subjects with frequent muscle contraction headaches. *Headache,* 16:313–317.
68. Welch, K. M. A., Gaudet, R., Wong, T. P. F., and Chabi, E. (1977): Transient cerebral ischemia and brain serotonin: Relevance to migraine. *Headache,* 17:145–147.

Mechanisms of Pain and Analgesic Compounds,
edited by R. F. Beers, Jr., and E. G. Bassett.
Raven Press, New York © 1979.

28. Site of Analgesic Action of Aspirin-like Drugs and Opioids

Sergio H. Ferreira

Department of Pharmacology, Faculty of Medicine of Ribeirão Preto, São Paulo, Brazil

INTRODUCTION

Aspirin-like drugs (nonsteroidal antiinflammatory agents) act as analgesics peripherally by blocking the generation of impulses at the chemoreceptors for pain, while narcotic analgesics block synaptic transmission in the central pathways for pain. This statement summarizes Lim's views (33,34,47) and is currently acceptable to most pharmacologists. It is supported by two recent findings: (a) prostaglandins, at concentrations found in inflammatory exudates, sensitize pain receptors to mechanical or chemical stimulation (14), and (b) the synthesis of prostaglandins is inhibited *in vivo* by therapeutic doses of aspirin-like drugs. However, this general view may no longer be true when one considers that aspirin-like drugs also have a central antialgesic action (16,17) and morphine, as well as morphine antagonists, have a peripheral analgesic action (20); these points will be discussed below.

Antialgesic Effect of Aspirin-like Drugs

The evidence supporting the theory that the antialgesic effect of aspirin-like drugs is related to an effect on the synthesis of prostaglandins can be summarized as follows:

(a) Prostaglandins or their metabolites are found in inflammatory exudates (Table 1).

(b) The key enzyme mediating the biosynthesis of prostaglandins, cyclooxygenase, is inhibited both *in vitro* and *in vivo* by drugs known to have antiinflammatory, antipyretic, or antialgesic activity. All the drugs which inhibit cyclooxygenase activity *in vivo* show at least one of these activities (37).

(c) Prostaglandins, at concentrations found in inflammatory exudates, are able to reproduce two basic inflammatory events: erythema and hyperalgesia (14). When prostaglandins are associated with other inflammatory mediators such as bradykinin or histamine, they strongly potentiate their edematogenic effect (51,63,64).

Prostaglandins are released by a variety of inflammatory stimuli (Table 1).

TABLE 1. *Detection of prostaglandins in inflammation*

Inflammatory stimuli	Site	Species	Reference
Chemical			
Carrageenin	Skin	Rat	66,67
	Pleural cavity	Rat	70
	Knee joint	Dog	52
Urate crystals	Knee joint	Pigeon	27
Endotoxin	Knee joint	Dog	36
Cantharidin	Skin	Man	28
Immunological			
Anaphylaxis	Lung	Guinea pig	9,10,35,46,54–57
	Eyes	Rabbit	3,12,13
	Knee joint	Rabbit	4
Contact eczema	Skin	Man	31
Arthus reaction	Pleural cavity	Rat	70
Cell-mediated	Pleural cavity	Rat	70
Rheumatoid arthritis	Knee joint	Man	38,53,62
Physical			
Ultraviolet	Skin	Man	30
Heat	Paw, hand	Dog, man	1,39,40

The current view is that those stimuli that disrupt cell integrity induce the release of prostaglandins. The basic events related to this release are (a) an activation of phospholipase A (which mediates generation of the substrate arachidonic acid) and (b) a functional loss of cell compartmentalization, that permits access of the substrate to cyclooxygenase. Detailed discussion of these events can be found elsewhere (22,23,25).

This review is mostly concerned with observations thought to be relevant to the relationship between prostaglandins and inflammatory pain. Before starting, however, I would like to emphasize that pain, susceptible to treatment with aspirin-like drugs, results from the release of inflammatory mediators and is not primarily due to the occurrence of structural tissue changes (such as edema or arrival of migrating cells). This is discussed further in ref. 16.

OBSERVATIONS AND DISCUSSION

Prostaglandin Hyperalgesia

The discovery that the synthesis of prostaglandins was inhibited *in vitro* and *in vivo* by aspirin-like drugs (18,60,62) stimulated our interest in the role of prostaglandins as mediators of inflammatory pain. At that time there was conflicting evidence concerning the pain-producing activity of prostaglandins in man. Hyperalgesia induced by intradermal injections of prostaglandins had already been described (50,61), and it was known that their intravenous administration caused headaches (2) and pain along the veins into which they were infused.

Intramuscular injection caused intense, lasting pain (43). Prostaglandins were described as the most powerful inducer of writhing in mice (7). In contrast, prostaglandins failed to induce pain in man when instilled on a blister base, and there was no mention of a hyperalgesic effect in a study on dermal vasodilation (14). Most probably, those painful effects of prostaglandins were not considered relevant because scientists were looking for a proper pain mediator and failed to recognize the importance of the hyperalgesia induced by prostaglandins.

Bradykinin or histamine, when administered intradermally, was observed to cause overt pain (the subject did suffer pain) which quickly subsided even in the presence of pronounced edema and erythema, without inducing hyperalgesia (i.e., a state in which overt pain can be aroused by painless mechanical or chemical stimulation). In fact, the immediate, overt pain-producing effect of intradermally administered prostaglandins was equivalent to that shown by other mediators, but was observed only at concentrations higher than those found in inflammatory exudates. This overt pain effect, however, was short-lived and gave place to long-lasting hyperalgesia. When infused subdermally at concentrations likely to be found at inflamed sites, prostaglandins did not cause overt pain but only hyperalgesia (14).

Our experiments with subdermal infusions, conducted so as to mimic the continuous release of a mediator that would occur at the site of an injury, revealed two important features of the action of prostaglandins: (a) prostaglandins sensitize the pain receptors to mechanical and chemical stimulation and (b) this effect is cumulative (14). This cumulative effect was demonstrated by infusing for 2 hr a concentration of prostaglandin that was ineffective for a 30-min period. Thus, a slow rate of release of prostaglandins during a long period of time (as might occur in inflammation) is capable of causing hyperalgesia. In these experiments there was no overt pain during separate infusions of prostaglandin E_1, bradykinin, histamine, or a mixture of bradykinin and histamine. However, when PGE_1 was added to bradykinin or histamine (or a mixture of both), strong pain developed. Furthermore, in areas made hyperalgesic by an infusion of prostaglandins (tested by pressure), a second infusion of either histamine or bradykinin caused overt pain. At the site where bradykinin or histamine has been previously infused (without producing hyperalgesia), a second infusion of prostaglandin caused little or no pain.

Another important observation concerned pruritus. Neither histamine, bradykinin, nor PGE_1, infused subdermally, caused itch (14). However, when PGE_1 was infused with bradykinin, there was pain rather than itch. This role of prostaglandins in potentiating the itching effects of histamine was later confirmed by Greaves and McDonald-Gibson (29).

The demonstration of sensitization of human pain receptors by prostaglandins helped to interpret the results obtained by Lim and colleagues (33,34,47) with respect to nociception induced by intraarterial injection of bradykinin into the dog spleen. In this preparation, they showed that aspirin-like drugs, acting peripherally as analgesics, blocked the nociceptive action of bradykinin. We showed that bradykinin caused the release of prostaglandins from the spleen and that this release was blocked by aspirin-like drugs. In those animals, infusion of prostaglandins into the spleen restored the nociceptive action of bradykinin (19). The fact that adrenaline, much weaker than bradykinin as a pain-producing substance in this system, releases similar amounts of prostaglandins *in vitro* and *in vivo*, suggests that prostaglandins cannot be considered as the mediator of the pain-producing activity of bradykinin. Thus, at least in the dog spleen preparation, the mechanism seems to be a bradykinin-induced release of prostaglandin, which sensitizes the nerve endings.

This unique ability of prostaglandins to sensitize pain receptors is also demonstrable in the rat. One hour after injection of carrageenin into the rat paw no hyperalgesia can be detected; at 2 to 4 hr, however, a marked hyperalgesia is observed. Bradykinin, histamine, or 5-hydroxytryptamine cause little or no hyperalgesia 1 hr following injection when given alone or together with carrageenin. But prostaglandins (which cause a mild effect by themselves), added to carrageenin induce a marked hyperalgesic, possibly due to a synergistic action in conjunction with other mediators that are released (15).

Additional studies in our and other laboratories have extended these observations. The sensitizing action of prostaglandins to nociceptive stimulation has been observed in the dog knee joint (52,59), in rat paw (68) and in rabbit ear preparations (41,42). From these experiments one can conclude that aspirin-like drugs do not interfere directly with the sensitizing action of prostaglandins or with the effect of nociceptive stimuli. They seem to act by blocking the local release of prostaglandins induced by inflammatory stimuli, thus preventing the development of hyperalgesia.

Hyperalgesic Effect of Prostaglandins and Prostacyclin

A long-lasting hyperalgesic effect of prostaglandins E_1 or E_2 has been shown in several models, as previously discussed. It is a common clinical observation, in various pathological conditions such as rheumatoid arthritis or special types of headaches, that the antialgesic effect of aspirin-like drugs requires a few hours to develop. This can be explained by the long-lasting hyperalgesic effect of prostaglandins. However, it is of general knowledge that for some acute pains, aspirin-like drugs have a relatively rapid effect. The hyperalgesic effect of prostaglandins in the rat paw is long-lasting (21,68) but aspirin-like drugs are capable of reducing an existing hyperalgesia within an hour (71). An explanation for this discrepancy has been recently obtained in our laboratories. Using two experimental models, a modification of the Randall-Selitto method (58) and the dog incapacitation test (59), it was shown that prostacyclin was a more potent hyperalgesic agent than PGE_2 (21). Furthermore, the hyperalgesia induced by prostacyclin was more immediate and of a much shorter duration (Fig. 1). Prostacyclin (PGI_2), like PGE_1 and PGE_2, is a product of the oxidation of arachidonic acid by cyclooxygenase; therefore, its release is also blocked by

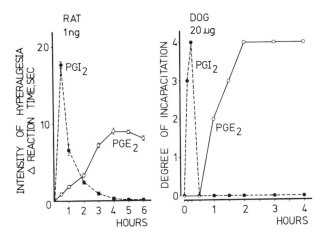

FIG. 1. Left: Hyperalgesic effect of PGI_2 and PGE_2 in the rat paw. Rats were treated with indomethacin 2 mg/kg, i.p., 30 min before the intraplantar injection of prostaglandins. The values indicate the mean and SEM of 6 rats in each group. **Right:** Incapacitation induced in dogs by intra-articular injection of PGI_2 and PGE_2. The dogs were treated with indomethacin 2 mg/kg., i.v., just before the intra-articular injection. Each curve was plotted with the median value of three experiments. (From Ferreira et al., ref. 21.)

aspirin-like drugs. The presence of a stable prostacyclin metabolite, 6-keto prostaglandin F_1, has been demonstrated in the exudate of carrageenin granuloma (5).

An alternative explanation is that aspirin-like drugs are blocking the release of substances sharing the pain-producing activity of fatty acid hydroperoxides. Intradermal injections of hydroperoxides of arachidonic, linoleic, and linolenic acids induced a much more intense, immediate overt pain than the original fatty acids or acetylcholine, bradykinin, histamine, or PGE_1 (14). Thus, it is conceivable that the endoperoxides, intermediates in the biosynthesis of prostaglandins, might be responsible for the type of pain that is quickly blocked by aspirin-like drugs.

Central Effect of Aspirin-like Drugs

Flower and Vane (25) explained the antialgesic or antipyretic activity of paracetamol and phenacetin by selectively blocking the prostaglandin synthetases of the CNS. This explains why these agents [as well as dipyrone (11)] display an antialgesic effect without conspicuous local antiinflammatory (antiedematogenic) action. Such interpretation presupposes that the prostaglandins responsible for causing hyperalgesia are generated at the sensory nerves by the same group of cyclooxygenases found in the CNS, in contrast to prostaglandins responsible for the edema and vasodilatation, which would be of vascular origin. Recently, we have proposed an additional interpretation (17).

Using carrageenin-induced hyperalgesia tests in rats, we have observed that hyperalgesia developed much faster when the contralateral paw had been previously treated with carrageenin. This was taken as an indication that the local inflammation evoked a central mechanism that facilitated local hyperalgesia. We have also studied the effects of aspirin, indomethacin, paracetamol, and phenacetin injected into the paw and into the cerebral ventricles. There was a synergistic antialgesic effect between central and peripheral administration of these agents. Administration of a specific prostaglandin antagonist (SC-19220), either into the cerebral ventricles or into the paw, significantly inhibited carrageenin-evoked hyperalgesia. This hyperalgesia in the rat paw could be mimicked only by a combined central and peripheral administration of prostaglandin. These results suggest that, in the rat, carrageenin-induced inflammatory hyperalgesia has two components resulting from prostaglandin release: a peripheral one, due to the local sensitizing action of pain receptors and a central one, possibly due to the participation of central pain circuits. The antialgesic effect of paracetamol or phenacetin may be partially related to an action on this central component. We do not know if this concept can be extended to other models of inflammation, but it is plausible that it will be applicable to those models in which fever due to prostaglandin release in CNS occurs during the development of inflammation.

Peripheral Action of Morphine and Its Antagonists

Recently we presented evidence that both morphine and enkephalins have a peripheral analgesic effect. At this site the pure opioid antagonist, naloxone, does not antagonize morphine but is an analgesic itself (20). In these experiments, hyperalgesia was measured by our modification of the Randall–Selitto test (9) in which instead of increasing pressure, a constant pressure of 20 mm Hg was applied to the rat paw. Hyperalgesia due to intraplantar injection of PGE_2 is fully developed by about 3 hr and remains constant for up to 6 hr. Intraplantar injection of 10 μg of morphine given when hyperalgesia had fully developed greatly reduced its intensity for 2½ hr. Met-enkephalin had a similar effect, but of shorter duration at the dose used (50 μg). Both substances cause hypoalgesia when injected into control saline-treated paws. Morphine treatment of the contralateral paw did not affect the intensity of hyperalgesia induced by prostaglandin or the threshold of saline-treated paws. This result excludes a possible central component in the analgesia that was observed.

To characterize further this peripheral site of action of morphine, we investigated the effects of naloxone, a pure morphine antagonist. The results showed, unexpectedly, that naloxone by itself had an agonist, morphine-like effect in reducing hyperalgesia. Furthermore, naloxone given at the same time as morphine did not show any antagonism of the analgesia but caused an effect greater than that attained by each substance given separately. Although naloxone is generally accepted as a pure antagonist, it might have partial agonistic activity at this peripheral site. One of the characteristics of a partial agonist is that antagonistic activity lasts longer than its agonist effect. However, morphine still displayed an analgesic effect when given 2 hr after naloxone, thus excluding this possible interpretation.

We estimated the potency of opioids and enkephalins at this peripheral site, relative to a standard, locally acting analgesic agent, lidocaine. From the results obtained (Fig. 2), two important points emerge. First, lidocaine is about one hundred times less potent than the opioid agonists and antagonists. Therefore, the effect observed cannot be explained by a local anesthetic effect. Second, although enkephalins are rapidly inactivated by plasma, Met-enkephalin was only four times less potent than morphine. The comparatively low potency of Leu-enkephalin is in accord with its potency in other systems. From these results, we calculated (by linear regression analysis) the ID_{50} value in nmoles for these substances to be: morphine, 14.3; nalorphine, 17.8; naloxone, 20.4; pentazocine, 22.4; Met-enkephalin, 74.5; Leu-enkephalin, 126.6; and lidocaine, 1,774.

Our experiments thus far had established the analgesic agonist effect of a morphine-antagonist injected intraplantarly. In the next series of experiments, we looked for this activity after systemic (intraperitoneal) injection of morphine antagonists in an attempt to evaluate the contribution of peripheral analgesia to the total analgesic effect. For comparative purposes, we included morphine and pentazocine. The doses used have been shown to be effective in the original Randall–Selitto test but are generally ineffective in tests based on reaction to thermal stimuli (71). All agents cause analgesia 30 min after systemic administration. However, with nalorphine and naloxone, the analgesic activity was short-lived and by 1 hr has been replaced by a hyperalgesic effect manifested in prostaglandin and saline-treated paws, which further increased by the second

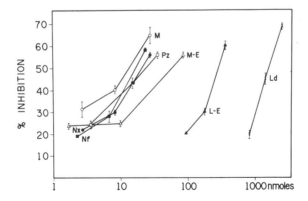

FIG. 2. Peripheral analgesic effect and its dose-dependence. Both hind paws were treated with PGE$_2$ and 2 hr later one received saline and the other the substance under investigation. Measurements were made at the third hour after PGE$_2$ injection. The hyperalgesia of the former paw was taken at 100%. The substances investigated were: morphine (M), naloxone (Nx), nalorphine (Nf), pentazocine (Pz), Met- and Leu-enkephalins (M-E and L-E) and lidocaine (Ld). Values are the mean and SEM for five animals at each concentration. (From Ferreira and Nakamura, ref. 20.)

hour. This hyperalgesic effect is most likely due to a central effect since these agents have only analgesic activity when given intraplantarly. At 30 min the analgesic activity of pentazocine and of a lower dose of morphine (0.1 to 0.5 mg/kg) is probably due to a peripheral action since they have little influence on saline-treated paws.

The observed peripheral analgesic agonist activity of morphine antagonists suggests the presence of a receptor different from those already postulated in the CNS (44,49) and in the periphery. At this peripheral analgesic receptor (N receptor), naloxone and nalorphine are agonists as potent as morphine, pentazocine, or Met-enkephalin, in contrast to their antagonist effect on central analgesic morphine (M) receptors. We have shown that enkephalins are analgesic at the N receptors and, because endorphins last longer in the circulation (32,48), one should expect them to be a more potent analgesic at the periphery. A possible physiological function of circulating endorphins is to maintain a lower peripheral pain threshold.

Our results would link PGE_2-induced hyperalgesia to an interference with release (or synthesis) of an endogenous opioid substance which regulates the threshold sensitivity at the various levels of the nociceptive system (Fig. 3). Perhaps the analgesic action of aspirin-like drugs is, through their inhibition

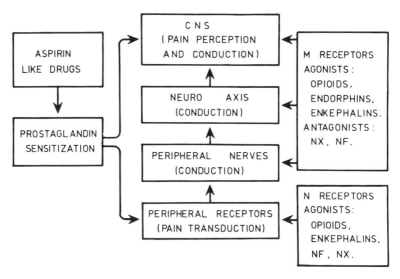

FIG. 3. General scheme of the nociceptive system. Prostaglandins are released at inflammatory sites. In some models of inflammation, a release of PG in the CNS may probably occur. This release enhances the local hyperalgesia induced by prostaglandins. The antialgesic effect of aspirin-like drugs is explained by an inhibition of prostaglandin synthesis which prevents the development of hyperalgesia. Opioids and endogenous opioid-like substance show a depressor effect at several levels of CNS. Naloxone (Nx) and Nalorphine (Nf) antagonize the analgesic effect of morphine at M receptors. Pentazocine, naloxone and nalorphine cause analgesia at peripheral site (N receptors). Morphine analgesia is due to its general depressor effect on the nociceptive system.

of PG synthesis, similarly related to a diminished release of an endogenous opioid substance at the periphery. A link between PGE_2 and the central analgesic effects of morphine has been proposed by Collier and Roy (6). However, in their system naloxone behaved as an antagonist to morphine.

Action on peripheral N receptors might also explain the analgesic effects of the systemically administered nalorphine described here and those observed previously in a similar test in rats (71) and on postsurgical pain in man (45). These analgesic effects were only transient and were replaced by a hyperalgesia probably of central origin, contrasting with the persistent analgesic seen when these drugs were injected locally. Preliminary experiments with intracerebroventricular injection of pentazocine, naloxone, and nalorphine supports our explanation of the situation. Naloxone and nalorphine produced hyperalgesia, while pentazocine had no effect when the intraplantar ID_{50} doses were given into the cerebral ventricles. Opioid antagonist hyperalgesia is probably a consequence of an antagonism at central M receptors by an endogenous opioid substance. Our results also suggest that a peripheral action may contribute to the analgesia shown by morphine given systemically; this contribution may be relatively large with low doses of morphine.

SUMMARY

Prostaglandins are inflammatory mediators, as evidenced by (a) they have been detected in several types of inflammation, (b) drugs which inhibit their *in vivo* synthesis diminish the intensity of inflammatory signs and symptoms, and (c) prostaglandins cause vasodilation, fever, and act synergistically with other mediators to cause inflammatory edema.

Prostaglandins E_1 and E_2 cause a long-lasting hyperalgesia in several animal models. PGI_2 causes an intense but short-lived hyperalgesia. Aspirin-like drugs, at therapeutic doses, block the *in vivo* synthesis of prostaglandins.

The term antialgesic, rather than analgesic, should be used to describe the effect of an aspirin-like drug. These agents do not directly block the hyperalgesic effect of prostaglandins or the direct action of nociceptive stimuli. By inhibiting cyclooxygenase, they prevent the development of hyperalgesia induced by PGE_2 previously released by inflammatory stimuli. If prostaglandin is released within the CNS, parallel to its release at the inflammatory site, it will enhance the local hyperalgesia. In such instance, a central effect of aspirin-like drugs, in addition to their local effect, would also be expected.

The direct peripheral hyperalgesic effect of prostaglandins is blocked by opioids and opioid antagonists. It was suggested that an endogenous opioid substance(s) (endorphins or enkephalins) regulated the threshold sensitivity at several levels of the nociceptive system. Prostaglandins may cause hyperalgesia by offsetting this mechanism. An important practical consequence of the peripheral analgesic action of the opioids and their antagonists is the possibility of developing a new class of morphine-like analgesics with selective peripheral action. Many of the presently used assays primarily measure analgesia at a central site, with selection based on pain relieving properties, as well as addiction liability. However, the ideal analgesic should have high activity in the peripheral assays and no effect in the central assays. Such a compound might be excluded from the CNS by virtue of its physicochemical properties. This analgesic would constitute a major therapeutic advance, lacking both the unwanted central effects of opioids and the peripheral side effects of aspirin-like drugs.

The interrelationship between prostaglandins, aspirin-like drugs and opioids provides a unifying hypothesis to interpret the mechanism of action of different types of pain killers.

REFERENCES

1. Arthurson, F., Hamberg, M., and Jonsson, C. E. (1973): Prostaglandins in human blister fluid. *Acta Physiol. Scand.,* 87:270–276.
2. Bergström, S., Duner, H., von Euler, U. S., Pernow, B., and Sjovall, J. (1959): Observations on the effects of infusions of prostaglandin E in man. *Acta Physiol. Scand.,* 45:145–151.
3. Bhattarcherjee, P., and Phylactos, A. (1977): Increased prostaglandin synthetase activity in inflamed tissues of the rabbit eye. *Eur. J. Pharmacol.,* 44:75–80.
4. Blackham, A., Farmer, J. B., Radziwonik, H., and Westwick, J. (1974): The role of prostaglandins in rabbit monoarticular arthritis. *Br. J. Pharmacol.,* 51:45–53.
5. Chang, W. C., Murota, A., Matsuo, M., and Tsurufuji, S. (1976): A new prostaglandin transformed from arachidonic acid in carrageenin-induced granuloma. *Biochem. Biophys. Res. Commun.,* 72:1259–1264.
6. Collier, H. O. J., and Roy, A. C. (1974): Hypothesis: Inhibition of prostaglandin E sensitive adenyl cyclase as the mechanism of morphine analgesia. *Prostaglandins,* 7:361–376.
7. Collier, H. O. J., and Schneider, C. (1972): Nociceptive response to prostaglandins and analgesic actions of aspirin and morphine. *Nature [New Biol.],* 236:141–143.
8. Collier, J. G., Karim, S. M. M., Robinson, B., and Somers, K. (1972): Action of prostaglandins A_2, B_1, and E_2 and $F_{2\alpha}$ on superficial hand veins of man. *Br. J. Pharmacol.,* 44:374P–375P.
9. Crutchley, D. J., Piper, P. J., and Seale, J. P. (1977): The nature of prostaglandin-like substances released from guinea-pig lungs in anaphylaxis. *Eur. J. Pharmacol.,* 44:319–323.
10. Dawson, W., Boot, J. R., Cockerill, A. F., Mallen, D. N. B., and Osborne, D. J. (1976): Release of novel prostaglandins and thromboxane after immunological challenge of guinea-pig lung. *Nature,* 262:699–702.
11. Dembinska-Kiec, A., Zmuda, A., and Krupinska, J. (1976): Inhibition of prostaglandin synthetase by aspirin-like drugs in different microsomal preparations. In: *Advances in Prostaglandin and Thromboxane Research, Vol. 1,* edited by B. Samuelsson and R. Paoletti, pp. 99–103. Raven Press, New York.
12. Eakins, K. E., Whitelock, R. I. F., Bennett, A., and Martenet, A. C. (1972): Prostaglandins in ocular inflammation. *Br. Med. J.,* 3:452–453.
13. Eakins, K. E., Whitelock, R. I. F., Perkins, E. S., Bennett, A., and Ungar, W. C. (1972): Release of prostaglandin E-like activity into the aqueous humour in experimental immunogenic uveitis. *Nature [New Biol.],* 239:248–249.
14. Ferreira, S. H. (1972): Prostaglandins, aspirin-like drugs and analgesia. *Nature [New Biol.],* 240:200–203.
15. Ferreira, S. H. (1976): Prostaglandins and immunological trauma. In: *The Role of Prostaglandins in Inflammation.* Edited by G. P. Lewis, pp. 75–87. Hans Huber Publishers, Vienna.
16. Ferreira, S. H., Lorenzetti, B. B., and Correa, F. M. A. (1977): Blockade of central and peripheral generation of prostaglandins explains the antialgic effect of aspirin-like drugs. *Pol. J. Pharmacol. Pharm.,* 30:133–140.
17. Ferreira, S. H., Lorenzetti, B. B., and Correa, F. M. A. (1978): Central and peripheral antialgesic action of aspirin-like drugs. *Eur. J. Pharmacol.* 53:39–48.

18. Ferreira, S. H., Moncada, S., and Vane, J. R. (1971): Indomethacin and aspirin abolish prostaglandin release from the spleen. *Nature* [*New Biol.*], 231:237–239.
19. Ferreira, S. H., Moncada, S., and Vane, J. R. (1973): Prostaglandins and the mechanism of analgesia produced by aspirin-like drugs. *Br. J. Pharmacol.,* 49:86–97.
20. Ferreira, S. H., and Nakamura, M. (1978): Peripheral analgesic activity of morphine, enkephalins and morphine-antagonists *(submitted)*.
21. Ferreira, S. H., Nakamura, M., and Castro, M. S. A. (1978): The hyperalgesic effects of prostacyclin and prostaglandin E_2. *Prostaglandins,* 16:31–37.
22. Ferreira, S. H., and Vane, J. R. (1974): Aspirin and prostaglandins. In: *The Prostaglandins, Vol. 2,* edited by P. W. Ramwell, pp. 1–39. Plenum Press, New York.
23. Ferreira, S. H., and Vane, J. R. (1978): Anti-inflammatory agents which are prostaglandin synthetase inhibitors. In: *Inflammation and Anti-inflammatory Drugs, Vol. II,* edited by J. R. Vane and S. H. Ferreira, pp. 348–398. Springer-Verlag, Berlin.
24. Ferreira, S. H., Zanin, M. T., and Lorenzetti, B. B. (1978): Relationships between increased vascular permeability, oedema, hyperalgesia and the effect of non-steroid anti-inflammatory drugs. In: *Perspectives in Inflammation,* edited by D. A. Willoughby, J. P. Giroud, and G. P. Velo, pp. 507–518. MTP Press, London.
25. Flower, R. J., and Blackwell, G. J. (1976): The importance of phospholipase A_2 in prostaglandin biosynthesis. *Biochem. Pharmacol.,* 25:285–291.
26. Flower, R. J., and Vane, J. R. (1972): Inhibition of prostaglandin synthetase in brain explains the anti-pyretic activity of paracetamol (4-acetamido-phenol). *Nature,* 240:410–411.
27. Glatt, M., Peskar, B., and Brune, K. (1974): Leukocytes and prostaglandins in acute inflammation. *Experientia,* 30:1257–1259.
28. Goldyne, M. E., Winkelmann, R. K., and Ryan, R. J. (1973): Prostaglandin activity in human cutaneous inflammation: Detection by radioimmunoassay. *Prostaglandins,* 4:737–748.
29. Greaves, M. W., and McDonald-Gibson, W. (1973): Itch: Role of prostaglandins. *Br. Med. J.,* 3:608–609.
30. Greaves, M. W., and Søndergaard, J. (1970): Pharmacological agents released in ultraviolet inflammation studied by continuous skin perfusion. *J. Invest. Dermatol.,* 54:365–367.
31. Greaves, M. W., Sødergaard, J., and McDonald-Gibson, W. (1971): Recovery of prostaglandins in human cutaneous inflammation. *Br. Med. J.,* 2:258–260.
32. Guillemin, R., Ling, N., Lazarus, L., Burgus, R., Minick, S., Bloom, F., Nicoll, R., Siggins, G., and Segal, D. (1977): The endorphins, novel peptides of brain and hypophysial origin, with opiate-like activity: biochemical and biologic studies. *Ann. NY Acad. Sci.,* 297:131–157.
33. Guzman, F., Braun, C., and Lim, R. K. S. (1962): Visceral pain and the pseudaffective response to intra-arterial injection of bradykinin and other algesic agents. *Arch. Int. Pharmacodyn. Ther.,* 136:353–384.
34. Guzman, F., Braun, C., Lim, R. K. S., Potter, G. D., and Rodgers, D. W. (1964): Narcotic and non-narcotic analgesics which block visceral pain evoked by intra-arterial injection of bradykinin and other algesic agents. *Arch. Int. Pharmacodyn. Ther.,* 149:571–588.
35. Hamberg, M., Svensson, J., Hedqvist, P., Strandberg, K., and Samuelsson, B. (1976): Involvement of endoperoxides and thromboxanes in anaphylactic reactions. In: *Advances in Prostaglandin and Thromboxane Research, Vol. 1,* edited by B. Samuelsson and R. Paoletti, pp. 495–501. Raven Press, New York.
36. Herman, A. C., and Moncada, S. (1975): Release of prostaglandins and incapacitation after injection of endotoxin in the knee joint of the dog. *Br. J. Pharmacol.,* 53:465P.
37. Higgs, G. A., Harvey, E. A., Ferreira, S. H., and Vane, J. R. (1976): The effects of anti-inflammatory drugs on the production of prostaglandins *in vivo*. In: *Advances in Prostaglandin and Thromboxane Research, Vol. 1,* edited by B. Samuelsson and R. Paoletti, pp. 105–110. Raven Press, New York.
38. Higgs, G. A., Vane, J. R., Hart, F. D., and Wojtulewski, J. A. (1974): Effects of anti-inflammatory drugs on prostaglandins in rheumatoid arthritis. In: *Prostaglandin Synthetase Inhibitors,* edited by H. J. Robinson and J. R. Vane, pp. 165–173. Raven Press, New York.
39. Jonsson, C. E. (1971): Smooth muscle stimulating lipids in peripheral lymph after experimental burn injury. *Scand. J. Plast. Reconstr. Surg.,* 5:1–5.
40. Jonsson, C. E., and Hamberg, M. (1972): Prostaglandin in burn injury. In: *Advances in Biosciences, Vol. 9,* edited by S. Bergström, pp. 441–445. Pergamon Press, London.
41. Juan, H., and Lembeck, F. (1974): Inhibition of action of E-prostaglandins (PGs) on paravascular pain receptors. *Naunyn Schmiedebergs Arch. Pharmacol.,* 284:R36.

42. Juan, H., and Lembeck, F. (1976): Release of prostaglandins from the isolated perfused rabbit ear by bradykinin and acetylcholine. *Agents Actions,* 6:642–645.
43. Karim, S. M. M. (1971): Action of prostaglandin in the pregnant woman. *Ann. NY Acad. Sci.,* 180:483–498.
44. Knoll, J., Furst, S., and Makleits, S. (1977): The pharmacology of N-substituted azido-morphines. *Arch. Int. Pharmacodyn Ther.,* 228:268–292.
45. Lasagna, L. (1968): The clinical pharmacology of analgesics and analgesic antagonists. In: *The Pharmacology of Pain, Vol. 9,* edited by R. K. S. Lim, pp. 113–120. Pergamon Press, New York.
46. Liebig, R., Bernauer, W., and Peskar, B. A. (1974): Release of prostaglandin metabolite, slow-reacting substances and histamine from anaphylactic lungs, and its modification by catecholamines. *Naunyn Schmiedebergs Arch. Pharmacol.,* 284:279–293.
47. Lim, R. K. S., Guzman, F., Rodgers, D. W., Goto, K., Braun, G., Dickerson, G. D., and Engle, R. J. (1964): Site of action of narcotic analgesics determined by blocking bradykinin-evoked visceral pain. *Arch. Int. Pharmacodyn. Ther.,* 152:25–59.
48. Loh, H. H., and Li, C. H. (1977): Biological activities of β-endorphin and its related peptides. *Ann. NY Acad. Sci.,* 297:115–130.
49. Martin, W. R. (1967): Opioid antagonists. *Pharmacol. Rev.,* 4:463–521.
50. Michaelsson, G. (1970): Effects of antihistamines, acetylsalicylic acid and prednisone on cutaneous reactions to kallikrein and prostaglandin E_1. *Acta. Derm. Venereol. (Stockh.),* 30:31–36.
51. Moncada, S., Ferreira, S. H., and Vane, J. R. (1973): Prostaglandins, aspirin-like drugs and the oedema of inflammation. *Nature,* 246:217–219.
52. Moncada, S., Ferreira, S. H., and Vane, J. R. (1975): Inhibition of prostaglandin biosynthesis as the mechanism of analgesia of aspirin-like drugs in the dog knee joint. *Eur. J. Pharmacol.,* 31:250–260.
53. Patrono, C., Bombardieri, S., Di Munno, O., Pasero, G. P., Greco, F., Grossi-Belloni, D., and Ciabattoni, G. (1976): Radioimmunoassay measurement of prostaglandin $F_{1\alpha}$ and $F_{2\alpha}$ in human synovial fluids and in superfusates of human synovial tissue. In: *The Role of Prostaglandins in Inflammation,* edited by G. P. Lewis, pp. 122–137. Hans Huber, Vienna.
54. Piper, P. J., and Vane, J. R. (1969): The release of prostaglandins during anaphylaxis in guinea-pig isolated lungs. In: *Prostaglandins, Peptides and Amines,* edited by P. Mantegazza and E. W. Horton, pp. 15–19. Academic Press, London.
55. Piper, P. J., and Vane, J. R. (1969): Release of additional factors in anaphylaxis and its antagonism by anti-inflammatory drugs. *Nature,* 223:20–35.
56. Piper, P. J., and Vane, J. R. (1971): The release of prostaglandin from lung and other tissue. *Ann. NY Acad. Sci.,* 180:363–385.
57. Piper, P. J., and Walker, J. L. (1973): The release of spasmogenic substances from human chopped lung tissue and its inhibition. *Br. J. Pharmacol.,* 47:291–304.
58. Randall, L. O., and Selitto, J. J. (1957): A method for measurement of analgesic activity on inflamed tissue. *Arch. Int. Pharmacodyn. Ther.,* 111:409–419.
59. Rosenthale, M. E., Dervinis, A., Kassarich, J., and Singer, S. (1972): Prostaglandins and anti-inflammatory drugs in the dog knee joint. *J. Pharm. Pharmacol.,* 24:149–150.
60. Smith, J. B., and Willis, A. L. (1971): Aspirin selectively inhibits prostaglandin production in human platelets. *Nature [New Biol.],* 231:235–237.
61. Solomon, L. M., Juhlin, L., and Kirschenbaum, M. B. (1968): Prostaglandin on cutaneous vasculature. *J. Invest. Derm.,* 51:280–282.
62. Swinson, D. R., Bennett, A., and Hamilton, E. B. D. (1976): Synovial prostaglandins in joint disease. In: *The Role of Prostaglandins in Inflammation,* edited by G. P. Lewis, pp. 41–46. Hans Huber, Vienna.
63. Vane, J. R. (1971): Inhibition of prostaglandin synthesis as a mechanism of action for aspirin-like drugs. *Nature [New Biol.],* 231:232–235.
64. Williams, T. J. (1977): Potentiation of bradykinin-induced exudation following intradermal injection of particulate or colloidal materials in the rabbit: evidence for prostaglandin release and action in inflammation. *Br. J. Pharmacol.,* 60:291P–292P.
65. Williams, T. J., and Morley, J. (1973): Prostaglandins as potentiators of increased vascular permeability in inflammation. *Nature,* 246:215–217.
66. Willis, A. L. (1969): Release of histamine, kinin and prostaglandin during carrageenin-induced inflammation in the rat. In: *Prostaglandins, Peptides and Amines,* edited by P. Montegazza and E. W. Horton, pp. 31–38. Academic Press, London.

67. Willis, A. L. (1969): Parallel assay of prostaglandin-like activity in rat inflammatory exudate by means of cascade superfusion. *J. Pharm. Pharmacol.,* 21:126–128.
68. Willis, A. L., and Cornelsen, M. (1973): Repeated injection of prostaglandin E_2 in rat paws induces chronic swelling and marked decrease in pain threshold. *Prostaglandins,* 3:353–357.
69. Willis, A. L., Davidson, P., Ramwell, P. W., Smith, J. B., and Brocklehurst, W. E. (1972): Release and actions of prostaglandins in inflammation and fever: inhibition by anti-inflammatory and antipyretic drugs. In: *Prostaglandins in Cellular Biology,* edited by P. W. Ramwell and B. B. Pharriss, pp. 227–259. Plenum Press, New York.
70. Willoughby, D. A., and Dieppe, P. (1976): Prostaglandins in the inflammatory response—pro or anti? In: *The Role of Prostaglandins in Inflammation,* edited by G. P. Lewis, pp. 14–25. Hans Huber, Vienna.
71. Winter, C. A., and Flataker, L. (1965): Reaction thresholds to pressure in edematous hindpaws of rats and responses to analgesic drugs. *J. Pharmacol. Exp. Ther.,* 150:165–171.

Mechanisms of Pain and Analgesic Compounds,
edited by R. F. Beers, Jr., and E. G. Bassett.
Raven Press, New York © 1979.

29. Discussion

Moderator: Sergio H. Ferreira

H. W. Kosterlitz: Dr. Ferreira, I was most interested in your observation of the peripheral effects of enkephalins. Did you try isomers, like levorphanol or dextrorphan, to see whether the particular effect you observed is specific, as if mediated by receptors? I would think that these effects are not stereospecific.

The second question is: What is the concentration of morphine and naloxone in the peripheral tissue in your experiments?

S. H. Ferreira: I can't answer the first question because we have yet to experiment with isomers. I believe it will be an important experiment.

In response to your question about concentration, it is difficult to express it precisely when a drug is administered locally. The ID_{50} for morphine was 5 µg, 42 µg for Met-enkephalin, 8 µg for nalorphine, about the same for naloxone, and 153 µg for Leu-enkephalin. We were impressed by these responses following local administration of microgram quantities.

I don't know of any other analgesic test that can measure an effect following local administration of 5 to 20 µg of a compound. Intraventricular injection of smaller doses of morphine may produce an analgesic effect; with pentazocine no effect is observed and with naloxone there is only hyperalgesia.

A. Gringauz: Dr. Ferreira, there seems to be a lot of controversy about acetaminophen (paracetamol) in the literature. Is it antiinflammatory or isn't it? And if it is, why has it escaped clinical realization during the last 60 or 70 years?

My second question deals with the concomitant and patent ulcerogenicity of aspirin and aspirin-like drugs in clinical use. Would it be possible to develop drugs which are inhibitors of prostaglandin synthesis, or prostaglandin antagonists, and that lack an ulcerogenic effect?

There seems to be evidence in the literature that prostaglandins are also involved in the ulcerogenic process; K. D. Rainsford (University of Tasmania) published recently on several compounds which he found to be nonulcerogenic, yet had an antiinflammatory effect.

S. H. Ferreira: I will ask R. Vinegar to respond to your first question.

R. Vinegar: Insofar as acetaminophen is concerned, it is antiinflammatory but it does not inhibit prostaglandin synthesis. At the International Congress[1] we are presenting a paper on its mechanism of action. I suggest that it inhibits the migration of inflammatory cells into the inflammatory site. It is not to be

---

[1] *Seventh International Congress of Pharmacology,* July 1978, Brussels, Belgium.

used in arthritis and similar diseases because it is too weak; for chronic inflammation in an arthritic, a dose of 15 to 20 g would be required. To treat an acute inflammation, it could still be used at dosages of 650 mg.

S. H. Ferreira: We administered paracetamol to rats, measured the prostaglandin content of carrageenin-containing sponges that had been subcutaneously implanted, and observed that prostaglandin levels were reduced. It is known that paracetamol is a very potent inhibitor of prostaglandin synthesis in brain tissue and it is possible the same mechanism is operative peripherally. This does not exclude that the other peculiar characteristics of this drug might also be responsible for its antiinflammatory activity.

With regard to the ulcerogenic properties of aspirin-like drugs, I just want to say that I don't understand why aspirin causes ulcers. This effect seems to be related to the inhibition of prostaglandin synthesis, or perhaps to the inhibition of other products of the cyclooxygenase pathway. If the second alternative is correct, it might be possible to find drugs that antagonize prostaglandin E_2 but lack ulcerogenic activity.

S. Kaymakcalan: Dr. Ferreira, how can you differentiate local anesthetics from analgesics by this method? More than 60 years ago a publication in France described some local anesthetic effects in guinea pigs following administration of morphine and some other opiates. I would appreciate your comments on this finding.

S. H. Ferreira: I can't differentiate a local anesthetic from an analgesic by this method. I believe the small doses that I am giving produce locally a concentration that is possibly reached in the circulation during therapy. As a result, we may have created a peripheral anesthetic effect. To obtain the same effect in our test, one would need 100 times more lidocaine—a local anesthetic—than morphine. Maybe it is a specific anesthetic effect on the sensory nerve endings. I am just describing an effect that I think may be of relevance.

R. Vinegar: I think that a word of caution is needed in considering that Sergio's experiments show a local effect of morphine. I have done many hyperalgesic experiments myself. I cannot get morphine or codeine to work locally, but lidocaine will. When his experimental details are published, the situation may be clarified; but, I think at this time it is a little dangerous to generalize on what Sergio says.

S. Kaymakcalan: I agree. What I am trying to do is provoke discussion. Your method of measuring hyperalgesia is completely different from mine. You mentioned a pressure of over one kg. Normally, what pressure do you use?

R. Vinegar: Two to 3 kg.

S. Kaymakcalan: I use 20 mm of mercury so I think we are measuring different things.

K. L. Casey: I am not familiar with the details of this testing method. How, in using this behavioral technique, can you determine that the action is central or peripheral? How is hyperalgesia validated? These points seem to be an issue here.

S. H. Ferreira: It is very simple. You compress the paw of the rat and the rat displays a behavioral response. If it is a normal paw, the latency of the response is 40 sec, while only 10 sec is required if the paw is made hyperalgesic by inflammation or by administration of prostaglandin. The rat, having two hind paws, enables us to make both of them hyperalgesic and treat only one of them with morphine. Giving morphine to the left paw, for example, did not affect the hyperalgesia of the other paw. However, when we gave it locally in the hyperalgesic paw, we did have an effect. Thus, we could completely exclude the central effect.

F. Sicuteri: I am wondering about the possibility of participation of the mast cell and serotonin. The release of the serotonin from the mast cell could be provoked by the injection of prostaglandin. Could morphine, in some way, be inhibiting the action of serotonin? This is only an idea. Have you used antiserotonin drugs?

S. H. Ferreira: Not in this experiment; but in other experiments, they did interfere with the hyperalgesic activity of prostaglandin. I believe this effect is not mediated by serotonin, but is a direct effect of prostaglandin that has been observed in animals treated with aspirin-like drugs.

J. H. Hu: Dr. Chahl, do you think it is useful to test pain-inducing compounds, such as acetylcholine and histamine, so as to differentiate between the afterdischarge of the nociceptor and the sensitization? Do you think it is useful to separate the two effects for different kinds of substance?

L. A. Chahl: Perl's group has looked at sensitization in polymodal receptors quite recently. They have tested a number of compounds to see whether they will mimic heat-induced sensitization of polymodal nociceptors. They feel that they have excluded the substances I talked about as being mediators of sensitization.

Whether they distinguished between sensitization and afterdischarge, I am not sure. Maybe someone else might speak to this point.

J. H. Hu: After sensitization with noxious heat, some nociceptors will afterdischarge and others will not. I am suggesting that it might be useful to differentiate these factors for different mediators.

L. A. Chahl: I think that most workers use the one term, sensitization, for both an increased response to a stimulus and afterdischarge. But I agree— these are two things that might be different.

J. H. Hu: In the painful sensation, these are quite different. If afterdischarge is there, you continue to feel it. If there is no afterdischarge, the subject has no sensation unless the receptor fields are being tested, even though thresholds are lowered and very sensitive to noxious stimuli. Afterdischarge has quite profound effects on the secondary or more central neural mechanisms as well as on the pain sensation.

L. A. Chahl: I agree that they are probably two different things. I don't know that it is really known whether any of the substances differentially alter threshold and afterdischarge. I am not aware of any information on this.

J. H. Hu: I feel that this point should be thoroughly examined.

L. A. Chahl: Yes, I would agree.

H. O. J. Collier: Several authors have described an antiinflammatory action of morphine. I think it was nonspecific. Have you taken this into account in estimating peripheral analgesic action in experiments using your inflammatory pain model?

S. H. Ferreira: I must point out that, to avoid any inflammatory response due to injection trauma, all animals were treated with indomethacin. Second, I am not using carrageenin but prostaglandin E_2, which causes hyperalgesia with a very mild edema. So I don't believe that an inflammatory effect could be the cause of the observed analgesia.

L. A. Chahl: How do you measure edema?

S. H. Ferreira: By immersing the paw into a unit that measures volumetric displacements.

F. W. L. Kerr: I recall Dr. Olgart saying that sensation from tooth pulp is either discomfort or pain. I think that it is probably incorrect, but I am not an expert on teeth. I believe temperature sensation on the teeth is a very important part of sensation if you don't get the threshold above. Of course, if you increase the temperature enough, it becomes painful. One can feel warmth or cold on your teeth without any pain; these, then, are non-painful sensations.

L. Olgart: Different opinions are expressed as to whether a painful sensation is the only experience when teeth are stimulated. There are two aspects of stimulation that I would like to comment on. First, there is no question that when human teeth are electrically stimulated, a nonpainful sensation is experienced, provided the stimulus intensity is close to or below the pain threshold. Such a stimulus may be regarded as an unnatural one, and results in a prepain sensation. On the other hand, when teeth are exposed to daily life situations—such as eating ice cream or drinking hot coffee—thermoreceptors in the lips and gingiva are also activated and provide additional information about the type of stimulus, making it possible to differentiate between heat and cold.

H. O. J. Collier: This is true if ice cream is taken into the mouth. However, if by using forceps, the ice cream is applied only to the tooth—or a hot metallic rod is applied to the tooth enamel—one gets a cold or warm sensation.

L. Olgart: Such a statement can be explained by associative learning from previous exposures to hot and cold stimuli. This is possible because the two types of thermal stimuli give different pain qualities. For example, the pain response of an isolated tooth to cold is rapid and sharp, whereas that produced by heat is slow in onset and dull in nature. Both stimuli activate the nerve endings by displacement of the tubular contents of dentin, which is dependent on the temperature gradient across the dentin rather than on effects of temperature directly on the nerve endings. Cold is more efficient than heat in this respect, as are airblasts. The different pain experiences elicited by heat and cold, together with prior experiences, helps one to decide which stimulus was used and the verbal response would be either hot discomfort or cold discomfort. No conclusive evidence that applies directly to the comments by Drs. Kerr and Collier is available.

A recent finding by B. Matthews (University of Bristol) relates to nerve fibers in the pulp that respond exclusively to heat stimulation of the tooth surface. This may explain the different pain sensations of heat and cold.

F. W. L. Kerr: Dr. Sicuteri, there are obviously important ways to objectively demonstrate that, during the venomotor response observed in the periphery, there are changes that can be measured without any subjective inputs by the patient.

Without any doubt, migraine and these severe headaches are distressful. Aren't you really measuring a result of stress over a period of time, whereby there is some sort of sensitization? Unquestionably, release can be obtained from many substances if the patient is under a stressful situation. Are you measuring a response rather than a primary effect? Did I make myself clear?

F. Sicuteri: Theoretically, it is possible for adrenalin released during pain to sensitize vessels to spasmogenic substances, such as noradrenaline and 5-HT. Others have reported, however, that during migraine attacks catecholamines do not increase but rather decrease. This intermittent supersensitivity to 5-HT and noradrenaline has been found to be 1,000-fold in some patients suffering from "central panalgesia," that is, systemic pains that are central in nature. Since this supersensitivity can persist after an interval of several months, it is difficult to attribute it to adrenaline sensitization.

B. Scoville: Dr. Sicuteri, are there therapeutic implications from your findings, for example, of the young woman with a headache who seemed to be so sensitive to small amounts of 5-HT? Are there drugs, such as serotonin-depleting agents, that might be useful?

F. Sicuteri: It is apparently incongruous to consider a deficiency of serotonin when the most active drugs used for treating migraine headache are antiserotonin drugs. However, in only large doses do the antiserotonin drugs act as antagonists in animals; when tested in small doses, as we have demonstrated in man and Drs. Schonbaum and Fozard in animals, antiserotonin drugs potentiate 5-HT activity. In the recent paper of Haigler and Aghajanan (*Nature,* 1977), such drugs in high doses are claimed to be antagonists of peripheral receptors in animals; the same substances, for example, ergotamine and methysergide, act as agonists on 5-HT receptors in the brain. Since 5-HT is a neurotransmitter, the antimigraine effect of ergotamine and methysergide could be attributed to the capacity of 5-HT receptors of the antinociceptive system.

F. W. L. Kerr: I have a question for the panel as a whole. For 40 or more years investigators have been looking for substances that would mediate pain. During this search, various substances such as bradykinin, histamine, and potassium and hydrogen ions and so forth have been considered as mediators. Is it not possible that in any normal pain situation caused by, for example, mechanical crushing or heating, there is a mixture of compounds of which any one would act as a sensitizing agent or potentiator for other compounds? In other words, have past investigations overemphasized the role of a single substance?

S. H. Ferreira: I believe that each kind of trauma releases a special set of mediators. For example, compound 40/80 or dextran introduced into the rat will release a group of mediators; carrageenin will release another group of mediators. Either group may play an important role because, if antihistaminics are given, you effectively block the effect of the dextran and if prostaglandins are administered, you block the effect of carrageenin. This indicates the importance of histamine in dextran-induced inflammation and of prostaglandin in carrageenin-induced inflammation.

It is important to understand that different traumas will cause the predominant release of one kind of mediator. On traumatizing with ultraviolet light, an erythema quite sensitive to aspirin is formed, perhaps involving prostaglandins as mediators. Later on, depending on the intensity of the ultraviolet trauma, you can get an erythema that is resistant to aspirin-like drugs. This happens because other mediators overcome the prostaglandins. The release of different sets of mediators depends on the intensity, locale, and type of the trauma.

L. A. Chahl: I tend to agree with what you say. The interactions between the mediators are extremely complex and until recently received little prominence. The original attempts were to show that they produced nociception on their own; even if they don't produce nociception by themselves, when they are combined with one or more other mediators, there might be a tremendous and complicated potentiation of their actions. Other workers and myself have studied the interactions between mediators. Now that substance P appears to be a candidate for the mediator of antidromic vasodilation, perhaps we might have to consider a possibility that the nerve terminal release of a substance or substances might also affect the inflammatory response.

I have found that substance P potentiated 5-HT, bradykinin, prostaglandin E_1, and adenosine triphosphate. I don't think anyone has mentioned ATP today, but it has been implicated in antidromic dilatation by Holton who found that it was released from sensory nerves.

Whether it plays a role in antidromic edema, we don't know. Interestingly, substance P itself was potentiated by prostaglandin E_1 and ATP.

Our potentiation studies utilized a wide range of dosages. Substance P in low dose did not produce edema but, when combined with 5-HT or bradykinin or PGE_1 or ATP, produced a great potentiation of the edema. A high dose of substance P, however, was edematogenic by itself. On the other hand, bradykinin had completely different interactions and was tested because I wanted to know if it was a peptide type of phenomenon: that the same substances potentiated all peptides. I was impressed with the complexity of the different activities shown by substances that might participate in the inflammatory response.

F. Sicuteri: Dr. Chahl, we saw in your slide that the viscera do not have the most receptive nociceptors. However, ischemic pain can be evoked by trauma and probably involves pain-producing substances. On the other hand, if we inject bradykinin into the humeral artery—this is an experiment I did myself—during local circulatory arrest and ischemia, intense pain will arise. This may have importance in ischemic pain evocation and weakness in angina pectoris.

On another matter, I have a suggestion for testing animal responses: the squeaking flight reaction due to intracisternal injection of bradykinin, as I have described many years ago. This test has a stronger correlation with the clinical situation; that is, the release of kinin into the intracranial and cerebral spinal fluid. When cerebral spinal fluid is contaminated with plasma, we have dilution and the release of kinin by this dilution. This is the pathogenic mechanism by which pain is produced in subarachnoid hemorrhage. The squeaking flight test is quite reproducible.

L. A. Chahl: The difference, I think, between the visceral nociceptors and the cutaneous ones is that there is, in the skin, a very well-defined set of fibers which respond to only high threshold stimuli, whereas the presence of such fibers in the viscera is not known.

There must be visceral nociceptors because this type of pain is such a common occurrence. But it is not yet known whether they are the same fibers which are normally involved in reflex control of the tissue and which respond to a greater than normal stimulus, producing pain.

I think no one would doubt the existence of visceral chemical nociceptors; however, evidence for a specific, high-threshold type of receptor is lacking.

A. Goldstein: Dr. Sicuteri, I did not hear and have not read in your published work if migraine headaches are made worse by naloxone. Have you used naloxone in this regard?

F. Sicuteri: I have tested the naloxone during migraine attacks but I have not seen important modifications. A very nice effect was observed in only two cases of migraine with visual hallucination, that is, visual scotomata, treated with two doses of 0.8 mg naloxone. The scintillation before the attack persists for about 20 to 30 min. After naloxone introduction, the scintillation period was reduced to 2 to 4 min; the placebo was ineffective. This can be related to the possibility that hallucination occurs with activation of opiate sigma receptors, according to the suggestion of Martin. No convincing effects of naloxone were observed in other symptoms; it was effective only on visual scotomata.

A. Goldstein: I want to ask Dr. Ferreira about this peripheral local anesthetic effect of morphine or whatever it is. What other compounds have you tried in the opiate series? For example, does codeine or levorphanol produce the same effect?

S. H. Ferreira: We have not tested other compounds yet.

A. Goldstein: I would like to comment on a topic Dr. Kosterlitz mentioned earlier. I would normally be the first person to ask about stereospecificity because, in our opiate receptor program, if a substance or an effect is not stereospecific, we are not really interested in it. But I think we have to begin to recognize that there are activities of these compounds that are not stereospecific and yet they are real pharmacological effects.

The first of the latter sort was a peculiar kind of behavioral activity in a rat which was produced by morphine and related compounds. It was not stereo-specific, as it turned out, and it was not blocked by naloxone. But levorphanol, which lacks the phenolic hydroxyl group and several other features of the morphine molecule, had no effect. There is certainly a receptor that mediates those effects, but it is not the receptor we are used to working with.

Now, we see that Spector's compound (MLC), a morphine-like substance of unknown composition, characteristically is not blocked by naloxone. Thus, there are receptors that have to be defined by a structure-activity relationship and they turn out to be different in some way.

I asked specifically about codeine and levorphanol because if one looks at the model of morphine, some of its stereospecificity involves the relative positioning of two groups, that is, the phenolic hydroxyl group and the basic nitrogen. If there is not a phenolic hydroxyl group as, for example, some of the benzomorphans, then it is quite conceivable that the two stereoisomers would fit into a receptor that is relatively similar, but not identical, to the receptors we work with.

J. E. Villarreal: There is a large body of literature, most of it old, dealing with peripheral actions of substances chemically related to morphine, and not regarded as opioids, that have some very interesting pharmacology. For instance, a cross-tolerance between thebaine and morphine when tested on vascular smooth muscles. Much of the early work has a wealth of pharmacological information that we should review in the light of our current investigations with endogenous or exogenous substances having opioid-like (in the classical sense) activities or with other behavioral effects.

This is a symposium on pain and much of the emphasis has been on analgesic actions or the actions of opiate substances on neurotransmission of pain. For me, the most important pharmacological effect is something totally different, because I work with the effects of narcotics as related to chronic administration— we will be talking about that tomorrow. I will offer the general comment that a lot of the data appearing in the recent literature is perhaps a reflection of not being well-read in that which we have accumulated over the past 50 or 60 years.

H. W. Kosterlitz: Since Avram Goldstein raised the question about the importance of the stereospecificity, I would like to add that we have known for a long time that all the narcotic analgesics have effects other than the one we expect and those effects are usually not blocked by naloxone. It is very characteristic of most of these effects that naloxone acts as a agonist—in the same way as morphine does. Even in a simple model like the guinea pig ileum, if one has a sufficiently high concentration of naloxone, the same effects are observed. It is not surprising that in dealing with a complicated molecule like morphine, interaction of receptors is to be expected.

The point I tried to make earlier was whether the effect you observed was an effect on the classic opiate receptor. I think this is very important because we wish to know if the effects of plasmosin—which A. Goldstein mentioned— are similar to those effects observed in experiments with endorphin opiate peptides.

After all, the plant alkaloids are not made for the mammalian body; they are used by deviates for other purposes. The peptides will be very different. I think we must not start to confuse the issue.

S. H. Ferreira: I am of the opinion that an experiment is one thing; the interpretation of the experiment is quite another thing.

Having worked with our testing system for about 5 years, I can speak from experience. I found a very interesting effect that I have never observed with other drugs, such as aspirin-like drugs. So I decided to stimulate this kind of discussion. For example, what is the explanation for the analgesic action of nalorphine? If nalorphine is introduced into the brain, you have hyperalgesia but not analgesia. Given peripherally, one observes algesia. It is difficult to understand. It may well be that the problem is that we have to think along other lines, not central receptor sites, to explain nalorphine analgesia.

A. Goldstein: The point I wanted to make as a reply to Hans Kosterlitz is very similar to the point that Julian Villarreal was making. Ultimately, we need to know if these peripheral receptors conform to the concept of the classical opioid receptor we have been discussing these two days. I am certain there are other receptors that, in their own way, will exhibit stereospecificity too, and one might predict that other receptors will also have endogenous ligands— perhaps peptides—which will conform to that particular specificity. Historically it happens that we have chosen to look into, and to move farthest with, a particular subclass of receptors that respond to opiates, which have those properties that we have described as classical opioid properties.

I think that there are perhaps many other receptors and, therefore, many other ligands that in some way or other resemble opiates but have detectable differences. I am sure we don't disagree with that.

L. S. Harris: Since it has been raised twice now, I would like to tell Dr. Ferreira something I found rather strange. Morphine, like almost every organic base, has some local anesthetic properties. But, as shown many years ago, morphine is a very weak local anesthetic.

Certainly, the doses that you were introducing directly into the limb would have no local anesthetic effect—as we classically describe local anesthesia. In addition to that, the data very clearly show that compounds many hundred times more potent than morphine as a local anesthetic were less effective than morphine in blocking this particular response.

L. A. Chahl: It would seem to me that the problem of naloxone is that it is behaving as a partial agonist. If one increased the dose, then the blocking action might be observed. Would this be likely?

S. H. Ferreira: No. You can increase the dose several times and still have an analgesic effect. Furthermore, given long before morphine, a partial agonist will usually be an antagonist to morphine in most tests. However, introducing naloxone 2 hr before morphine, I did not observe such a reversal; on the contrary, it added effects.

F. Sicuteri: I am perplexed about your paper describing this activity. Is it a prostaglandin effect or is it generally a peripheral anesthetic? Does it show any effect in other pain tests?

S. H. Ferreira: The main point about the test is that you need a contralateral paw to ensure that you don't have a central effect. In most of the tests, you don't find such a design. I believe it is an effect against the hyperalgesia induced by prostaglandins.

F. W. L. Kerr: I am going to make a pharmacological comment from a nonpharmacologist. I will probably be shot down in flames very fast.

It seems to me that pharmacologists are enamored of the idea of receptors everywhere. I have no belief at all in receptors in the peripheral nerve. Yet, you are getting marked effects on peripheral nerves, and you are talking about receptors where there are no synaptic contacts.

I would like to suggest that instead of getting an effect on the receptor, you are getting some kind of interference with sodium channels. It is a nonspecific effect and it is specific only to the extent that you are interfering with the channel and nothing else. This in turn would take you into central nonspecific effects of drugs that have nothing to do with receptors. Maybe that is an uninformed comment but I would like to offer it.

S. H. Ferreira: I would agree with you. Maybe I should just say that it has a peripheral site action. I am trying to emphasize the fact of whether a receptor is involved is, for me, almost irrelevant at this stage. I think there is an effect, a peripheral effect, at a site where prostaglandins are able to cause hyperalgesia, which is counteracted by morphine, nalorphine, pentazocine, etc.

F. W. L. Kerr: As a pharmacologist, you say it really doesn't make much difference whether we talk about receptor or a site. At least to me, the definition of receptor includes very specific characteristics and many of them are stereospecific characteristics which have to be answered. So, this is why we have to keep the terminology very clear, at least for us who are not pharmacologists but try to understand what is going on.

S. H. Ferreira: So we have to investigate stereospecificity. Give us time.

L. A. Chahl: Dr. Kerr, one should hesitate to state that there are no receptors unless there are synaptic contacts. There is one very good example, and that is the peripheral terminal of the adrenergic nerves: norepinephrine itself can act presynaptically with specific receptors on the nerve terminals. There are also specific acetylcholine receptors, and perhaps specific prostaglandin receptors on the terminals of adrenergic nerves.

I think that it is not necessary for there to be neuron to neuron contacts for pharmacological receptors to be present.

F. W. L. Kerr: Dr. Halstead, right here at Hopkins at the beginning of the century, pointed out one didn't have to inject cocaine into the skin. An injection of saline would suffice to produce a pretty good analgesic effect and the skin could be cut. That, again, is a disruptive effect, totally nonspecific, not related to any receptor.

S. H. Ferreira: But we had a control with saline, isn't that correct?

J. E. Villarreal: I hope this is the last word on this very interesting pharmacology session. The vascular effects of thebaine and morphine seem to be specific in that cross-tolerance between phenane and morphine and nalorphine has been observed.

In 1928 when nalorphine was not yet available, Schmidt and Livingston, and some papers by Jane Haggard, mentioned a specificity different from the specificity we have been concentrating on. But, nevertheless, there is something that is not just like the action of ethanol or something on sodium channels.

Mechanisms of Pain and Analgesic Compounds,
edited by R. F. Beers, Jr., and E. G. Bassett.
Raven Press, New York © 1979.

30. Introduction to Section E: Mechanisms of Opioid Analgesia and Dependence

H. O. J. Collier

Miles Laboratories, Ltd., Stoke Poges, Slough SL2 4LY, England

In this section, we try to probe into the molecular mechanisms by which opioid substances act. Not only does morphine produce analgesia and dependence, as the title of the section indicates, but it has so many and so paradoxical an assemblage of other pharmacological actions that few, if any of us, could list from memory all that have been described. Enough actions were known, however, more than a century ago, for Claude Bernard to describe them as a mixture or a succession of the depressant and the stimulant. The same description would apply to the actions of the many opioids, both exogenous and endogenous, that have since been discovered.

Many of the actions of opioids are not well understood and will provide work for future generations of pharmacologists; but we can reduce the number of opioid actions to consider by excluding those that are not the result of interaction between an opioid drug and a neuronal receptor that can be blocked by naloxone.

The use of naloxone to define the type of opioid-receptor interaction, now called specific, with which we are concerned is based on two findings from Kosterlitz's laboratory: First, naloxone is a "pure" competitive antagonist of the inhibition by morphine of the neurally evoked contraction of the longitudinal muscle of the guinea pig ileum (4). In other words, naloxone is without appreciable morphine-like agonist activity. Second, the potency of opioids in this test on the ileum correlates excellently with their potencies as inhibitors of pain sensation and as ligands of the opioid receptor in brain homogenates (3).

Figure 1 illustrates the use of naloxone to exclude an action of morphine as nonspecific. It shows the increased production of prostaglandins (PG) by a homogenate of bull seminal vesicles that results from adding morphine, or naloxone, or both, to the incubate. This nonspecific action is probably due to both compounds being phenols, since other phenols also stimulate PG synthetase, whereas codeine, in which the phenolic hydroxyl group is modified, does not (1,2).

These considerations enable us to define an "opioid" as any substance, whether derived from opium, or of synthetic origin, or produced within the body, having morphine-like actions that are potently and competitively blocked by naloxone.

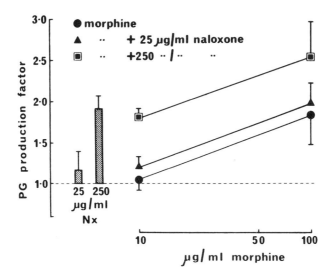

FIG. 1. Effect of morphine, naloxone, and their mixture on PG production by bull seminal vesicle homogenate. The PG production factor is the ratio of total PG-like activity in test incubate to that in reference incubate (basal), assayed on rat stomach strip. The incubates contained added substrate (61 μM arachidonic acid), but no added cofactors. Nx, naloxone. (Refs. 1,2.)

Since naloxone blocks these morphine-like actions, we may assume that they are mediated by interaction of drug molecule with opioid receptor on the neuron. We can then define an "opioid-sensitive neuron" as one possessing opioid receptors blocked by naloxone.

We are concerned with the molecular mechanisms by which opioids affect the behavior of opioid-sensitive neurons after interacting with the specific opioid receptor; in short, we are concerned with "postreceptor reactions." These include not only the acute specific actions of opioids, but also the induction of tolerance and dependence, which naloxone also antagonizes, although we do not know if the antagonism is competitive.

In this section, we have four chapters, covering four different experimental approaches to the analysis of the acute and subacute specific actions of opioids; all of these approaches have yielded useful insights. In Chapter 31, I discuss direct and indirect studies of the reactions to opioids of the cyclic AMP system in the brains of whole animals and in preparations of brain and myenteric plexus *in vitro*. In Chapter 32, Werner Klee discusses reactions to opioids of adenylate cyclase in a model of the opioid-sensitive neuron—the neuroblastoma x glioma hybrid cell, strain 108–15 (NG 108–15 cells). Then, in Chapter 33, Dr. Alan North discusses the effects of opioids on nerve impulse production by single neurons *in situ*. Finally, in Chapter 34, Albert Herz et al. consider changes in sensitivity of the opioid-sensitive neuron that arise in response to the subacute action of opioids.

REFERENCES

1. Collier, H. O. J., Francis, D. L., McDonald-Gibson, W. J., Roy, A. C., and Saeed, S. A. (1975): Prostaglandins, cyclic AMP and the mechanism of opiate dependence. *Life Sci.,* 17:85–90.
2. Collier, H. O. J., McDonald-Gibson, W. J., and Saeed, S. A. (1976): Stimulation of prostaglandin biosynthesis by drugs: Effects *in vitro* of some drugs affecting gut function. *Br. J. Pharmacol.,* 58:193–199.
3. Kosterlitz, H. W., and Waterfield, A. A. (1975): In vitro models in the study of structure-activity relationships of narcotic analgesics. *Annu. Rev. Pharmacol.,* 15:29–47.
4. Kosterlitz, H. W., and Watt, A. J. (1968): Kinetic parameters of narcotic agonists and antagonists, with particular reference to *N*-allylnoroxymorphone (naloxone). *Br. J. Pharmacol.,* 33:266–276.

Mechanisms of Pain and Analgesic Compounds,
edited by R. F. Beers, Jr., and E. G. Bassett.
Raven Press, New York © 1979.

31. Consequences of Interaction Between Opioid Molecule and Specific Receptor

H. O. J. Collier

Miles Laboratories, Ltd., Stoke Poges, Slough SL2 4LY, England

INTRODUCTION

When an opioid molecule binds with its specific receptor, events happen at two rates, one measurable in seconds or minutes and one in hours or days. The faster are the acute, immediate, or primary actions; the slower are the subacute, delayed, or reactive, expressed as tolerance and dependence. The acute actions that concern us are those that occur within the opioid-sensitive neuron itself. But do the subacute actions also occur within one neuron? There is evidence of four kinds that they do.

First, tolerance and dependence can be induced in the neuroblastoma x glioma hybrid cell by simply exposing it for more than 12 hr to morphine (75,83; W. A. Klee, *this volume*). Second, individual postganglionic neurons of the isolated guinea pig ileum can develop tolerance and dependence through exposure to morphine or normorphine for 18 to 24 hr *in vitro* (32,60,86; R. A. North, *this volume*). Third, single cortical neurons of the rat, studied *in situ* by means of micropipettes and microelectrodes, can exhibit tolerance and dependence (68). Fourth, in dependent rats, heroin inhibits all withdrawal signs, whereas inhibitors of the synthesis or action of humoral messengers decrease some signs but increase others (14).

These findings show that tolerance and dependence can be induced within the opioid-sensitive neuron. This means that changes in enzymes, hormones, transmitters, or neural pathways outside the opioid-sensitive cell can be regarded as secondary in the mechanism of cellular tolerance/dependence toward opioids, even though such outside influences may affect the cellular induction process. That opioid tolerance and dependence occur within the opioid-sensitive neuron also means that they are part of the postreceptor reaction. I have referred to tolerance and dependence in the plural, but, since they seem to arise within the cell as expressions of one process, we can sometimes refer to opioid tolerance/ dependence as a single entity, with two observable aspects.

Three main acute, specific, inhibitory effects of opioids on opioid-sensitive neurons have been observed. First, opioids inhibit cyclic adenosine monophosphate (cyclic AMP) formation (15,16,77,82); second, they inhibit transmitter release (54,62,69); third, they inhibit the production of nerve impulses, either spontaneously or in response to excitatory messenger substances (3,4,20,68,93).

As a result of the subacute action of opioids, the neuron loses its ability to respond in these three ways. Thus it develops a changed and greater capacity to form cyclic AMP (9,36,55,75,76,83), it becomes less responsive to opioids or other inhibitors (29,32,60,68), and it reacts excessively to excitatory messengers (68,72,73) and to naloxone (32,60,68,86).

In this chapter I want to discuss the reactions to opioids of the cyclic AMP system in normal neurons, which I plan to discuss under four main heads: first, the inhibition by opioids of adenylate cyclase; second, the antagonism between opioids and substances believed to act by stimulating adenylate cyclase, particularly E prostaglandins (PGEs); third, the interactions between opioids and inhibitors of phosphodiesterase, particularly methylxanthines; and finally, I want to integrate these first three aspects by making a model of opioid action in the neuron.

INHIBITION OF CYCLIC AMP FORMATION

In 1974, we reported that morphine and other opioids inhibit PGE-stimulated cyclic AMP formation in rat brain homogenate, probably by inhibiting an adenylate cyclase (15,16). The opioids did not inhibit basal cyclic AMP formation, nor that stimulated by sodium fluoride. The effect was specific and stereospecific. In a group of opioids, potency in inhibiting PGE-stimulated cyclic AMP formation correlated with analgestic potency and affinity for the opioid receptor (16,64). The enkephalins and β-endorphin (C-fragment) also inhibited PGE_1-stimulated cyclic AMP formation, as shown in Fig. 1.

The experiments in Fig. 1 are unfinished, but they provide a mean dose-response line for morphine of slope 48.1 ($p < 0.001$) giving an IC_{50} value for morphine of 4.98 μM (limits 3.86 to 6.77). It is noteworthy that the opioid peptides to some extent inhibit basal cyclic AMP formation also, although with less potency and a dose-response line of lower slope than PGE-stimulated formation.

Several workers have been unable to repeat our experiments (70,81,85), although Laduron (13,51) has done so. This difficulty arises largely because prostaglandins (PGs) cannot easily be induced to stimulate adenylate cyclase in brain homogenates. We are now exploring better ways to do such experiments. In the meantime, however, Havemann and Kuschinsky (34) have shown, in certain conditions, that morphine and Met-enkephalin specifically inhibit the formation of cyclic AMP stimulated by PGE_2 in rat brain striatal slices *in vitro*. These investigators, however, have not been able to show the same effect in striatal homogenate. Figure 2 summarizes their findings in striatal slices.

Several investigators have shown that, in micromolar concentrations, opioids specifically inhibit the stimulation with catecholamines of cyclic AMP formation

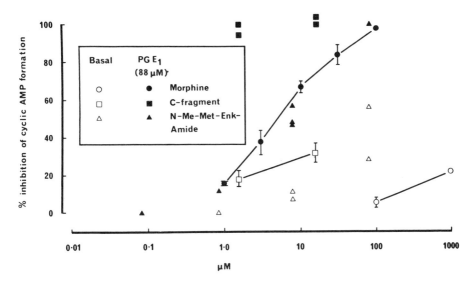

FIG. 1. Inhibition by morphine and opioid peptides of basal and PGE$_1$-stimulated cyclic AMP formation in rat brain homogenate. ^{3}H-cyclic AMP formation from ^{3}H-ATP was measured in the presence or absence of PGE$_1$ (88 μM) in various concentrations of test drug, using the method of Collier and Roy (15), modified by replacement of EDTA and 2-mercaptoethanol with 0.1 mM EGTA and 0.1 mM dithiothreitol, and by use of a total concentration of 106.25 μM ATP in the reaction mixture.

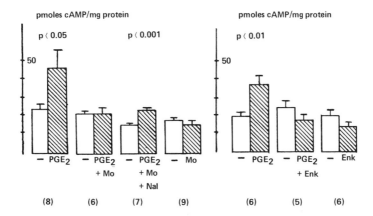

FIG. 2. Effects of opiates on the elevation of cyclic AMP (cAMP) (pmoles/mg protein, mean values ± SEM) induced by 10 μM PGE$_2$ in slices of rat striata, which were incubated for 5 min in the absence or presence of PGE$_2$, or opioid, or both. The striatum of one side of the brain was used as control *(white columns)* and the contralateral striatum was incubated with test drug *(hatched columns)*. Numbers of experiments in parentheses. Concentrations: Morphine (Mo), 2 μM; naloxone (Nal), 2 μM; Met-enkephalin (Enk) in the presence of 0.2 mM bacitracin, 100 μM. (From Havemann and Kuschinsky, ref. 34.)

in preparations of various brain regions *in vitro.* Thus morphine (56) and β-endorphin (58) inhibit stimulation with dopamine of cyclic AMP formation in slices and homogenates, respectively, of rat striatum. Again, morphine and Met-enkephalin inhibit stimulation with norepinephrine of cyclic AMP formation in homogenates of rat cortex and hypothalamus (84). Yet again, morphine inhibits stimulation with dopamine in homogenates of primate brain amygdaloid nucleus (91). In some of these and other experiments, basal cyclic AMP formation was also, but less strongly, inhibited (57,58,91).

Although catecholamines stimulate cyclic AMP formation in these preparations, and opioids specifically block this stimulation, it must be remembered that, in neuroblastoma x glioma hybrid cells, strain 108–15 (NG 108–15 cells) in culture, catecholamines, like morphine, inhibit adenylate cyclase (W. A. Klee, *this volume*) and, in the isolated guinea pig ileum, catecholamines, again like morphine, inhibit the neurally evoked contraction of the longitudinal muscle (50).

In dependent brain, after withdrawal, increased cyclic AMP formation has been observed (7,12,36,55). Moreover, cyclic AMP, injected into a lateral cerebral ventricle of the morphine-dependent rat, just before naloxone challenge, intensifies withdrawal effects (9), as shown in Fig. 3.

Inhibition by opioids of adenylate cyclase has also been demonstrated and explored in NG 108–15 cells in culture (77,82), as discussed by Klee *(this volume).*

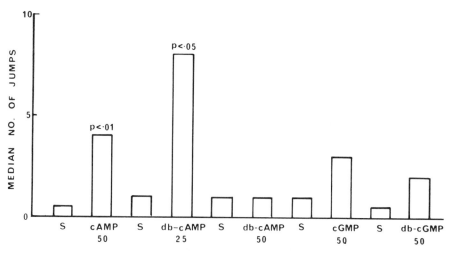

FIG. 3. Effect on morphine withdrawal jumping of injection of cyclic AMP (cAMP), dibutyryl cyclic AMP (db-cAMP), cyclic guanosine monophosphate (cGMP), or dibutyryl cyclic GMP (db-cGMP) into a lateral cerebral ventricle of dependent rats, 1 hr before challenge with naloxone. Rats were made dependent by a single subcutaneous injection of a sustained-release preparation of morphine (14) 24 hr before withdrawal was precipitated with naloxone, I mg/kg subcutaneously. S, saline. (Ref. 9.)

ANTAGONISM BETWEEN OPIOIDS AND PGEs

I have already mentioned evidence that PGEs can stimulate brain adenylate cyclase (15,34). There is some evidence that 5-hydroxytryptamine (5-HT) does so also, at least in newborn rats (87). I would now like to outline the evidence that these substances, particularly PGEs, antagonize opioids. Let me begin by saying that there is no evidence of antagonism between PGEs and opioids at the opioid receptor, but there is good evidence of antagonism between them elsewhere in the responding cell.

Acute Effects on Guinea Pig Ileum

Antagonism between PGEs and opioids was first reported in 1969 by Jaques. Jaques (45) showed that several opioids, but not drugs of the aspirin group, inhibit the contraction of the guinea pig ileum elicited by PGE_1; whereas, as he had previously reported (44), both opioids and aspirin-like drugs inhibit the contraction owing to arachidonic acid, the precursor of PGs of the 2 series. Later, Rüegg and Jaques (65) found that nine of 10 ligands of the opioid receptor inhibited contractions of the guinea pig jejunum to PGE_1. The 10th, naloxone, was inactive, but effectively blocked the inhibitory action of morphine.

Sanner (66) confirmed the main finding of Jaques and extended it to PGE_2. More recently, Jaques (46) showed that Leu- and Met-enkephalin also antagonize the ileal contraction to PGE_1. Whereas Jaques showed that opioids specifically inhibit the stimulant effect of PGE on the ileum, Ehrenpreis et al. (22) found that PGEs reverse the inhibitory effect of morphine on the ileal response to electrical stimulation.

We have confirmed Ehrenpreis's observation and shown that it occurs downstream of the ganglia of the myenteric plexus (32). Although PGE_1 sensitizes the longitudinal muscle of the ileum to acetylcholine (71), several investigators have shown that, at the concentrations used in these experiments, PGE_1 stimulates shortening of the ileum largely through enhancing the release of acetylcholine by motoneurons of the myenteric plexus (23,31,71). These findings therefore indicate that the effect of PGE_1 on the myenteric plexus can be compared with that of electrical stimulation, that the antagonism of the effect of PGE_1 is an acute specific action of opioids, and that it occurs within the opioid-sensitive neurons.

Tolerance/Dependence in the Ileum

When the isolated ileum is incubated overnight at 4°C or at room temperature in Krebs solution containing morphine, the postganglionic neurons supplying the longitudinal muscle develop a measurable degree of tolerance and dependence (32,60,86). This effect occurs in the myenteric plexus, since hexamethonium does not prevent tolerance induction (32) and since the contractile response

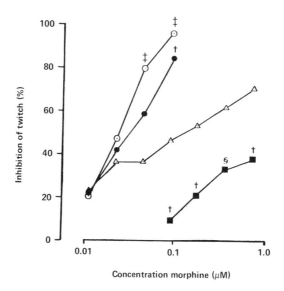

FIG. 4. Effects of PGE_2 or caffeine on the induction of tolerance to morphine in isolated guinea pig ileum. Pieces of ileum were incubated for 18 to 22 hr at 4°C in Krebs solution containing 17.5 μM morphine with or without test drug. All experiments were done with pairs of pieces of ileum, each pair being taken from one ileum and one of each pair being the control. ⊙, Krebs solution (control); ●, morphine + PGE_2, 6.6 μM; △, morphine; ■, morphine + caffeine, 0.5 mM. §, $p < 0.05$; †, $p < 0.01$; ‡, $p < 0.001$, compared with effect of morphine in the absence of test drug. (From Hammond et al., ref. 32.)

to naloxone is prevented by hyoscine. When, however, PGE_2 is added to the morphine solution to which the preparation is exposed, no tolerance develops. In other words, PGE_2 inhibits tolerance development in the opioid-sensitive neuron, as shown in Fig. 4. This figure also shows an interesting effect of caffeine, which I discuss below. We have also found that 5-HT inhibits the induction of tolerance/dependence in the ileum (H. O. J. Collier et al., *unpublished observations*). Consistent with these findings, the morphine-dependent ileum exhibits a nonspecific supersensitivity to PGEs and 5-HT (73,74; A. Herz et al., *this volume*).

Intestinal Function

Another instance of an antagonism between PGEs and opioids comes from intestinal function, particularly in the struggle between diarrhea and constipation. Opioids specifically contract the circular muscle of the rat colon (37). E prostaglandins antagonize the contractile effect of morphine but not of acetylcholine on the circular muscle of the dog intestine (19,30). E prostaglandins also induce diarrhea by increasing the salt and water content of the intestinal lumen. Opioids, including loperamide and diphenoxylate, which Wüster and Herz (92) have shown to bind with the opioid receptor, readily antagonize this effect of PGEs

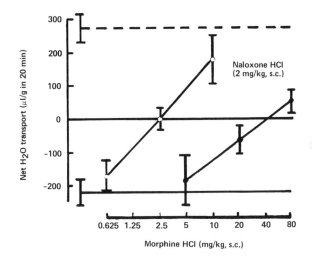

FIG. 5. Inhibition by naloxone of the antisecretory effect of morphine in the rat jejunum *in situ.* The bottom continuous line represents the mean maximal fluid secretion stimulated by PGE₁, 2 μg/min. The top broken line represents the mean value of net fluid absorption in the control group infused with saline into the carotid artery and pretreated with indomethacin (10 mg/kg s.c., 1 hr before). The vertical bars represent the standard error of the mean. Number of animals = 7 at each point. O, morphine; ●, morphine and naloxone mixture. (From Coupar, ref. 17.)

(47,52,53,79). These observations, however, do not constitute a study of the antagonism of PGEs in intestinal function as a specific action of morphine. Such a study has recently been reported by Coupar (17).

In rat jejunum, prepared for measurement of fluid secretion into the lumen *in situ,* Coupar (17) has shown that intraarterial infusion of PGEs increases the fluid content, whereas morphine and other opioids specifically inhibit this effect. Figure 5, from Coupar's recent paper, shows a dose-response line for morphine, in the absence and presence of naloxone, for inhibition of the increased water content of the lumen induced by intraarterial infusion of PGE_1.

The precise site of this specific antisecretory action of morphine remains to be determined. It is usually said to be in the mucosa, but, since atropine blocks the diarrhea elicited by PGE_1 in the mouse (79), we may suppose that PGE acts on the neurons supplying the mucosal cell. It remains to be determined if there are opioid receptors on these neurons, but we may expect to find them there. It also remains to be determined if PGE and opioids interact through a neuronal cyclic AMP, although it is believed that PGEs elicit diarrhea by stimulating a mucosal adenylate cyclase (49).

Central Nervous System in Whole Animals

In the central nervous system of the whole rat, the antagonism between PGEs and opioids has been explored by several workers. Ferri et al. (25) reported that injection of PGE_1 into a cerebral ventricle of rats briefly reversed the antinociceptive action of morphine, previously given intraperitoneally. Oltmans et al. (61) pursued this observation by infusing morphine and then PGE_2 or 16,16-dimethyl PGE_2, through an indwelling cannula, into the periaqueductal gray matter of the brain, which is a central site of antinociceptive action in the rat (42,43). In the experiments of Oltmans et al., both PGE_2 and its derivative reversed, as potently as did naloxone, the unresponsiveness to noxious stimulation of the paws induced by the intracerebral injection of morphine.

These experiments in the rat are supported by some observations indicating that PGs can mediate nociception within the brain. Thus injection of PGE_2 into a cerebral ventricle of the rat heightens hyperalgesia in an inflamed paw, whereas intracerebroventricular injection of an inhibitor of PG synthesis, such as aspirin or indomethacin, diminishes hyperalgesia in the paw (24; S. H. Ferreira, *this volume*). Again, the experiments of Sicuteri (78) and Dubas and Parker (21) suggest that systemic injection of PG synthetase inhibitors can block nociception attributable to a central release of PGs.

It cannot be said that all experiments support the idea that opioids act as antagonists of PGEs. For example, Vonvoightlander and Losey (88) were able to raise the level of cyclic AMP in the striatum of rats by intravenous administration of PGE_2, but systemic administration of morphine (up to 10 mg/kg i.v.) did not lower the raised level. Again, the dependent rat, which showed increased jumping in response to 5-HT, apomorphine, or dopamine injected into a cerebral ventricle, did not exhibit this response to PGE (74).

Moreover, it has been reported that PGEs themselves exhibit antinociceptive action (63,67) and that they are even synergistic with morphine (2). Before we accept these findings at face value, however, we should exclude the possibility that PGE may liberate endogenous opioids.

In the dependent rat some participation of PG in withdrawal effects can be recognized, since diclofenac, a powerful inhibitor of PG synthetase, which penetrates the brain well, given shortly before naloxone challenge, inhibits withdrawal jumping and diarrhea, although not other withdrawal effects (26). Furthermore, the dependent rat reacts excessively to intravenous PGE_1 (90).

INTERACTIONS BETWEEN OPIOIDS AND METHYLXANTHINES

Antagonism of Opioids by Methylxanthines

Bellville, in 1964, was, I believe, the first to establish experimentally that methylxanthines antagonize opioids. He showed, by experiments in man, that caffeine lessens the respiratory depression induced by morphine (1). Next, Ho, Loh and Way (35) reported that theophylline antagonizes the antinociceptive effect of morphine in mice. More recently, Grubb and Burks (30) have shown that theophylline antagonizes the stimulatory effect of morphine, but not of acetylcholine, on the circular muscle of the isolated small intestine of the dog.

In the guinea pig ileum, after ganglionic blockade, caffeine antagonizes the inhibition by morphine of the neurally evoked contraction (32), although caffeine does not stimulate the muscle directly, when tested in the presence of hyoscine. This indicates that the antagonism occurs within the opioid-sensitive neuron.

Antagonism of Methylxanthines by Opioids

We have mainly studied the converse relationship between opioids and methylxanthines—that is, the antagonism by opioids of the behavioral effects of methylxanthines and like-acting drugs in the rat (8,11,28). In this species, methylxanthines elicit behavioral excitation, in which a number of acts or states of behavior recur. These include jumping, rearing on the hind legs, restlessness, head or body shaking, teeth chattering, paw tremor, squeak on touch or handling, aggressiveness, salivation, diarrhea, ptosis, and penis licking. Moreover, low doses of naloxone intensify the behavior pattern induced by methylxanthines, and the result so closely resembles the precipitated withdrawal syndrome in morphine-dependent rats that we have termed it the "quasi–morphine withdrawal (or abstinence) syndrome" (QMWS). Opioids readily suppress all these behavioral responses to methylxanthines, except salivation. This suppression is stereospecific, as we showed some years ago for levorphanol and dextrorphan, given subcutaneously (10), and have recently confirmed (D. L. Francis et al., *unpublished observations*), by injecting into a lateral cerebral ventricle of rats, treated subcutaneously with 3-isobutyl-1-methylxanthine (IBMX), 10 μg of either the natural (−) enantiomer or the (+) enantiomer of morphine, recently synthesized by Rice and colleagues (38,40,41).

The suppression by opiates of the behavioral responses to methylxanthine is also specific, since it is reversed by naloxone, given either subcutaneously or into a cerebral ventricle (8,11). We have recently shown that this reversal is, moreover, stereospecific (D. L. Francis et al., *unpublished observations*), since 3 mg of the usual (−) enantiomer of naloxone was effective, when given intracerebroventricularly, whereas this dose of the recently synthesized (+) enantiomer (39) was wholly ineffective.

Another feature of this effect of opioids on behavioral responses to methylxanthines is that the potencies of opioids in suppressing the behavior pattern correlates well with their potency in other agonist actions, such as analgesia, binding with opioid receptors in brain homogenates, and inhibition of the neurally evoked contraction of the guinea pig ileum (8; D. L. Francis et al., *unpublished observations*).

These observations on the specific and stereospecific effects of opioids would be much more meaningful if we knew what biochemical action of the methylxanthines was causing the behavior. To determine this, we have correlated, in a group of seven xanthines, potencies in eliciting behavioral excitation with potencies in inhibiting low K_m cyclic AMP phosphodiesterase in rat brain homogenate *in vitro* (D. L. Francis et al., *unpublished observations*). The correlation obtained ($r = 8.6$; $p < 0.01$) strongly supports the argument that the behavioral effects of the methylxanthines are the result of their ability to inhibit brain phosphodiesterase, which would be expected to raise the level of a neuronal cyclic AMP.

The conclusion that the QMWS is the result of raising the level of a neuronal cyclic AMP is supported by the work of Chiu et al. (5), who showed that, in the rat, theophylline and the nonxanthine phosphodiesterase inhibitor ICI 63,197, which also induces a QMWS, significantly raise the brain cyclic AMP level.

Another phosphodiesterase inhibitor, Ro 20–1724, also produces quasi–morphine withdrawal behavior, but papaverine does not. Papaverine, however, administered systemically, does not raise the cyclic AMP level of the rat cerebrospinal fluid, although theophylline does (48).

Methylxanthines and Dependence

Quasi-withdrawal Behavior

The relationship between methylxanthines and opioid dependence is intriguing for several reasons. First, there is the curious observation I have mentioned—that the pattern of behavior elicited in opioid naive rats by systemic treatment with a methylxanthine plus naloxone is almost indistinguishable from the precipitated withdrawal syndrome of dependent rats (28). This quasi–withdrawal behavior is not only suppressed by opioids, but it is also diminished by lanthanum, which Harris et al. (33) have shown to possess morphine-like analgesic action. Lanthanum is interesting because it not only interacts with calcium, but also inhibits rat brain adenylate cyclase independently of calcium (59). The state of quasi–morphine dependence induced by methylxanthines differs from true morphine dependence in only two ways, as far as we have so far been able to determine: (a) It is rapid in onset—it is evident within 30 min of injection—and (b) its onset is not blocked by cycloheximide.

Intensification of True Withdrawal Signs

Another aspect of the relationship between methylxanthines and dependence is that these phosphodiesterase inhibitors, administered to morphine-dependent rats shortly before naloxone challenge, intensify the true withdrawal syndrome (9), as shown in Fig. 6. Not only do the methylxanthines, given systemically, intensify the true morphine withdrawal syndrome, but imidazole, which stimulates phosphodiesterase, has the opposite effect (9), as shown in Fig. 7.

Rapid Intensification of Responsiveness to Naloxone

Another phenomenon of quasi-dependence that appears to have a parallel in true dependence is what we have termed "methylxanthine-accelerated opiate dependence" (27). In the course of experiments on the QMWS, we noticed

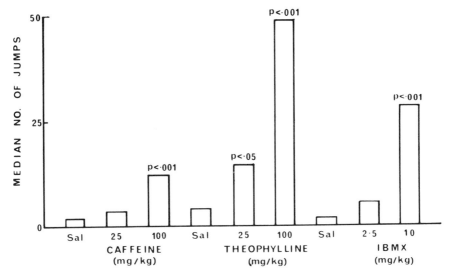

FIG. 6. Intensification of morphine withdrawal jumping by methylxanthines, administered to dependent rats before challenge with naloxone, 1 mg/kg subcutaneously. Rats were made dependent as in Fig. 3; caffeine and theophylline were administered orally 2 hr before and IBMX was administered subcutaneously 1 hr before challenge. (Ref. 9.)

that, if rats made quasi-dependent with IBMX were given heroin, not only was their behavioral excitation suppressed, but they quickly developed a higher sensitivity to naloxone. Figure 8 shows that, in rats made quasidependent with IBMX, treatment with heroin 20 to 40 min before naloxone challenge greatly intensifies the subsequent withdrawal syndrome.

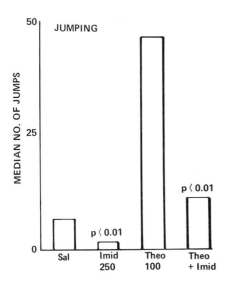

FIG. 7. Reduction by imidazole of morphine withdrawal jumping, with or without intensification by theophylline, in dependent rats. Imidazole (250 mg/kg) and theophylline (100 mg/kg) were given orally in water 2 hr before naloxone challenge. (Ref. 9.)

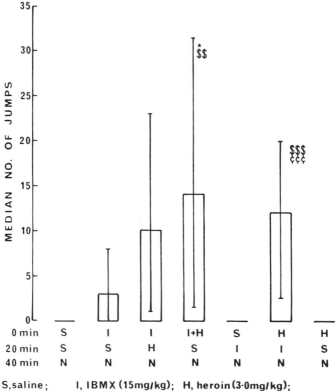

FIG. 8. Rapid intensification by heroin of jumping in response to naloxone in quasi-dependent rats. S, saline; I, IBMX; H, heroin; N, naloxone. Drugs were given subcutaneously in the sequence and at the times indicated. ★, $p < 0.05$ for difference from I + S + N; §§, $p < 0.01$ and §§§ $p < 0.001$ for difference from H + S + N; ¢¢¢, $p < 0.001$ for difference from S + I + N. (Ref. 27.)

As shown in Fig. 9, cycloheximide blocked the intensified jumping, after rats that had received heroin and IBMX were challenged with naloxone (27). The total withdrawal score was also reduced.

These experiments show that opioid drugs, against a background of brain phosphodiesterase inhibition, very quickly induce supersensitivity to naloxone. This remarkable phenomenon appears to have parallels in true tolerance/dependence. For example, when tolerance to morphine is being induced in the guinea pig ileum *in vitro,* addition of caffeine to the incubation fluid increases the amount of tolerance produced (Fig. 4). Again, the isolated ileum, derived from a highly dependent guinea pig, retains its responsiveness to naloxone challenge in the presence of normorphine, but loses responsiveness quickly when the opiate is withdrawn (73). The responsiveness to naloxone is quickly restored by reexpo-

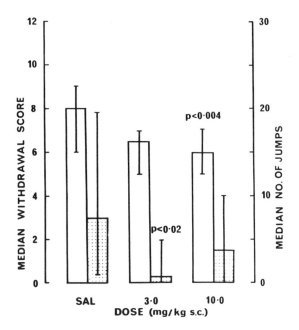

FIG. 9. Blockade by cycloheximide of the rapid intensification by heroin of responsiveness to naloxone in quasi-dependent rats. One hour after treatment with saline (SAL) or cycloheximide (3 or 10 mg/kg), rats were treated with IBMX (15 mg/kg) plus heroin (3 mg/kg); 30 min later, the rats were challenged with naloxone (3 mg/kg). All treatments were subcutaneous. The withdrawal score was obtained by counting 1 for the presence and 0 for the absence of each withdrawal sign. White columns, median withdrawal score; dotted columns, median number of jumps. (Ref. 27.)

sure to normorphine. Likewise, in mice made dependent on morphine after withdrawal of drug, the responsiveness to naloxone wanes, but this can be restored by a single dose of 30 mg/kg morphine (89).

These experiments suggest that there is an underlying, long-lasting state of dependence that is distinct from responsiveness to naloxone. This is also indicated by the experiments of Cox et al. (18). If this underlying state is present, then exposure to opiate quickly restores responsiveness to naloxone. It seems that methylxanthines produce in opioid-naive rats a comparable underlying state of quasi-dependence, in which responsiveness to naloxone can quickly be increased by treatment with an opioid (27). These observations support the proposition that opioid dependence is a state of increased potential for raising cyclic AMP in appropriate neurons (9,12).

MODEL OF OPIOID ACTION

The foregoing experiments and their interpretation, coupled with the work described by other writers in this section, provide us with material for making a model of the mechanism of the specific action of an opioid on an opioid-sensitive neuron. In so doing, we must also take account of the following considerations.

When an opioid molecule binds with the recognition site of the receptor, the neuron reacts; but when naloxone binds, no overt reaction follows. We can therefore assign two parts to the receptor—the recognitive and the reactive. It is necessary to suppose that these parts are linked in some way. Hence, we can postulate a third part, coupling these two.

The evidence I have outlined, together with that from NG 108–15 cells, suggests that the reactive part of the opioid receptor may be the catalytic unit of an adenylate cyclase; but the coupling between this unit and the recognition site of the receptor may be complex, for various reasons. For example, as reported by R. A. North *(this volume)*, neither cyclic AMP nor methylxanthines have yet been shown to antagonize the inhibitory effect of opioids on nerve impulse production by the neuron. We do not yet know, however, if our expectation that these drugs should so antagonize opioids is valid, since their effectiveness in antagonizing the action of opioids in the NG 108–15 cell has not been reported, although methylxanthines appear to antagonize opioids in rat brain preparations *in vitro* (8,57). In constructing our model, therefore, we must build some vagueness into the coupling between the recognition site and the reactive unit.

The opioid actions with which we are concerned are inhibitory. Since inhibition is meaningless without excitation, we may suppose that the neuron can be excited by some other humoral messenger substance or substances. There is evidence that one of these may be a PGE, but the evidence indicates that other excitatory messengers may be involved additionally or alternatively. Some evidence suggests that one of these other messengers might be 5-HT; it would therefore be interesting to know if 5-HT stimulated the adenylate cyclase of NG 108–15 cells. It is possible, even likely, that yet other endogenous substances may also stimulate the cyclase of opioid-sensitive neurons. To indicate these possibilities, the model is given two excitatory receptors.

There is also evidence that, in the opioid-sensitive cell, there can be inhibitory receptors other than that for opioids (50; W. A. Klee, *this volume*). A second inhibitory receptor is therefore also incorporated in the model. It would be economical to suppose that the inhibitory and excitatory couplings will converge on a single reactive unit; but it has been proposed that, in dependence in the NG 108–15 cell, another, more active, form of adenylate cyclase takes over (76). For the present, therefore, we should keep an open mind about the nature of the catalytic part of the enzyme and of its coupling to the receptors.

Since methylxanthines and other phosphodiesterase inhibitors intensify, and the phosphodiesterase stimulant, imidazole, diminishes the morphine withdrawal syndrome (9), we should also build into our model receptors for inhibitors and stimulants of phosphodiesterase.

Since there is evidence that cyclic AMP may be involved in at least some forms of transmitter release from neurons (80), we can incorporate in our model the possibility that the effect of inhibiting cyclic AMP formation would be to

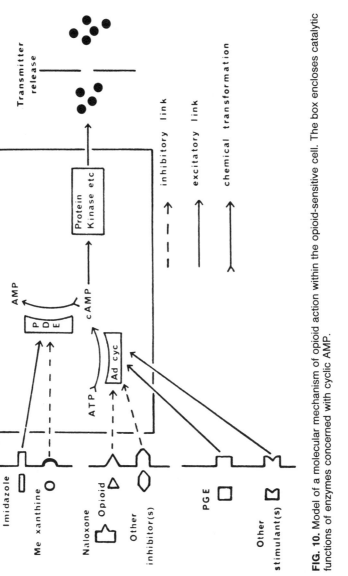

FIG. 10. Model of a molecular mechanism of opioid action within the opioid-sensitive cell. The box encloses catalytic functions of enzymes concerned with cyclic AMP.

reduce the ultimate release of transmitter, which is an established effect of opioids on opioid-sensitive neurons (54,62,69).

The known principles of cyclic nucleotide action, coupled with the finding that protein kinase markedly increases in the brain of morphine-dependent rats (6), suggests that protein kinase should also be incorporated into our model.

Figure 10 illustrates the model that can be built from the foregoing considerations. In this model, I have placed in a box the catalytic units of the enzymes concerned with the formation, destruction, and action of cyclic AMP. The couplings between the receptors and the units inside this box, and between these units and the ultimate release of transmitter must for the present be left vague.

SUMMARY AND CONCLUSIONS

The evidence I have reviewed suggests that a decisive action of opioids on the opioid-sensitive neuron is to inhibit an adenylate cyclase, and that opioid tolerance and dependence constitute a state in which, through a feedback mechanism, the capacity of the neuron to raise its cyclic AMP level is increased. Furthermore, the withdrawal syndrome is an expression of raised cyclic AMP levels in appropriate neurons. These concepts stand much as we first proposed some years ago; they have been greatly supported and extended by work on NG 108–15 cells.

The following evidence suggests that the adenylate cyclase that opioids inhibit can be stimulated by PGEs, or other endogenous substances, of which 5-HT may be one, or both. E prostaglandins can act centrally to enhance peripheral hyperalgesia and it is possible that other PGs do likewise. Acutely, PGEs and opioids antagonize one another on opioid-sensitive neurons of the ileum on which both act, although there is no evidence that the two substances interact at the same receptor. E prostaglandins and 5-HT inhibit the induction of morphine tolerance and dependence in these neurons of the ileum. The dependent ileum is supersensitive to PGEs and 5-HT. The dependent rat is supersensitive to PGE and some withdrawal effects are suppressed by the PG synthetase inhibitor, diclofenac.

Acutely, the methylxanthines antagonize opioids. They also produce quasi–withdrawal behavior to an extent that parallels their ability to inhibit brain phosphodiesterase. The opioids, to a degree that is directly related to their agonist potencies, specifically and stereospecifically suppress these behavioral effects of the methylxanthines and quickly convert the state of quasi-dependence into a state of still higher sensitivity to naloxone. Given to morphine-dependent animals before challenge with naloxone, methylxanthines also intensify the true withdrawal syndrome. These observations support and extend the conclusions on the role of cyclic AMP in opioid dependence stated above.

Finally, a model is constructed for a specific inhibitory action of opioids on the opioid-sensitive neuron. In this model, opioids act specifically by inhibiting adenylate cyclase, which is also susceptible to excitation and inhibition by other humoral messengers, acting at other receptors and coupled through an undefined mechanism to the catalytic part of adenylate cyclase. The inhibition of adenylate cyclase leads in turn to (a) blockade of transmitter release and (b) a compensating biochemical hypertrophy of the enzyme system, expressed as tolerance and dependence. The model thus provides intracellular mechanisms for the acute specific actions of opioids and for the induction of tolerance and dependence. It also provides a mechanism for the interaction with opioids of phosphodiesterase stimulants and inhibitors.

ACKNOWLEDGMENTS

I gratefully acknowledge the help of many colleagues who have participated in the work included in this review. These include Mr. N. M. Butt, Mr. N. J. Cuthbert, Mr. L. C. Dinneen, Mr. D. L. Francis, Dr. M. D. Hammond, Dr. G. Henderson, Mrs. Jane Marshall, Mr. Ivan Richards, Mrs. Wendy McDonald-Gibson, Dr. A. C. Roy, Dr. S. A. Saeed, and Dr. C. Schneider. I also thank Dr. K. C. Rice for (+)-morphine and (+)-naloxone and Dr. D. G. Smyth for β-endorphin (C-fragment) and *N*-methyl-Met-enkephalinamide. The following companies have kindly supplied the substances indicated: Ciba-Geigy, diclofenac; Imperial Chemical Industries Pharmaceuticals, ICI 63197; Miles-Yeda, Leu-and Met-enkephalin; Roche Products, Ro 20–1724, dextrorphan, and levorphanol.

REFERENCES

1. Bellville, J. W. (1964): Interaction of caffeine and and morphine on respiration. *J. Pharmacol. Exp. Ther.*, 143:165–168.
2. Bhattacharya, S. K., Reddy, P. K. S. P., Debnath, P. K., and Sanyal, A. K. (1975): Potentiation of antinociceptive action of morphine by prostaglandin E_1 in albino rats. *Clin. Exp. Pharmacol. Physiol.*, 2:353–357.
3. Bramwell, G. J., and Bradley, P. B. (1974): Actions and interactions of narcotic agonists and antagonists on brain stem neurones. *Brain Res.*, 73:167–170.
4. Calvillo, O., Henry, J. L., and Neuman, R. S. (1974): Effects of morphine and naloxone on dorsal horn neurones in the cat. *Can. J. Physiol. Pharmacol.*, 52:1207–1211.
5. Chiu, A., Eccleston, D., and Palomo, T. (1977): A model to test the relative potencies of phosphodiesterase inhibitors in brain *(in vivo)*. *Br. J. Pharmacol.*, 61:119P–120P.
6. Clark, A. G., Jovic, R., Ornellas, M. R., and Weller, M. (1972): Brain microsomal protein kinase in the chronically morphinized rat. *Biochem. Pharmacol.*, 21:1989–1990.
7. Clouet, D. H., Gold, G. J., and Iwatsubo, K. (1975): Effects of narcotic analgesic drugs on the cyclic adenosine 3'5'-monophosphate-adenylate cyclase system in rat brain. *Br. J. Pharmacol.*, 54:541–548.
8. Collier, H. O. J., Butt, N. M., Francis, D. L., Roy, A. C., and Schneider, C. (1978): Mechanism of opiate dependence elucidated by analysis of the interaction between opiates and methylxanthines. In: *Proceedings 10th Congress Collegium Internationale Neuropsychopharmacologicum*, edited by P. Deniker, C. Radouco-Thomas, and A. Villeneuve, pp. 1331–1338. Pergamon, Oxford.
9. Collier, H. O. J., and Francis, D. L. (1975): Morphine abstinence is associated with increased brain cyclic AMP. *Nature*, 255:159–162.
10. Collier, H. O. J., and Francis, D. L. (1976): Stereo-specific suppression by opiates of the quasi-morphine abstinence syndrome elicited by 3-isobutyl-1-methylxanthine (IBMX). *Br. J. Pharmacol.*, 56:382P.

11. Collier, H. O. J., Francis, D. L., Henderson, G., and Schneider, C. (1974): Quasi morphine-abstinence syndrome. *Nature,* 249:471–473.
12. Collier, H. O. J., Francis, D. L., McDonald-Gibson, W. J., Roy, A. C., and Saeed, S. A. (1975): Prostaglandins, cyclic AMP and the mechanism of opiate dependence. *Life Sci.,* 17:85–90.
13. Collier, H. O. J., Francis, D. L., and Roy, A. C. (1976): Opiates, cyclic nucleotides, and xanthines. *Adv. Biochem. Psychopharmacol.,* 15:337–345.
14. Collier, H. O. J., Francis, D. L., and Schneider, C. (1972): Modification of morphine withdrawal by drugs interacting with humoral mechanisms: Some contradictions and their interpretation. *Nature,* 237:220–223.
15. Collier, H. O. J., and Roy, A. C. (1974): Morphine-like drugs inhibit the stimulation by E prostaglandins of cyclic AMP formation by rat brain homogenate. *Nature,* 248:24–27.
16. Collier, H. O. J., and Roy, A. C. (1974): Hypothesis: Inhibition of E prostaglandin-sensitive adenyl cyclase as the mechanism of morphine analgesia. *Prostaglandins,* 7:361–376.
17. Coupar, I. M. (1978): Inhibition by morphine of prostaglandin-stimulated fluid secretion in rat jejunum. *Br. J. Pharmacol.,* 63:57–63.
18. Cox, B. M., Ginsburg, M., and Willis, J. (1975): The offset of morphine tolerance in rats and mice. *Br. J. Pharmacol.,* 53:383–391.
19. Dajani, E. Z., Roge, E. A. W., and Bertermann, R. E. (1975): Effects of E prostaglandins, diphenoxylate and morphine on intestinal motility in vivo. *Eur. J. Pharmacol.,* 34:105–113.
20. Davies, J., and Duggan, A. W. (1974): Opiate agonist-antagonist effects on Renshaw cells and spinal interneurones. *Nature,* 250:70–71.
21. Dubas, T. C., and Parker, J. M. (1971): A central component in the analgesic action of sodium salicylate. *Arch. Int. Pharmacodyn. Ther.,* 194:117–122.
22. Ehrenpreis, S., Greenberg, J., and Belman, S. (1973): Prostaglandins reverse inhibition of electrically-induced contractions of guinea-pig ileum by morphine, indomethacin and acetylsalicylic acid. *Nature (New Biol.),* 245:280–282.
23. Ehrenpreis, S., Greenberg, J., and Comaty, J. E. (1976): Block of electrically induced contractions of guinea-pig longitudinal muscle by prostaglandin synthetase and receptor inhibitors. *Eur. J. Pharmacol.,* 39:331–340.
24. Ferreira, S. H., Lorenzetti, B. B., and Correa, F. M. A. (1978): Antialgesic effect of non-steroid anti-inflammatory drugs and the synergism between central and local hyperalgesic effects of prostaglandins. *Prostaglandins,* 15:703–704.
25. Ferri, S., Santagostino, A., Braga, P. C., and Galatulas, I. (1974): Decreased antinociceptive effect of morphine in rats treated intraventricularly with prostaglandin E_1. *Psychopharmacologia,* 39:231–235.
26. Francis, D. L., Cuthbert, N. J., and Collier, H. O. J. (1978): Inhibition by diclofenac of morphine withdrawal diarrhea in the rat. In: *Proceedings of International Narcotic Research Conference,* edited by J. M. Van Ree and L. Terenius, pp. 59–60. Elsevier/North Holland, Amsterdam.
27. Francis, D. L., Cuthbert, N. J., Dinneen, L. C., Schneider, C., and Collier, H. O. J. (1976): Methylxanthine-accelerated opiate dependence in the rat. In: *Opiates and Endogenous Opioid Peptides,* edited by H. W. Kosterlitz, pp. 177–184. Elsevier/North Holland, Amsterdam.
28. Francis, D. L., Roy, A. C., and Collier, H. O. J. (1975): Morphine abstinence and quasi-abstinence effects after phosphodiesterase inhibitors and naloxone. *Life Sci.,* 16:1901–1906.
29. Goldstein, A., and Schulz, R. (1973): Morphine-tolerant longitudinal muscle strip from guinea-pig ileum. *Br. J. Pharmacol.,* 48:655–666.
30. Grubb, N. M., and Burks, T. F. (1975): Selective antagonism of the intestinal stimulatory effects of morphine by isoproterenol, prostaglandin E_1 and theophylline. *J. Pharmacol. Exp. Ther.,* 193:883–891.
31. Hall, W. J., O'Neill, P., and Sheehan, J. D. (1975): The role of prostaglandins in cholinergic neurotransmission in the guinea pig. *Eur. J. Pharmacol.,* 34:39–47.
32. Hammond, M. D., Schneider, C., and Collier, H. O. J. (1976): Induction of opiate tolerance in isolated guinea-pig ileum and its modification by drugs. In: *Opiates and Endogenous Opioid Peptides,* edited by H. W. Kosterlitz, pp. 169–176. Elsevier/North Holland, Amsterdam.
33. Harris, R. A., Loh, H. H., and Way, E. L. (1976): Antinociceptive effects of lanthanum and cerium in nontolerant and morphine tolerant-dependent animals. *J. Pharmacol. Exp. Ther.,* 196:288–297.
34. Havemann, U., and Kuschinsky, K. (1978): Interactions of opiates and prostaglandins E with

regard to cyclic AMP in striatal tissue of rats in vitro. *Naunyn Schmiedebergs Arch. Pharmacol.,* 302:103–106.

35. Ho, I. K., Loh, H. H., and Way, E. L. (1973): Cyclic adenosine monophosphate antagonism of morphine analgesia. *J. Pharmacol. Exp. Ther.,* 185:336–346.
36. Hosein, E. A., and Lau, A. (1977): Adenyl cyclase activity during tolerance and dependence to morphine. *Trans. Am. Soc. Neurochem.,* 8:83 (Abstr. No. 39).
37. Huidobro-Toro, J. P., and Way, E. L. (1976): The effect of narcotic agonists and antagonists on the rat colon. *Proc. West. Pharmacol. Soc.,* 19:278–281.
38. Iijima, I., Minamikawa, J., Jacobson, A. E., Brossi, A., and Rice, K. C. (1978): Studies in the (+)-morphinan series. 4. A markedly improved synthesis of (+)-morphine. *J. Org. Chem.,* 43:1462–1463.
39. Iijima, I., Minamikawa, J., Jacobson, A. E., Brossi, A., and Rice, K. C. (1978): Studies in the (+)-morphinan series. 5. Synthesis and biological properties of (+)-naloxone. *J. Med. Chem.,* 21:398–400.
40. Iijima, I., Rice, K. C., and Silverton, J. V. (1977): Studies in the (+)-morphinan series. 1. An alternative conversion of (+)-dihydrocodeinone into (+)-codeine. *Heterocycles,* 6:1157–1165.
41. Jacquet, Y. F., Klee, W. A., Rice, K. C., Iijima, I., and Minamikawa, J. (1977): Stereospecific and nonstereospecific effects of (+)- and (−)-morphine: Evidence for a new class of receptors. *Science,* 198:842–845.
42. Jacquet, Y. F., and Lajtha, A. (1974): Paradoxical effects after microinjection of morphine in the periaqueductal gray matter in the rat. *Science,* 185:1055–1057.
43. Jacquet, Y. F., and Lajtha, A. (1976): The periaqueductal gray: Site of morphine analgesia and tolerance as shown by 2-way cross tolerance between systemic and intracerebral injections. *Brain Res.,* 103:501–513.
44. Jaques, R. (1965): Suppression by morphine and other analgesic compounds of the smooth-muscle contraction produced by arachidonic acid peroxide. An in vitro method for detecting potential analgesics. *Helv. Physiol. Pharmacol. Acta,* 23:156–162.
45. Jaques, R. (1969): Morphine as an inhibitor of prostaglandin E_1 in the isolated guinea-pig intestine. *Experientia,* 25:1059–1060.
46. Jaques, R. (1977): Inhibitory effect of methionine- and leucine-enkephalin on contractions of the guinea-pig ileum elicited by PGE_1. *Experientia,* 33:374–375.
47. Karim, S. M. M., and Adaikan, P. G. (1977): The effect of loperamide on prostaglandin induced diarrhoea in rat and man. *Prostaglandins,* 13:321–331.
48. Kiessling, M., Lindl, T., and Cramer, H. (1975): Cyclic adenosine-monophosphate in cerebrospinal fluid. Effects of theophylline, L-dopa, and a dopamine receptor stimulant in rats. *Arch. Psychiatr. Nervenkr.,* 220:325–333.
49. Kimberg, D. V., Field, M., Johnson, J., Henderson, A., and Gershon, E. (1971): Stimulation of intestinal mucosal adenyl cyclase by cholera enterotoxin and prostaglandins. *J. Clin. Invest.,* 50:1218–1230.
50. Kosterlitz, H. W., Lydon, R. J., and Watt, A. J. (1970): The effects of adrenaline, noradrenaline and isoprenaline on inhibitory α- and β-adrenoceptors in the longitudinal muscle of the guinea-pig ileum. *Br. J. Pharmacol.,* 39:398–413.
51. Laduron, P. (1975): Adenyl cyclase: A possible target for morphine-like compounds and neuroleptics. *Abstracts of the 6th International Congress of Pharmacology,* p. 612 (Abstr. No. 1477).
52. Lange, A. P., Secher, N. J., and Amery, W. (1977): Prostaglandin-induced diarrhoea treated with loperamide or diphenoxylate. *Acta Med. Scand.,* 202:449–454.
53. Lippes, J., and Hurd, M. (1975): The use of chlorpromazine and lomotil to prevent and/or reduce the side effects of prostaglandin E_2 used for abortion. *Contraception,* 12:569–577.
54. Macdonald, R. L., and Nelson, P. G. (1978): Specific-opiate-induced depression of transmitter release from dorsal root ganglion cells in culture. *Science,* 199:1449–1451.
55. Mehta, C. S., and Johnson, W. (1974): Elevation of brain cyclic adenosine $3':5'$ monophosphate during naloxone precipitated withdrawal in morphine dependent rats. *Fed. Proc.,* 33:493 (Abstr. No. 1594).
56. Minneman, K. P. (1977): Morphine selectively blocks dopamine-stimulated cyclic AMP formation in rat neostriatal slices. *Br. J. Pharmacol.,* 59:480P–481P.
57. Minneman, K. P., and Iversen, L. L. (1976): Enkephalins and opiate narcotics increase cyclic GMP accumulation in slices of rat neostriatum. In: *Opiates and Endogenous Opioid Peptides,* edited by H. W. Kosterlitz, pp. 137–142. Elsevier/North Holland, Amsterdam.
58. Motomatsu, T., Lis, M., Seidah, N., and Chretien, M. (1977): Inhibition by beta-endorphin

of dopamine-sensitive adenylate cyclase in rat striatum. *Biochem. Biophys. Res. Commun.,* 77:442–447.

59. Nathanson, J. A., Freedman, R., and Hoffer, B. J. (1976): Lanthanum inhibits brain adenylate cyclase and blocks noradrenergic depression of Purkinje cell discharge independent of calcium. *Nature,* 261:330–332.

60. North, R. A., and Karras, P. J. (1978): Opiate tolerance and dependence induced *in vitro* in single myenteric neurones. *Nature,* 272:73–75.

61. Oltmans, G. A., Comaty, J. E., and Ehrenpreis, S. (1977): Antagonism by prostaglandin (PG) of morphine-induced effects in the periaqueductal gray (PAG). *Abstracts, 7th Meeting, Society for Neuroscience, Anaheim,* 3:299 (Abstr. No. 957).

62. Paton, W. D. M. (1957): The action of morphine and related substances on contraction and on acetylcholine output of coaxially stimulated guinea-pig ileum. *Br. J. Pharmacol.,* 12:119–127.

63. Poddubiuk, Z. M. (1976): A comparison of the central actions of prostaglandins A_1, E_1, E_2, $F_{1\alpha}$ and $F_{2\alpha}$ in the rat. I. Behavioral, antinociceptive and anticonvulsant actions of intraventricular prostaglandins in the rat. *Psychopharmacology,* 50:89–94.

64. Roy, A. C., and Collier, H. O. J. (1975): Prostaglandins, cyclic AMP and the biochemical mechanism of opiate agonist action. *Life Sci.,* 16:1857–1862.

65. Rüegg, M., and Jaques, R. (1972): A simple *in vitro* method of characterizing narcotic antagonists. *Experientia,* 28:1525–1526.

66. Sanner, J. (1971): Prostaglandin inhibition with a dibenzoxazepine hydrazide derivative and morphine. *Ann. NY Acad. Sci.,* 180:396–409.

67. Sanyal, A. K., Bhattacharya, S. K., Keshary, P. R., Srivastava, D. N., and Debnath, P. K. (1977): Prostaglandins: Antinociceptive effect of prostaglandin E_1 in the rat. *Clin. Exp. Pharmacol. Physiol.,* 4:247–255.

68. Satoh, M., Zieglgänsberger, W., and Herz, A. (1976): Actions of opiates upon single unit activity in the cortex of naive and tolerant rats. *Brain Res.,* 115:99–110.

69. Schaumann, W. (1957): Inhibition by morphine of the release of acetylcholine from the intestine of the guinea-pig. *Br. J. Pharmacol.,* 12:115–118.

70. Schmidt, W. K., and Way, E. L. (1976): Does morphine inhibit prostaglandin-stimulated adenylate cyclase in the rat brain? *Proc. West. Pharmacol. Soc.,* 19:55–59.

71. Schulz, R., and Cartwright, C. (1976): Sensitization of the smooth muscle by prostaglandin E_1 contributes to reversal of drug-induced inhibition of the guinea-pig ileum. *Naunyn Schmiedebergs Arch. Pharmacol.,* 294:257–260.

72. Schulz, R., and Goldstein, A. (1973): Morphine tolerance and supersensitivity to 5-hydroxytryptamine in the myenteric plexus of the guinea-pig. *Nature,* 244:168–170.

73. Schulz, R., and Herz, A. (1976): Aspects of opiate dependence in the myenteric plexus of the guinea-pig. *Life Sci.,* 19:1117–1128.

74. Schulz, R., and Herz, A. (1977): Naloxone-precipitated withdrawal reveals sensitization to neurotransmitters in morphine tolerant/dependent rats. *Naunyn Schmiedebergs Arch. Pharmacol.,* 299:95–99.

75. Sharma, S. K., Klee, W. A., and Nirenberg, M. (1975): Dual regulation of adenylate cyclase accounts for narcotic dependence and tolerance. *Proc. Natl. Acad. Sci. USA,* 72:3092–3096.

76. Sharma, S. K., Klee, W. A., and Nirenberg, M. (1977): Opiate-dependent modulation of adenylate cyclase. *Proc. Natl. Acad. Sci. USA.,* 74:3365–3369.

77. Sharma, S. K., Nirenberg, M., and Klee, W. A. (1975): Morphine receptors as regulators of adenylate cyclase activity. *Proc. Natl. Acad. Sci. USA.,* 72:590–594.

78. Sicuteri, F. (1970): Bradykinin and intracranial circulation in man. In: *Bradykinin, Kallidin and Kallikrein,* edited by E. G. Erdos, pp. 482–515. Springer-Verlag, Berlin.

79. Sohji, Y., Kawashima, K., Nakamura, H., and Shimizu, M. (1978): Pharmacological studies of loperamide, an anti-diarrheal agent. I. Effects on diarrhea induced by castor oil and prostaglandin E_1. *Folia Pharmacol. Jpn.,* 74:145–154.

80. Standaert, F. G., Dretchen, K. L., Skirboll, L. R., and Morgenroth, V. H. (1976): A role of cyclic nucleotides in neuromuscular transmission. *J. Pharmacol. Exp. Ther.,* 199:553–564.

81. Tell, G. P., Pasternak, G. W., and Cuatracasas, P. (1975): Brain and caudate nucleus adenylate cyclase: Effects of dopamine, GTP, E prostaglandins and morphine. *FEBS Lett.,* 51:242–245.

82. Traber, J., Fischer, K., Latzin, S., and Hamprecht, B. (1975): Morphine antagonizes action of prostaglandin in neuroblastoma and neuroblastoma × glioma hybrid cells. *Nature,* 253:120–122.

83. Traber, J., Gullis, R., and Hamprecht, B. (1975): Influence of opiates on the levels of adenosine 3′:5′-cyclic monophosphate in neuroblastoma × glioma hybrid cells. *Life Sci.,* 16:1863–1868.
84. Tsang, D., Tan, A. T., Herny, J. L., and Lal, S. (1977): Effect of Met-enkephalin and morphine on *l*-noradrenaline-stimulated cyclic AMP formation in rat cortex and hypothalamus. *Can. J. Neurol. Sci.,* 4:234.
85. Van Inwegen, R. G., Strada, S. J., and Robison, G. A. (1975): Effects of prostaglandins and morphine on brain adenylyl cyclase. *Life Sci.,* 16:1875–1876.
86. Villarreal, J. E., Martinez, J. N., and Castro, A. (1977): Validation of a new procedure to study narcotic dependence in the isolated guinea-pig ileum. In: *Problems of Drug Dependence 1977,* pp. 305–314. Committee on Problems of Drug Dependence. National Academy of Sciences, Washington, D.C.
87. Von Hungen, K., Roberts, S., and Hill, D. F. (1974): Developmental and regional variations in neurotransmitter-sensitive adenylate cyclase systems in cell-free preparations from rat brain. *J. Neurochem.,* 22:811–819.
88. Vonvoigtlander, P. F., and Losey, E. G. (1977): Prostaglandin E_2, cyclic adenosine monophosphate and morphine analgesia. *Brain Res.,* 128:275–283.
89. Way, E. L., and Loh, H. H. (1976): Responsivity to naloxone during morphine dependence. *Ann. NY Acad. Sci.,* 281:252–261.
90. Weeks, J. R., and Collins, R. J. (1976): Changes in morphine self-administration in rats induced by prostaglandin E_1 and naloxone. *Prostaglandins,* 12:11–19.
91. Wilkening, D., Mishra, R. K., and Makman, M. H. (1976): Effects of morphine on dopamine-stimulated adenylate cyclase and on cyclic GMP formation in primate brain amygdaloid nucleus. *Life Sci.,* 19:1129–1138.
92. Wüster, M., and Herz, A. (1978): Opiate agonist action of anti-diarrheal agents *in vitro* and *in vivo*—Findings in support for selective action. *Naunyn Schmiedebergs Arch. Pharmacol.,* 301:187–194.
93. Zieglgänsberger, W., and Bayerl, H. (1976): The mechanism of inhibition of neuronal activity by opiates in the spinal cord of cat. *Brain Res.,* 115:111–128.

Mechanisms of Pain and Analgesic Compounds,
edited by R. F. Beers, Jr., and E. G. Bassett.
R: ● i Press, New York © 1979.

32. Molecular Mechanisms of Opioid Action in Neuroblastoma x Glioma Cells

Werner A. Klee

Laboratory of General and Comparative Biochemistry, National Institute of Mental Health, National Institutes of Health, Bethesda, Maryland 20014

INTRODUCTION

The neuroblastoma x glioma hybrid cell line, NG108–15, was originally prepared by Hamprecht et al. (11) by fusion of a rat glioma cell with a mouse neuroblastoma cell. Although this particular clone was originally selected on morphological grounds (Fig. 1), it soon became apparent that NG108–15 cells have many interesting properties that make them a very useful model system for neurobiological studies. After having examined a number of neuronally derived cell cultures for the presence of opiate receptors, Klee and Nirenberg (17) concluded that NG108–15 cells were more richly endowed with these receptors than were all other cell lines studied, including the two parental clones. In the past few years, this cell line has been used in a large number of studies of opiate action (19,31,33,35,37) as well as in many other neurobiological investigations (23–25,29). The hybrid cells carry a number of receptors in addition to those for the opioids. The receptors which are best characterized to date are those that are functionally coupled to adenylate cyclase either as stimulators (PGE and adenosine), or as inhibitors (opioids, α-adrenergic agonists, and acetylcholine); see Table 1.

Another important property of NG108–15 cells is their ability to synthesize, store, and release acetylcholine. Choline acetyl transferase can readily be demonstrated in these cells (7) and the levels of this enzyme can be greatly enhanced by inducing the cells to differentiate by starving the cells for serum or adding cyclic AMP (7). Acetylcholine release, on depolarization of the cell membranes with K^+, has recently been demonstrated in an elegant series of experiments by McGee et al. (23). Acetylcholine release, at a rate well in excess of spontaneous release, can be seen in differentiated cells (treated with dibutyryl cyclic AMP for 3 to 5 days) as shown in Fig. 2B, but not in control cells (Fig. 2A). Choline release, which is also stimulated by KCl, is not dependent on the state of differentiation of the cells (Fig. 2C and D). These simple and yet incisive experiments go a long way toward demonstrating the relevance of work with NG108–15 cells to our understanding of the nervous system.

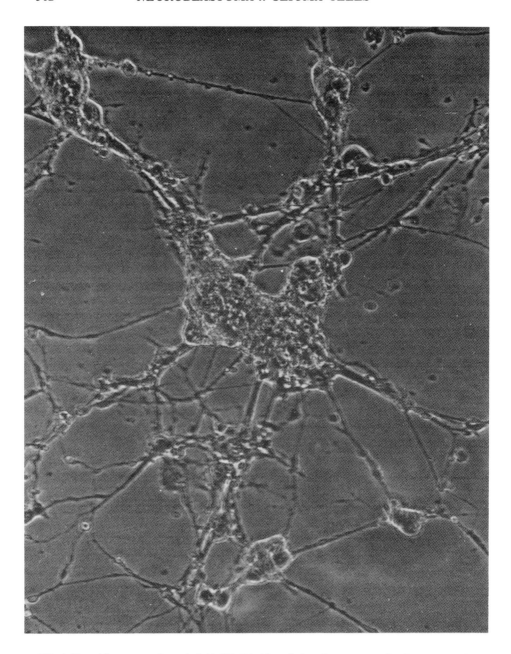

FIG. 1. Neuroblastoma x glioma hybrid, NG108–15, cells in culture as seen in phase contrast. Note the many long processes extending from cell to cell.

TABLE 1. *Effectors of NG108–15 cell adenylate cyclase activity*

Compound	Concentration (μM)	Adenylate cyclase activity	Antagonist
Control	—	40	—
Etorphine	1	28.6	Naloxone
Norepinephrine	100	35.9	Dihydroergotamine
Carbachol	100	33.9	Atropine
PGE$_1$	10	185	—
2-Chloroadenosine	10	80	Theophylline

Communication among cells is almost certainly the basis of nervous system function. The recent demonstration by Nelson et al. (25) of synapse formation between NG108–15 cells and muscle cells in culture therefore represents a giant step forward in the application of cultured cell lines to neurobiological problems.

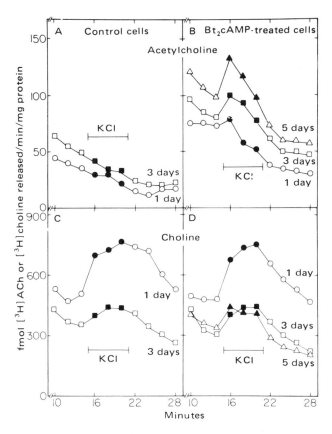

FIG. 2. Acetylcholine (**A** and **B**) or choline (**C** and **D**) release from NG108–15 cultures perfused with medium or with 80 mM KCl, as shown. In **B** and **D,** cells had been induced to differentiate by culture with dibutyryl cyclic AMP for the times indicated. (From McGee et al., ref. 23.)

Figure 3 shows the kinds of data that were used to demonstrate the formation of a functional synapse between these two cultured cell types. In part A of the figure, an NG108–15 cell, with its cell body at N is seen to send out long processes and appears to contact a muscle cell fiber at M. In part B, action potentials are recorded from the muscle fiber (lines 1 to 4) after electrical stimulation of the NG108–15 cell, as shown in line 6. The record in line 5 shows the shape of the action potential of the NG108–15 cell. In part C, a control experiment shows that direct electrical stimulation of the muscle cell produces an action potential profile which is easily distinguishable from that produced by transsynaptic stimulation. The chemical coupling of NG108–15 cells to a number of different types of muscle cells in culture has now been demonstrated (2,27), and these studies are clearly harbingers of many more studies that will be performed of cell communication in culture. The degree to which integrated nervous system function can be mimicked by interacting cell lines in culture is not known, but at present there are no clear constraints other than technical ones. Certainly, these exciting experiments show that NG108–15 cells can function

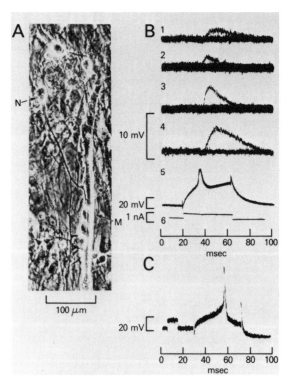

FIG. 3. A: Demonstration of synapse formation between NG108–15 cells (N) and cultured muscle fibers (M). **B:** Action potentials generated in muscle fiber M on stimulation of NG108–15 cell N. Recording from the cell N produces the trace shown in curve 5. **C:** Action potential of muscle cell M included by direct electrical stimulation. (From Nelson et al., ref. 25.)

as neurons and that they are therefore a valid model system with which to study the biochemistry of neurons.

RESULTS AND DISCUSSION

An important advance in our understanding of the mechanism of opiate action was the reports of Collier and Roy (4,5) of the inhibition of the accumulation of cyclic AMP in rat brain homogenates by opiates. These reports were rapidly supported by experiments that showed that the adenylate cyclase of NG108–15 cell homogenates is inhibited by opiates in a receptor-mediated fashion (33), and that cyclic AMP levels in NG108–15 cells are lowered by opiates as well (35). With the aid of cultured cell lines, it was possible to show that opiate inhibition of adenylate cyclase is seen only in cells carrying opiate receptors (33). The hybrid cells are particularly sensitive to the influence of the endogenous opioid peptides (18). As shown in Fig. 4, methionine enkephalin has more than 100 times the potency of morphine as an inhibitor of either the PGE_1-stimulated, or the basal adenylate cyclase, activity of NG108–15 homogenates (18). Although not shown in the figure, inhibition due to enkephalin (as well as that due to the alkaloid opiates, such as morphine) is completely reversed by naloxone. Recently, as a result of the chemical synthesis of the enantiomeric (+)-naloxone, it has been possible to show that naloxone antagonism is stereospecific (13).

All opioid peptides studied so far inhibit the adenylate cyclase activity of

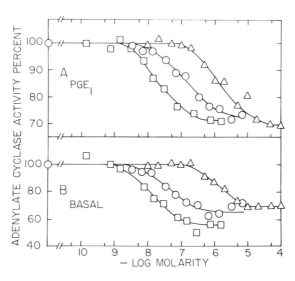

FIG. 4. Basal and PGE_1-stimulated adenylate cyclase activity of NG108–15 homogenates as a function of concentration of Met-enkephalin (□), Leu-enkephalin (O), or morphine (△). (From Klee and Nirenberg, ref. 18.)

TABLE 2. *Concentrations of endorphins required for half-maximal inhibition of adenylate cyclase activity of NG108–15 cell homogenates*

Compound	K_i (nM)
Met-enkephalin	10
α-Endorphin	250
γ-Endorphin	300
β-Endorphin	150
Morphine	1,500
Etorphine	10

NG108–15 cells (1,16,38). Interestingly, the relative potencies of the naturally occurring endogenous opioid peptides, the endorphins, are different from one another and also differ from those found in many other assays. Thus, as shown in Table 2, methionine enkephalin is much more potent than either α-, β-, or γ-endorphin in this assay, whereas the opposite is true *in vivo* (15) or in the guinea pig ileum assay (6). However, in the mouse vas deferens, enkephalin is more active than the longer chain endorphins (21). It is the author's opinion that whether these potency differences reflect different classes of receptors (21) or only differences in the accessibility of receptors to different ligands, is still an open question.

Exposure of NG108–15 cells to opiates for 12 hr or more results in an increase in adenylate cyclase activity that effectively compensates for the inhibition of activity observed as an immediate effect of opiate action (31). Lampert et al. (20) have recently shown that methionine enkephalin behaves as an opiate in this respect as well. When cells are cultured for many hours in the presence of either methionine enkephalin or etorphine (a potent analog of morphine), comparable increases in adenylate cyclase activity are observed, as shown in Fig. 5. The figure illustrates the fact that both basal (part A) and hormone-stimulated (part B) adenylate cyclase activities are increased as a result of chronic opioid treatment. Thus, changes in hormone coupling are not exclusively responsible for this phenomenon. These experiments led to a model for opiate tolerance and dependence, which is summarized in Fig. 6. The figure shows that opiates produce an immediate drop in cellular cyclic AMP levels, due to an inhibition of adenylate cyclase activity. On continued exposure of the cells to opiates, cellular cyclic AMP levels return to the normal state (31), as a result of the slow increase in adenylate cyclase activity elicited by the opiates. At this stage, the cells are tolerant to opiates since cyclic AMP levels are normal even in their presence. The cells are also in a dependent state, because rapid withdrawal of opiates, by addition of naloxone for example, results in an immediate, large rise in cyclic AMP due to the expression of the hitherto masked enzymic activity (31). Continued culture of the cells in the absence of opiates for a few hours leads to a loss of adenylate cyclase activity until normal levels are reached. It is thus possible to account for the major features of opiate action in animals by this simple, dual regulation model. Very similar proposals have been put

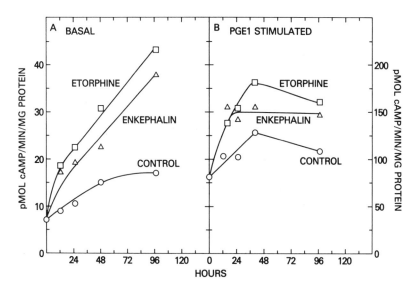

FIG. 5. Basal and PGE$_1$-stimulated adenylate cyclase activity of homogenates of NG108–15 cells cultured for the times shown in the presence of 10 μM Met-enkephalin (△), 1 μM etorphine (□), or in the absence of these compounds. (From Lampert et al., ref. 20.)

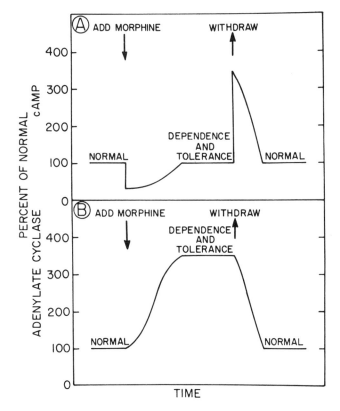

FIG. 6. A model of the role of changes in adenylate cyclase in the development of opiate tolerance and dependence in NG108–15 cells. (From Sharma et al., ref. 31.)

forward by Collier and his colleagues (3), and the general features of this model conform to the homeostatic regulation first proposed by Himmelsbach (12) and expressed in more modern form by Goldstein and Goldstein (10) and Shuster (34) almost 20 years ago.

What is the mechanism that couples the initial inhibition of adenylate cyclase with the subsequent increase in enzymic activity? This question can presently be answered only in part and only with reservations. Since basal and hormone stimulated enzyme activity are both increased in opiate-conditioned cells, hormone receptor coupling does not seem to be appreciably changed in the process. Interestingly, however, Sharma et al. (32) found that when the enzyme assays are performed in the presence of F^- or the stable GTP analog guanylylimidodiphosphate (agents that activate the enzyme but also uncouple it from receptors), there were no differences between enzyme prepared from control or from opiate-conditioned cells. Although an unequivocal interpretation of these experiments is not possible, the data imply that the increased enzymic activity elicited by opiates is due to an activation of preexisting enzyme rather than to the production of new enzyme. Consistent with this interpretation is the observation that cycloheximide, a protein-synthesis inhibitor, blocks only a portion of the increase in enzymic activity.

Scheme 1 is consistent with the presently available data and may be a useful working hypothesis.

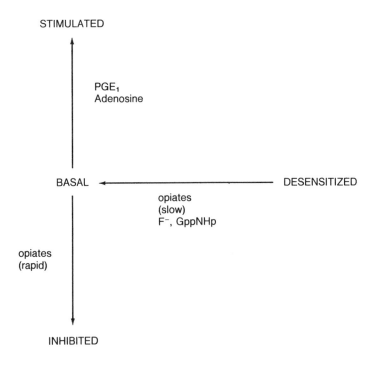

The scheme postulates two forms of adenylate cyclase, an active form, which can be stimulated or inhibited by the appropriate receptor-coupled effectors, and an inactive form, which can be called desensitized. It is postulated that the opiate-dependent, slow increase in adenylate cyclase activity is the result of the conversion of some of the enzyme from the desensitized to the active state. It is also proposed that F^- and guanylylimidodiphosphate effect the same conversion, but essentially completely. Thus, the latter two agents will eliminate all differences between control cells and opiate-treated cells by activating all of the enzyme present. Clearly this model should be considered to be only a guide for further experiments, especially since it leaves unanswered the interesting question of how the partition between the two types of enzyme is arrived at.

Recent work with NG108–15 cells has made it clear that dual regulation of adenylate cyclase activity is not a unique property of opiates. To the contrary, it has been found that agents which act as agonists at each of the three inhibitory receptors listed in Table 1 induce a slow compensatory increase in adenylate cyclase activity (24,30,31,36). Representative data from separate experiments, with α-adrenergic, muscarinic, and opiate agonists, are compiled in Table 3. Thus, dual regulation of the enzyme is a general property of inhibitory receptors. A degree of tolerance to and dependence on neuroeffectors may be the normal state of the organism and may therefore play an important role in controlling adenylate cyclase activity and cyclic AMP levels. If this view is correct, then drug dependence can be considered to be only an exaggeration of a normal state rather than a qualitatively new, pathological state. It would seem to be no easy task to demonstrate a small degree of tolerance and dependence in normal organisms. Certainly, however, the experiments of Jacob et al. (14) showing hyperalgesia associated with naloxone administration to naive animals points in this direction, as do the experiments of Francis et al. (8), which demonstrate some abstinence signs in naive rats after administration of naloxone.

Adenylate cyclase estimations, in homogenates of NG108–15 cells, are easy to perform in large numbers, and give reproducible results over long periods of time. The enzyme preparations may be stored for years at $-80°C$ without

TABLE 3. *Effects of long-term exposure of NG108–15 cells to inhibitory receptor agonists*

Agonist	Concentration (μM)	Adenylate cyclase activity	Growth period (hr)	Ref.
Control		13.9		
Norepinephrine	1	23.8	16	30
Control		5	48	24
Carbachol	100	16		
Control		10.5	25	20
Etorphine	1	18.5		
Met-enkephalin	10	19.3		

change in properties. Thus, the assay lends itself well to the study of opioid activities in tissue and other extracts. The enzyme preparation is half-maximally inhibited by 10^{-8} M enkephalin and can therefore reliably measure 250 fmoles or less of the peptide. An important attribute of this assay for opioid activity is its complete antagonism by naloxone. Thus, specificity of effect can readily be demonstrated. For these reasons, NG108–15 adenylate cyclase has been used by a number of workers to characterize opioid activity. For example, Giagnoni et al. (9) have used this assay in a study of opioid peptide production by cultured cell lines. Similarly, Mata et al. (22) measured changes in pituitary endorphin levels associated with changes in vasopressin levels in normal rats and in rats genetically lacking vasopressin. Recently Zioudrou et al. (39) have used the adenylate cyclase assay to help characterize a new class of opioid peptides, the exorphins, which are derived from food proteins after breakdown by the gastric protease, pepsin. These peptides behave as opiates in a number of assay systems. One of them appears to exhibit a potency similar to the most active of the endogenous opioid peptides. The physiological significance of the exorphins remains to be determined.

The many hundreds of enkephalin analogs so far synthesized have not all been tested in the adenylate cyclase assay. The potencies of some of those that have been examined are listed in Table 4, which is representative of a larger body of data obtained in our laboratory. A number of interesting conclusions can be drawn from the structure-activity profile of these analogs. First, no peptide has been found whose potency exceeds that of methionine enkephalin in this assay. Since proteolytic degradation is apparently negligible in this assay system (at least in assays of 5 min or less duration), it may be that the enhanced activity of peptides 10 and 12 in some assays (26,28) reflects primarily their relative stability toward proteolysis. Second, the free carboxyl group of methionine (or leucine) apparently contributes favorably to receptor interaction, although it may also help degradation in other systems and *in vivo*. Third, in

TABLE 4. *Concentrations of enkephalin analogs required for half-maximal inhibition of adenylate cyclase in homogenates of neuroblastoma x glioma hybrid cells*

	Analog	K_i (nM)
1	Tyr Gly Gly Phe Met	12
2	Tyr Gly Gly Phe Met Thr	30
3	Arg Tyr Gly Gly Phe Met	1,000
4	Phe Gly Gly Phe Met	10,000
5	Tyr Gly Gly Phe Leu	25
6	Tyr Ala Gly Phe Leu	1,500
7	Tyr Gly Ser Phe Leu	2,400
8	Tyr Gly Phe Leu	6,500
9	Tyr Ser Gly Phe Leu	30,000
10	Tyr D-Ala Gly Phe Met-NH$_2$	12
11	Tyr L-Ala Gly Phe Met-NH$_2$	400
12	Tyr-D-Ala Gly *N*-Me-Phe Met(O)-ol	200

agreement with other assay systems, any L-amino acid residue in position 2 is unfavorable, whereas D-amino acids seem easily tolerated. Fourth, unsubstituted tyrosine at the amino terminus is clearly necessary for a high potency peptide. Finally, in view of the extraordinary potency of methionine enkephalin, analogs with only 1/1,000 of the activity of the natural peptide can still be potent pharmacological agents in the appropriate circumstances.

SUMMARY

The neuroblastoma x glioma hybrid cell line, NG108–15, is a stable and homogeneous system that displays a number of the morphological, functional, and biochemical properties expected of neurons. In particular, these cells are found to be richly endowed with opiate receptors that are coupled, as inhibitory modulators, to adenylate cyclase. The cells have thus proven to be useful models for studies of the biochemical mechanism of the acute and chronic actions of opiates. Interestingly, the cells exhibit a homeostatic regulation of adenylate cyclase activity, which compensates for short-term inhibition by opiates as well as other receptor-coupled inhibitors, such as norepinephrine and carbamylcholine. Thus, tolerance and dependence may be general and normal regulatory mechanisms in the nervous system.

REFERENCES

1. Brandt, M., Buchen, C., and Hamprecht, B. (1977): Endorphins exert opiate-like action on neuroblastoma x glioma hybrid cells. *FEBS Lett.,* 80:251–254.
2. Christian, C. N., Nelson, P. G., Peacock, J., and Nirenberg, M. (1977): Synapse formation between two clonal cell lines. *Science,* 196:995–998.
3. Collier, H. O. J., Francis, D. L., McDonald-Gibson, W. J., Roy, A. C., and Saeed, S. A. (1975): Prostaglandins, cyclic AMP, and the mechanism of opiate dependence. *Life Sci.,* 17:85–90.
4. Collier, H. O. J., and Roy, A. C. (1974): Morphine-like drugs inhibit stimulation by E prostaglandins of cyclic AMP formation by rat brain homogenate. *Nature,* 248:24–27.
5. Collier, H. O. J., and Roy, A. C. (1974): Hypothesis: Inhibition of E prostaglandin-sensitive adenyl cyclase as the mechanism of morphine analgesia. *Prostaglandins,* 7:361–376.
6. Cox, B. M., Goldstein, A., and Li, C. H. (1976): Opioid activity of a peptide, β-lipotropin (61–91), derived from β-lipotropin. *Proc. Natl. Acad. Sci. USA,* 73:1821–1823.
7. Daniels, M. P., and Hamprecht, B. (1974): The ultrastructure of neuroblastoma glioma somatic cell hybrids. *J. Cell. Biol.,* 63:691–699.
8. Francis, D. L., Roy, A. C., and Collier, H. O. J. (1975): Morphine abstinence and quasi-abstinence effects after phosphodiesterase inhibitors and naloxone. *Life Sci.,* 16:1901–1906.
9. Giagnoni, G., Sabol, S. L., and Nirenberg, M. (1977): Synthesis of opiate peptides by a clonal pituitary tumor cell line. *Proc. Natl. Acad. Sci. USA,* 74:2259–2263.
10. Goldstein, D. B., and Goldstein, A. (1961): Possible role of enzyme inhibition and repression in drug tolerance and addiction. *Biochem. Pharmacol.,* 8:48.
11. Hamprecht, B., Amano, T., and M. Niremberg *(in preparation);* Hamprecht, B. (1976): Neuron models. *Angew. Chem. [Engl.],* 15:194–206.
12. Himmelsbach, C. K. (1943): The morphine abstinence syndrome. *Fed. Proc.,* 2:201–203.
13. Iijima, I., Minamikawa, J., Jacobson, A. E., Brossi, A., Rice, K. C., and Klee, W. A. (1978): Studies in the (+)-morphinan series. 5. Synthesis and biological properties of (+)-naloxone. *J. Med. Chem.,* 21:398–400.
14. Jacob, J. J., Tremblay, E. C., and Colombel, M-C. (1974): Facilitation de reactions nociceptives par la naloxone chez le souris et chez le rat. *Psychopharmacologia,* 37:217–223.

15. Jacquet, Y. F., and Marks, N. (1976): C-Fragment of beta-lipotropin: Endogenous neuroleptic or antipsychotogen? *Science,* 194:632–635.
16. Klee, W. A. (1977): Endogenous opiate peptides. In: *Peptides in Neurobiology,* edited by H. Gainer, pp. 375–396. Plenum Press, New York.
17. Klee, W. A., and Nirenberg, M. (1974): Neuroblastoma x glioma hybrid cell line with morphine receptors. *Proc. Natl. Acad. Sci. USA,* 71:3474–3477.
18. Klee, W. A., and Nirenberg, M. (1976): Mode of action of endogenous opioid peptides. *Nature,* 263:609–612.
19. Klee, W. A., Sharma, S. K., and Nirenberg, M. (1975): Opiate receptors as regulators of adenylate cyclase. *Life Sci.,* 16:1869–1874.
20. Lampert, A., Nirenberg, M., and Klee, W. A. (1976): Tolerance and dependence evoked by an endogenous opiate peptide. *Proc. Natl. Acad. Sci. USA,* 73:3165–3167.
21. Lord, J. A. H., Waterfield, A. A., Hughes, J., and Kosterlitz, H. W. (1977): Endogenous opioid peptides: Multiple agonists and receptors. *Nature,* 267:495–499.
22. Mata, M. M., Gainer, H., and Klee, W. A. (1977): Effect of dehydration on the endogenous opiate content of the rat neurointermediate lobe. *Life Sci.,* 21:1159–1162.
23. McGee, R., Simpson, P., Christian, C., Mata, M., Nelson, P., and Nirenberg, M. (1978): Regulation of acetylcholine release from neuroblastoma x glioma hybrid cells. *Proc. Natl. Acad. Sci. USA,* 75:1314–1318.
24. Nathanson, N. M., Klein, W. L., and Nirenberg, M. (1978): Regulation of adenylate cyclase activity mediated by muscarinic acetylcholine receptors. *Proc. Natl. Acad. Sci. USA,* 75:1788–1791.
25. Nelson, P., Christian, C., and Nirenberg, M. (1976): Synapse formation between clonal neuroblastoma x glioma hybrid cells and striated muscle cells. *Proc. Natl. Acad. Sci. USA,* 73:123–127.
26. Pert, C. B., Pert, A., Chang, J. R., and Fong, B. T. W. (1976): [D-Ala^2]-Met-enkephalinamide: A potent long-lasting synthetic pentapeptide analgesic. *Science,* 194:330–332.
27. Puro, D. G., and Nirenberg, M. (1976): On the specificity of synapse formation. *Proc. Natl. Acad. Sci. USA,* 73:3544–3548.
28. Roemer, D., Buescher, H. H., Hill, R. C., Pless, J., Bauer, W., Cardinaux, F., Closse, A., Hauser, D., and Huguenin, R. (1977): A synthetic enkephalin analogue with prolonged parenteral and oral analgesic activity. *Nature,* 268:547–549.
29. Sabol, S. L., and Nirenberg, M. (1979): Regulation of adenylate cyclase of neuroblastoma x glioma hybrid cells by α-adrenergic receptors. I. Inhibition of adenylate cyclase mediated by α-receptors. *J. Biol. Chem. (in press).*
30. Sabol, S. L., and Nirenberg, M. (1979): Regulation of adenylate cyclase of neuroblastoma x glioma hybrid cells by α-adrenergic receptors. II. Long-lived increase of adenylate cyclase activity mediated by α-receptors. *J. Biol. Chem. (in press).*
31. Sharma, S. K., Klee, W. A., and Nirenberg, M. (1975): Dual regulation of adenylate cyclase accounts for narcotic dependence and tolerance. *Proc. Natl. Acad. Sci. USA,* 72:3092–3096.
32. Sharma, S. K., Klee, W. A., and Nirenberg, M. (1977): Opiate-dependent modulation of adenylate cyclase. *Proc. Natl. Acad. Sci. USA,* 74:3365–3369.
33. Sharma, S. K., Nirenberg, M., and Klee, W. A. (1975): Morphine receptors as regulators of adenylate cyclase activity. *Proc. Natl. Acad. Sci. USA,* 72:590–594.
34. Shuster, L. (1961): Repression and de-repression of enzyme synthesis as a possible explanation of some aspects of drug action. *Nature,* 189:314–315.
35. Traber, J., Fischer, K., Latzin, S., and Hamprecht, B. (1975): Morphine antagonizes action of prostaglandin in neuroblastoma and neuroblastoma x glioma hybrid cells. *Nature,* 253:120–122.
36. Traber, J., Gullis, R., and Hamprecht, B. (1975): Influence of opiates on the levels of adenosine 3′:5′ cyclic monophosphate in neuroblastoma x glioma hybrid cells. *Life Sci.,* 16:1863–1868.
37. Traber, J., Reiser, G., Fischer, K., and Hamprecht, B. (1975): Measurements of adenosine 3′:5′ cyclic monophosphate and membrane potential in neuroblastoma x glioma hybrid cells: Opiates and adrenergic agonists cause effects opposite to those of prostaglandin E$_1$. *FEBS Lett.,* 52:327–332.
38. Wahlström, A., Brandt, M., Moroder, L., Wünsch, E., Lindeberg, G., Raguarsson, U., Terenius, L., and Hamprecht, B. (1977): Peptides related to β-lipotropin with opioid activity. *FEBS Lett.,* 77:28–32.
39. Zioudrou, C., Streaty, R. A., and Klee, W. A. (1979): Opioid peptides derived from food proteins: The exorphins. *J. Biol. Chem. (in press).*

Mechanisms of Pain and Analgesic Compounds,
edited by R. F. Beers, Jr., and E. G. Bassett.
Raven Press, New York © 1979.

33. Mechanism of Action of Opiates on Single Myenteric Neurons

R. Alan North

Department of Pharmacology, Loyola University Stritch School of Medicine, Maywood, Illinois 60153

INTRODUCTION

Electrophysiological studies of opiate action in the central nervous system have recently been reviewed (1,31,52). These studies provide evidence for three distinct sites and mechanisms of action of opiates and opioid peptides. These are, first, a direct inhibitory postsynaptic action on the neuron whose activity is recorded; second, a presynaptic action to inhibit release of (excitatory) transmitters; third, a direct interference at the level of the ionophore with the postsynaptic action of a conventional transmitter. None of these effects has yet been demonstrated unequivocally at the level of the single neuron (31). The reasons for this are the limitations of the *in vivo* technique: When the opiate is applied by iontophoresis the concentration at the receptor site is unknown, and when the opiate is administered systemically the locus of action is unknown. It is fortunate that sites in the peripheral nervous system exist that are also sensitive to morphine and where two of the above opiate actions are manifest. These sites offer relatively simple experimental models with which to study the mechanism of action of opiates. One of these, the guinea pig ileum, has been extensively employed for this purpose since the initial observations of Trendelenburg (48), Schaumann (44), Paton (38), and Kosterlitz and Robinson (20).

The myenteric plexus contains large amounts of acetylcholine (ACh) that can be released on nerve stimulation (39), and both the output of ACh following nerve stimulation and the nerve-mediated contraction of the longitudinal muscle layer are depressed by narcotics. That these actions of narcotics are mediated by opiate receptors is substantiated by several pieces of evidence. Briefly, these are as follows:

(a) The potency of narcotic agonists in depressing the nerve-mediated contractile response of the longitudinal muscle correlates closely with their analgesic potency in man; this relationship holds for a potency range of 10,000 times and for more than 20 different agonists (21).

(b) The relative affinities of narcotic agonists and antagonists for binding sites in the myenteric plexus correlate extremely well with their binding in rat brain, which in turn correlates with antinociceptive potency (4).

(c) The actions of narcotic agonists in depressing acetylcholine output or in inhibiting the contractile response are stereospecific (19).

(d) Narcotic antagonist such as naloxone prevents the actions of narcotics on the acetylcholine output or on the contractile response (22); both actions are inhibited in a strictly competitive manner, and the experiments indicate a dissociation constant similar to that determined from the binding studies and compatible with the antagonism in the central nervous system.

(e) Tolerance occurs to the effects of repeated administration of narcotics, as well as cross-tolerance among narcotics (38). The preparation also produces signs that appear to be manifestations of withdrawal when it is removed from an animal previously made physically dependent on morphine (8,45).

The evidence outlined above indicates clearly that the myenteric plexus of the guinea pig ileum contains neurons that bear opiate receptors. It therefore offers the possibility of recording the activity of single neurons and studying the effects of opiates on their properties. Such an *in vitro* system offers a way of avoiding the major difficulties inherent in *in vivo* studies because drugs can be applied in precisely known concentrations, the ionic environment can be manipulated to block synaptic transmission, and both extracellular and intracellular recordings can be made. On the other hand, it must always be borne in mind that although the opiate receptors in the myenteric plexus appear to be identical to those responsible for the production of analgesia in the central nervous system, the immediate electrophysiological or biochemical consequences of opiate receptor occupation need not necessarily be the same at the two sites.

The myenteric plexus contains several different types of neuron. There is considerable physiological evidence for the presence of afferent cells, interneurons, cholinergic excitatory efferents to the muscle layers, and nonadrenergic inhibitory efferents to the muscle layers. The cholinergic efferents could be considered the postganglionic elements in the parasympathetic outflow, although it was realized as long ago as 1921 (24) that it was better to regard the enteric nervous system as distinct from either the sympathetic or the parasympathetic systems. For example, the intestine receives adrenergic fibers from the postganglionic elements of the sympathetic outflow, but in the guinea pig ileum these fibers end predominantly within the myenteric plexus rather than directly on the smooth muscle layers. The principal effect of the sympathetic nerves appears to be presynaptic inhibition of cholinergic transmission within the myenteric plexus (14,27). More recently, considerable evidence has accrued for the presence within the plexus of neuroactive substances other than noradrenaline and acetylcholine [these include 5-hydroxytryptamine (5-HT) (41), substance P (40), enkephalin (11,46), somatostatin (2), and vasoactive intestinal peptide (25)], although there is no *a priori* reason to believe that these are all in neurons subserving physiologically distinguishable roles.

The relative complexity of the preparation suggested the possibility that opiates acted on one kind of neuron which then, by a transsynaptic effect, led to a depression of acetylcholine release from the cholinergic neurons. The only way to distinguish the site and mechanism of action of the opiates more clearly was to record the activity of single myenteric neurons.

OBSERVATIONS AND DISCUSSION

Extracellular Recording

The first test of morphine on unit activity in the myenteric plexus of the guinea pig ileum was by Sato et al. (42). They showed that morphine (10 to 30 μM) inhibited the firing of neurons that discharged "spontaneously," and firing was probably not the result of ongoing synaptic activity because it was unaffected by hexamethonium. This group subsequently (43) showed that 5-HT, sodium picrate, pentagastrin, and cerulein all increased the firing rate of the myenteric neurons and, in each case, the increase was prevented by morphine. The inference from this study was that the morphine was acting directly on the cell whose activity was being recorded, but the concentrations of morphine were high and the specificity of the action was not demonstrated.

Dingledine et al. (7) studied the effects of opiates on unit activity by similar techniques. Narcotics depressed both the spontaneous firing rate of the neurons and the increase produced by 5-HT. Like the Japanese group, Dingledine also described units that could be distinguished by their distinct firing patterns and their insensitivity to morphine [similar to the burst units described by Wood (51) at other sites in the intestine]. Dingledine and Goldstein (5,6) made a very complete study of this action of morphine, showing it to occur at concentrations closely similar to those required to inhibit the nerve-mediated contractile response of the preparation, showing it to be antagonized by rather low concentrations of naloxone and, most important, showing it to be mimicked by levorphanol but not by dextrorphan. They suggested that morphine might inhibit ongoing excitatory activity at synapses utilizing 5-HT; this seemed somewhat unlikely at that time because intracellular recording had indicated that all the fast synaptic potentials were blocked by d-tubocurarine or hexamethonium and were therefore believed to be cholinergic.

However, Dingledine and Goldstein subsequently made good advantage of the *in vitro* technique by repeating their experiments under conditions in which all synaptic transmission was blocked by a low-calcium, high-magnesium solution. Morphine was equally effective in such conditions; it was therefore concluded that morphine probably acted by stabilization or hyperpolarization of the membrane of the neurons whose activity was being recorded. Since morphine in similar concentrations depressed the release of acetylcholine from the plexus, the likelihood was that the morphine-sensitive neurons from which they recorded were the cholinergic efferents to the muscle. Furthermore, because intracellular recording from the neuronal somata had not (at that time) provided any evidence for a direct membrane effect of the opiates, these investigators concluded that the extracellular electrodes might be recording neuronal activity at or near nerve terminals; they pointed out that their data were consistent with the concept of morphine acting to block impulse invasion into the terminal varicosities of the cholinergic neuron. The difficulty that remained for this interpretation of the action of morphine was that intracellular recording had failed to reveal any effect of morphine, and revealed very little spontaneous activity in neuronal somata. It was therefore considered that the extracellular electrodes were inducing the neuronal firing, probably by direct mechanical deformation of the cell membrane.

The experiments of North and Williams (36) supported this interpretation, but failed to distinguish unequivocally whether the extracellular electrodes recorded activity in nerve processes (from which transmitter is released) or neuron somata. Although such a distinction cannot be made conclusively, it seemed likely that the extracellular electrodes are recording electrical activity in the cell soma, since spontaneous activity was never recorded from the interconnecting strands of the plexus (although evoked propagating neuronal activity can be recorded) and the spontaneous activity could only be recorded by relatively large electrodes with tip sizes similar to or larger than the size of the neuronal somata. However, the recording suction electrodes are so large that it is quite likely that the activity is generated by mechanical deformation of a cell process but actually recorded after it is propagated to the soma and generates a greater transmembrane current flow.

There is considerable evidence suggesting that inhibition of adenylate cyclase is a primary consequence of the occupation of the opiate receptor. However, it seems not to be an essential intermediate step in the inhibition of firing of myenteric neurons brought about by opiates. The ability of morphine to inhibit neuronal firing was unchanged in three conditions in which intraneuronal cyclic adenosine $3',5'$-monophosphate (cyclic AMP) levels might be expected to be markedly elevated (16). These were prior and concurrent administration of cyclic AMP or dibutyryl cyclic AMP, of prostaglandin E_2, and of the phosphodiesterase inhibitor 3-isobutyl-1-methylxanthine. These findings do not address the possibility that inhibition of adenylate cyclase may be an important intermediate step in the inhibition of acetylcholine release brought about by the opiates, for the evidence that the same primary mechanism underlies both the inhibition of firing and the depression of transmitter release is inconclusive (see below). The possibility also exists that the inhibition of adenylate cyclase may be unrelated to either of these two *acute* effects of the opiates, but may be more relevant to the long-term changes underlying the development of tolerance and dependence. Since such changes can be readily induced in myenteric neurons (33,37), this possibility can be tested experimentally.

The more recent suggestion by the Sato group (10) that there are two sites of action of opiates in the myenteric plexus—those responsible for blockade of acetylcholine release and those responsible for inhibition of firing—is interesting. Such a hypothesis is not economical and is not strongly supported by the available evidence. Their finding that morphine is less effective in inhibiting firing than in depressing the contractile response is not in agreement with the work of North and Williams (36) or Dingledine and Goldstein (6), which indicated that the ED_{50} for morphine is very similar in both cases. More important, the dose ratio for naloxone versus morphine and enkephalin (50) is similar for reversal of the inhibition of firing and reversal of the depression of the contractile response (which is a measure of acetylcholine release).

Intracellular Recording

Intracellular recording from the myenteric neurons indicates that the cells rarely show any spontaneous activity. The fast synaptic potentials of these neurons are typical of autonomic ganglia elsewhere and are abolished by d-tubocurarine (13) or hexamethonium (28). They are also depressed by noradrenaline (27) and 5-HT (12); however, these agents are acting presynaptically to depress acetylcholine output since they do not depress the amplitude of the depolarization obtained by applying acetylcholine directly to the soma membrane. Some myenteric neurons do exhibit a slow depolarizing synaptic response—especially after repetitive presynaptic stimulation—that is unaffected by hexamethonium or atropine. The transmitter responsible for this slow synaptic potential has not been identified conclusively but the response can be closely simulated by iontophoretic application of substance P (17).

The first experiments on the effect of morphine showed no consistent effects on the resting membrane potential, input resistance, or amplitude of the excitatory postsynaptic potential (32). Hyperpolarizations were sometimes observed but these were generally small and often passed off while the morphine was still present. A subsequent analysis with lower concentrations of the more rapidly acting narcotic normorphine indicated that a substantial number of myenteric neurons were hyperpolarized (29,34). The hyperpolarization was mimicked by levorphanol and not by dextrorphan, and it was reversed or prevented by naloxone (34,35). Subsequent experiments have shown that the effect is also produced by enkephalin (18,30). The synaptic potentials recorded from the myenteric neurons are not affected by morphine or enkephalin and it therefore seems that the action is the one proposed by Dingledine and Goldstein: namely, a direct one on the membrane of the cholinergic neuron that innervates the muscle.

Is the hyperpolarization recorded by the intracellular studies the reason why the neuronal firing is inhibited in the extracellular studies? The obvious answer is affirmative, since the effective concentrations and the time course of the responses are closely similar. But it should be pointed out that there remains one discrepancy between the results of intracellular and extracellular recordings. The majority of cells sampled by extracellular electrodes are sensitive to morphine, whereas only a small proportion of them exhibit sensitivity in studies with intracellular electrodes. There are two probable reasons for this: Type 1 cells [which are more likely to be sensitive to morphine (35)] are more excitable than type 2 cells, and the extracellular electrodes preferentially sample the more excitable cell population; second, the intracellular electrodes record events taking place on or close to the soma membrane, whereas the extracellular electrodes detect changes taking place (or at least originating) further out on the cellular processes. The latter possibility, that the site of action is nonsomatic, is now supported by three other pieces of evidence (18). First, the hyperpolarization may or may not be associated with a change of resistance in the myenteric neuron. This suggests that a resistance change is occurring in all cases, but whether or not it is detected in the soma depends chiefly on the distance from the soma at which it is taking place. Second, iontophoretic application of enkephalin or morphine to the neuronal somata rarely produces any effect (except when very high currents are used and the flow of perfusate is stopped, thus allowing diffusion to distant nonsomatic sites). Third, application of enkephalin by iontophoresis to regions of the ganglion away from the soma produces a naloxone-reversible hyperpolarization, whereas application of the same iontophoretic current directly to the soma membrane does not cause any hyperpolarization (18). In summary, it seems that the membrane hyperpolarization is the probable reason for the inhibition of firing when using extracellular electrodes, but the main site of the cell's hyperpolarization is the nonsomatic membrane, and this contributes to the variability in expression of the effect recorded in the soma.

A second question seeks to determine if the membrane hyperpolarization might also be the reason why the acetylcholine output evoked by nerve stimulation is reduced. The hypothesis is that the membrane hyperpolarization and increase of conductance prevents the neuronal excitation by the brief pulse (1 msec or less) applied by field stimulation. Intracellular recording provides direct evidence that this occurs (35). Furthermore, this interpretation accounts for two observations that are otherwise difficult to explain. First, the depression of the contractile response by morphine can be overcome by raising the stimulus strength, even though the stimulus strength was already supramaximal before the addition of morphine (35). This indicates that morphine has prevented some neurons from being excited but that they can be reexcited by a higher stimulating current. Second, it has been well observed that the contractile response is much more sensitive to inhibition by morphine when submaximal stimulation is used than when supramaximal stimulation is used (3,9,15). One interpretation of this discrepancy is that with submaximal stimulation, even a low concentration of morphine will hyperpolarize some neurons and prevent their excitation, whereas with supramaximal stimulation a relatively greater hyperpolarization (i.e., a greater concentration of morphine) will be required before the first neurons are prevented from being excited. Since the hyperpolarization is taking place away from the soma membrane, it seems reasonable to conclude that the sites affected are the nervous processes from which acetylcholine is normally released. These findings therefore support the original suggestion of Dingledine and Goldstein that morphine is acting by blocking impulse propagation into the nerve terminals. There is evidence that such a propagation block has rather widespread occurrence in the nervous system and may be a more important mechanism of presynaptic inhibition than hitherto realized (49).

Any explanation that purports to account for the inhibition of the contractile response by opiates must also take cognizance of one other important phenomenon: that the effects of opiates are manifest only at low frequencies of stimulation.

Indeed, it is characteristic of morphine-sensitive transmitter release that the inhibition is greater at low than at high frequencies of stimulation (26). Similarly, it is known that morphine-sensitive junctions are characterized by a relatively high release of transmitter per pulse at low frequencies of stimulation. The possibility exists that, at higher frequencies of stimulation, impulse propagation into the nerve terminals is normally intermittent; the apparent output of transmitter per pulse would be less than at lower frequencies, and morphine would have less effect because fewer action potentials are invading nerve terminals. At low frequencies of stimulation, each stimulus invades the nerve terminals, and it would therefore become sensitive to propagation block by a slight membrane hyperpolarization or increase of conductance caused by morphine. It is interesting to observe that as long ago as 1967 morphine was thought to act by such a mechanism (23).

SUMMARY

Opiates inhibit neuronal firing and reduce the output of transmitter from the neurons of the myenteric plexus, thus providing a model system for two of the best-known actions of opiates in the central nervous system. The inhibition of neuronal firing appears to be brought about by a direct action of opiates on the neuronal membrane at sites distant from the soma; this action represents an increase of conductance, or a membrane hyperpolarization, or both. The inhibition of transmitter release evoked by field stimulation could have a similar explanation, namely, hyperpolarization of fine nerve processes or nerve terminals leading to a block of invasion by the action potential; however, other mechanisms of interference with transmitter release are possible. It is not yet clear if these mechanisms of action also operate in the central nervous system, but there is encouraging evidence that there might be similarities in some circumstances. In the first place, the central effects of opiates on cell firing are almost always inhibitory (1,31,52). Second, the depression of the dorsal root potential by opiates in the neonatal rat spinal cord seems to be associated with a hyperpolarization of the fine nerve terminals (47).

ACKNOWLEDGMENT

Work carried out in the author's laboratory was supported by grants NS06672, DA01730, and the Schweppe Foundation.

REFERENCES

1. Bradley, P. B. (1978): Electrophysiological effects of opiates and opioid peptides. In: *Centrally Acting Peptides,* edited by J. Hughes, pp. 215–229. University Park, Baltimore.
2. Costa, M., Patel, Y., Furness, J. B., and Arimura, A. (1977): Evidence that some intrinsic neurons of the intestine contain somatostatin. *Neurosci. Lett.,* 6:215–222.
3. Cox, B. M., and Weinstock, M. (1966): The effect of analgesic drugs on the release of acetylcholine from electrically stimulated guinea-pig ileum, *Br. J. Pharmacol. Chemother.,* 27:81–92.

4. Creese, I., and Snyder, S. H. (1975): Receptor binding and pharmacological activity of opiates in the guinea-pig intestine. *J. Pharmacol. Exp. Ther.*, 194:205–219.
5. Dingledine, R., and Goldstein, A. (1975): Single neuron studies of opiate action in the guinea pig myenteric plexus. *Life Sci.*, 17:57–62.
6. Dingledine, R., and Goldstein, A. (1976): Effect of synaptic transmission blockade on morphine action in the guinea-pig myenteric plexus. *J. Pharmacol. Exp. Ther.*, 196:97–106.
7. Dingledine, R., Goldstein, A., and Kendig, J. (1974): Effects of narcotic opiates and serotonin on the electrical behavior of neurons in the guinea pig myenteric plexus. *Life Sci.*, 14:2299–2309.
8. Ehrenpreis, S., Greenberg, J., and Comaty, J. E. (1975): Mechanism of development of tolerance to injected morphine by guinea pig ileum. *Life Sci.*, 17:49–54.
9. Ehrenpreis, S., Light, I., and Schonbuch, G. H. (1973): Use of electrically stimulated guinea-pig ileum to study potent analgesics. In: *Drug Addiction: Experimental Pharmacology*, edited by J. M. Singh, L. H. Miller, and H. Lal, pp. 319–342. Futura, New York.
10. Ehrenpreis, S., Sato, I., Takayanagi, I., Comaty, J. E., and Takagi, K. (1976): Mechanism of morphine block of electrical activity in ganglia of Auerbach's plexus. *Eur. J. Pharmacol.*, 40:303–311.
11. Elde, R., Hökfelt, T., Johansson, O., and Terenius, L. (1976): Immunohistochemical studies using antibodies to leucine-enkephalin: Initial observations on the nervous system of the rat. *Neuroscience*, 1:349–351.
12. Henderson, G., and North, R. A. (1975): Presynaptic action of 5-hydroxytryptamine in the myenteric plexus of the guinea-pig ileum. *Br. J. Pharmacol.*, 54:265P.
13. Hirst, G. D. S., Holman, M. E., and Spence, I. (1974): Two types of neurons in the myenteric plexus of the guinea-pig duodenum. *J. Physiol. (Lond.)*, 236:303–326.
14. Hirst, G. D. S., and McKirdy, H. C. (1974): Presynaptic inhibition at a mammalian peripheral synapse. *Nature*, 250:430–431.
15. Johnson, S. M., Westfall, D. P., Howard, S. A., and Fleming, W. W. (1978): Sensitivities of the isolated ileal longitudinal smooth muscle–myenteric plexus and hypogastric nerve–vas deferens of the guinea pig after chronic morphine pellet implantation. *J. Pharmacol. Exp. Ther.*, 204:54–66.
16. Karras, P. J., and North, R. A. (1979): Inhibition of neuronal firing by morphine: Evidence against the involvement of cyclic nucleotides. *Br. J. Pharmacol. (in press)*.
17. Katayama, Y., and North, R. A. (1978): Does substance P mediate slow synaptic excitation within the myenteric plexus? *Nature*, 274:387–388.
18. Katayama, Y., North, R. A., and Williams, J. T. (1979): On the mechanisms and site of action of enkephalin on single myenteric neurones. *Brain Res. (in press)*.
19. Kosterlitz, H. W., Lord, J. A. H., and Watt, A. J. (1973): Morphine receptor in the myenteric plexus of the guinea-pig ileum. In: *Agonist and Antagonist Actions of Narcotic Analgesic Drugs*, edited by H. W. Kosterlitz, H. O. J. Collier, and J. E. Villareal, pp. 45–61. University Park, Baltimore.
20. Kosterlitz, H. W., and Robinson, J. A. (1957): Inhibition of the peristaltic reflex of the isolated guinea-pig ileum. *J. Physiol. (Lond)*, 136:249–262.
21. Kosterlitz, H. W., and Waterfield, A. A. (1975): In vitro models in the study of structure-activity relationships of narcotic analgesics. *Annu. Rev. Pharmacol.*, 15:29–47.
22. Kosterlitz, H. W., and Watt, A. J. (1968): Kinetic parameters of narcotic agonists and antagonists, with particular reference to N-allylnoroxy-morphone (naloxone). *Br. J. Pharmacol. Chemother.*, 33:266–276.
23. De La Lande, I. S., and Porter, R. B. (1967): Factors influencing the action of morphine on acetylcholine release in the guinea-pig intestine. *Br. J. Pharmacol. Chemother.*, 29:158–167.
24. Langley, J. N. (1921): *The Autonomic Nervous System, Part I.* Meffer, Cambridge.
25. Larsson, L. I., Fahrenkrug, J., Schaffalitzky de Muckadell, O., Sundler, F., Hakanson, R., and Rehfeld, J. F. (1976): Localization of vasoactive intestinal polypeptide (VIP) to central and peripheral neurons. *Proc. Natl. Acad. Sci. USA*, 73:3197–3200.
26. Lees, G. M., Kosterlitz, H. W., and Watt, A. J. (1973): Characteristics of morphine sensitive release of neurotransmitter substances. In: *Agonist and Antagonist Actions of Narcotic Analgesic Drugs*, edited by H. W. Kosterlitz, H. O. J. Collier, and J. E. Villareal, pp. 142–152. University Park, Baltimore.
27. Nishi, S., and North, R. A. (1973): Presynaptic action of noradrenaline in the myenteric plexus. *J. Physiol. (Lond.)*, 231:29P–30P.

28. Nishi, S., and North, R. A. (1973): Intracellular recording from the myenteric plexus of the guinea-pig ileum. *J. Physiol. (Lond.)*, 231:471–491.
29. North, R. A. (1976): Effects of morphine on myenteric plexus neurons. *Neuropharmacology*, 15:719–721.
30. North, R. A. (1977): Hyperpolarisation of myenteric neurons by enkephalin. *Br. J. Pharmacol.*, 59:504P–505P.
31. North, R. A. (1979): Opiates, opioid peptides and single neurones. *Life Sci. (in press)*.
32. North, R. A., and Henderson, G. (1975): Action of morphine on guinea-pig myenteric plexus and mouse vas deferens studied by intracellular recording. *Life Sci.*, 17:63–66.
33. North, R. A., and Karras, P. J. (1978): Opiate tolerance and dependence induced *in vitro* in single myenteric neurones. *Nature*, 272:73–75.
34. North, R. A., and Tonini, M. (1977): Hyperpolarisation by morphine of myenteric neurones. In: *Opiates and Endogenous Opioid Peptides*, edited by H. W. Kosterlitz, pp. 205–211. Elsevier, Amsterdam.
35. North, R. A., and Tonini, M. (1977): The mechanism of action of narcotic analgesics in the guinea-pig ileum. *Br. J. Pharmacol.*, 61:541–549.
36. North, R. A., and Williams, J. T. (1977): Extracellular recording from the guinea-pig myenteric plexus and the action of morphine. *Eur. J. Pharmacol.*, 45:23–33.
37. North, R. A., and Zieglgänsberger, W. (1978): Opiate withdrawal signs in single myenteric neurones. *Brain Res.*, 144:208–211.
38. Paton, W. D. M. (1957): The action of morphine and related substances on contraction and on acetylcholine output of coaxially stimulated guinea-pig ileum. *Br. J. Pharmacol. Chemother.*, 12:119–127.
39. Paton, W. D. M., and Zar, M. A. (1968): The origin of acetylcholine released from guinea-pig intestine and longitudinal strips. *J. Physiol. (Lond.)*, 194:13–33.
40. Pearse, A. G. E., and Polak, J. (1975): Immunocytochemical localization of substance P in mammalian intestine. *Histochemistry*, 41:373–375.
41. Robinson, R. G., and Gershon, M. D. (1971): Synthesis and uptake of 5-hydroxytryptamine by the myenteric plexus in the guinea-pig ileum: A histochemical study. *J. Pharmacol. Exp. Ther.*, 179:311–324.
42. Sato, T., Takayanagi, I., and Takagi, K. (1973): Pharmacological properties of electrical activities obtainable from neurones in Auerbach's plexus. *Jpn. J. Pharmacol.*, 23:665–671.
43. Sato, T., Takayanagi, I., and Takagi, K. (1974): Effects of acetylcholine releasing drugs on electrical activities obtained from Auerbach's plexus in the guinea-pig ileum. *Jpn. J. Pharmacol.*, 24:447–451.
44. Schaumann, W. (1957): Inhibition by morphine of the release of acetylcholine from the intestine of the guinea-pig. *Br. J. Pharmacol. Chemother.*, 12:115–118.
45. Schulz, R., and Herz, A. (1976): Aspects of opiate dependence in the myenteric plexus of the guinea-pig. *Life Sci.*, 19:1117–1128.
46. Smith, T. W., Hughes, J., Kosterlitz, H. W., and Sosa, R. P. (1976): Enkephalins: Isolation, distribution and function. In: *Opiates and Endogenous Opioid Peptides*, edited by H. W. Kosterlitz, pp. 57–62. Elsevier/North Holland, Amsterdam.
47. Suzue, T., and Jessell, T. M. (1979): Morphine and endorphins inhibit rat dorsal root potential *in vitro:* A CNS bioassay for opiate analgesics. *Brain Res. (in press)*.
48. Trendelenburg, P. (1917): Physiologische und pharmakologische Versuche über die Dünndarmperistaltik. *Naunyn Schmiedebergs Arch. Exp. Pathol. Pharmakol.*, 81:55–129.
49. Van Essen, D. C. (1973): The contribution of membrane hyperpolarisation to adaptation and conduction block in sensory neurones of the leech. *J. Physiol. (Lond.)*, 230:509–534.
50. Williams, T. J., and North, R. A. (1979): Effects of endorphins on single myenteric neurons. *Brain Res. (in press)*.
51. Wood, J. D. (1975): Neurophysiology of Auerbach's plexus and control of intestinal motility. *Physiol. Rev.*, 55:307–325.
52. Zieglgänsberger, W., and Fry, J. P. (1978): Actions of opioids on single neurones. In: *Developments in Opiate Research*, edited by A. Herz, pp. 193–239. Marcel Dekker, New York.

Mechanisms of Pain and Analgesic Compounds,
edited by R. F. Beers, Jr., and E. G. Bassett.
Raven Press, New York © 1979.

34. Changes in Neuronal Sensitivity in Opiate Tolerance/Dependence

Albert Herz, Rüdiger Schulz, and Julia Bläsig

*Department of Neuropharmacology, Max-Planck-Institut für Psychiatrie,
D-8000 München 40, Federal Republic of Germany*

INTRODUCTION

Drug addiction, a phenomenon characterized by tolerance, physical dependence, and compulsive drug abuse, reflects the adaptation of nerve cells to an altered environment owing to continuous presence of the drug. The adaptive changes compensate for the biochemical effects of the drugs causing, in turn, a new homeostatic equilibrium. Disturbance of the newly established homeostasis by withdrawal of the addictive drug again causes pathophysiological changes that manifest themselves as withdrawal signs.

Several theories have been advanced to explain the compensatory mechanisms leading to tolerance and dependence. The theories proposed by Collier (6,7) and by Jaffe and Sharpless (23) particularly emphasize changes in neuronal sensitivity—although the other theories (32) also implicate such changes. Collier postulated that postsynaptically located receptors become supersensitive on prolonged opiate-induced inhibition of a presynaptically released excitatory neurotransmitter, a concept closely resembling the phenomenon of denervation- or disuse-supersensitivity (23). The theory implies that the ability to induce changes in neuronal sensitivity is not specific to opiates or other addictive drugs, but, rather, that such changes reflect a general regulatory mechanism of cells to adapt to the altered functional state.

MODELS FOR TESTING ADAPTIVE MECHANISMS TO OPIATES

The complexity of the central nervous system creates serious problems for the analysis of changes in neuronal sensitivity in the whole animal. Most available evidence concerning the occurrence of supersensitivity during chronic opiate action is based on behavioral observations. Additional information is provided by isolated organs containing less complicated nervous structures, such as the longitudinal muscle–myenteric plexus preparation of the guinea pig. Neurophysiological aspects of opiate-induced changes in neuronal sensitivity have been studied in single neurons *in vivo* (34), whereas biochemical aspects of such

changes have been thoroughly investigated in cultured cells bearing opiate receptors (19). In this chapter only data obtained in isolated organs and intact animals
are discussed in more detail.

Isolated Organs

It has been shown that preparations from tolerant/dependent guinea pigs
are supersensitive to the excitatory actions of 5-hydroxytryptamine (5-HT) and
prostaglandin E_1 (PGE_1), as indicated by a shift of the dose-response curve
to the left (34). At the same time, the inhibitory activities of epinephrine and
dopamine were found to be reduced, whereas the sensitivity to acetylcholine,
the neurotransmitter acting mainly at the smooth muscle, remained unchanged
(36). Although these preparations are highly tolerant, naloxone failed to precipitate a visible withdrawal phenomenon. This finding seemed to contradict the
postulated unitary theory of tolerance and dependence. Most likely, withdrawal
is induced when the tissue is removed from the chronically morphinized guinea
pig and set up in Krebs-Ringer solution lacking any opiate. Such a mechanism
was suggested by subsequent experiments in which withdrawal was prevented
by exposure of the preparations to an adequate opiate concentration outside
the animal. Those conditions enabled not only precipitation of a withdrawal
sign by naloxone, indicated by a contracture of the muscle, but also investigations
of the relationship between supersensitivity, tolerance, and withdrawal signs
(37). It appears that as long as morphine is in contact with opiate receptors
of tolerant/dependent preparations, the sensitivity to 5-HT and PGE_1 is similar
to that of naive preparations. Figure 1 shows that displacement of morphine
from the receptor by naloxone causes a withdrawal contracture and reveals
supersensitivity. On continuous washing, supersensitivity diminishes, as does
tolerance, although even after 3 hr of washing a normal sensitivity is not yet
reached. One hour after starting the wash procedure, naloxone fails to precipitate
a withdrawal contracture, although tolerance and altered sensitivity to 5-HT
and PGE_1 still exists. These results emphasize the importance of differentiating
between the manifestation of the dependent state (that is, the withdrawal sign),
and the tolerant/dependent state itself. Thus a withdrawal sign may not be
inducible although supersensitivity still exists. This altered sensitivity is suggested
to be the actual cause of tolerance and dependence.

In the mouse vas deferens, another *in vitro* preparation widely used for testing
opioids, the relationship between tolerance, change in neuronal sensitivity, and
withdrawal signs is difficult to demonstrate. Employing experimental conditions
comparable to those described for the tolerant/dependent guinea pig ileum,
naloxone fails to precipitate a withdrawal sign, although some tolerance to morphine is seen (R. Schulz, *unpublished observations*). At present, no explanation
for these differences between the two preparations can be given. From the guinea
pig ileum it is known, however, that axonal conduction is essential for exhibition
of the withdrawal contracture. In the mouse vas deferens preparation, the somata

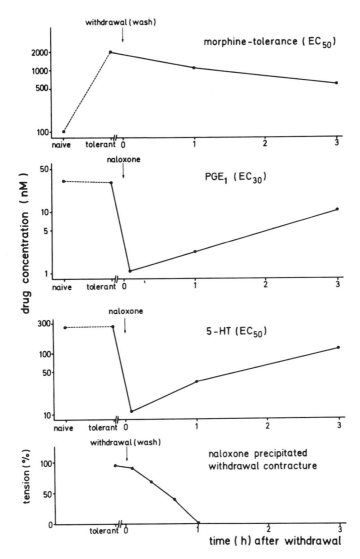

FIG. 1. Demonstration of tolerance, neuronal supersensitivity, and withdrawal contracture of the isolated longitudinal muscle–myenteric plexus preparation from morphine-tolerant/dependent guinea pigs. The strips were set up *in vitro* in the presence of 200 nM normorphine. Tests were conducted either before or after induction of withdrawal *(arrows)*. The median effective concentration (EC_{50} or EC_{30}) is plotted against time on a logarithmic scale. The intensity of withdrawal contracture precipitated by naloxone (50 nM) is expressed as percent of the twitch tension evoked by electrical stimulation (0.1 Hz, 60 V, 0.5 msec pulse duration). (Adapted from Schulz and Herz, ref. 37.)

of the neurons impinging on the muscle are cut off. Whether or not these differences are responsible for the inability of naloxone to precipitate a visible withdrawal sign in the vas deferens remains to be seen.

Experiments with Intact Animals

The existence of a general increase in neuronal excitability during opiate abstinence is obvious from the lowered seizure threshold observed in withdrawn animals (1,17). More detailed information on the location and nature of neuronal pathways undergoing a state of latent supersensitivity during opiate intake is obtained from behavioral studies showing an increased sensitivity of the central nervous system to certain specific effects of individual neurotransmitters or transmitter receptor agonists.

Thus there are several reports pointing to an increase in the effectiveness of catecholamine receptor agonists during opiate withdrawal to induce aggression (28,33), stereotypies (12), increased motor activity (41), circling (18), or dyskinesias (11). Also, some reports indicate an increased response to cholinergic agents (44) during abstinence from morphine.

In accord with data obtained from studies of abruptly withdrawn rats are recent observations showing remarkable alterations in the responsiveness to intracerebroventricularly administered neurotransmitters or neurotransmitter receptor agonists after interruption of morphine effects by naloxone (38). In these experiments, the test substances were injected after naloxone-induced withdrawal jumping had ceased (Fig. 2). Contrary to naloxone, transmitters such as dopamine (DA), norepinephrine, 5-HT (as well as the DA receptor agonist apomorphine, or the adrenoceptor agonist clonidine) were able to reinitiate jumping in a dose-dependent manner. Since all these substances, even at higher dosages, failed to induce jumping when applied to naive rats or to tolerant/dependent animals before precipitation of withdrawal, it seems appropriate to speak of "sensitization" to the test drugs, rather than to use the strictly defined term "supersensitivity" to describe the above phenomenon.

Of all transmitter receptor agonists tested, DA and apomorphine proved to be most effective to reinitiate jumping. These compounds proved to be effective even after 3 hr of continuous exposure of the animals to naloxone. After this time, however, norepinephrine, clonidine, and 5-HT had no effect. Acetylcholine and PGE_1 completely failed to reinitiate jumping.

Interestingly, the time course of decline of altered responsiveness to DA agonists after initiation of withdrawal shows some similarity to the time course at which supersensitivity to 5-HT disappears in the longitudinal muscle–myenteric plexus preparation of guinea pig. Nevertheless, one has to consider that, in contrast to the effect determined in the isolated tissue, the behavioral response observed in the intact animal does not strictly fulfill the pharmacological criteria for supersensitivity, that is, a shift to the left of the dose-response curve.

In an attempt to further investigate the mechanism of sensitization to neuro-

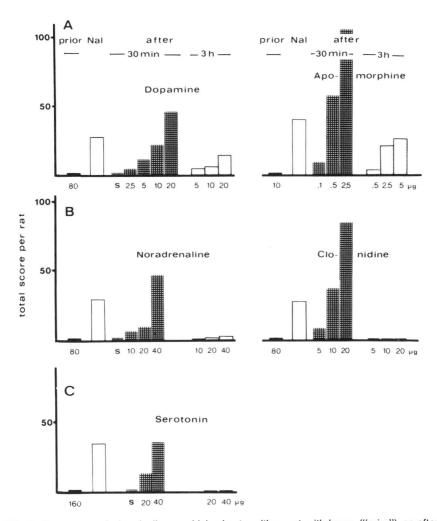

FIG. 2. Responses of chronically morphinized rats, either not withdrawn ("prior") or after naloxone (10 mg/kg, i.p.) -precipitated withdrawal, to intracerebroventricular (i.c.v.) administration of neurotransmitters or their receptor agonists. Naloxone-induced jumping *(open columns)* ceased after 20 to 40 min. Five minutes after cessation of jumping, the first i.c.v. injection of a drug or the vehicle (saline, S) was performed *(hatched columns)*. The second i.c.v. injection was conducted 3 hr *(stippled columns)* after the initial naloxone treatment. Each column represents the mean total score for jumping. Rats not withdrawn failed to respond to i.c.v. drug injection. *Abscissa,* doses (μg free base) given i.c.v. (From Schulz and Herz, ref. 38.)

transmitters and their agonists, experiments were performed to localize the site of action at which such sensitivity changes occurred (35). Previous experiments with rats revealed that the structures in which naloxone is most effective in precipitating withdrawal jumping (in addition to other withdrawal signs) are located periventricularly in the anterior part of the fossa rhomboidea, or the

posterior part of the periaqueductal gray, or both (29). It was interesting to
see if the same sites also represented the substrate for reinitiation of withdrawal
jumping by transmitters. This question is answered by findings presented in
Fig. 3. In these experiments, the spread of the drugs injected into the various
parts of the ventricular system (VS) was restricted by a plug placed in the
anterior part of the aqueductus mesencephali. The figure illustrates that apomorphine was highly effective in reinducing withdrawal jumping when injected
into the lateral ventricle and allowed to spread into the third ventricle, but
failed when injected into the fourth ventricle. In contrast, naloxone was highly
effective when injected into the fourth ventricle and rather ineffective in the
restricted anterior parts of the VS.

This dissociation between the sites of action of apomorphine and naloxone
for inducing jumping is an unexpected result. It may be discussed in relation
to Fig. 4 which represents various possibilities for the location of opiate and
DA receptors involved in these experiments.

In Fig. 4A, the opiate receptors (where naloxone acts after tolerance/depen-
dence development) and the receptors for neurotransmitters (or neuromodulators), for which supersensitivity (or sensitization) develops, are located on the

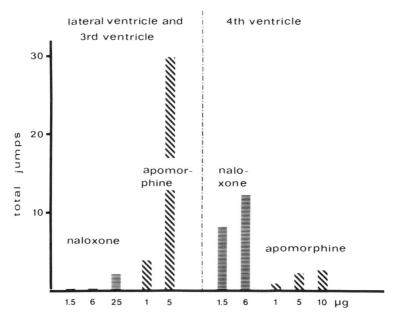

FIG. 3. Response of morphine-tolerant/dependent rats to intracerebroventricular (i.c.v.) injection of naloxone, or to apomorphine given i.c.v. 30 min after systemically applied naloxone
(2 mg/kg, i.p.). Intracerebroventricular injection was performed either into the anterior or posterior part of the ventricular system. Spread of the drug was prevented by insertion of an eucerine
plug into the mesencephalic aqueduct immediately before the i.c.v. drug injection. *Ordinate,*
mean total jumps per rat; *abscissa,* dose (μg free base) given i.c.v. (From Schulz et al., ref.
35.)

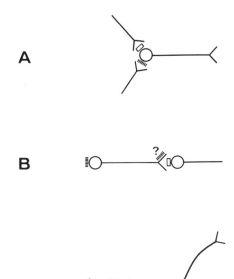

FIG. 4. Schematic representation of DA-morphine interactions discussed in an attempt to explain withdrawal jumping of tolerant/dependent rats caused either by naloxone or by apomorphine in previously withdrawn rats. Question marks indicate alternative locations of receptors. For details see text. (From Schulz et al., ref. 35.)

same neuron. Such a model seems to be applicable to opiate sensitivity in cultured neuroblastoma x glioma hybrid cells that develop supersensitivity for PGE_1 on chronic opiate treatment (19). Our observation of a dissociation in the sites of action of naloxone and DA excludes such a DA-morphine interaction at the same neuron as far as the withdrawal sign jumping is concerned.

Figure 4B simulates a situation induced by so-called "denervation supersensitivity" (23). In this case, a neuron "downstream" of that bearing the opiate receptors becomes supersensitive to neurotransmitters.

In Fig. 4C, the neuron(s) through which apomorphine acts is/are located "upstream" of those neurons involved in jumping and bearing the opiate receptors. Such apomorphine-affected neurons do not represent links in the neuronal circuit through which the withdrawal sign is mediated. In this case, dopaminergic mechanisms have, instead, a facilitatory function on the actions of the neurons that are "disinhibited" by naloxone and are thus probably in a state of hyperexcitation. The view of only a facilitatory influence of dopaminergic mechanisms on jumping is supported by previous experiments that showed that neuroleptics only partially block withdrawal jumping, even at high dosages (4).

Thus the results do not oppose the concept that neuronal supersensitivity is induced at the site of morphine action. Rather, the finding suggests that the altered response to apomorphine induced at naloxone-insensitive sites cannot be explained by the existence of specific supersensitivity to DA at this site. Instead, it is assumed that apomorphine might have activated some "normal" input to "dependent" neurons located at a remote site.

This close interrelationship between "normal" and "hyperreactive" neurons in the brain during opiate withdrawal seems also to have therapeutic consequences insofar as unexpected and altered responses may occur to all kind of drugs during withdrawal, independently of whether or not specific supersensitivity has occurred at the transmitter whose mechanism of action is affected by these drugs.

POSSIBLE MECHANISMS UNDERLYING CHANGES IN NEURONAL SENSITIVITY

An increase in responsiveness to a specific transmitter can be caused either by a qualitative or quantitative change of transmitter binding sites or by any of the mechanisms through which coupling of the transmitter is translated into a given effect. Preliminary data concerning opiate-induced changes in transmitter sensitivity support the latter possibility.

Changes at the Receptor Level

There is no evidence that development of opiate tolerance/dependence is associated with an altered binding of neurotransmitters to their receptors or with an increase in the number of transmitter receptors, at least as far as DA is concerned. Figure 5 compares the displacement of ^{3}H-spiroperidol, a DA receptor antagonist with high receptor affinity, by either DA or haloperidol from striatal membranes of naive rats, with that of tolerant/dependent rats (A. Czlonkowski and V. Höllt, *unpublished observations*). The curves obtained in both groups do not significantly differ from each other, indicating that neither the number nor the affinity of the DA receptors seemed to have changed during chronic opiate treatment. Thus the mechanism underlying opiate-induced dopaminergic supersensitivity apparently differs from that of neuroleptic-induced supersensitivity, which has been shown to be associated with an increase in the number of DA binding sites (5). This difference between opiates and neuroleptics might be explained by the fact that neuroleptics block DA receptors directly, whereas opiates seem to influence dopaminergic activity in some indirect way (3). On the other hand, the fact that the observed increase in binding sites after neuroleptic treatment was rather low (20%) suggested that mechanisms other than an increase in binding sites might be responsible for the observed increase in sensitivity to DA.

Any consideration of the possibility that changes in transmitter receptors may be responsible for the increased or altered transmitter responses during opiate withdrawal has to account for the existence of presynaptic or so-called

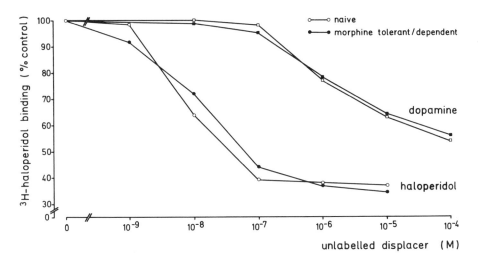

FIG. 5. Displacement of binding of ³H-haloperidol (2.5 nM) to rat striatal membranes of naive and morphine-tolerant rats by increasing amounts of unlabeled haloperidol and DA. Rats were rendered morphine-tolerant/dependent by s.c. implantation of six morphine pellets (75 mg) within 10 days. Each point represents the mean of three experiments. (From A. Czlonkowski and V. Höllt, *unpublished observations*.)

"auto-receptors" (39,42). Activation of such receptors leads to decreased neuronal activity, or reduction of transmitter output, or both, and thereby to the effects that counteract those induced by activation of postsynaptic receptors. The observed increase in response to transmitters or their agonists during withdrawal may theoretically be the result of reduction of such presynaptic receptors rather than the result of an increase in postsynaptic receptors (39). The occurrence of such supersensitivity has recently been suggested to be the underlying mechanism of so-called "agonist-induced supersensitivity" (30). The theory of this kind of supersensitivity is based on the concept that, after administration of a receptor agonist that possesses higher affinities for presynaptic than for postsynaptic receptors, the occupation of the former outlasts the occupation of the latter. Such long-lasting presynaptic inhibitory effects of agonists are thought to be compensated for by a reduction in the number of presynaptic receptors. The increasing evidence for a presynaptic location of opiate receptors (which, of course, does not exclude the additional possibility of postsynaptically located receptors) as well as the independently obtained evidence for inhibitory effects of opiates on transmitter release, favors the hypothesis that neurons affected in this way by opiates will compensate for the opiate action by reduction of a "redundant" inhibitory presynaptic mechanism. Preliminary findings have supported this idea by showing that the sedative effects of clonidine (thought to be the result of an action at presynaptic receptors to which clonidine has a higher affinity than to postsynaptic receptors) are converted into excitatory effects during withdrawal (45).

Besides the changes in sensitivity of pre- and postsynaptically located transmitter receptors on chronic drug exposure discussed above, great interest has been focused on the question: What happens to opiate receptors during the process of development of opiate tolerance and dependence? Do changes in the number or the affinity of opiate receptors represent a major factor in narcotic tolerance and dependence? Evidence available to date suggests that neither the number nor the binding affinities of opiate receptors are altered during chronic opiate exposure (22,26,40). Rather, it appears that the cell adapts to the prolonged inhibitory action of opiates, not with a reduction of opiate receptors, but with a reduction in the response of the cell to opiate binding. As discussed above, an enhanced sensitivity of such opiate-affected cells to excitatory transmitters may represent one of the mechanisms by which opiate effectiveness is reduced. The question then arises: Is prolonged blockade of opiate receptors by the opiate antagonist naloxone paralleled by changes opposite to those occurring after prolonged opiate receptor activation, e.g., an increased responsiveness to opiates coupled with unchanged opiate binding and decreased effectiveness of excitatory transmitters? Unexpectedly this was not the case. Figure 6 demonstrates that electrically stimulated longitudinal muscle-myenteric plexus preparations taken from guinea pigs chronically treated with naloxone develop supersensitivity to Met-enkephalin (Fig. 6A), whereas no change in sensitivity to 5-HT, PGE, or epinephrine was observed. This increase in response to enkephalin is paralleled by a 25 to 30% increase in the number of binding sites (Fig. 6B). Thus, as might be expected from the above considerations, the myenteric plexus responds to prolonged blockade of opiate receptors with an increase in efficacy of the opiate receptor system. However, this increase is associated with an increase in opiate binding sites and with an unaltered sensitivity to transmitters.

Cyclic Nucleotides

It is well established that adenosine $3',5'$-monophosphate (cyclic AMP) and guanosine $3',5'$-monophosphate (cyclic GMP) act as "second messengers" in synaptic transmission (16) and thus represent immediate links between coupling of transmitter and mediation of cell responses. It is suggested that changes in the function of these second messengers are closely related to supersensitivity phenomena (13). Clear evidence exists from opiate studies performed in neuroblastoma x glioma hybrid cells for an altered activity of adenylate cyclase during chronic opiate action in tolerant/dependent cells undergoing withdrawal (25). This increased activity manifests itself in supersensitivity to PGE_1, expressed by increased cyclic AMP formation. Again, this supersensitivity is thought to reflect compensatory processes (i.e., dependence) to the inhibitory effects of opiates on adenylate cyclase activity. The observation that the adenylate cyclase system of cells *in vitro* is apparently able to adapt not only to opiate-induced inhibition but also to adrenergic and cholinergic inhibitory effects (19) suggested that this system might represent a general homeostatic principle of the cell.

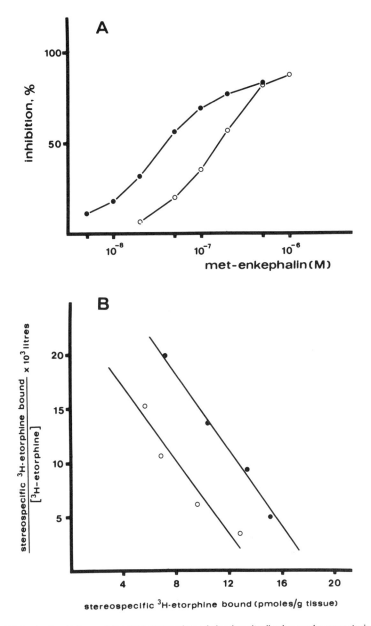

FIG. 6. Biological activity and binding properties of the longitudinal muscle–myenteric plexus preparation of the ileum taken from guinea pigs chronically treated with naloxone. **A:** The effect of Met-enkephalin to inhibit electrically evoked twitches of preparations from naive (○) and naloxone-treated (●) animals. The strips were washed, after set-up, for 3 hr (5-min intervals) before conducting the tests. **B:** The Scatchard plot of stereospecific ³H-etorphine binding of strips from naive (○) and naloxone-treated (●) animals undergoing the wash procedure described above. (From R. Schulz et al., *unpublished data.*)

However, findings obtained with rat brains concerning adaptive changes of the adenylate cyclase system to chronic opiate treatment conflict (8). Thus it seems difficult at present to evaluate the role of cyclic nucleotides in the behavioral correlates of neuronal supersensitivity accompanying chronic opiate action in the whole animal. For a more detailed discussion of this problem see the chapters by Collier and Klee, *this volume.*

Changes in the Neuronal Membrane

Biochemical changes in the "effector system" of cells, as described in the previous chapter, may manifest themselves electrophysiologically in a change of membrane potentials. Such connections have recently been stressed by the hypothesis that opiate-induced supersensitivity phenomena may reflect a partial depolarization of neuronal membranes (13,24). Such proposed changes in the resting potential of membranes would account for the apparently unspecific nature of the sensitivity changes observed during withdrawal.

The fact that the acutely induced changes of opiates at cell membranes are thought to be mediated by influences on the permeability or binding of ions, such as Na^+ and Ca^{2+}, suggests that opposite changes in such ionic mechanisms are responsible for the reversal of such acute effects during withdrawal. The possible involvement of ions in electrophysiological processes on the one hand, and in biochemical enzymatic activities on the other hand (15), suggests that the neurophysiologically determined changes in membrane stability during withdrawal are a reflection of the biochemically established changes in the cyclic AMP system.

Thus, in an attempt to elucidate the mechanism underlying opiate-induced changes in neuronal excitability, information obtained from different research levels has to be integrated, and the intimate relationship between phenomena established on the neurobiochemical or neurophysiological levels has to be considered. For instance, as recently pointed out (27), not only the binding of neurotransmitters to a receptor, which changes membrane properties, and the activity of the adenylate cyclase, but also functional changes in the cyclic AMP system might influence the binding of transmitters.

GENERAL DISCUSSION AND CONCLUSIONS

There is undisputed evidence from behavioral data as well as from pharmacological and biochemical *in vitro* findings that prolonged exposure to opiates is associated with a latent development of increased neuronal sensitivity (20). However, the capability to induce such changes in neuronal sensitivity is not specific to opiates but seems to be a common characteristic of both addictive and nonaddictive drugs that disrupt neuronal transmission by various mechanisms. Thus supersensitivity phenomena are observed after prolonged administration of addictive central depressants such as alcohol and barbiturates (21) as well as after continued exposure to nonaddictive depressants such as neuroleptics (5,14), catecholamine synthesis inhibitors (31), or drugs that affect transmission in noradrenergic or cholinergic systems (2,10,43).

The way in which such differently induced changes in neuronal sensitivity are manifested is dependent on the specificity of the individual drugs. Thus withdrawal from drugs, like alcohol and barbiturates, that unspecifically depress more or less the whole central nervous system, leads to a more general hyperexcitation, expressed in a lowering of the seizure threshold and in the occurrence of spontaneous convulsions (21). On the other hand, interruption of chronic treatment with neuroleptic drugs that predominantly disrupt dopaminergic transmission leads to a specific diskinetic syndrome, probably owing to increased neuronal sensitivity in restricted brain regions involved in extrapyramidal motor functions. A most differentiated and complex symptomatology is seen when chronic opiate exposure is interrupted. In addition to signs such as increased susceptibility to seizures (a sign that opiate withdrawal has in common with alcohol and barbiturate withdrawal), a great variety of distinct signs occur, suggesting participation of all individual brain sites that possess specific opiate receptors.

From this it follows that cellular supersensitivity to neurotransmitters might represent one basic mechanism underlying the development of tolerance to and dependence on opiates and other drugs. However, the property of opiates to induce such mechanisms cannot, by itself, explain the phenomenon of "drug addiction." The important point seems to be in what brain site or functional systems the changes in neuronal sensitivity take place. Thus the fact that neuronal systems involved in the regulation of mood and drive are primarily affected by opiates may be important for the highly addictive properties of these drugs, as well as for the highly aversive character of the syndrome following withdrawal of these drugs.

Recent theories go so far as to consider the occurrence of changes in neuronal sensitivity as no longer a pathophysiological phenomenon and to suggest that a normal regulatory mechanism for physiological functioning of the brain lies behind such phenomenon (9,25).

REFERENCES

1. Adler, M. W., Lin, C., Smith, K. P., Tresky, R., and Gildenberg, P. L. (1974): Lowered seizure threshold as a part of the narcotic abstinence syndrome in rats. *Psychopharmacologia,* 35:243–247.
2. Baudry, M., Martres, M. P., and Schwartz, J. C. (1976): Modulation in the sensitivity of noradrenergic receptors in the CNS studied by the responsiveness of the cyclic AMP system. *Brain Res.,* 116:111–124.
3. Bläsig, J. (1978): On the role of brain catecholamines in acute and chronic opiate action. In: *Developments in Opiate Research,* edited by A. Herz, pp. 279–356. Marcel Dekker, New York.
4. Bläsig, J., Gramsch, C., Laschka, E., and Herz, A. (1976): The role of dopamine in withdrawal jumping in morphine dependent rats. *Arzneim. Forsch.,* 26:19–21.
5. Burt, D. R., Creese, I., and Snyder, S. H. (1977): Antischizophrenic drugs: Chronic treatment elevates dopamine receptor binding in brain. *Science,* 196:326–328.

6. Collier, H. O. J. (1965): A general theory of the genesis of drug dependence by induction of recepto.*. Nature, 205:181–182.
7. Collier, H. O. J. (1968): Supersensitivity and dependence. Nature, 220:228–231.
8. Collier, H. O. J., and Francis, D. L. (1979): A pharmacological analysis of opiate tolerance/ dependence. In: The Basis of Addiction, edited by J. Fishman, pp. 281–298. Dahlem Konferenzen, Berlin.
9. Deguchi, T., and Axelrod, J. (1973): Supersensitivity and subsensitivity of the β-adrenergic receptor in pineal gland regulated by catecholamine transmitter. Proc. Natl. Acad. Sci., USA, 70:2411–2414.
10. Dix, R. K., and Johnson, E. M., Jr. (1977): Withdrawal syndrome upon cessation of chronic clonidine treatment in rats. Eur. J. Pharmacol., 44:153–159.
11. Eibergen, R. D., and Carlson, K. R. (1975): Dyskinesias elicited by methamphetamine: Susceptibility by former methadone-consuming monkeys. Science, 190:588–590.
12. Eibergen, R. D., and Carlson, K. R. (1976): Behavioral evidence for dopaminergic supersensitivity following chronic treatment with methadone or chlorpromazine in the guinea pig. Psychopharmacology, 48:139–146.
13. Fleming, W. W. (1976): Variable sensitivity of excitable cells: Possible mechanism and biological significance. In: Reviews of Neuroscience, Vol. 2, edited by S. Ehrenpreis and I. J. Kopin, pp. 43–90. Raven Press, New York.
14. Gianutsos, G., Drawbaugh, R. B., Hynes, M. D., and Lal, H. (1974): Behavioral evidence for dopaminergic supersensitivity after chronic haloperidol. Life Sci., 14:887–898.
15. Gnegy, M. E., Lucchetti, A., and Costa, E. (1977): Correlation between drug-induced supersensitivity of dopamine dependent striatal mechanisms and the increase in striatal content of the Ca^{2+} regulated protein activator of the cAMP phosphodiesterase. Naunyn Schmiedebergs Arch. Pharmacol., 301:121–127.
16. Greengard, P. (1976): Possible role for cyclic nucleotides and phosphorylated membrane proteins in postsynaptic actions of neurotransmitters. Nature, 260:101–108.
17. Greer, C. A., Alpern, H. P., and Collins, A. C. (1976): Increased CNS sensitivity to flurothyl as a measure of physical dependence in mice following morphine, phenobarbital, and ethanol treatment. Life Sci., 18:1375–1382.
18. Halliwell, J. V., and Kumar, R. (1977): Influence of morphine dependence and withdrawal on circling behavior in rats with unilateral nigral lesions. Br. J. Pharmacol., 59:454P.
19. Hamprecht, B. (1978): Opiates and cyclic nucleotides. In: Developments in Opiate Research, edited by A. Herz, pp. 357–406. Marcel Dekker, New York.
20. Herz, A., and Schulz, R. (1978): Changes in neuronal sensitivity during addictive processes. In: The Basis of Addiction, edited by J. Fishman. Dahlem Konferenzen, Berlin (in press).
21. Herz, A., Zieglgänsberger, W., Schulz, R., Fry, J. P., and Satoh, M. (1977): Neuronal aspects of opiate dependence and tolerance in comparison to central depressants. In: Alcohol Intoxication and Withdrawal, Vol. 3B, edited by Milton M. Gross, pp. 117–140. Plenum, New York.
22. Höllt, V., Dum, J., Bläsig, J., Schubert, P., and Herz, A. (1975): Comparison of in vivo and in vitro parameters of opiate receptor binding in naive and tolerant/dependent rodents. Life Sci., 16:1823–1828.
23. Jaffe, J. H., and Sharpless, S. K. (1968): Pharmacological denervation supersensitivity in the central nervous system: A theory of physical dependence. Res. Publ. Assoc. Res. Nerv. Ment. Dis., 46:226–246.
24. Johnson, S. M., Westfall, D. P., Howard, S. A., and Fleming, W. W. (1978): Sensitivities of the isolated ileal longitudinal smooth muscle-myenteric plexus and hypogastric nerve-vas deferens of the guinea pig after chronic morphine pellet implantation. J. Pharmacol. Exp. Ther., 204:54–66.
25. Klee, W. A. (1979): Dual regulations of adenylate cyclase: A biochemical model for opiate tolerance and dependence. In: The Basis of Addiction, edited by J. Fishman, pp. 431–440. Dahlem Konferenzen, Berlin.
26. Klee, W. A., and Streaty, R. A. (1974): Narcotic receptor sites in morphine-dependent rats. Nature, 248:61–63.
27. Kolata, G. B. (1977): Hormone receptors: How are they regulated? Science, 196:747–748, 800.
28. Lal, H. (1975): Narcotic dependence, narcotic action and dopamine receptors. Life Sci., 17:483–496.
29. Laschka, E., Teschemacher, H., Mehraein, P., and Herz, A. (1976): Sites of action of morphine involved in the development of physical dependence in rats. Psychopharmacologia, 46:141–147.

30. Martres, M. P., Costentin, J., Baudry, M., Marcais, H., Protais, P., and Schwartz, J. C. (1977): Long-term changes in the sensitivity of pre- and postsynaptic dopamine receptors in mouse striatum evidenced by behavioral and biochemical studies. *Brain Res.,* 136:319–337.

31. Moore, K. E., and Thornburg, J. E. (1975): Drug-induced dopaminergic supersensitivity. In: *Advances in Neurology, Vol. 9: Dopaminergic Mechanisms,* edited by D. B. Calne, T. N. Chase, and A. Barbeau, pp. 93–104. Raven Press, New York.

32. Platt, J. J., and Labate, C. (1976): *Heroin Addiction: Theory, Research and Treatment.* Wiley-Interscience, New York.

33. Puri, S. K., and Lal, H. (1974): Reduced threshold to pain induced aggression specifically related to morphine dependence. *Psychopharmacologia,* 35:237–241.

34. Schulz, R. (1978): The use of isolated organs to study the mechanism of action of narcotic analgesics. In: *Developments in Opiate Research,* edited by A. Herz, pp. 241–277. Marcel Dekker, New York.

35. Schulz, R., Bläsig, J., Laschka, E., and Herz, A. (1978): Site of naloxone-precipitated opiate withdrawal dissociates from that at which apomorphine reinitiates this phenomenon. *Naunyn Schmiedelbergs Arch. Pharmacol.,* 305:1–4.

36. Schulz, R., and Goldstein, A. (1973): Morphine tolerance and supersensitivity to 5-hydroxytryptamine in the myenteric plexus of the guinea-pig. *Nature,* 244:168–170.

37. Schulz, R., and Herz, A. (1976): Aspects of opiate dependence in the myenteric plexus of the guinea-pig. *Life Sci.,* 19:1117–1128.

38. Schulz, R., and Herz, A. (1977): Naloxone precipitated withdrawal reveals sensitization to neurotransmitters in morphine tolerant/dependent rats. *Naunyn Schmiedebergs Arch. Pharmacol.,* 299:95–99.

39. Seeman, P., Tedesco, J. L., Lee, T., Chau-Wong, M., Muller, P., Bowles, J., Whitaker, P. M., McManus, C., Tittler, M., Weinreich, P., Friend, W. C., and Brown, G. M. (1978): Dopamine receptors in the central nervous system. *Fed. Proc.,* 37:130–136.

40. Simon, E. J., and Hiller, J. M. (1978): In vitro studies on opiate receptors and their ligands. *Fed. Proc.,* 37:141–146.

41. Smee, M. L., and Overstreet, D. H. (1976): Alterations in the effects of dopamine agonists and antagonists on general activity in rats following chronic morphine treatment. *Psychopharmacology,* 49:125–130.

42. Starke, K. (1977): Regulation of noradrenaline release by presynaptic receptor systems. *Rev. Physiol. Biochem. Pharmacol.,* 77:1–124.

43. Sulser, F., Vetulani, J., and Mobley, P. L. (1978): Mode of action of antidepressant drugs. *Biochem. Pharmacol.,* 27:257–261.

44. Vasquez, B. J., Overstreet, D. H., and Russel, R. W. (1974): Psychopharmacological evidence for increase in receptor sensitivity following chronic morphine treatment. *Psychopharmacologia,* 38:287–302.

45. Zebrowska-Lupina, I., Przegalinski, E., Sloniec, M., and Kleinrok, Z. (1977): Clonidine-induced locomotor hyperactivity in rats: The role of central postsynaptic α-adrenoceptors. *Naunyn Schmiedebergs Arch. Pharmacol.,* 297:227–231.

Mechanisms of Pain and Analgesic Compounds,
edited by R. F. Beers, Jr., and E. G. Bassett.
Raven Press, New York © 1979.

35. Discussion

Moderator: H. O. J. Collier

J. N. Johannessen: I have two comments for Drs. Collier and Klee. In light of what has been said this morning, I would like to suggest a theoretical possibility and ask for your comments. The possibility is: that the opiate receptor itself is one of the membrane proteins that can be phosphorylated by cyclic AMP and protein kinase, and phosphorylation is necessary for the receptor to be viable.

In this case, it would be a nice feedback mechanism so that a large pulse of an opiate would decrease cyclic AMP levels and consequently the number of viable receptors, thus eventually decreasing the overstimulative effect of that opiate, and release the adenylate cyclase from inhibition, tending to restore the cyclic AMP levels to normal, which I think is part of the model Dr. Klee presented.

Is there any evidence for any phosphorylation of membrane proteins that might be receptors?

W. Klee: I think it is an interesting idea that phosphorylation might play a role in the adaptation. But I am not so sure it is all that reasonable to postulate that it is phosphorylation of the receptors because most workers who have looked at receptors in cells of tolerant animals have not found any qualitative or quantitative changes in receptor binding properties.

It is perhaps more likely that there is a phosphorylation of the adenylate cyclase or a coupling protein involved in that system. I don't know of any good evidence one way or the other.

H. O. J. Collier: I do not see how an opiate receptor could be both a part of adenylate cyclase and a protein that is phosphorylated by cyclic AMP and protein kinase. The evidence that we have supports the former role for the opiate receptor. There is evidence, however, that there is a compensating increased activity of protein kinase in morphine dependence [Clark et al. (1972), *Biochem. Pharmacol.,* 21:1989; and Kuriyama et al. (1978), *Jpn. J. Pharmacol.,* 28:73].

J. N. Johannessen: There is some recent evidence that short bursts of stimulation, either electrical or chemical, in nerve tissue, can cause long-term changes in cyclic AMP levels. Has Dr. Klee subjected his cells to a short burst of opiates and looked for time-dependent changes in the cyclic AMP levels?

W. Klee: We haven't really done that kind of experiment. We have done short-term exposures of cells to opiates and find in general that you do need a number of hours of single exposures to see an effect. We haven't done multiple short bursts, if that is your question.

J. J. Feigenbaum: Dr. North, you mentioned that the effect of microiontophoretic applications of opiates in the region of single neurons almost always inhibits activity in such neurons and that this is less likely to be due to inhibition than to release of postsynaptic inhibitory effect. Why do you feel that inhibition release is less likely?

R. A. North: No, I think I said that in most of these experiments the site of action cannot be determined unequivocally. Many people interpret the results as a direct action on the neuron whose activity is being recorded. There are possibilities that it is acting presynaptically to depress the chronic, ongoing release of an excitatory transmitter.

The best evidence offered against this is the fact that opiate blocks the excitation of these cells by glutamate. Glutamate, of course, may be acting directly postsynaptically or may itself be acting to cause release of an excitatory transmitter. However, glutamate seems to be acting, in most circumstances, directly on the neuron whose activity is being recorded, because glutamate always causes an excitation, whereas if glutamate itself were acting on other neurons and thereby affecting the cell whose activity is being recorded, then you would not expect it always to excite.

So I think the evidence is reasonably good that, if morphine inhibits the glutamate-induced excitation, this is likely to be a direct inhibitory action on the cell from which you recorded.

F. Sicuteri: I would like to comment on Dr. Herz's paper. We have also observed, in clinical pharmacology, the phenomenon of supersensitivity toward 5-HT after a few days of treatment with morphine.

We have observed a 20-fold increase in sensitivity to serotonin and a five- to tenfold increase in sensitivity to dopamine. This supersensitivity occurs after only 3 days of treatment with clinical doses of morphine. It is very singular that in those patients who are serious migraine sufferers, after abstinence from morphine, severe systemic pain arises, as has been described in an intense abstinence syndrome.

H. O. J. Collier: May I ask, are these reactions you observed mediated centrally or is the action of 5-HT on the nerves supplying the veins?

F. Sicuteri: On the vein, but by which mechanism I don't know.

F. W. L. Kerr: I have two questions, one for Dr. Klee, and that concerns the work you showed by Sharma et al. in 1975. You didn't have time to discuss it, I know.

I was most intrigued by the enormous change in activity of the enkephalins caused by small changes in the structure of the molecule, resulting in increases up to 10,000- and 30,000-fold. Has it been determined whether this correlates with changes in pain and its effectiveness on pain responses?

W. Klee: I don't believe I can answer that question. In general, enkephalins have not been found to have very good analgesic activity. At least they are very short-acting analgesics in general. I don't know enough about the testing that has been done with these analogs; perhaps someone here knows more about it than I do. But I wouldn't expect that there is a great deal of analgesic activity in any of those compounds shown except perhaps in the bottom one, which is the Sandoz compound that shows oral analgesic activity. That one is a good deal weaker than enkephalin in our adenylate cyclase assay and yet it is a more potent analgesic compound. So, there is no obvious correlation.

F. W. L. Kerr: Does anybody else on the panel have an answer to that question? It seems very important if you can get an increase in effectiveness up to 30,000 times. John Hughes, do you have a comment?

J. Hughes: I think the point is, you can't relate analgesic potency to receptor activity. Analgesia is a result of a collection of effects. You are dealing with the crossing of the molecules across various barriers, particularly the blood brain barrier; and, even injecting intracerebrally, you have problems of distribution and metabolism. I think it would be very unwise to compare these *in vitro* models directly with analgesia. Analgesia really doesn't tell you too much about the direct receptor interactions, so unless you are dealing with a molecule about which you know the pharmacodynamics very well, I don't think you can draw any conclusions at all.

A. Herz: I think there are some data that show a rather close relationship between receptor affinities of stable enkephalin derivatives and analgesic potency after intraventricular injection in rats.

For example, the extremely potent Sandoz compound is 10 times more active in analgesia then beta endorphin, and, I think, 10 times more active than D-alanine amide, so there is some correlation in spite of the fact that there are not enough data to compare effects directly.

H. W. Kosterlitz: I think this compound is very interesting. I was very intrigued by one of Klee's findings because, on his neuroblastoma cells, this compound has completely different receptor affinities from those of methionine-enkephalin. It is very potent in the guinea pig ileum and has a high affinity for the naltrexone binding sites of the guinea pig brain, but has lost a great deal of its affinity for the leucine-enkephalin sites just as it has lost its affinity to the receptor of the neuroblastoma cell. But I don't think that this is necessarily the only explanation for the high analgesic activity of this compound, which is very resistant to the degrading activities of enzymes. This fact may facilitate the passage of a greater proportion through the blood brain barrier.

A. Herz: No. The Sandoz compound has great difficulty entering the brain and, if one compares the relative potency of analgesics, including enkephalins, for instance, with compounds such as fentanyl, one finds that one needs only about a 10-fold dose to get an effect after systemic application in relation to intraventricular application. In morphine this ratio is about 100 to 1, but in the case of the Sandoz compound, the ratio between the effective doses of systemic and intraventricular application is 20,000 to 1. It means that this compound has great difficulty entering the brain. The reason why it is effective at all after systemic application is that it has an extremely high receptor affinity and so a very small amount is sufficient to get an effect.

H. W. Kosterlitz: It has a very high affinity to the binding site which is presented by naltrexone and relatively low affinity to the enkephalin binding site.

P. R. Myers: Dr. Klee, were the data you discussed on the effects of PGE_1 and morphine on NG 108–15 cells taken from exponential growth phase or from differentiated cells, and also, did you find a difference between the two growth states?

W. Klee: That is a good question. Most of our work is done with cells following their exponential growth phase. The long-term culture experiments with opiates were done both with exponentially growing cells and with stationary type cells. We haven't found any differences in dependence related to growth rates.

Most of the experiments were not done with dibutyryl cyclic AMP–treated cells, if that is what you are asking. So no, they are not the most highly differentiated possible cells.

P. R. Myers: Dr. North, in your studies on postsynaptic effects of morphine, have you ever noted a biphasic effect of morphine where one dose is excitatory and another dose inhibitory?

R. A. North: Yes, it is the other way around. The inhibitory effect, which is sensitive to naloxone, occurs at a lower concentration. If you increase the concentration, you sometimes find excitatory effects that are not antagonized by naloxone; but naloxone-sensitive effects appear to be always inhibitory.

H. W. Kosterlitz: I would like to ask Dr. Herz one more point about the Sandoz compound. What is the basis for your statement that it doesn't penetrate the brain easily? Is it based on direct estimation of the entry of the labeled compound?

A. Herz: May I repeat what I have tried to say? In the case of a lipophilic compound, which we know enters the brain easily, the relationship between intraventricular and systemically applied dosages is in the range of 10. That means that it easily penetrates the brain. Morphine is a rather hydrophilic compound. It has difficulty entering the brain. There is a relationship between equipotent doses in the range of 100 or 200. In the case of the Sandoz compound, this relationship is in the range of 20,000, indicating very great difficulty entering the brain.

H. W. Kosterlitz: That could be due to the very high distribution in the periphery. I think it is a terribly important point, the entry into the brain. I think we really should have direct evidence of the rate of entry of the labeled compound into the brain before we can be certain about this particular question.

F. W. L. Kerr: Dr. Klee, you briefly mentioned some of the effects of cycloheximide on the development of tolerance to morphine. I wonder if you could expand on that?

The second part of the question is if acetylcholine or epinephrine will induce further changes on the adenylate cyclase activity in morphine-dependent cells?

W. Klee: I am not sure I understand the second question, but we have done a number of experiments that have shown that cycloheximide, at concentrations that almost completely inhibit protein synthesis in general, does not inhibit the acquisition or the increase in adenylate cyclase activity, or at least when they do so, it is only a partial inhibition and it usually takes place only in very long-term experiments, where we often see a clear indication of cycloheximide toxicity in the paradigm.

F. W. L. Kerr: Are the changes in cyclic AMP in the morphine-dependent cells comparable with those that you get in the cells exposed to the actions of acetylcholine and norepinephrine?

W. Klee: If I understand you correctly, I think the answer is yes. I believe I showed a slide with some data from the work of Sabol and Nirenberg, and of Nathanson, Kline, and Nirenberg, in which they showed the same kind of increases in the adenylate cyclase activity. I didn't show you cyclic AMP levels in the cells. They also change in the same way as in the opiate-treated cells.

P. S. Lietman: Since opiates suppress the behavioral excitation in rats caused by methylxanthines, I would like to ask Dr. Collier if he thinks that the opiates could be used to treat aminophylline poisoning. This is characterized by convulsions and is not uncommon.

H. O. J. Collier: I think that is an interesting suggestion for use in emergencies. Only relatively small doses of morphine are needed to suppress the excitatory effects of methylxanthines in rats. Naloxone should probably be avoided as an antagonist of morphine, however, because in the presence of 3-isobutyl-1-methylxanthine (IBMX), morphine tends to readily induce sensitivity to naloxone.

Mechanisms of Pain and Analgesic Compounds,
edited by R. F. Beers, Jr., and E. G. Bassett.
Raven Press, New York © 1979.

36. Introduction to Section F: New Leads for the Development of Analgesics

Julián E. Villarreal

Instituto Miles de Terapéutica Experimental México, D. F., México

Much of the work presented in this volume owes a great deal to the impetus provided by a systematic research program started in 1929 under the auspices of the then called Committee on Drug Addiction of the National Research Council (U.S.A.). One of the primary objectives of this research program was the synthesis of drugs "having little tendency to cause addiction, which may serve to replace morphine, heroin, and other dangerous narcotics in their therapeutic applications" (1). A parallel objective of this program was to find better methods for the prevention and treatment of narcotic dependence through "research into the true nature of addiction." One leading figure in this program was Nathan B. Eddy who was one of the initiators of the enterprise and who, until his recent death, provided not only much of the drive for all of the work involved but also accurate direction, together with the recruitment into the objectives of the program of chemists, pharmacologists, and clinical investigators from universities, the drug industry, and governmental research institutions. This program has been exemplary of the type of team effort that our society is capable of integrating. The program started with a clear and distinct problem that led not only to the synthesis of a very large number of new compounds but also to the development of animal models in which to assess the desirable and undesirable effects of the new compounds, as well as the development of clinical procedures that could yield quantitative evaluations of the effects of the new drugs in man.

Quite independently of its actual or potential achievements, the search for dependence-free analgesics has contributed enormously to our understanding of the nature of the actions of opioids and related drugs, including the nature of opioid dependence. Studies on the biological actions of the many chemical classes of compounds so far synthetized have produced a vast body of knowledge that permits solid pharmacological generalizations. This body of knowledge has made possible the valuable recent studies of the actions of opioids and their antagonists at the level of molecular biology. The efforts to develop biological preparations that would allow the evaluation of new drugs led to the discovery of endogenous substances with opioid-like actions. The overall effect of the program of search for dependence-free morphine substitutes is an outstanding example that contradicts a notion that unfortunately is very widespread; i.e., that the transfer of information and the origin of new knowledge is unidirectional from the so-called basic sciences to applied sciences. The flow of new knowledge and of the mechanisms that test its general validity is multidirectional between all the levels and disciplines that bear on the issue.

In spite of the preparation of large numbers of new analgesics, no significant separation between analgesic activity and physiological dependence production was achieved until the 1950s, when opioid antagonists began receiving attention as potential analgesics. An almost accidental clinical discovery revealing that the opioid antagonist nalorphine has pain-relieving properties was followed by a study finding no dependence capacity for this drug. Strong dysphoric effects precluded the clinical use of nalorphine as an analgesic, but the interest created by its unprecedented lack of dependence capacity led to the synthesis and study of many other narcotic-antagonist analgesics.

The narcotic-antagonist analgesics first studied were found to have a set of apparently distinct pharmacological properties. Physical dependence capacity was found to be low in those antagonists that were tested on chronic administration. Soon, however, the picture of the pharmacology of the antagonist-analgesics changed considerably. An increasing diversity of patterns of action emerged. Some of the newer antagonists produce significant degrees of physical dependence. Some chemical analogs of the antagonist-analgesics do not act as antagonists and do not substitute for morphine in morphine-dependent monkeys. There is a drug, buprenorphine, that has clear morphine-like effects on single dose administration, yet its chronic administration leads to only minimal signs of physiological dependence.

Adding to the richness of leads in the field of compounds related to the opioids, analgesic properties have been discovered in structures related to the cannabinoids.

The transfer of promising new analgesics from the stages of preclinical and clinical pharmacology to the possibility of use in medicine requires the prior identification of potential for compulsive self-administration and for morphine-like dependence capacity. The methodologies to accomplish this and the problems presented by the newer compounds with peculiar profiles of action will make up a considerable portion of the present section.

The title of "New Leads" employs the term lead in a general sense—not in the restricted sense in which a lead is a clue that gives insight into the solution of one problem. In this section, leads are presented as clues for action or as objectives for focusing effort. Such leads come from theory, from puzzling new findings, from methodology, and from clearly defined medically and socially desirable objectives.

REFERENCE

1. Small, L. F., Eddy, N. B., Mosettig, E., and Himmelsbach, C. K. (1938): Studies on drug addiction. *Public Health Rep.,* Suppl. No. 138, U.S. Government Printing Office, Washington, D.C.

Mechanisms of Pain and Analgesic Compounds,
edited by R. F. Beers, Jr., and E. G. Bassett.
Raven Press, New York © 1979.

37. A Reformulation of the Dual-Action Model of Opioid Dependence: Opioid-Specific Neuronal Kindling

Julián E. Villarreal and Antonio Castro

Instituto Miles de Terapéutica Experimental, México, D.F., México

INTRODUCTION

The discovery of endogenous substances with morphine-like actions has brought about the most consequential change in our entire perspective about the pharmacology of the drugs traditionally designated as narcotic analgesics. Even a casual onlooker can no longer fail to perceive the rich pharmacological possibilities of drugs derived from morphine and from its pharmacological relatives. Also, no longer can anyone afford to regard phenomena associated with acute or chronic treatment with morphine and related drugs as simply queer reactions without broad physiological meaning and consider them as simply the result of chance interactions of certain foreign chemicals with organisms. Finally, no longer can anyone afford to regard the actions of the numerous compounds related to the classical opioids—but that possess significantly different pharmacological profiles—as the actions of peculiar, nonclassical substances with little fundamental meaning. Many of these special drugs are not only potential or actual therapeutic tools but are also instruments that are helping in the identification and dissection of basic neural physiological and biochemical mechanisms.

This chapter is written in the spirit of search for new and basic significance in the accumulated knowledge we possess about the pharmacology of "exogenous" morphines. This knowledge has clear pertinence to the study of endogenous substances with morphine-like actions and to the mechanisms of pain and other neural functions. The intention is also that the concepts and results presented here may clarify certain pharmacological puzzles and stimulate interest as well in the development of preparations and strategies that may help the identification of new analgesics with patterns of action that may render them advantageous for clinical use.

No attempt will be made to cover even a considerable part of the material on the pharmacology of synthetic morphine-like substances. The focus will be on phenomena related to physiological dependence. This chapter has been arranged to deal first with a reformulation of the dual-action model of opioid dependence, initially proposed by Tatum et al. in 1929 (23), and now revised in the light of evidence accumulated over the last 15 years. Dependence is proposed to consist of the activation of an opioid-specific kindling mechanism that, when triggered, gives rise to abstinence or abstinence-like effects. The second section reviews important abstinence-like phenomena of large magnitude, which have been generally overlooked and which cannot be accounted for on the assumption that they result from the removal of a narcotic from its sites of action. Analysis of the nature of these peculiar abstinence-like phenomena gives support to the present formulation of the mechanism of opioid dependence and such phenomena are thereby integrated in a single ensemble with the more conventionally known facts about dependence. A third section presents some new findings about opioid dependence *in vitro,* which also support the views on the mechanisms of dependence presented here and which may stimulate a widening of vision about the mechanisms and possible physiological roles of what we still, by tradition, call dependence.

Difficulties have risen in a progressively increasing fashion with the use of terms such as dependence and abstinence or withdrawal syndrome. These terms originate from an historical sequence of events in the development of knowledge in the field. There are tolerated instances of syntactic awkwardness like the expression "antagonist-precipitated withdrawal." A more important reason for concern is that these traditional expressions may impose restrictions on our thinking about the subject. Since the mechanisms of what we call dependence and abstinence are activated by endogenous substances with morphine-like actions, such mechanisms are likely to play parts in physiological phenomena, for which terms like dependence and abstinence may be wholly inappropriate. Therefore, in this chapter we will move in a direction that may help remedy this problem. In order not to lose contact with historical or clinical contexts, most of the time we will use expressions such as "naloxone-precipitated abstinence." However, we will also use more descriptive expressions with precedence in the general physiological or pharmacological literature; for instance, "superreactivity to naloxone." The term superreactivity was proposed by Cannon and Rosenblueth in 1949 (2) to designate the state of a tissue (organism) that responds to certain stimuli with responses that exceed the maxima obtained under basal or control conditions.

Physical or physiological dependence has presented outstanding difficulties for clean and precise experimental analysis. Physiological dependence is generally conceived as an abnormal physiological condition induced by chronic administration of narcotics that remains *covert* as long as continuous drug exposure is maintained, but that on drug withdrawal leads to a series of gross physiopathological events known as the abstinence syndrome. Thus, physical dependence is a term designating an "intervening" variable that remains covert and inaccessible to direct measurement.

For purposes of clinical management and for the assessment of the degree of dependence capacity of new drugs, the covert nature of physical dependence presents no major difficulties. The objectives of those dealing with these problems can be met by the qualitative identification of the abstinence syndrome and by the assessment of its magnitude. However, for the purposes of experimental analysis, the covert nature of physical dependence and the current impossibility of its direct measurement present serious problems that too often have gone unrecognized and thus have caused some naive laboratory work and also a good share of inadequate interpretations and inferences. The model of dependence advanced here proposes a basic mechanism about its nature that is verifiable and that we think will improve the possibilities of clean experimental analysis of the phenomenon.

A simple listing of a few of the different possible ways of indirectly measuring physical dependence brings out some of the questions that investigators in this field must face. At least four types of variables can be mentioned that could be considered as possible "measures" of narcotic physical dependence.

(a) How much physiological disorder occurs after drug withdrawal (i.e., the intensity of the abstinence syndrome).

(b) How much narcotic is being administered (i.e., the maintenance dose).

(c) The intensity of the abstinence syndrome precipitated by the administration of narcotic antagonists.

(d) How much narcotic is needed to relieve abstinence at the time when the maintenance drug has been reasonably well eliminated from tissues (i.e., abstinence-suppression dose-response curves). This last procedure would determine how much drug is needed in an abstinent system or organism to restore it to its base-line level of function.

There is almost no information available generated by procedures of type (d), but it is known that measurements obtained in procedures of types (a) and (c) yield results that are not necessarily congruent. Two cases in point here are given by the effects of methadone in man, and by those of diphenoxylate in the monkey. High levels of physiological dependence during chronic exposure to these drugs are revealed by abstinence syndromes of high intensity precipitated by narcotic antagonists; yet, termination of drug treatment leads to abstinence syndromes of only mild or minimal intensity, probably because of the long washout constants of these drugs.

Further, the severity of the abstinence syndrome does not increase indefinitely with increments in the dosage level of chronically administered narcotic. In the rhesus monkey, using gross observations of the intact animal, the abstinence syndrome obtained after withdrawal from a regimen of 150 mg/kg/day of morphine (9) is not significantly more severe than that obtained after withdrawal from a regimen of 12 mg/kg/day of the same drug (3). In confirmation of this, it has been found that the magnitude of abstinence hypothermia of monkeys maintained on 12 mg/kg/day of morphine (7) is of exactly the same order of magnitude as the abstinence hypothermia obtained in monkeys maintained on 200 mg/kg/day of the drug (12). As with any other indirect measurement of drug action, questions immediately arise on whether the limitations of the response observed represent the limits of the terminal response system or the limits of the primary basic change in the causal chain that drives the overt response system. It must be noted, however, that in spite of the fact that the maximal level for the severity of morphine abstinence in the monkey is reached with dosages as low as 12 mg/kg/day, other phenomena related to dependence do not have the same ceiling. Most deserving of attention is the fact that increases in the daily dose of morphine beyond 12 mg/kg/day, although they do not lead to abstinence syndromes of greater severity, continue to produce increases in the sensitivity of the monkey to the abstinence-precipitating effects of narcotic antagonists (13).

Way et al. (29) were the first to suggest that increases in sensitivity to the abstinence-precipitating effects of naloxone represent a measurement of the magnitude of morphine physical dependence. Villarreal and Dummer (25) extended this concept and suggested that shifts to the left and increases in the maxima of dose-response curves to naloxone measure the magnitude of physical dependence in the isolated guinea pig ileum. Further work on mouse intestinal peristalsis (17) has demonstrated the usefulness of this convention. Quantitative analysis of the dose-response curves for antagonists avoids the problems of interpretation of the indirect measurements of dependence discussed above. Quantitative comparisons of dose-response curves allow the formal types of analysis carried out in other areas of pharmacology. Further, the model of physiological dependence presented in this paper suggests strongly that the key action of opioids that is the basis for dependence is the setting up of a kindling mechanism that can be triggered by narcotic antagonists and certain other substances. Therefore, under the reasonable supposition that the changes in responsiveness to naloxone represent to date the closest and cleanest measure of dependence, in this paper we will place emphasis on the changes in dose-response curves to naloxone as quantitative indicators of the magnitude of dependence.

REFORMULATION OF THE DUAL-ACTION MODEL OF OPIOID DEPENDENCE: OPIOID-SPECIFIC NEURONAL KINDLING

It is clear from a careful analysis of the literature on chronic effects of opioids that no single mechanism will account for the totality of their known effects. However, there is an impressive set of commonalities in the nature of the dependence-producing effects of drugs of widely different chemical classes. There are also commonalities in the nature of the response that we call dependence in different organisms and in different preparations such as the chronic spinal dog and the isolated guinea pig ileum. These commonalities strongly suggest the existence of a nodal mechanism being the keystone of the action of opioids that is their most specific effect, namely physiological dependence. We propose here a model for such a mechanism.

We regard physiological dependence as the most specific effect of opioids, because as has been pointed out elsewhere (24), these effects are in fact the defining characteristics of this class of drugs. Analgesia, respiratory depression, presynaptic inhibition of neurotransmitter release, etc. are actions shared by many other classes of drugs. Therefore, a pharmacological analysis of the dependence-producing actions of the opioids appears to be one of the most specific approaches to the basis of their actions available to us at present.

Even tolerance to the opioids is known to be a complex phenomenon involving different mechanisms operating at different levels of integration (i.e., cellular, neurophysiological, and behavioral). Therefore, opioid tolerance is essentially left out of the present model of dependence although we assume, as have many others, that the "latent hyperexcitability" of dependence is likely to be involved in the reduction in magnitude of most of the primary effects of opioids during chronic administration.

A few words are necessary to describe the spirit in which the new model is offered. Models have to be taken carefully because they may help or hinder real understanding. The model is, of course, proposed as an object for further articulation or change as new evidence arises. The *literal* truth of the components proposed and their interactions is not the most important part of it. The components and their interactions are there for the known facts and phenomena that they symbolize. The value of the model resides in the variety and number of facts that it puts together into a single plausible ensemble

The experimental findings presented in this chapter are only a part of the body of information that authorize us to speak of it. Other facts are those that led to the first version of the dual nature of morphine's action (23). Others yet may be found in reviews by Seevers and Woods (22), Seevers (19), Seevers and Deneau (21), Wikler (30), and Villarreal (24).

The first version (23) of the dual nature of morphine's actions postulated that:

   (a) Morphine simultaneously stimulates certain parts of the brain and depresses others.
   (b) Irritability increases with repeated administration of morphine because the stimulant actions increment progressively due to the fact that they outlast the narcotic's depressant effects.
   (c) Dependence is largely a question of physiological balance between stimulation and depression.
   (d) Abstinence effects are due to the fact that stimulation of the nervous system, manifested as increased irritability, outlasts the depressant effects of morphine.

Seevers and Deneau (20,21) rejected the previous hypothesis after the finding that narcotic antagonists fail to block the direct stimulant actions of narcotics in the monkey; yet on chronic administration concurrently with opioids, the antagonists prevent the development of opioid dependence. Hence, they concluded that the direct stimulant actions of opioids are not the cause of physiological dependence nor of the abstinence syndrome.

The model for opioid dependence proposed here differs from the first version of the dual action of morphine in that it does not assign hyperexcitability or abstinence to the direct stimulant actions which morphine and other narcotics exert at high doses on the central nervous system. The model proposes that the so-called latent hyperexcitability of dependence results from the activation by the dependence-producing opioids of a pathway (mechanism B in Fig. 1) that sets up or sensitizes a kindling mechanism within morphine-sensitive neurons. Such a mechanism, when kindled, can be triggered by various procedures (right portion, Fig. 1), and its triggering then results in the overt disturbances seen as abstinence or abstinence-like effects.

The scheme in Fig. 1 borrows from Pert and Snyder (16) their conception of two conformations for the opioid receptor: one with more affinity for opioid agonists, and the other with more affinity for opioid antagonists. In the present model, the interaction of an opioid agonist with its receptor has a dual action. One operates through the pathway of mechanism A resulting in the acute, overt opioid effects such as analgesia or inhibition of neurotransmitter release in morphine-sensitive neurons. The other action operates through mechanism B by setting up or sensitizing the opioid-specific kindling mechanism. The chronic activation of mechanism B results in a progressive buildup of sensitivity to certain triggering agents and a progressive increase in the capacity of the enkindled mechanism to respond to triggers leading to abstinence effects of a progressively larger, up to a limit, magnitude.

There is ample precedence in neurophysiology for neural phenomena in which chronic stimulation of certain brain structures results in a progressive sensitization to stimuli and also to a progressively increasing capacity for explosive epileptic responses. The term kindling has been used for this phenomenon. Epileptogenic kindling was discovered in 1958 (1) and has been reviewed recently (27). The term has so far been used mainly to describe the condition generated by chronic, intermittent, subthreshold electrical or chemical stimulation of the brain which consists of a progressive increase in stimulatory effects, eventually resulting in a state in which normally subthreshold stimuli produce major convulsions. Such kindling effects can persist beyond the period of application of the

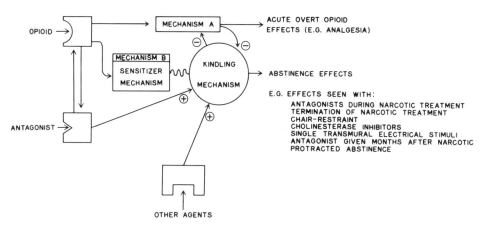

FIG. 1. Schematic representation of a dual-action model for the mechanisms of action of dependence-producing opioids.

stimulation that originally brought them about; sometimes the kindling effect is permanent.

The progressive sensitization with chronic treatment and the progressive capacity of the kindled structures to respond with explosive disturbances have led us to borrow the term kindling for the covert changes in the organism that take place during chronic opioid treatment and which have been traditionally designated as latent hyperexcitability.

The proposition that we use the concept of kindling is not, of course, a suggestion that we simply change old terms for new. The concept of kindling as the basis of opioid dependence gives an explanatory unification or at least a unified organization to a wide variety of facts whose possible interrelationships have been so far overlooked.

In epileptogenic kindling, the hyperexcitability outlasts the period of stimulation that produced it originally. Analogously, in opioid dependence, we know of effects that outlast the period of drug administration. There are the long-lasting disturbances designated as protracted abstinence (15,31), and there are the reports of the production of abstinence-like effects by narcotic antagonists given weeks or months after termination of opioid treatment (6,10,28).

As we shall see in the next section, agents or interventions other than the administration of narcotic antagonists can trigger abstinence-like phenomena in opioid-dependent organisms or tissues. It is difficult to conceive of an explanation for these abstinence-like phenomena other than the triggering of an explosive mechanism already kindled by chronic treatment with opioids.

Further, during opioid dependence the interaction of opioids and antagonists ceases to be one of competitive interaction. The abstinence syndrome precipitated by antagonists cannot be reversed or reduced by opioids except under very special circumstances (9,26). In fact, the presence of narcotic facilitates the production of abstinence-like phenomena by antagonists (see Fig. 2 and ref. 18). An opioid-kindled mechanism that is sensitive to triggering by antagonists can account for the previous phenomena. The scheme of Fig. 1 presents a direct arrow from the antagonist receptor to the kindling mechanism suggesting that there may be a direct link between these two structures.

The type of kindling mechanism proposed here for opioid dependence differs from epileptogenic kindling in three ways:

(a) Epileptogenic kindling occurs with chronic intermittent stimulation, whereas the kindling of latent hyperexcitability of opioid dependence requires the continual presence of the drug (21).

(b) The kindling of opioid latent hyperexcitability is topographically different; it is specific to dependence-producing opioids and to morphine-sensitive neurons (there is no known structure that is responsive to the acute specific effects of narcotics which does not show abstinence effects).

(c) Under certain circumstances, the triggered kindled mechanism can be turned off by opioid administration (e.g., relief of abstinence after termination of narcotic treatment and relief of those abstinence-like phenomena that are produced in monkeys either by chair restraint or by cholinesterase inhibitors).

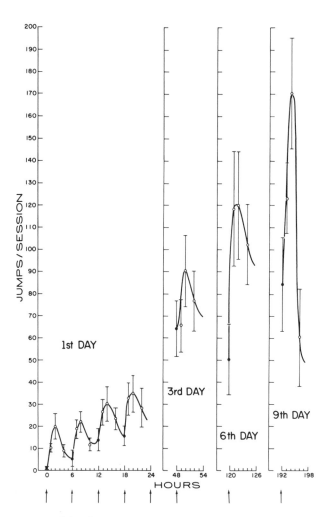

FIG. 2. Time course of development of superreactivity to naloxone (kindling, dependence) with morphine treatment. Each point represents the mean number of jumps in 20 min produced by 30 mg/kg of naloxone given to separate groups of 10 mice each. Morphine (100 mg/kg) given every 6 hr.

This last point of difference between epileptogenic kindling and opioid kindling deserves elaboration. In epileptogenic kindling, there appears to be a single type of action: repeated excitatory subthreshold stimuli lead to increases in excitability. In the model of opioid kindling that we present here, the opioids are proposed to have a dual action: one (mechanism A) that, under certain circumstances, is capable of turning off or stabilizing the kindling mechanism, and the other (mechanism B) that sets up and maintains the kindled mechanism. If opioid kindling, like epileptogenic kindling, outlasts for an extensive time the period in which kindling was developed, we may have in opioid kindling an account of the abstinence syndrome that occurs after termination of chronic opioid treatment. If the firing of the opioid-kindling mechanism is held in check by the presence of opioid, the reduced concentration of opioid or its absence will make the kindled mechanism more prone to fire in response to triggering stimuli—or even spontaneously. As we shall see in the next section, abstinence-like hypothermia produced by the stress of chair restraint in morphine-dependent monkeys occurs most consistently when morphine is beginning to wear off. Also, frequently observed, although not formally reported, morphine-dependent monkeys with partial abstinence will suffer a marked increase in the severity of their abstinence syndrome when handled by observers or when attacked by other monkeys.

It seems appropriate to clarify the present model for opioid dependence by contrasting it with other views about the basis of dependence. As pointed out by Wikler (30), most hypotheses about the nature of opioid physiological dependence postulate one or another sort of counter-adaptation by the organism to the acute agonist actions of narcotics. Such counter-adaptation mechanisms are supposed to overshoot when the opioid is absent and thus cause abstinence effects. These views—that dependence is the result of counter-responses to the acute agonist actions of narcotics—carry as a necessary corollary the prediction that all compounds with acute agonist effects will necessarily produce dependence. This has been shown not to be the case for a number of compounds which share with the classical narcotics strong, acute agonist actions (14,24–26). These are not facts that can be discounted as minor anomalies for the counter-adaption theories of dependence. They are in frank contradiction with them. One outstanding example of a strong agonist devoid of morphine-like dependence capacity is cyclazocine. Villarreal (24) has reported on the effects of chronic treatment with high doses of cyclazocine in the rhesus monkey and of its lack of morphine-like dependence capacity. To illustrate the differences between cyclazocine and morphine, the results of attempts to precipitate abstinence with naloxone in monkeys under chronic cyclazocine treatment are presented in Fig. 3. Elsewhere in this chapter it will be seen that the morphine abstinence syndrome in the monkey courses with hypothermias of a magnitude greater than 4°C. Figure 3 presents rectal temperature measurements of monkeys that received cyclazocine for 30 days in four daily doses that reached levels 16 times higher than the dose initially producing such strong central nervous depression that the monkeys would lay on the floor in a state of almost complete immobility. This figure also shows that an 8 mg/kg dose of naloxone (40 times higher than the dose needed to precipitate an abstinence syndrome of maximal severity in morphine-dependent monkeys) produced only minimal effects in monkeys treated chronically with the above-mentioned high doses of cyclazocine.

The separation of the acute agonist from the dependence-producing actions of drugs related to morphine is strikingly apparent in the isolated guinea pig

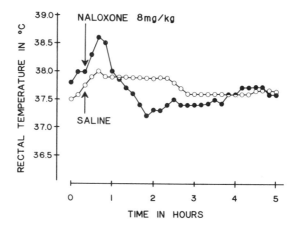

FIG. 3. An attempt to precipitate abstinence with a very large dose of naloxone in monkeys previously treated with cyclazocine for 30 days (24). Average values of rectal temperatures from three rhesus monkeys are shown. In one session, the monkeys were injected with saline (○), and in another they received subcutaneous naloxone (●). This effect of naloxone should be contrasted with the observation that doses of 0.1 or 0.2 mg/kg of this narcotic antagonist given to morphine-dependent monkeys produces drops in body temperature greater than 4°C.

ileum. Drugs with strong, acute agonist actions such as nalorphine and cyclazocine do not produce dependence (25,26).

In the kindling model of opioid dependence presented here, cyclazocine and other dependence-free agonists are thought to act either on the same opioid receptor as the classic dependence-producing opioids (but without setting up the kindling mechanism), or to act on different receptors not linked to a kindling structure.

Besides the counter-adaption hypothesis of opioid dependence, there have been proposals that a mechanism analogous to supersensitivity due to pharmacological denervation underlies opioid physiological dependence. Since opioids have been shown to inhibit neurotransmitter release at certain neuroeffector junctions, it has been thought that the lower levels of neurotransmitter in the junction might lead to supersensitivity toward the neurotransmitter. Such a mechanism cannot account for opioid dependence and abstinence. One reason for this conclusion is the same as that employed against the counter-adaptation hypothesis; namely, the lack of dependence production by certain drugs with strong agonist actions. Further, the increases in sensitivity produced during pharmacological denervation by strong antagonists such as scopolamine (5) or transmitter depleting agents (4,11) are very modest compared to the changes in sensitivity to naloxone *(vide infra)* and to cholinesterase inhibitors generated by opioid dependence (8).

In denervation supersensitivity, there is a shift to the left in the dose-response curve to drugs but no increase in the maximal effect (2). Figure 4 (left) presents

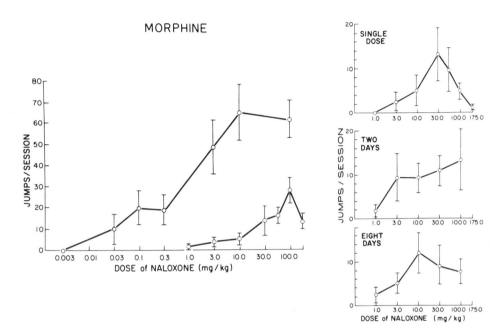

FIG. 4. Dose-response curves to the jump-eliciting effects of naloxone under different treatments during 20-min sessions. Each point represents the mean of separate groups of 10 mice each. **Left:** the lower curve shows the effects of naloxone administered 2 hr after a single injection of 100 mg/kg morphine. The upper curve represents the effects of naloxone given 2 hr after the last of eight injections of 100 mg/kg morphine given every 6 hr for 2 days. **Right:** The effects of naloxone after a single dose of 10 mg/kg *d*-amphetamine (upper), after 2 days (middle), and after 8 days (lower) of treatment with the same dose of *d*-amphetamine repeated at 6-hr intervals.

dose-response curves to naloxone after a single dose of morphine and after a 2-day treatment with morphine, given every 6 hr. The dose-response curve for naloxone shifted markedly to the left after the two day morphine treatment, accompanied by a very marked increase in the maximal effect. This type of change in dose-response configuration corresponds to what Cannon and Rosenblueth (2) termed superreactivity in distinction with supersensitivity.

Figure 4 also shows that pretreatment with 10.0 mg/kg *d*-amphetamine sensitizes mice to the jump-eliciting effects of naloxone. However, the dose-response curves of naloxone remain essentially the same after a single *d*-amphetamine dose as after two or eight days of treatment with the same dose of *d*-amphetamine given every 6 hr. Therefore, chronic *d*-amphetamine administration does not produce the naloxone superreactivity that we assign to opioid specific kindling.

The development of superreactivity to naloxone and, by inference, kindling, following chronic morphine treatment is seen in Fig. 2. The effects of naloxone increased nearly 10-fold over the course of the experiment. The marked increase in reactivity to naloxone, coupled with the fact that peak naloxone effects are observed when tissue levels of morphine should be higher, are further evidence of the operation of a kindling mechanism that is set up by morphine and triggered by naloxone.

APPARENTLY ANOMALOUS ABSTINENCE-LIKE PHENOMENA THAT SUPPORT THE VIEW OF OPIOID-SPECIFIC KINDLING IN OPIOID DEPENDENCE

There are certain phenomena occurring in opioid-dependent organisms and tissues that seem to be special forms of precipitated abstinence but are produced by neither narcotic antagonists nor opioid withdrawal. Analysis of these phenomena strongly suggest the existence of an opioid-kindled mechanism that can be triggered by agents of interventions not previously considered.

The first series of these phenomena were discovered and analyzed by Holtzman and Villarreal (7,8) and until now these phenomena have not been integrated with the better known facts about dependence. The first peculiarity these authors observed were large falls in body temperature on placing morphine-dependent monkeys in standard restraining chairs a few hours after one of their regular morphine injections (Fig. 5). Evidence that these restraint-induced hypothermias are a special form of precipitated abstinence consisted of the following:

(a) Hypothermia is a component of the morphine abstinence syndrome, either when precipitated by nalorphine or by termination of morphine treatment.

(b) Restraint-induced hypothermia occurs regularly only if restraint is imposed after a few hours following a regular morphine injection.

(c) After hypothermia has been produced by chair restraint, administration of morphine causes the body temperature to return to base-line levels.

(d) Dependence-producing opioids of different chemical classes other than morphine also reverse restraint-induced hypothermia (levorphanol reverses the hypothermia but dextrorphan does not).

(e) The reversal of hypothermia by morphine cannot be attributed to a nonspecific hyperthermic effect of morphine since d-amphetamine given in doses producing mild hyperthermia in nondependent monkeys failed to reverse the restraint-induced hypothermia produced in dependent monkeys.

With the exception of the administration of cholinesterase inhibitors to dependent monkeys (Table 1), we are not aware of any other procedure that causes decreases of body temperature in monkeys as large as those seen following chair restraint in morphine dependence. It has been pointed out (7) that monkeys and dogs with neurological lesions that seriously interfere with thermoregulation are capable of maintaining their body temperatures in the environmental temperatures at which restraint-induced hypothermia in dependent monkeys is observed.

Attempts at a pharmacological analysis of restraint-induced hypothermia led

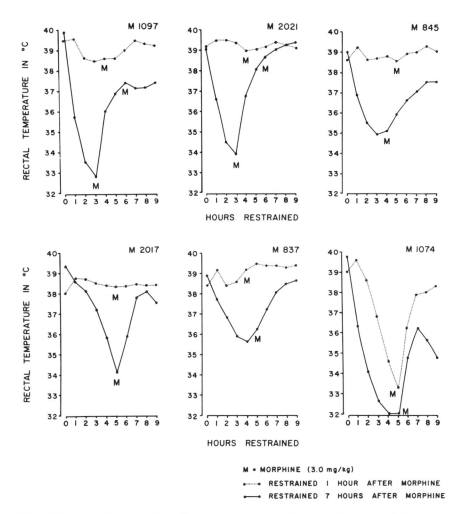

FIG. 5. Effects of chair restraint on the body temperature of six morphine-dependent monkeys in a cross-over study. Each monkey was twice subjected to the restraining procedure, once 7 hr after a regular maintenance dose of morphine (———) and once 1 hr after a regular morphine injection (· · · ·). Administration of the maintenance dose of morphine (3 mg/kg) during the recording session is indicated by M. (From ref. 7.) (From Holtzman and Villarreal, ref. 7.)

to other observations that are summarized in Table 1. The cholinesterase inhibitors physostigmine (Fig. 7) and neostigmine also produced falls in body temperature of more than 4°C in morphine-dependent monkeys, while causing only modest hypothermias in nondependent monkeys. The hypothermias produced by the cholinesterase inhibitors were reversed by the maintenance dose of morphine.

Table 1 also contains comparisons of the hypothermic effects of anesthetic

TABLE 1. *Hypothermic effects of drugs and chair restraint in morphine-dependent and nondependent monkeys*

Treatment	Temperature fall (°C)		Difference between dependent and nondependent
	Morphine-dependent	Nondependent	
Nalorphine (1 mg/kg)	4.04 ± 0.38 (7)[a]	0.06 ± 0.09 (6)	$p < 0.001$
Physostigmine (0.2 mg/kg)	4.87 ± 0.22 (5)	0.74 ± 0.25 (6)	$p < 0.001$
Neostigmine (0.2 mg/kg)	4.31 ± 0.25 (4)	1.21 ± 0.41 (4)	$p < 0.01$
Chair restraint	4.72 ± 2.01 (5)[b]	0.53[c]	
Chlorpromazine (4 mg/kg)	1.36 ± 0.19 (5)	0.66 ± 0.13 (6)	$p < 0.05$
Pentobarbital (30 mg/kg)	2.37 ± 0.50 (6)	1.61 ± 0.34 (6)	NS

[a] Number of animals indicated parenthetically.
[b] Value from experiments in which chair restraint was started 7 hr after the last dose of morphine.
[c] Value represents the difference between mean values and not the mean of differences (see Fig. 1 of ref. 7).

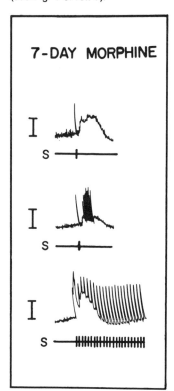

7-DAY MORPHINE

FIG. 6. Tracings of longitudinal isometric tension from three segments of isolated ileum from guinea pigs previously injected with 60 mg/kg morphine sulfate every 6 hr for 7 days. The marks on the lines labeled S indicate the application of 0.5 msec transmural electrical pulses of an intensity 30% over the maxima. Bars at left indicate the calibration tension (1 g).

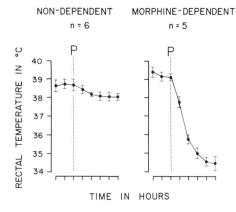

NON-DEPENDENT   MORPHINE-DEPENDENT
      n = 6   n = 5

FIG. 7. Effects of physostigmine (P) administration (0.2 mg/kg) on the body temperature of nondependent and morphine-dependent monkeys 3 hr after a maintenance dose of morphine. Points represent means and bars standard errors. (From ref. 8.)

doses of pentobarbital and high doses of chlorpromazine in nondependent and dependent monkeys. These drugs were examined to learn whether the hypothermias produced by restraint or by the cholinesterase inhibitors were due to a general incompetence of the thermoregulatory mechanisms in morphine-dependent monkeys. This does not appear to be the case.

A further point of interest is that the hypothermia produced by cholinesterase inhibitors is due to the peripheral actions of these drugs and not to effects on the central nervous system (8). It seems likely that the large hypothermias produced by these drugs result from nonspecific stress through their peripheral actions that is mediated by a mechanism analogous to that of restraint-induced hypothermia: the triggering of an opioid kindling mechanism.

Another instance of abstinence-like phenomenon not related to opioid withdrawal or to the administration of opioid antagonists is illustrated in Fig. 6. The figure presents tracings of longitudinal isometric tension of isolated segments of ilea taken from guinea pigs treated with 60 mg/kg morphine every 6 hr for 7 days. Single transmural electrical pulses elicited the commonly observed single muscle twitch. However, in these segments of ileum taken from animals made morphine-dependent, the single longitudinal twitch was followed by an "afterdischarge" contraction. This is another item of evidence supporting the view that there is operating, in opioid dependence, a kindling mechanism that can be triggered by interventions other than the removal of morphine or the administration of narcotic antagonists.

ULTRA-RAPID *IN VITRO* DEVELOPMENT OF SUPERREACTIVITY TO NALOXONE IN THE PRESENCE OF DEPENDENCE-PRODUCING OPIOIDS

This section will describe some recent experiments in which dependence-producing opioids were shown to generate superreactivity to naloxone within minutes of exposure to the opioid. This ultrarapid development of superreactivity was observed *in vitro* with isolated segments of guinea pig ileum maintained at 40°C. The degree of superreactivity to naloxone observed under these conditions is comparable to that obtained after a 2-day treatment *in vitro* with morphine (25) or after a 24-hr incubation with several opioids (26). This very rapid development of superreactivity to naloxone is remarkable because it represents a marked departure from previous experiences with the time course for the development of dependence. Opioid dependence in intact organisms generally requires weeks, or at least several days (Fig. 2), for its full development (8,21). The finding that at elevated temperatures opioids can set up the opioid kindling mechanism and make it capable of operating at its full capacity leads to a strong inference and to some speculations. This observation strongly suggests that the entity kindled by the opioids is already present in the tissue and not something the chronic presence of the opioid generates *de novo*. If such is indeed the case, we may be allowed to speculate that certain conditions operating in the intact organism might also accelerate opioid-specific kindling; also that endogenous substances with opioid-like actions could set up such a mechanism and that yet other endogenous substances or physiological events could trigger the opioid-kindled mechanism. Other experiments of ours, not discussed here, have shown that low levels of opioids can evoke, within 1 hr, superreactivity to naloxone in tissue bathed in solutions containing low concentrations of calcium. The rapid *in vitro* development of superreactivity to naloxone contrasted with its slow *in vivo* development suggests that, if there are counter-responses of the organism to exogenous opioids, these are in the direction of opposing the manifestations of dependence and abstinence. This is the exact opposite of what the counter-adaptation hypothesis of dependence proposes: that the counter-responses of the organism are the mechanism of abstinence.

The experiments on ultra-rapid development of opioid-induced superreactivity to naloxone were carried out with the same *in vitro* procedures used to generate dependence in guinea pig ilea at low temperatures (26). Fresh ilea incubated with levorphanol at 40°C respond to naloxone with the same type of abstinence contractions as ilea incubated for 24 hr with levorphanol at 4°C (Fig. 8). Table 2 compares the responses of the ileum to naloxone under different conditions. Naloxone produces minimal or no responses in ilea incubated in 40°C solutions lacking opioid or in ilea incubated with levorphanol at 36°C. Large responses of a similar magnitude were obtained after a 30-min incubation with levorphanol at 40°C, after a 24-hr incubation at 4 to 6°C, and a 48-hr levorphanol treatment *in vivo*.

Figure 9 presents tracings of longitudinal tension of fresh segments of guinea pig ileum maintained at 40°C. When the segments were being stimulated with supramaximal transmural stimuli (left half), levorphanol, nalorphine, and cyclazocine produced inhibition of the neurogenic contraction. In the absence of transmural stimulation (right half), naloxone produced a very large contraction in the segment treated with the dependence-producing opioid levor-

ILEA PREINCUBATED AT 4°C FOR
24 HRS IN LEVORPHANOL

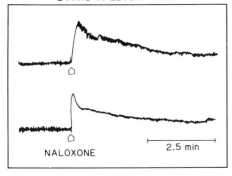

NALOXONE   2.5 min

FIG. 8. Comparison of naloxone-precipitated abstinence contractions shown by segments of isolated guinea-pig ileum incubated at 4°C for 24 hr with levorphanol **(top)** with the responses to naloxone obtained in fresh segments of guinea pig ileum incubated at 40°C with levorphanol for 30 min **(bottom).**

ILEA AT 40°C FOR 30 MIN IN LEVORPHANOL

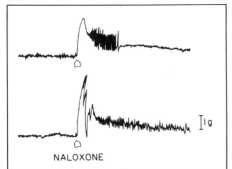

NALOXONE

LEVORPHANOL : 64 nM
NALOXONE : 300 nM

TABLE 2. *Naloxone-induced contraction of isolated guinea pig ilea under different conditions[a]*

Preparation	Peak increase in tension (g)
30-min incubation at 40°C in Krebs solution	0.12 ± 0.05
30-min incubation at 36°C with levorphanol	0.32 ± 0.05
30-min incubation at 40°C with levorphanol	2.60 ± 0.40
24-hr incubation at 4–6°C with levorphanol	2.80 ± 0.38
48-hr levorphanol administration, *in vivo*	2.18 ± 0.33

[a] *In vitro* concentrations: levorphanol, 64 nM; naloxone, 300 nM.

GUINEA PIG ILEA AT 40°C

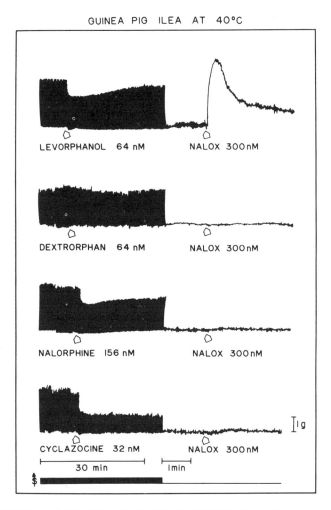

FIG. 9. Comparison of the acute effects and the capacity of several drugs to create the opioid kindling mechanism in freshly isolated segments of guinea pig ileum incubated at 40°C. At left the ilea are being transmurally stimulated at 0.1 Hz with single stimuli; because the recorder ran at a slow rate, the single longitudinal twitches are superimposed. Levorphanol, nalorphine, and cyclazocine, but not dextrorphan, inhibit the neurogenic contractions. At right, there was no transmural stimulation and the recorder ran at a higher rate. Naloxone is seen to produce abstinence contractions only in the segment exposed to levorphanol. A 30-min exposure to the drugs preceded the application of naloxone. The bar indicates calibration tension. To compose the figure, segments of the faster speed tracings were eliminated and the remaining portion joined to the slower speed tracings in order to make level the points of naloxone administration.

phanol but none in segments treated with nalorphine and cyclazocine—both agonists devoid of morphine-like dependence capacity. The effect is stereospecific as can be seen by comparing the effects of levorphanol with those of dextrorphan.

TABLE 3. *Naloxone-induced contractions of isolated guinea pig ilea[a,b]*

Compound	Concentration (nM)	Peak increase in tension (g)	Area under contraction curve[c]
Krebs solution		0.12 ± 0.05	0.38 ± 0.06
Levorphanol	64	2.60 ± 0.40	12.03 ± 1.34
Morphine	480	1.83 ± 0.27	10.24 ± 0.90
Meperidine	1,715	1.00 ± 0.52	3.57 ± 0.94
Pentazocine	1,715	0.89 ± 0.70	2.21 ± 0.82
Nalorphine	156	0.40 ± 0.09	1.30 ± 0.13
Cyclazocine	24	0.03 ± 0.003	0.29 ± 0.07
Dextrophan	64	0.02 ± 0.001	0.09 ± 0.008

[a] Induction by 300 nM naloxone.
[b] Exposure, 30 min at 40°C.
[c] Calculated as $g \times min$.

The average responses to naloxone after a 30-min, 40°C exposure to a series of opioids and related drugs is shown in Table 3. The rank order of magnitude of the responses to naloxone in the presence of different drugs closely parallels their physiological dependence capacity in monkeys and man.

Figure 10 depicts naloxone dose-response curves in ilea extensively preincubated with levorphanol at a low temperature and briefly exposed to levorphanol at 40°C. The two curves have approximately the same maxima and ED_{50} values that differ only by a factor of about two.

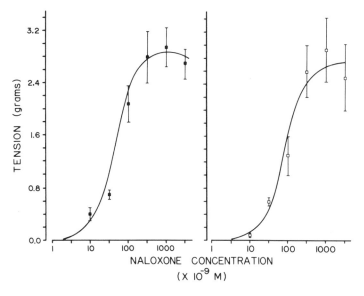

FIG. 10. Dose-response curves of naloxone-induced abstinence contractions in segments of isolated guinea pig ileum under two conditions of preincubation with levorphanol. **Left:** 24 hr at 4°C. **Right:** 30 min at 40°C.

It is not yet possible to state unequivocally that the rapid development of superreactivity to naloxone induced by opioids in these experiments is an exact reproduction of that superreactivity observed following an *in vivo* opioid treatment or a 24-hr preincubation with dependence-producing opioids. The high incubative temperature may, in part, lead to the strong responses to naloxone through sensitization of the ileal smooth muscle to substances released by the triggering of the kindling mechanism. Unfortunately, we do not yet know what such substances are in order to be able to test directly whether high temperature increases the sensitivity of the intestinal muscle to them. However, the experiments examining the rapid superreactivity to naloxone of tissue bathed in low calcium solutions at 36°C provide converging evidence that the opioid kindling mechanism is an entity already present in tissues and not synthetized *de novo*.

POSSIBLE PHYSIOLOGICAL SIGNIFICANCE OF THE OPIOID-SPECIFIC KINDLING MECHANISM

It is tempting to speculate on the possible physiological role of the opioid-specific kindling mechanism. Possibly, certain painful stimuli, like those of renal colic or of coronary occlusion, may provoke an excessive release of endogenous substances having morphine-like activity and such an excess could set up the opioid kindling mechanism. This would permit other agents released during the stress of the pathological condition to trigger the kindled mechanism and produce certain opioid abstinence-like effects (such as restlessness, disquiet, anxiety, and apprehension) that seem to be out of proportion to the pain stimulus itself. It appears to be too much of a coincidence that morphine-like analgesics not only relieve the pain of renal colic and coronary occlusion but also relieve all the concurrent symptoms.

It would be clearly unwise to abandon the term "opioid dependence" because of its clear clinical and pharmacological usefulness. However, it might be profitable to think of what we still call the "mechanisms of dependence" using concepts that are not restricted to their classical connotations. If the opioid-specific kindling mechanism operates in a form analogous to that suggested in the above paragraph, the entity involved in opioid-specific kindling might play the role of a "reverse-sign amplifier" when painful stimuli exceed a certain intensity or duration.

REFERENCES

1. Alonso-de-Florida, F., and Delgado, J. M. R. (1958): Lasting behavioral and EEG changes in cats induced by prolonged stimulation of amygdala. *Am. J. Physiol.,* 193:223–229.
2. Cannon, W. B., and Rosenblueth, A. (1949): *The Supersensitivity of Denervated Structures.* Macmillan, New York.
3. Deneau, G. A. (1956): An Analysis of Factors Influencing the Development of Physical Dependence to Narcotics with Methods for Predicting Physical Dependence Liability in Man. Doctoral Dissertation, The University of Michigan, Ann Arbor.

4. Fleming, W. W., and Trendelenburg, U. (1961): The development of supersensitivity to norepi-nephrine after pretreatment with reserpine. *J. Pharmacol. Exp. Ther.,* 133:41–51.
5. Friedman, M. J., Jaffe, J. H., and Sharpless, S. K. (1969): Central nervous system supersensitivity to pilocarpine after withdrawal of chronically administered scopolamine. *J. Pharmacol. Exp. Ther.,* 167:45–55.
6. Goldberg, S. R., and Schuster, C. R. (1969): Nalorphine: Increased sensitivity of monkeys formerly dependent on morphine. *Science,* 166:1548–1549.
7. Holtzman, S. G., and Villarreal, J. E. (1969): Morphine dependence and body temperature in rhesus monkeys. *J. Pharmacol. Exp. Ther.,* 166:125–133.
8. Holtzman, S. G., and Villarreal, J. E. (1971): Pharmacologic analysis of the hypothermic re-sponses of the morphine-dependent rhesus monkey. *J. Pharmacol. Exp. Ther.,* 177:317–325.
9. Irwin, S. (1953): Characteristics of Depression, Antagonism and Development of Tolerance, Physical Dependence and Neuropathology to Morphine and Morphine-like Agents in the Mon-key. Doctoral Dissertation, The University of Michigan, Ann Arbor.
10. Irwin, S., and Seevers, M. H. (1956): Altered response to drug in the post-addict Macaca mulatta. *J. Pharmacol. Exp. Ther.,* 116:31–32.
11. Kirpekar, S. M., Cervoni, P., and Furchgott, R. F. (1962): Catecholamine content of the cat nictitating membrane following procedures sensitizing it to norepinephrine. *J. Pharmacol. Exp. Ther.,* 135:180–190.
12. Kolb, L., and DuMez, A. G. (1931): Experimental addiction of animals to opiates. *Public Health Rep.,* 46:698–726.
13. MacCarthy, D. A. (1958): Pharmacologic Analysis of Mechanism in the Morphine Dependent State. Doctoral Dissertation, The University of Michigan, Ann Arbor.
14. Martin, W. R. (1967): Opioid antagonists. *Pharmacol. Rev.,* 19:463–521.
15. Martin, W. R., and Jasinski, D. R. (1969): Physiological parameters of morphine dependence in man—tolerance, early abstinence, protracted abstinence. *J. Psychiatr. Res.,* 7:9–17.
16. Pert, C. B., and Snyder, S. (1974): Opiate receptor binding of agonists and antagonists affected differentially by sodium. *Mol. Pharmacol.,* 10:868–879.
17. Rodriguez, R., and Villarreal, J. E. (1974): Graded quantitation of morphine tolerance and dependence on the same physiological system in the mouse. In: *Report of the 36th Meeting of the Committee on Problems of Drug Dependence,* pp. 453–459.
18. Schulz, R., and Herz, A. (1976): The guinea-pig ileum as an in vitro model to analyse dependence liability of narcotic drugs. In: *Opiates and Endogenous Opioid Peptides,* edited by H. W. Koster-litz, pp. 319–326. Elsevier, Amsterdam.
19. Seevers, M. H. (1954): Adaptation to narcotics. *Fed. Proc.,* 13:672–684.
20. Seevers, M. H., and Deneau, G. A. (1962): A critique of the dual action hypothesis of morphine physical dependence. *Arch. Int. Pharmacodyn. Ther.,* 140:514–520.
21. Seevers, M. H., and Deneau, G. A. (1963): Physiological aspects of tolerance and physical dependence. In: *Physiological Pharmacology, Vol. 1,* edited by W. S. Root and F. G. Hofmann, pp. 565–640. Academic Press, New York.
22. Seevers, M. H., and Woods, L. A. (1953): The phenomena of tolerance. *Am. J. Med.,* 14:546–557.
23. Tatum, A. L., Seevers, M. H., and Collins, K. H. (1929): Morphine addiction and its physiological interpretation based on experimental evidence. *J. Pharmacol. Exp. Ther.,* 36:447–475.
24. Villarreal, J. E. (1973): The effects of morphine agonists and antagonists on morphine-dependent rhesus monkeys. In: *Agonist and Antagonist Actions of Narcotic Drugs Analgesic,* edited by H. Kosterlitz, H. O. J. Collier, and J. E. Villarreal, pp. 73–93. University Park Press, Baltimore.
25. Villarreal, J. E., and Dummer, G. E. (1973): Separation of the dependence-producing actions from the direct actions of narcotics on guinea pig ileum. *Fed. Proc.,* 32:688 (Abstr. No. 2678).
26. Villarreal, J. E., Martinez, J. N., and Castro, A. (1977): Validation of a new procedure to study narcotic dependence in the isolated guinea pig ileum. In: *Report of the 39th Meeting of the Committee on Problems of Drug Dependence,* pp. 305–314.
27. Wada, J. A., and Ross, R. T., editors (1976): *Kindling.* Raven Press, New York.
28. Way, E. L., Brase, D. A., Iwamoto, E. T., Shen, J., and Loh, H. H. (1976): A possible test for protracted abstinence. In: *Opiates and Endogenous Opioid Peptides,* edited by H. W. Koster-litz, pp. 311–318. Elsevier, Amsterdam.
29. Way, E. L., Loh, H. H., and Shen, F. (1969): Simultaneous quantitative assessment of morphine tolerance and physical dependence. *J. Pharmacol. Exp. Ther.,* 167:1–8.

30. Wikler, A. (1972): Theories related to physical dependence. In: *Chemical and Biological Aspects of Drug Dependence,* edited by J. Mule and H. Brill, pp. 359–377. CRC Press, Cleveland.
31. Wikler, A., and Pescor, F. T. (1967): Classical conditioning of a morphine abstinence phenomenon, reinforcement of opioid-drinking behavior and "relapse" in morphine-addicted rats. *Psychopharmacologia,* 10:255–284.

Mechanisms of Pain and Analgesic Compounds,
edited by R. F. Beers, Jr., and E. G. Bassett.
Raven Press, New York © 1979.

38. Preclinical Testing of New Analgesic Drugs

James H. Woods, Charles B. Smith, Fedor Medzihradsky, and
Henry H. Swain

Department of Pharmacology, University of Michigan, Ann Arbor, Michigan 48109

INTRODUCTION

Since morphine has many different actions on living organisms, drugs can be "morphine-like" in many different ways, and morphine-like drugs can be quite different from one another. Since some of the actions of morphine can be dissociated from one another, it is reasonable to search for substances that have any particular subset of morphine-like properties. The quest for a potent analgesic that does not have morphine's liability for abusive self-administration is an example of such a search.

The abuse liability of a drug is difficult to assess accurately by any procedure that is less direct than exposing a large human population to its use; nevertheless, a number of experimental techniques have been developed in the hope that prehuman testing can have predictive value in assessing the abuse potential of a new analgesic compound. In this chapter, we describe the procedures used in the Department of Pharmacology at the University of Michigan to predict abuse liability of new narcotic drugs.

As illustrative examples, several compounds are described in terms of their appearance from the vantage points provided by the different test procedures. We have selected (a) nalorphine, (b) cyclazocine, (c) ketazocine and the analogous ethylketazocine, (d) UM 909 and the isomeric UM 911, and (e) UM 1070 and the enantiomorphic UM 1072. This progression of compounds can be viewed as a series of steps away from morphine toward what might become a significant new class of dependence-free analgesic drugs. Nalorphine is the classic example of a substance that shares some actions with morphine but is strikingly different in its most obvious feature, its narcotic antagonist action. Cyclazocine shares narcotic antagonist properties with nalorphine, but shows direct actions that are difficult to explain on the basis of interaction with the usual morphine receptor. Ketazocine and ethylketazocine, first described by Michne et al. (13,15), have agonist properties like those of cyclazocine but lack its antagonist actions. In turn, they possess striking similarities to the UM-numbered compounds, which are a series of *N*-furyl-substituted benzomorphans, described by Merz et al. (12). The structural formulas of these illustrative compounds are shown in Figs. 1 and 2.

Physical Dependence Evaluation

The development of physical dependence is a characteristic of morphine and related analgesic drugs, and of some, but not all, of the other drugs that are abusively self-administered by humans. To assess physical dependence of the morphine type, drugs can be tested for their ability to suppress the signs of abstinence that appear on the discontinuation of morphine administration in animals that have received the drug regularly over a period of time. The late M. H. Seevers, to whom this volume is dedicated, established and maintained a colony of rhesus monkeys that receive morphine sulfate (3 mg/kg) four times each day. At periodic intervals, morphine doses are withheld and the monkeys allowed to develop morphine withdrawal signs. Fourteen hours after their last dose of morphine, when their abstinence signs are approximately half-maximal, animals receive a dose of a test drug. If that drug is a narcotic agonist, the abstinence signs are promptly suppressed, in this so-called "Single Dose Suppression Test"; on the other hand, if the test drug is a narcotic antagonist, there will be a prompt enhancement of the severity of the abstinence syndrome. With this test, experienced observers can distinguish between the effects of a narcotic depressant, such as morphine, and those of a nonnarcotic depressant (e.g., a barbiturate, benzodiazepine, or phenothiazine).

Certain compounds having some morphine-like activity do not produce unequivocal effects in the Single Dose Suppression Test, and so additional procedures are used to evaluate their physical dependence liability. Nonwithdrawn, morphine-dependent monkeys are more responsive to the effects of narcotic antagonists than are animals that are already showing half-maximal abstinence signs before they receive the test drug. Physical dependence production can be demonstrated more directly, though more expensively, by a 30-day chronic-administration study in which monkeys originally nondependent receive the test drug on a regular basis at maximum tolerated doses; in these animals, dependence is shown by the precipitation of abstinence signs, either by the administration of a narcotic antagonist (e.g., naloxone) or by the abrupt cessation of treatment with the test drug.

The results of physical dependence evaluation of the selected illustrative compounds are as follows.

Nalorphine: Nalorphine is a narcotic antagonist that precipitates abstinence signs in morphine-dependent monkeys. On repeated administration to nondependent animals, tolerance to its depressant effects develops, but the physical dependence produced is of a low order; on abrupt withdrawal, the animals show a lot of body scratching but not the increased irritability and gastrointestinal disorders that characterize withdrawal from morphine-like drugs.

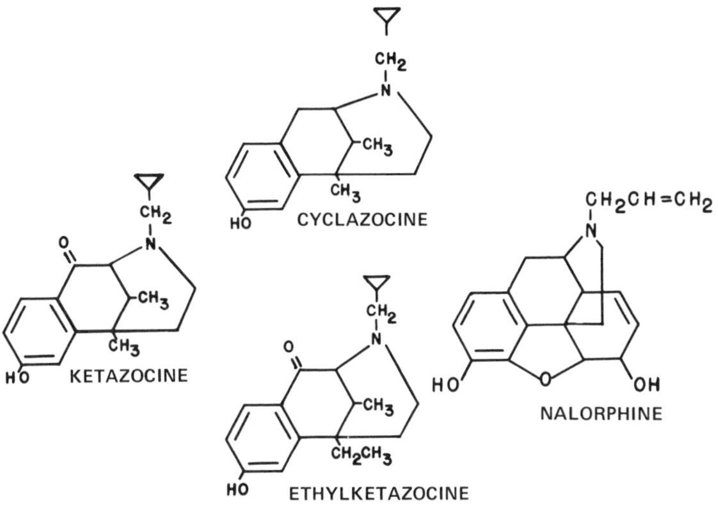

FIG. 1. Structural formulas of nalorphine, cyclazocine, ketazocine (ketocyclazocine), and ethylketazocine (ethylketocyclazocine, WIN 35,197–2).

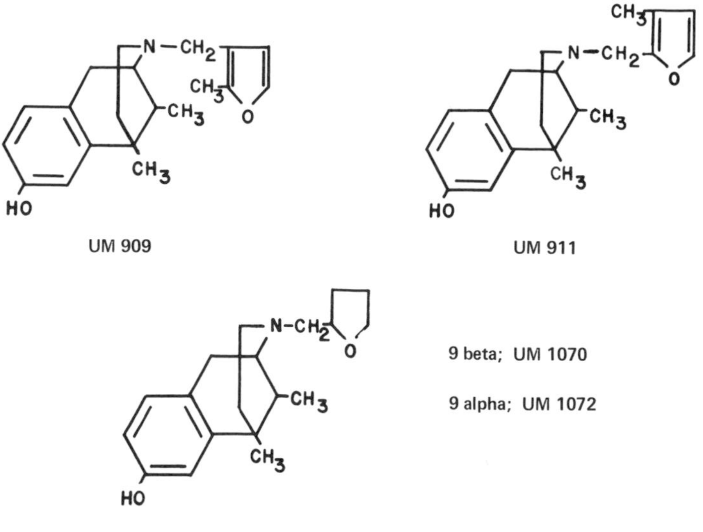

FIG. 2. Structural formulas of the UM-numbered compounds. UM 909 (also known as NIH 8735 and Mr 1268-MS) is 2-(2-methyl-3-furylmethyl)-2'-hydroxy-5,9α-dimethyl-6, 7-benzomorphan methanesulfonate. UM 911 (which has also been labeled NIH 8737 and Mr 1353-MS) is 2-(3-methylfurfuryl)-2'-hydroxy-5,9α-dimethyl-6,7-benzomorphan methanesulfonate. The compound UM 1070 has been known variously as MCV 4049, NIH 9100, and Mr 2184-CL, and has the structure (±)-(1R/S, 5R/S, 9S/R, 2"R/S)-5,9-dimethyl-2'-hydroxy-2-tetrahydrofurfuryl-6,7-benzomorphan hydrochloride. Differing from the previous compound only in the steric configuration of the 9-methyl group, UM 1072 (MCV 4051, NIH 9102, Mr 2033-CL) is (±)-(1R/S, 5R/S, 9S/R,-2"R/S)-5,9-dimethyl-2'-hydroxy-2 tetrahydrofurfuryl-6,7-benzomorphan hydrochloride.

Cyclazocine: In precipitating morphine withdrawal, cyclazocine is approximately equipotent to levallorphan and 3.5 times as potent as nalorphine; the duration of action of minimally effective doses is 10 to 12 hr. Following chronic administration of the drug, withdrawal signs are quite distinct from those of morphine: There is less abdominal rigidity than with morphine, and there is extensive scratching, peculiar postures and stretching motions, and a characteristic "half-yawn/half-retch" phenomenon.

Ketazocine: Ketazocine is a remarkable compound that neither suppresses nor precipitates abstinence in the morphine-dependent monkey, but in a dose of 1.6 mg/kg, it produces marked ataxia and muscle weakness, and these signs are reversed by 2 mg/kg of either nalorphine or naloxone.

Ethylketazocine: Like ketazocine, the effects of ethylketazocine are blocked by nalorphine or naloxone but ethylketazocine does not suppress morphine abstinence. Somewhat more potent than ketazocine, a dose of 0.4 mg/kg causes marked ataxia and muscle weakness, and bodily movements are somewhat more jerky than those of animals treated with ketazocine.

UM 909: This compound causes no suppression of the signs of morphine abstinence, nor does it precipitate abstinence in the dependent monkey. The least potent of the illustrative compounds, in a dose of 8 mg/kg it causes CNS depression characterized by a marked increase in the animals' response to their environment and to applied stimuli. Mildly ataxic, the animals tend to sit quietly in one place.

UM 911: Similar to UM 909 in its effects, in a dose of 4 mg/kg UM 911 causes CNS depression with some vomiting, which causes the monkeys to move about somewhat more than the UM 909–treated animals. UM 911 causes neither precipitation nor suppression of abstinence signs in the dependent monkeys.

UM 1070: More potent than the compounds listed above, UM 1070 neither suppresses nor precipitates abstinence signs in morphine-dependent monkeys. In a dose of 0.05 mg/kg it causes a short-lasting CNS depression, characterized by decreased bodily movement, glassy-eyed staring, and ataxia. Both tolerance and physical dependence develop on repeated administration. Abstinence signs from UM 1070 differ somewhat from those seen after repeated morphine administration, in that abdominal rigidity is not present, and the animals show a peculiar "half-yawn/half-retch" reaction, similar to that seen with cyclazocine.

UM 1072: UM 1072 is essentially identical to UM 1070, in that significant tolerance and physical dependence develop, but its actions are quite distinct from those of morphine. It neither suppresses nor precipitates the abstinence snydrome in morphine-dependent monkeys. The CNS depression it produces is only partially reversed by standard doses of nalorphine or naloxone, in that the monkeys appear somewhat less stuporous, but they continue their glassy-eyed staring. On repeated administration of this drug, the signs of depression become less severe and shorter-lasting. Challenge with narcotic antagonists or abrupt withdrawal of the drug precipitate an abstinence syndrome characterized more by CNS stimulation and less by abdominal cramping than is seen in animals withdrawing from the effects of morphine.

OBSERVATIONS

Self-Administration Studies

The study of physical dependence capacity of new narcotics has been complemented by the study of their ability to reinforce self-injection responding. Repeated self-injection is an invariant characteristic of the abuse of narcotics in man. The rhesus monkey self-injects many narcotic compounds abused by man (Hoffmeister, *this volume*), and therefore this method of evaluation may provide a framework for analyzing new narcotics that is different from dependence evaluation. Indeed, analysis of the compounds under consideration in this chapter shows that compounds that produce dependence are not necessarily self-injected.

Test compounds are evaluated in rhesus monkeys that have been conditioned to inject codeine phosphate intravenously. The schedule of intravenous drug delivery is a fixed-ratio 30 (FR-30): When a light above a lever is illuminated, the 30th response in its presence turns off the fixed-ratio light and delivers a 5-sec intravenous drug injection in the presence of another light that is always illuminated during drug delivery. After each injection, a 10-min time-out condition is in effect, during which responses have no programmed consequence and no lights are illuminated. Each of two daily sessions consists of 13 injections or 130 min, whichever occurs first.

Codeine was selected as the maintenance drug and 0.32 mg/kg/injection was selected as the dosage because this maintains a high, essentially constant rate of responding by the monkeys. Higher codeine doses produce lower rates of responding, probably owing to the carry-over of direct effects from drug self-administered previously. Periodically each animal receives saline instead of codeine solution on the FR-30 schedule for an experimental session, and after a very small number of such substitutions, the saline controls much lower rates of responding than codeine. Procedural details and a more complete description of codeine-reinforced responding are provided elsewhere (19).

For many of the standard narcotic agonists, the monkeys lever-press at rates similar to those seen with codeine for at least one of the doses of the test drug. The relative potencies of these drugs as reinforcers parallel their potencies for the suppression of abstinence signs in the physical dependence evaluation (H. H. Swain and J. H. Woods, *unpublished observations*). The effects of a morphine-like narcotic agonist on the rate of responding in the monkeys is shown in Fig. 3.

Many drugs in the narcotic family act both as agonists and as antagonists. These mixed agonist-antagonists, particularly those that have fairly prominent acute morphine-like actions, are self-injected by the monkeys, but the maximal

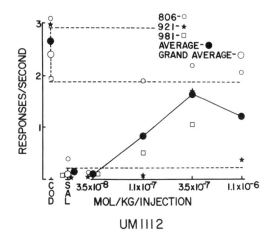

FIG. 3. Rates of fixed-ratio responding maintained by codeine (COD), saline (SAL), and various doses of UM 1112 (MCV 4096, NIH 9337, 2-cyclopropylmethyl-10-*m*-hydroxyphenyl-*trans*-decahydroisoquinoline). This drug is fully morphine-like in suppressing morphine abstinence signs in the rhesus monkey. Duplicate observations on codeine (7.5 × 10⁻⁵ moles/kg/injection=0.32 mg/kg/injection) and saline were obtained in each monkey. A saline substitution was conducted before and after the series of observations on UM 1112; the rates of codeine-reinforced responding were obtained by randomly selecting two of the many codeine sessions for each of the animals. These data are represented in the graph with individual symbols for each of the monkeys; in addition, using the same symbols, the mean of duplicate observations is given for the doses studied in each monkey. There are two additional types of averaged data. ●, averaged data for observations on the subset of monkeys used to study UM 1112 under each of the experimental conditions; ○, codeine and saline rate of responding of 20 monkeys under the same conditions. The brackets indicate ± 3 SEM.

rate of responding by the monkeys is sometimes below that maintained by codeine, and not a great deal above that sustained by saline (J. H. Woods, *unpublished observations*).

Of the drugs used here as illustrative examples, most are not self-administered by these monkeys whose lever-pressing activity is normally maintained with codeine. Figure 4 shows that nalorphine and cyclazocine do not maintain rates of drug-reinforced responding higher than those of saline. These findings are similar to those of other studies (3). In the cases of ketazocine and ethylketazocine (Fig. 4), it is possible that their failure to maintain self-injection was caused by doses too small to be effective; however, this seems unlikely, because direct effects of these drugs were observed in the dose range studied, and, with ethylketazocine, we have been able to establish drug-discrimination responding at these doses.

Figure 5 shows that the compounds UM 1070 and UM 1072 are also not injected at rates different from saline; on the other hand, UM 909 and UM 911 did control rates of self-injection slightly higher than saline. These results indicate that it is possible for a compound (e.g., UM 909) to be self-injected even though it neither suppresses nor precipitates the morphine abstinence syn-

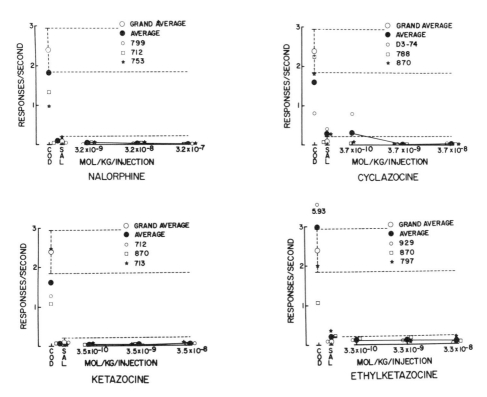

FIG. 4. Rates of fixed-ratio responding maintained by codeine (COD), saline (SAL), or the various doses of nalorphine, cyclazocine, ketazocine, or ethylketazocine. See legend to Fig. 3 for details pertaining to the symbols.

drome. Conversely, a drug (e.g., cyclazocine) can cause physical dependence but not serve as a reinforcer. As experience with these and similar compounds is accrued, it may be increasingly possible to divorce the reinforcing and the dependence-producing capabilities of narcotics. Whether or not the ketazocines and the N-furyl-substituted benzomorphans prove to be clinically satisfactory analgesics, they appear to be free of morphine-like abuse potential.

Guinea Pig Ileum and Mouse Vas Deferens Preparations

Morphine and related drugs decrease neurotransmitter release and thus depress the twitch of electrically driven smooth muscle from either the ileum of the guinea pig or the vas deferens of the mouse. Kosterlitz and his colleagues (8) pioneered in the utilization of these isolated tissue preparations to study drugs of this family, and recently we have begun to use the preparations for the evaluation of test drugs.

Male albino guinea pigs, weighing 300 to 500 g, are sacrificed by a blow to

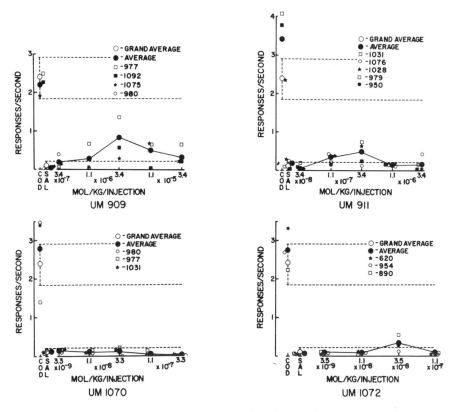

FIG. 5. The rates of fixed-ratio responding maintained by codeine (COD), saline (SAL), or the various doses of UM 909, UM 911, UM 1070, or UM 1072. See legend to Fig. 3 for details pertaining to the symbols. (From Woods et al., ref. 20.)

the head. The terminal portion of the ileum is removed after discarding a 10- to 15-cm segment nearest to the ileocecal junction. The ileum is placed immediately in Krebs physiological buffer, which contains: mepyramine maleate, 0.125 mM; hexamethonium bromide, 0.07 mM; NaCl, 118 mM; KCl, 4.75 mM; $CaCl_2$, 2.54 mM; $MgSO_4$, 1.19 mM; KH_2PO_4, 1.19 mM; glucose, 11 mM; $NaHCO_3$, 25 mM. The buffer is saturated with 95% O_2–5% CO_2 and kept at 37°C. Segments 3 cm in length are placed in a 15-ml organ bath and attached to a strain gauge transducer. The resting tension is adjusted to 0.5 g, and the tissues are equilibrated for 30 to 45 min with washes every 10 min. Tissues are stimulated coaxially at 1.5 times the voltage necessary to produce maximal twitch height, with single pulses, 0.5 msec in duration, delivered once every 10 sec. The tissues are equilibrated without stimulation for 15 min, after which the stimulator is turned on and the tissues equilibrated for an additional 40 min or until twitch height remains stable. Cumulative concentration-response curves for the drugs are determined.

TABLE 1. ED_{50} values of selected drugs in two preparations

	Mouse vas deferens		Guinea pig ileum		
Drug	ED_{50}	Relative potency	ED_{50}	Relative potency	Relative efficacy
Morphine	5.6×10^{-8}	1.0	3.0×10^{-8}	1.0	1.00
Nalorphine	4.5×10^{-8}	1.2	—	—	—
Cyclazocine	3.8×10^{-8}	1.5	—	—	—
Ketazocine	—	—	—	—	—
Ethylketazocine	1.8×10^{-10}	322.2	—	—	—
UM 909	5.5×10^{-9}	10.8	1.9×10^{-6}	0.02	0.96
UM 911	1.1×10^{-8}	5.1	3.9×10^{-7}	0.08	1.07
UM 1070	5.9×10^{-10}	95.2	6.5×10^{-10}	45.7	0.58
UM 1072	2.6×10^{-9}	21.9	3.3×10^{-9}	8.9	0.54

Male albino Swiss-Webster mice, weighing 25 to 30 g, are sacrificed by decapitation. The vasa deferentia are removed and 1.5-cm segments are suspended in organ baths that contain a modified Krebs physiological buffer. The buffer is constituted as described above for the guinea pig ileum except that mepyramine maleate is omitted and the following are added: 0.3 mM pargyline, 0.2 mM tyrosine, 0.1 mM ascorbic acid, and 0.03 mM disodium edetate. The buffer is saturated with 95% O_2–5% CO_2 and kept at 37°C. The segments are attached to a strain gauge transducer and suspended between two platinum electrodes. After a 15-min equilibration period, the segments are stimulated once every 10 sec with pairs of pulses of 1-msec duration, 1 msec apart, and at supermaximal voltage. The segments are stimulated for 30 min or until a stable twitch height is achieved. Cumulative concentration-response curves are determined for the various drugs.

Shown in Table 1 are ED_{50} values for the drugs tested in these two preparations. The relative potency is the ED_{50} for the tested drug divided by the ED_{50} for morphine. With the vas deferens preparation, the maximal drug effects are all approximately equal to that produced by morphine. With the ileal preparation the maximal effects varied greatly, and the efficacy of each drug relative to morphine (maximal response produced by the test drug divided by the maximal response produced by morphine) is given.

Hutchinson et al. (4) examined some of the compounds studied here and noted that they are relatively more potent in the vas deferens than in the guinea pig ileum. This relationship is also shown with the drugs studied in both preparations under our experimental conditions. It should also be noted that the relative potencies of these compounds correlate positively with their analgesic and locomotor activity–increasing effects in mice (20).

Receptor Binding

A membrane preparation isolated from rat cerebral cortex is used to investigate the stereospecific binding of drugs by observing their ability to compete with radioactive narcotic drugs (e.g., etorphine and naltrexone). Male Sprague-Dawley rats weighing 200 g are decapitated and the brains quickly excised and chilled to 2 to 4°C. The brains are washed briefly in 50 mM Tris-HCl, pH 7.4, blotted with filter paper, and the cerebrum dissected and weighed. The tissue is homogenized with 100 parts of the cold buffer for 1 min at 10^4 rpm in a Sorvall Omni Mixer. The homogenate is centrifuged at $20,000 \times g$ for 15 min in the cold. The pellet obtained is resuspended with the original amount of buffer, using a Dounce all-glass homogenizer. Aliquots of this suspension, sufficient for a set of experiments on one given day, are frozen at −70°C. Prior to use, the aliquots are quickly thawed and briefly homogenized in a Dounce homogenizer. The protein concentration of the homogenate is determined by the method of Lowry et al. (9).

The opiate receptor assay is carried out in 8–ml polyethylene tubes. In experiments with radiolabeled etorphine (11), the assay mixture consists of 400 μl membrane suspension, 50 μl H_2O or 1.6 M NaCl, 50 μl dextrorphan, levorphanol, or the narcotic drug being tested, and 25 μl [15,16(n)-^{3}H]etorphine (specific activity = 31 Ci/mmole, Amersham). The final concentration of NaCl, dextrorphan, levorphanol, and etorphine in the medium are 1.5×10^{-1} M, 6×10^{-7} M, and 3×10^{-9} M, respectively. Appropriate dilutions of the drugs are made daily from stock solutions kept either at −20°C (dextrorphan, levorphanol, test drugs) or at 4°C (^{3}H-etorphine).

During pipetting of the assay mixture, the tubes are kept on ice. After the addition of NaCl, the tubes are incubated for 10 min at 25°C. Subsequently, dextrorphan, levorphanol, or the test drug is added and the incubation continued for 15 min, at which time radiolabeled etorphine is added. After an incubation of 30 min, the tubes are placed in ice and their contents filtered through Whatman GF-C filters previously washed in H_2O. Prior to filtering the sample, the filter disc is washed on the assembly with 3×5 ml water saturated with n-amyl alcohol. The samples on the filter are washed with 3×4 ml of ice-cold 50 mM Tris-HCl, pH 7.4. Subsequently, the filters are placed in counting vials, 1 ml absolute ethanol and 10 ml dioxane-xylene-naphthalene scintillation mixture are added, and the vials are then subjected to liquid scintillation counting. The counting efficiency is determined by the use of ^3H_2O as internal standard.

The binding of ^{3}H-etorphine in the presence of a given drug is related to the maximal stereospecific etorphine binding, obtained as the difference between binding in the presence of excess dextrorphan and of excess levorphanol. The EC_{50} values are obtained graphically from log-probit plots of the binding data. Each drug is investigated at five or more concentrations, run in duplicate.

In order to determine the sodium response ratio, the receptor assay is carried out in the presence and in the absence of 150 mM NaCl in the medium. The sodium response ratio for a given drug is expressed as the ratio of the EC_{50} values obtained under these two experimental conditions. Results of these binding studies for the illustrative compounds are shown in Table 2.

The data show that the ketazocines and the N-furyl compounds bind to the

TABLE 2. *EC$_{50}$ values and sodium response ratios for selected drugs*

Drug	EC$_{50}$ (nM)		Sodium response ratio
	−NaCl	+NaCl	
Morphine	60.2	142.1	2.36
Naltrexone	8.57	2.34	0.27
Nalorphine	51.3	20.0	0.39
Cyclazocine	6.46	3.55	0.55
Ketazocine	45.7	63.1	1.38
Ethylketazocine	28.8	21.4	0.74
UM 909	87.8	141.1	1.61
UM 911	45.5	93.7	2.06
UM 1070	16.4	18.0	1.32
UM 1072	8.13	7.52	0.92

agonist conformation of the narcotic receptor, as indicated by their interaction with sodium. These data generally agree with previous work with the ketazocines, nalorphine, and cyclazocine (14). This is in keeping with the previously mentioned absence of precipitated withdrawal in morphine-dependent monkeys. In addition, the compounds demonstrate affinities in the order of potency that is appropriate for their behavioral actions, both in the monkey and in the mouse (i.e., the tetrahydrofurfuryl compounds are the most potent, the ketazocines are intermediate, and the furylmethyl compounds the least potent). Thus their *in vivo* potencies may reflect primarily their affinity for a narcotic receptor.

DISCUSSION

Table 3 summarizes the actions of the illustrative compounds as they appear from the different vantage points provided by these several different assays. It is apparent that the different measurements complement, rather than duplicate, one another.

The compounds we have selected here as illustrative examples are not a random collection of recently tested drugs; instead, they were selected quite specifically as compounds that are similar to one another in many of their properties, and that all differ from the prototype substance, morphine, in several important ways. All, like morphine, are potent analgesics, but none of them suppresses the signs of morphine abstinence in the rhesus monkey. Therefore, if the Single Dose Suppression Test were the only measure employed, all would be judged "not morphine-like." However, two of these drugs are specific antagonists of morphine, capable of precipitating morphine abstinence signs in dependent animals; two others are self-injected, though not to the extent that morphine is; and all show some activity on the smooth muscle preparations and bind to so-called morphine receptors of the membrane preparation.

Historically, it was from the studies of nalorphine that it first became apparent that different drugs of the narcotic family can be similar in some of their proper-

TABLE 3. *Various actions of selected compounds*

Drug	Mouse analgesia (ED50)	Morphine abstinence		Physical dependence		Self-injected (monkey)	Guinea pig ileum twitch depression	Mouse vas deferens depression	Receptor binding (−Na+)
		Suppress	Precipitate	Morphine-like	Cyclazocine-like				
Morphine	1.17	Yes	No	Yes	No	Yes	++	++	++
Nalorphine	36.3	No	Yes	No	Partially	No	(++)[a]	++	++
Cyclazocine	23.1	No	Yes	No	Yes	No	(++++)[a]	++	++++
Ketazocine	0.42	No	No	No	No	No	(++++)[a]	NT[c]	++
Ethylketazocine	0.18	No	No	NT[c]	NT	No	(++++)[a]	+++	+++
UM 909	2.2	No	No	NT	NT	Yes[b]	+	++++	+
UM 911	1.8	No	No	NT	NT	Yes[b]	+	++	++
UM 1070	0.06	No	No	Partially	Partially	No[b]	++++	+++	+++
UM 1072	0.09	No	No	Partially	Partially	No[b]	+++	+++	++++

+, ++, +++, ++++, original amounts of potency. The larger the number of symbols, the greater the potency.
[a]Data from Lord et al., ref. 8.
[b]Data from Woods et al., ref. 20.
[c]Not tested.

ties and radically different in others. It was 24 years ago that Lasagna and Beecher (6) made the important observation that nalorphine provides significant pain relief comparable to that provided by morphine. At analgesic doses, however, nalorphine also produces such disturbing side effects as racing thoughts and anxiety reactions. In animal studies, nalorphine precipitates abstinence signs in morphine-dependent monkeys, of course, and it is bound to membrane receptors with a low sodium ratio, which is characteristic of narcotic antagonists (14). Its analgesic action can be demonstrated in animals, but the drug is not self-administered by monkeys. On repeated administration of nalorphine, monkeys become tolerant to its depressant actions, but the physical dependence it produces is of a very low order and of a distinctly different character than that produced by morphine. The finding that this strong narcotic antagonist has significant analgesic activity was encouraging for the search to find drugs that were strong analgesics but that lacked some of the other characteristics of morphine.

Cyclazocine shares some, but not all, of the properties of nalorphine. In man, acute doses of cyclazocine induce sleepiness and drunkenness; knowledgeable ex–narcotic addicts are more likely to identify it as a barbiturate than as a narcotic (1). An important experiment with squirrel monkeys that has bearing on this subject has recently been reported. Schaefer and Holtzman (16) trained squirrel monkeys to make one particular response to avoid an electric shock in the presence of cyclazocine and another response in its absence. If the monkeys completed at least 22 trials of a 25-trial session on the appropriate lever after receiving the drug, their behavior was considered to be under stimulus control. Stimulus control of behavior, comparable to that produced by 0.1 mg/kg cyclazocine, was seen with ketazocine (0.1 mg/kg), butorphanol (1.0 mg/kg), oxilorphan (3.0 mg/kg), and levallorphan (3.0 mg/kg). Naloxone was capable of reversing the discriminative properties of cyclazocine and some of the drugs with which cyclazocine has common discriminative properties. The monkeys showed incomplete generalization to other drugs with activity as narcotic agonists, antagonists, or both (e.g., morphine, naloxone, or pentazocine), but little or no generalization to the nonopioid drugs *d*-amphetamine, mescaline, pentobarbital, and scopolamine.

The compounds reviewed here, as suggested by the results mentioned above with ketazocine, may have some partial or complete common discriminative properties with cyclazocine. Studies of the discriminative characteristics of these compounds are in progress in our laboratory. It would appear that these and other studies of the discriminative effects of narcotics may come as close to matching subjective reports of narcotics as any assessment technique yet devised with animals.

On chronic administration to human subjects, cyclazocine never becomes preferred; rather, subjects are quite indifferent to it. On abrupt withdrawal after chronic administration, the abstinence signs and symptoms are quite distinct from those of abrupt morphine withdrawal (1). In the monkey, there are differences between cyclazocine and morphine withdrawal, as mentioned above and as reported by Villarreal (18). Likewise, in the dog, as described by Martin and colleagues (2,10), the cyclazocine withdrawal syndrome differs from that of morphine in several ways: in the drugs that suppress it, in the different contributing signs, and in the larger amounts of narcotic antagonists necessary to elicit it. In man, cyclazocine withdrawal is not associated with requests for the drug—which is quite remarkable in subjects who have a history of drug-seeking behavior (1). Thus similar cyclazocine-like agonists might produce dependence not associated with abusive self-administration.

Like nalorphine, cyclazocine is quite capable of reversing morphine's actions in a number of situations and in a number of species.

Ketazocine and ethylketazocine represent an interesting development because they share many of the important actions of cyclazocine without having cyclazocine's morphine antagonist activity. They are potent analgesic agents in a variety of tests, but in mice they do not induce the Straub tail phenomenon or cause intense running, which is associated with morphine administration (17,20).

These drugs afford the possibility of examining cross-tolerance to narotics since they have no morphine antagonist activity. Tepper and Woods (17) used locomotor activity in mice to show that specific tolerance to ethylketazocine is not associated with cross-tolerance to morphine. Llewellyn (7) reported that, with food-reinforced operant behavior in the rhesus monkey, the chronic administration of ketazocine produced tolerance that showed little cross-tolerance with morphine. Conversely, morphine tolerance in this circumstance showed no cross-tolerance to ketazocine—if anything, there was a slight sensitization to ketazocine.

Llewellyn also found that physical dependence was not associated with repeated administration of ketazocine. When a three- to sixfold reduction in sensitivity had been induced over a 2-month period of drug administration, naloxone sensitivity was unchanged, and no withdrawal syndrome was induced by the abrupt cessation of the injection (five/day) routine. An equivalent degree of morphine tolerance would be associated with a significant amount of physical dependence, with obvious abstinence signs on withdrawal of the drug. It is possible that the absence of physical dependence is related to the fact that ketazocine and ethylketazocine are very short-acting drugs, in the monkey as well as in man, as W. F. Michne (personal communication) has reported.

We found both ketazocine and ethylketazocine not to suppress morphine abstinence in the rhesus monkey; they are bound to membrane receptors with sodium ratios of intermediate magnitude; they are more potent depressants of electrically induced twitches of the isolated vas deferens of the mouse than of those in the guinea pig ileum. All of these observations taken together support a strong distinction between these two drugs and the drugs of the conventional narcotic class.

The similarity of actions of the N-furyl compounds to those of ketazocine was first shown by Kosterlitz and his colleagues (4,8). Our results are in complete agreement with theirs, and offer considerable pharmacological and behavioral generality. The 2-methyl-3-furylmethyl compound, designated UM 909, is less potent than, but otherwise similar in action to, the isomeric 3-methylfurfuryl derivative, UM 911. Both of these drugs are active agonists in analgesic test procedures, but they neither precipitate nor suppress the morphine withdrawal syndrome in the rhesus monkey. Nevertheless, with affinities comparable to that of morphine, they both displace radiolabeled etorphine from receptors of the membrane preparation, where they have a high sodium response ratio, indicating that they bind to the "agonist conformation" of the receptor. Interestingly, both of these drugs are self-administered by rhesus monkeys, at rates above those for saline, but not as rapid as those for codeine. The spectrum of results in these assays suggests that the reinforcing action of these drugs has a different mechanism than that of others. The comparability of the isomers of the compounds in our assays suggests that the position of the methyl group is not critical for the mediation of the actions of the compounds.

The closely related tetrahydrofurfuryl-substituted benzomorphans we have studied differ structurally from one another only in the steric configuration of the methyl group in the 9 position of the benzomorphan nucleus: The methyl group is α in UM 1072 and β in UM 1070. These two tetrahydrofurfuryl derivatives are potent analgesics, and they neither precipitate nor suppress morphine abstinence in the monkey. On chronic administration in the monkey, they produce physical dependence, with withdrawal signs that somewhat resemble those of cyclazocine and somewhat resemble those of morphine; these abstinence signs can be precipitated by naloxone administration. The drugs have a high affinity for etorphine binding sites, and they show intermediate values for their sodium response ratios. Unlike UM 909 and UM 911, they are not self-administered by the monkeys. The steric configuration of the 9-methyl group in this pair of compounds does not appear to affect the actions of UM 1070 and UM 1072 in any of our preparations.

It is common pharmacological practice to propose that more than one type of receptor can exist in the body for a particular active substance. Thus the complexities of the responses to the autonomic mediators, acetylcholine and norepinephrine, become easier to understand when it is suggested that there are both muscarinic and nicotinic cholinergic receptors, and that there are alpha and beta adrenergic receptors. Martin et al. (10) have proposed, on the basis of experiments with chronic spinal dogs, that there are three different types of narcotic receptor, which he has designated mu, kappa, and sigma. More recently, Kosterlitz and his colleagues (4) have referred to mu and delta receptors to explain the fact that narcotic agonists can be separated into two groups on the basis of their potency, relative to morphine, when they are assayed on the two smooth muscle preparations described above. It appears that the mouse vas deferens preparation is richer than the guinea pig ileum preparation in the type of receptor that Kosterlitz calls delta (which is probably the type that Martin calls kappa). Furthermore, larger doses of naloxone are required to reverse the actions of the so-called kappa (delta) agonists than are needed to block the effects of the conventional mu agonists, such as morphine itself (5).

The illustrative compounds chosen for discussion in this chapter have actions that can be explained in terms of multiple narcotic receptors; if, in fact, kappa receptors actually exist, most of these drugs can be viewed as kappa agonists. We are continuing to examine these and other atypical narcotic drugs in an attempt to answer the moot question of whether or not there is more than one type of narcotic receptor. Thus far, all drugs that fit the kappa agonist pattern are in the chemical family of the 6,7-benzomorphans; it would be reassuring to discover substances from other chemical families that possess these properties. Whereas naloxone appears to be more effective against mu agonists than against kappa agonists, the discovery of an antagonist that is more effective against kappa actions would strengthen the multiple-receptor hypothesis. Possibly the availability of so-called kappa agonists radiolabeled with high specific activity will permit the use of the binding assay to identify a second family of membrane receptors. The behavioral actions of these drugs in animal preparations seem to offer us a sensitive assay for some of the subtle differences we are seeking. Finally, we will watch with great interest as these atypical analgesic drugs are tested in human populations, in pain clinics for example, because then it will be possible to assess which of the preclinically measurable factors contribute to the use and abuse of these drugs by man.

ACKNOWLEDGMENT

The studies described in this report were supported by grant DA00254 from the National Institute on Drug Abuse.

REFERENCES

1. Eddy, N. B., and Martin, W. R. (1970): Drug dependence of specific opiate antagonist type. *Pharmakopsychiatr. Neuropsychopharmakol.*, 3:73–82.
2. Gilbert, P. E., and Martin, W. R. (1976): The effects of morphine- and nalorphine-like drugs in the nondependent, morphine-dependent and cyclazocine-dependent chronic spinal dog. *J. Pharmacol. Exp. Ther.*, 198:66–82.
3. Hoffmeister, F., and Schlichting, U. U. (1972): Reinforcing properties of some opiates and opioids in rhesus monkeys with histories of cocaine and codeine self-administration. *Psychopharmacologia*, 23:55–74.
4. Hutchinson, M., Kosterlitz, H. W., Leslie, F. M., Waterfield, A. A., and Terenius, L. (1975): Assessment in the guinea-pig ileum and mouse vas deferens of benzomorphans which have strong antinociceptive activity but do not substitute for morphine in the dependent monkey. *Br. J. Pharmacol.*, 55:541–546.
5. Kosterlitz, H. W., Waterfield, A. A., and Berthoud, V. (1973): Assessment of agonist and antagonist properties of narcotic analgesic drugs by their actions on the morphine receptor in the guinea pig ileum. In: *Advances in Biochemical Psychopharmacology, Vol. 8, Narcotic Antagonists,* edited by M. C. Braude et al., pp. 319–334. Raven Press, New York.
6. Lasagna, L., and Beecher, H. K. (1954): The analgesic effectiveness of nalorphine and nalorphine-morphine combinations in man. *J. Pharmacol. Exp. Ther.*, 112:356–363.

7. Llewellyn, M. E. (1978): Acute and chronic effects of ketocyclazocine and morphine on operant behavior in rhesus monkeys. *Fed. Proc.,* 37:310 (Abstr. No. 525).
8. Lord, J. A. H., Waterfield, A. A., Hughes, J., and Kosterlitz, H. W. (1977): Endogenous opioid peptides: Multiple agonists and receptors. *Nature,* 267:495–499.
9. Lowry, O., Rosebrough, N. J., Farr, A. L., and Randall, R. J. (1951): Protein measurement with the Folin phenol reagent. *J. Biol. Chem.,* 193:265–275.
10. Martin, W. R., Eades, C. G., Thompson, J. A., Huppler, R. E., and Gilbert, P. E. (1976): The effects of morphine- and nalorphine-like drugs in the nondependent and morphine-dependent chronic spinal dog. *J. Pharmacol. Exp. Ther.,* 197:517–532.
11. Medzihradsky, F. (1976): Stereospecific binding of etorphine in isolated neural cells and in retina, determined by a sensitive microassay. *Brain Res.,* 108:212–219.
12. Merz, H., Langbein, A., Stockhaus, K., Walther, G., and Wick, H. (1973): Structure-activity relationships in narcotic antagonists with *N*-furylmethyl substituents. In: *Advances in Biochemical Psychopharmacology; Vol. 8, Narcotic Antagonists,* edited by M. C. Braude et al., pp. 91–107. Raven Press, New York.
13. Michne, W. F., Pierson, A. K., and Albertson, N. F. (1974): Ketocyclazocine, a narcotic antagonist with a new activity profile. *Report to the Committee on Problems of Drug Dependence,* pp. 524–532. National Academy of Sciences, Washington, D.C.
14. Pert, C. B., Snyder, S. H., and May, E. L. (1976): Opiate receptor interactions of benzomorphans in rat brain homogenates. *J. Pharmacol. Exp. Ther.,* 196:316–322.
15. Pierson, A. K., and Rosenberg, F. J. (1976): WIN 35,197-2, another benzomorphan with a unique analgesic profile. *Report to the Committee on Problems of Drug Dependence,* pp. 949–965. National Academy of Sciences, Washington, D.C.
16. Schaefer, G. J., and Holtzman, S. G. (1978): Discriminative effects of cyclazocine in the squirrel monkey. *J. Pharmacol. Exp. Ther.,* 205:291–301.
17. Tepper, P., and Woods, J. H. (1978): Changes in locomotor activity and naloxone-induced jumping in mice produced by WIN 35,197-2 (ethylketazocine) and morphine. *Psychopharmacology,* 58:125–129.
18. Villarreal, J. E. (1973): The effects of morphine agonists and antagonists on morphine-dependent rhesus monkeys. In: *Agonist and Antagonist Actions of Narcotic Analgesic Drugs,* edited by H. W. Kosterlitz, H. O. J. Collier, and J. E. Villarreal, pp. 73–93. University Park Press, Baltimore.
19. Woods, J. H. (1979): Narcotic-reinforced responding: A rapid evaluation procedure. *Drug Alcohol. Depend. (in press).*
20. Woods, J. H., Fly, C. L., and Swain, H. H. (1978): Behavioral actions of some *N*-furyl benzomorphans and ketazocines in rhesus monkeys and mice. In: *Characteristics and Function of Opioids, Vol. 4, Developments in Neuroscience,* edited by J. M. Van Ree and L. Terenius, pp. 404–411. Elsevier/North-Holland, Amsterdam.

Mechanisms of Pain and Analgesic Compounds,
edited by R. F. Beers, Jr., and E. G. Bassett.
Raven Press, New York © 1979.

39. Preclinical Evaluation of Reinforcing and Adversive Properties of Analgesics

Friedrich Hoffmeister

*Institut für Pharmakologie, Bayer AG, D-5600 Wuppertal 1,
Federal Republic of Germany*

INTRODUCTION

Current pharmacotherapy of pain is limited by side effects of analgesics rather than by their lack of pain-alleviating potency. If administered in appropriate doses, the most potent analgesics presently available extinguish, for a brief period, even the most severe states of pain.

Among the side effects that limit their utility are depression of respiratory function and reduction of vigilance and attention, which decrease the ability of a patient to perform. With chronic treatment almost all groups of strong analgesics lead to tolerance, resulting in the need for increasingly larger doses and the development of physical dependence. Although these effects of analgesics are clearly negative, appraisal of their psychic actions on mood, feeling, and self-esteem is less easy to achieve.

The pain to be treated is not simply the sum of the nociceptive input. It is a state of feeling in which certain patterns of impulses from the peripheral nervous system progressively govern the psychic state unless this input can be attenuated by the individual's appropriate behavior.

After experiencing the mood-depressive and panic-producing psychic reactions to pain, an individual becomes less and less able to judge the significance of pain relative to its meaning for survival. In addition, the euphorigenic, mood-elevating psychopharmacological properties of analgesics certainly contribute to the therapeutic effect. On the other hand, these psychopharmacological actions are the source of the danger inherent in our pain-killing agents, because they give rise to improper use, inducing drug-taking behavior and psychic dependence.

The recent discovery that the opiate receptor and its endogenous ligands constitute a system physiologically involved in the regulation of the psyche, beyond discrimination and psychic evaluation of nociceptive input, forms a new basis for the development of drugs, provided there is a way to interfere pharmacologically with structures that *specifically* permit only nociceptive input to excite mood regulatory systems. The demands, however, have not changed, and absence of dependence-producing effects is still the most important goal to be reached.

Preclinical evaluation of a drug's psychopharmacological properties that are possibly related to their dependence-producing liability is based on the behavior of animals that induces or deters administration of the drug under study.

Such behavioral activity is considered functional because it depends on the relationship between administration and response in which behavioral changes are further modified by environmental variables and the drug's behavioral effects persist beyond its active metabolic life. However, these functional effects depend on, or are mediated by, direct effects on behavior that are independent of environmental variables and limited to the drug's active metabolic life (17).

OBSERVATIONS AND DISCUSSION

Some Direct Effects of Analgesics on Behavior

Among the direct behavioral effects of analgesics are drug group–specific patterns of antinociceptive activities as well as physical dependence–producing effects.

For example, vocalization and vocalization afterdischarge (two nociceptive responses of the rat induced by electrical stimulation of the tail and mediated by different parts of the brain), are inhibited by increasing doses of opiates in a characteristic sequence as seen in Fig. 1. The patterns of agonist-antagonists of the pentazocine-cyclazocine type differ from those of the pure agonists. The former group inhibits vocalization afterdischarge in a dose-dependent manner but exerts only a moderate effect on vocalization which plateaus at low ceiling (4). Nalorphine, although an agonist-antagonist, exhibits a different type of action. Its dose-effect curves on the nociceptive reactions resemble those of morphine and codeine but have a less steep slope (4).

The effects of the antipyretic analgesic aminophenazone are opposite, i.e., vocalization is inhibited to a greater degree than is vocalization afterdischarge (5), whereas the effects of another antipyretic analgesic, phenacetin, are qualitatively closer to those of nalorphine or morphine than to those of aminophenazone. Paracetamol and acetylsalicyclic acid (not shown) do not influence these nociceptive reactions to a measurable degree.

Morphine agonists extinguish individual symptoms of the withdrawn, physically dependent rat with increasing doses in a group-specific sequence (Fig. 2). The agonist-antagonists pentazocine, cyclazocine, and nalorphine precipitate additional withdrawal symptoms at low doses, as expected; at high doses, however, they decrease the total withdrawal scores, thus mimicking morphine substitution (4).

In a corresponding manner, the antagonists cyclazocine and nalorphine precipitate, in nonwithdrawn dependent rats, a maximal withdrawal syndrome at low to medium dose levels and decrease the withdrawal score at high doses (Fig. 3).

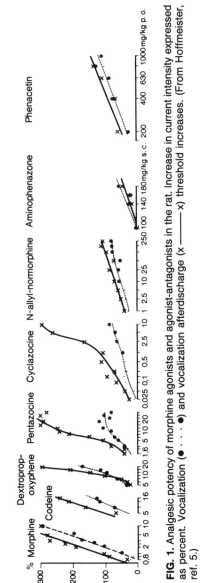

FIG. 1. Analgesic potency of morphine agonists and agonist-antagonists in the rat. Increase in current intensity expressed as percent. Vocalization (● · · · ●) and vocalization afterdischarge (x———x) threshold increases. (From Hoffmeister, ref. 5.)

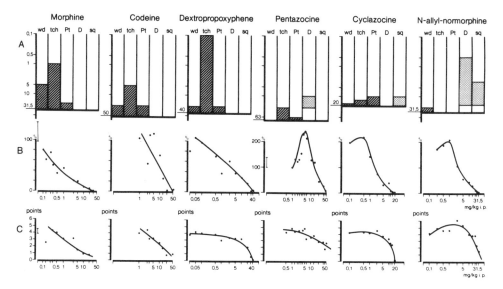

FIG. 2. Inhibition and precipitation of withdrawal symptoms by morphine agonists and agonist-antagonists in the withdrawn, morphine-dependent rat. **A:** Inhibition or precipitation of the different withdrawal symptoms (wd, wet dog; tch, teeth chatter; Pt, ptosis; D, diarrhea; sq, squealing) at the indicated mg/kg dose administered i.p.; ▨, Dose range inhibiting withdrawal symptoms; ▦, dose range precipitating withdrawal symptoms. **B:** Frequency of writhing symptoms in percent of control population; vertical bar indicates confidence limits. **C:** Influence on the total withdrawal symptoms (mean score, 5 animals/dose). (From Hoffmeister, ref. 4.)

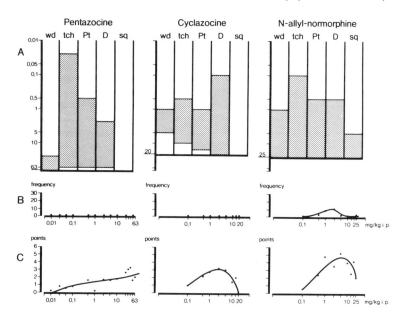

FIG. 3. Precipitation of withdrawal symptoms by morphine agonist-antagonists in the nonwithdrawn morphine-dependent rat. **A:** Inhibition or precipitation of different symptoms at the indicated mg/kg dose administered i.p. ▦, Dose range precipitating withdrawal symptoms. See legend to Fig. 2 for symptom code. **B:** Number of writhing reactions (mean values). **C:** Influence on the total withdrawal symptoms (mean score, 5 animals/dose). (From Hoffmeister, ref. 4.)

Some Functional Effects of Analgesics Controlling Self-Administration Behavior

The qualitatively different, direct behavioral effects of the individual analgesics are reflected, to some extent, in their effects on self-administration behavior.

If, for example, an animal is offered an opiate agonist (e.g., morphine) for self-administration, one observes that at least two different properties of the compound involve the occurrence of self-administration behavior. The initial responding for drug infusions is caused by the psychopharmacological properties of the compound and maintained by drug-seeking behavior which, in turn, is regulated by environmental (e.g., schedule-dependent) variables (Fig. 4).

The appearance of withdrawal symptoms following saline replacement demonstrates that the monkey has become physically dependent, a state in which his behavior is induced and governed primarily by the direct behavioral effects of the drug. Thus both types of effects contribute to self-administration.

The significance of functional behavioral effects relevant to the initiation and maintenance of self-administration behavior are more clearly assessed by the "cross–self-administration" procedure. This technique takes advantage of the finding that well-trained animals can be exposed to different drugs and dosages over the course of relatively few test sessions. The rate of self-administration

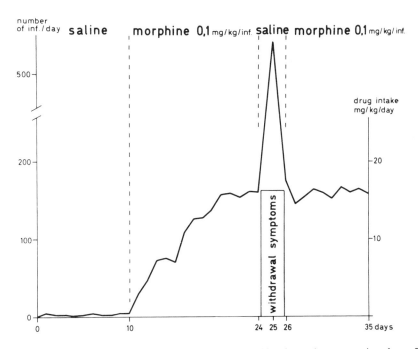

FIG. 4. Continuous self-administration of saline or morphine by a rhesus monkey for a 35-day period. Number of infusions/day = number of daily self-administered infusions of morphine at 100 μg/kg; drug intake, morphine intake/day in mg/kg i.v.

is stabilized and maintained by response-evoked infusions of a standard drug at dosages too low to produce severe physical dependence. The test drugs are then substituted for the original in several consecutive sessions to determine the extent to which a substituted drug becomes self-administered. The technique has recently been improved by application of schedules making drug delivery contingent on high as well as low rates of response in order to minimize the number of false positives (18). Thus, under the conditions of this procedure, it is comparatively easy to make self-administration of a drug contingent on a variety of operant schedules.

Further, the technique enables one to analyze the influence of previous and past drug histories on self-administration behavior. Rhesus monkeys with either a narcotic or a stimulant drug history self-administer narcotic analgesics such as morphine, codeine, and dextropropoxyphene, as well as the agonist-antagonists pentazocine and propiram fumarate (Fig 5).

Morphine is self-administered at low dosages under these conditions by monkeys. The number of self-administered infusions is, however, low compared to the rates at which the weaker agonists of the codeine-dextropropoxyphene type are self-administered. This is caused by the long duration of action of morphine in the rhesus monkey and by the consequence of the rate-depressing properties of this substance. Again, two effects of morphine not primarily related to its reinforcing properties are shown to modify self-administration behavior.

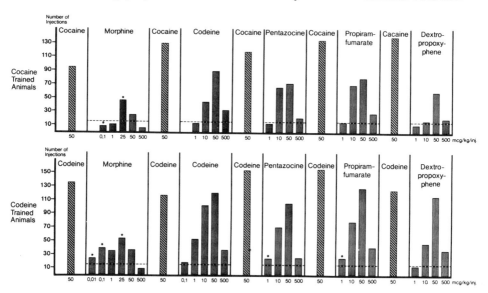

FIG. 5. Infusions of various drugs self-administered by monkeys at different dosages under the contingency of a fixed-ratio 10 schedule of reinforcement when replacing codeine, compared with infusions of standard drug and saline. ▨, Infusions of stabilizing drugs, averages of 3 animals and of the last two sessions before replacement of each new dose of the drug; ▥, infusions of replacement drugs, averages of 3 animals and six sessions; – – – –, saline infusions, averages of 15 animals and six sessions; *, average of 2 animals.

Monkeys with a narcotic history self-administer infusions of opiates and opioids more frequently than do animals with a stimulant cocaine history, as seen in Fig. 5. These differences become strikingly obvious in the experiments using morphine and dextropropoxyphene as replacement drugs. Moreover, the intraindividual differences in opiate drug intake at the unit dose of 50 μg/kg/ infusion are higher in the cocaine- than in the codeine-trained group of monkeys (Fig. 6). Thus the extent of the reinforcing property of opiates and opioids depends on whether the monkey had a history of self-administering opiates or central nervous system stimulants.

In contrast to pure agonists and weak agonist-antagonists, the strong agonist-antagonists nalorphine and cyclazocine are not self-administered and their dose-effect curves do not have the characteristic inverted V shape shown by self-administered drugs (see Fig. 7).

Generally, the cross–self-administration technique is the procedure most widely used for the screening of reinforcing properties of drugs: More than 20 laboratories worldwide, in submitting their results to the International Study Group Investigating Drugs as Reinforcers (ISGIDAR), have demonstrated the reliability and consistency of the method. Its main disadvantage, however, is the fact that it ranks drugs according to their potency rather than their relative reinforcement strength.

Among the procedures providing more quantitative results in this respect are the progressive ratio paradigm and the choice procedure. Both experimental approaches have been shown to be useful in assessing the relative reinforcement strength, especially of the psychomotor stimulants (3,15,19,20).

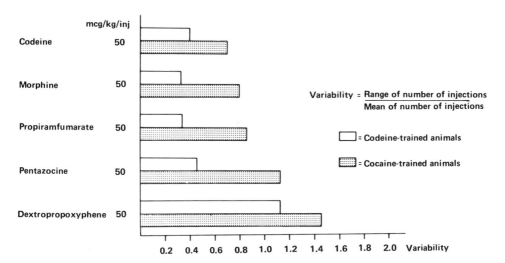

FIG. 6. Intraindividual differences during 6-day administration of various replacement drugs in cocaine- and codeine-trained monkeys. Differences are calculated from the indicated variability formula and averaged for the 3 animals involved in replacement by each drug in both groups. (From Hoffmeister and Schlichting, ref. 9.)

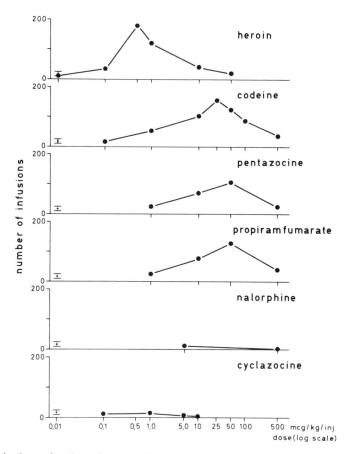

FIG. 7. Injections of various drugs at different dosages under the contingency of a fixed-ratio 10 schedule of reinforcement in a codeine replacement experiment. (From Hoffmeister and Wuttke, ref. 12.)

In the progressive ratio procedure, the so-called breaking point is measured, e.g., the ratio requirement for drug infusion at which the self-administration performance falls below a selected level of one or two injections per day (Fig. 8) (7).

Heroin motivates monkeys to fulfill a fixed-ratio (FR) 12800 requirement, whereas the breaking point with codeine is FR-6400 (Fig. 8). The dose breaking point curves of heroin and codeine are linear over a wide dose range; those for dextropropoxyphene and pentazocine indicate, however, that high doses of these drugs are less reinforcing than low and medium doses, possibly owing to toxic or antagonistic effects (Fig. 9) (7).

Among the strong analgesics, there are drugs that have *no* positive reinforcing properties in self-administration techniques. Without further knowledge, some of them, nalorphine and cyclazocine for example, would appear to be useful

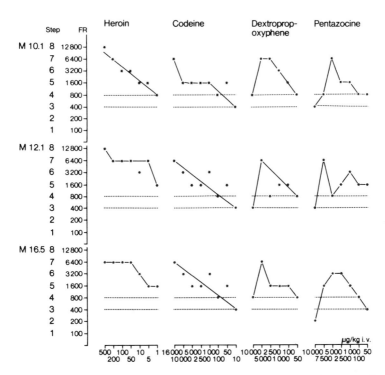

FIG. 8. Individual breaking points for drugs self-administered i.v. by 3 rhesus monkeys in a trial using the progressive ratio procedure. Each point represents a single breaking point observation. Fixed-ratio requirements are equated with steps; dosage indicated is µg/kg/infusion. :::::::, Range of saline effects. (From Hoffmeister, ref. 7.)

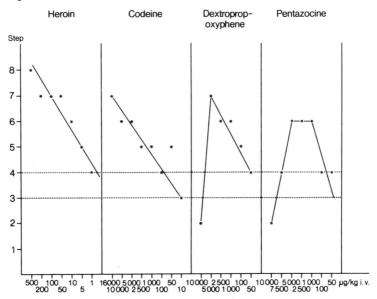

FIG. 9. Average breaking points for drugs self-administered i.v. by 3 rhesus monkeys. See legend to Fig. 8 for details. (From Hoffmeister, ref. 7.)

analgesics. Since it is known that strong agonist-antagonists are devoid of therapeutic value as analgesics on account of their aversive, negative reinforcing effects (16), the predictive value of self-administration experiments to determine the applicability of a substance as an analgesic in man is not complete unless the existence and the extent of negative reinforcing properties can be demonstrated. Certainly a decrease of the infusion rate of a drug below saline levels might permit the speculation that negative reinforcing properties are involved (2). On the other hand, a decrease in the rate of self-administration is very often caused by nonspecific, rate-depressing behavioral effects.

Results more clearly interpretable about the existence of negative reinforcement are achieved when scheduled drug injections give rise to avoidance or escape behavior, resulting in the preclusion of infusion. Here again, the drug history of an animal and the interference of direct with functional behavioral effects of a drug play an important role. Drug-naive animals will not avoid scheduled infusions of pentazocine, codeine, and propiram fumarate (Fig. 10),

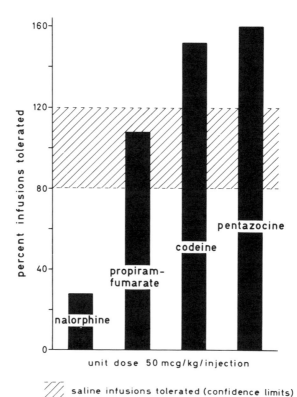

FIG. 10. Avoidance of and escape from drug injections by 7 naive rhesus monkeys. Drug infusions tolerated expressed as percent of saline infusions tolerated (with confidence limits) during a 6-day control period. Columns represent the means of at least 3 monkeys/substance. The mean number of saline infusions tolerated (with confidence limits) was assigned a value of 100%. (From Hoffmeister and Wuttke, ref. 12.)

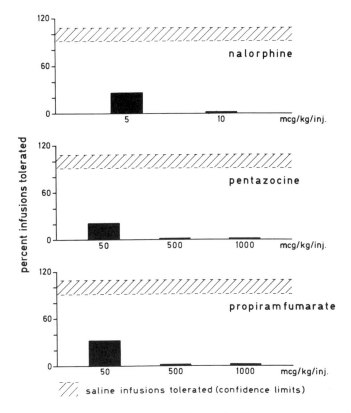

FIG. 11. A 6-day trial of avoidance and escape from nalorphine, pentazocine, and propiram fumarate in 3 rhesus monkeys physically dependent on morphine. Columns represent the means of 3 animals/substance. See legend to Fig. 10 for details. (From Hoffmeister and Wuttke, ref. 12.)

but will avoid nalorphine infusions (8). In contrast, monkeys physically dependent on morphine avoid infusions not only of nalorphine but also of propiram fumarate and of pentazocine, indicating that the latter compounds are positive reinforcers in normal individuals but aversive when administered to a dependent organism, as seen in Fig. 11 (2,8).

The negative reinforcing properties of agonist-antagonists of the nalorphine-cyclazocine type, however, become apparent in drug-naive monkeys also. Drug-naive rhesus monkeys with a past history of shock avoidance terminate the stimuli associated with infusions of nalorphine, indicating that nalorphine has negative reinforcing properties (Fig. 12) (14).

The intensity of avoidance-escape behavior depends on dose size of the scheduled nalorphine infusions (Fig. 13) (14). Since nalorphine does not influence avoidance responding maintained by electrical shock, drug avoidance responding is not caused by the behavioral effects of the administered drug (Fig. 13). Dose-dependent, negative reinforcing effects can also be demonstrated for cyclazocine (Fig. 14) (10). In contrast, the so-called pure antagonist naloxone is devoid,

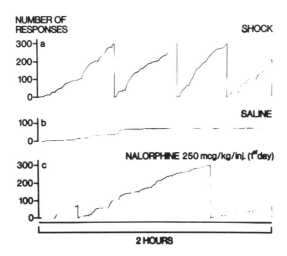

FIG. 12. Representative performance of a monkey pressing a key under schedules of termination of a stimulus associated with an electric shock, infusions of saline, or nalorphine. Electric shocks or infusions of 10-sec duration were scheduled every 30 sec in the presence of a white light. Each response terminated the light and the shock for a 60-sec period in which key pressing had no scheduled consequences. Diagonal strokes indicate periods during which the recording pen was offset during the shock or infusion.

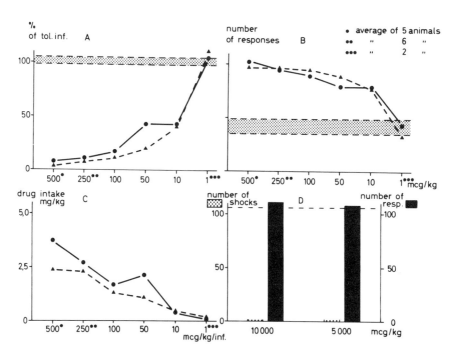

FIG. 13. A-C: Effects of different doses of nalorphine on percent of infusions tolerated, number of responses, and drug intake during a six-session trial. ●, Sessions 1 to 3; ▲, sessions 4 to 6; ▦, confidence limits of saline infusions tolerated and number of responses with saline infusions. **D:** Effects of nalorphine on mean of responses and shocks per session under a schedule of termination of a stimulus associated with electric shock.

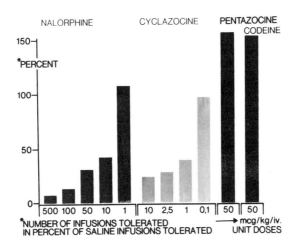

FIG. 14. Avoidance or tolerance of injections of nalorphine, cyclazocine, pentazocine, and codeine by naive rhesus monkeys performing under a discrete avoidance escape schedule. See legend to Fig. 11 for experimental details. (From Hoffmeister and Wuttke, ref. 10.)

at least under the experimental conditions described, of negative reinforcing properties in the drug-naive monkey (10).

The abuse of the potent psychoactive drugs, including strong analgesics, constitutes an overt hazard to public health. Naturally, extensive research has been focused on the prediction and analysis of the reinforcing capacity of these drug groups. Less attention has been devoted to possible psychoactive actions of the weak analgesics, despite a large nonmedical use, since these substances are easily available without legal restrictions to the public.

The subjective reasons for nonmedical use of weak analgesics are still obscure. The nonmedical use of antipyretic analgesics may be attributed, in part, to the fact that the act of drug taking per se, like other oral behaviors, may evolve into a conditioned reinforcement. On the other hand, the possibility of pharmacologically positive reinforcing effects as a cause for their expanded use cannot be excluded. Since most of these substances are prescribed in combination with psychoactive drugs or strong analgesics, the question arises to what extent drug interactions contribute to positive reinforcement.

Rhesus monkeys trained to self-administer codeine will not self-administer intravenous acetylsalicylic acid, phenylbutazone, or aminophenazone when these drugs are substituted for codeine. The number of self-administered infusions (see Fig. 15) is within or even below the saline level (11,13). When offered in combination with codeine, acetylsalicylic acid, phenylbutazone, and aminophenazone (Fig. 16) (6), the intake rate falls below the self-administration rate of codeine alone (11,13). Conversely (Fig. 17), the addition of codeine to these three drugs markedly increases their intake.

In other words, these antipyretic analgesics are devoid of positive reinforcing properties in animals with an opiate experience and seem to decrease the rein-

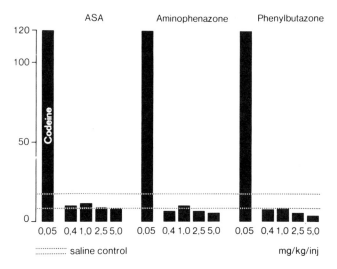

FIG. 15. Replacement of codeine by acetylsalicylic acid (ASA), aminophenazone, and phenylbutazone in rhesus monkeys trained in codeine self-administration. *Ordinate:* Mean number of infusions/3-hr session. Dosage: 0.05 to 5 mg/kg/infusion. Codeine column represents mean of 8 animals during a 6-day replacement period; other columns represent mean of 3 animals during replacement period of 6 days. ::::::::, Confidence limits of self-administered saline in 10 animals during a 6-day replacement period.

forcement strength of opiates. When added to opiates, they are self-administered in comparatively high doses, resulting in a drug intake that does not occur with the pure compounds (11,13).

There are also no positive reinforcing properties of acetylsalicylic acid when tested in the drug-naive rhesus monkey (Fig. 18) (13). Moreover, acetylsalicylic

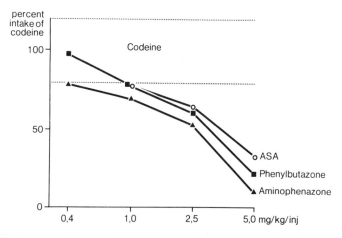

FIG. 16. Effect of acetylsalicylic acid (ASA), aminophenazone, and phenylbutazone on mean intake per session of codeine.

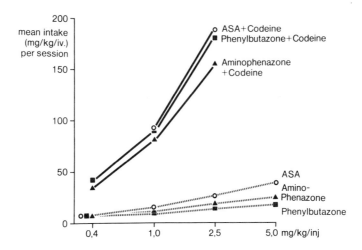

FIG. 17. Effect of self-administered codeine (0.05 mg/kg/infusion) on mean intake per session of acetylsalicylic acid (ASA), aminophenazone, and phenylbutazone.

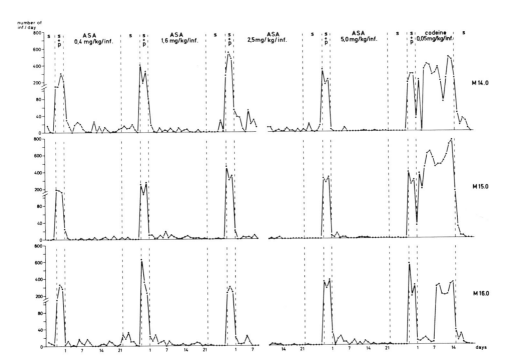

FIG. 18. Continuous self-administration of varying doses of acetylsalicylic acid (ASA) and codeine in 3 drug-naive rhesus monkeys. Saline infusion (S), saline infusion + food pellets (S+P). *Ordinate:* Averaged total number of infusions. (From Hoffmeister and Wuttke, ref. 13.)

acid does not maintain responding initiated by food reinforcement (13). If, however, acetylsalicylic acid is presented to drug-naive animals in combination with codeine, the combination of the two drugs (Fig. 19) is self-administered by monkeys (6). Surprisingly, animals under these conditions continue lever pressing even when they are in a state of severe salicylate intoxication. They continue to respond until lethal doses of acetylsalicylic acid have been administered. The behavior of the animal indicates that the state of salicylate intoxication per se does not represent a punishing event that would motivate the monkey to refrain from further responding when responding is reinforced by codeine infusions.

A

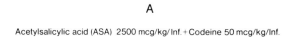

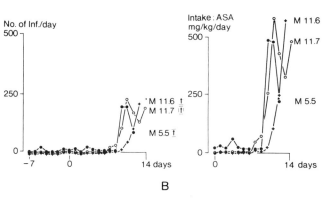

B

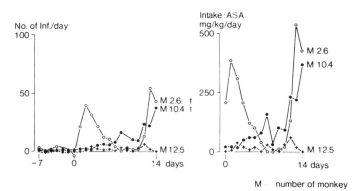

M   number of monkey

FIG. 19. A and B (left): Self-administered infusions of combinations of acetylsalicylic acid and codeine by 3 monkeys during a 14-day period. A and B (right): Daily acetylsalicylic acid intake (mg/kg) of the same monkeys. †, death.

The strength of reinforcing effects of drugs depends, to a large degree, on the route of administration. Delayed reinforcement (occurring necessarily with oral administration) is likely to attenuate the reinforcement capability markedly and, in some instances, to a significant degree. There are so-called "borderline drugs" which are strong reinforcers following parenteral administration but weak, or nonactive, reinforcers after intragastral administration. This observation is one of the reasons underlying the importance of self-administration experiments using the intragastric route.

It has been shown (19,20) that a number of sedative hypnotics are self-administered via the intragastric route. Our experience regarding the reinforcement capability of intragastrically administered analgesics, however, is still limited and restricts the interpretation and predictive value of such experiments. For example, the question has been raised of whether or not the antipyretic analgesic phenacetin and its active metabolite paracetamol have positive reinforcing properties that contribute to their nonmedical use. A pilot study on intragastric self-administration of the two compounds compared with that of codeine showed that there might be differences in their reinforcing properties. It is seen in Fig. 20 that codeine at a dosage of 0.5 mg/kg is self-administered at a

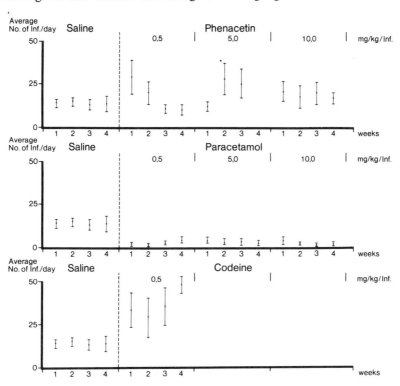

FIG. 20. Intragastric self-administration of phenacetin, paracetamol, and codeine in 3 drug-naive rhesus monkeys.

rate well above the saline range. Phenacetin seems to be self-administered by the drug-naive rhesus monkey. The rate of self-administration of 0.5 mg/kg phenacetin doses exceeds that of saline during the first two weeks of drug exposure; after that period, the rate decreases to the saline level. At 5 mg/kg dosages during weeks 2 and 3, the phenacetin intake rate surpasses the saline level. During all 4 weeks, the number of injections at 10 mg/kg is somewhat higher (Fig. 20) than during the saline periods. Paracetamol, however, is self-administered at rates much lower than those of saline.

Although this experiment is far from conclusive, the possibility that there may be measurable differences between the reinforcing properties of compounds otherwise pharmacologically related should stimulate the analysis of both strong and weak reinforcing properties.

SUMMARY

Figure 21 summarizes the reinforcing properties of representatives of the most important groups of analgesics as assessed by the methods discussed.

Although incomplete, this survey demonstrates that there is a way to differentiate analgesics according to their reinforcing properties in the monkey. The ranking shown, although far from complete and precise, nevertheless reflects the

Substance	Route of administration	Positive reinforcing Properties		Negative reinforcing Properties	
		Continuous Selfadministration	Cross Selfadministration	Drug Avoidance behavior	
				naive animals	morphine-dependent animals
Heroin	i. v.	+ + +	+ + + +	∅	∅
Morphine	i. v.	+ + +	+ +	∅	∅
Codeine	i.v.; i. g.	+ +	+ + +	∅	∅
Tilidine	i. v.	+ +	+	∅	∅
Profadol	i. v.	+ +	+ +	∅	(+)
Propiram	i. v.	+ +	+ +	∅	+ +
Pentazocine	i. v.	+ +	+ +	∅	+ +
Nalorphine	i. v.	∅	∅	+ + +	+ + + +
Cyclazocine	i. v.	∅	∅	+ + + +	+ + + +
Acetylsalicylic acid	i. v.	∅	∅	∅	∅
Aminophenazon	i. v.	∅	∅	∅	∅
Phenylbutazon	i. v.	∅	∅	∅	∅
Phenacetin	i. g.	(+)	−	−	−
Paracetamol	i. g.	∅	−	−	−

FIG. 21. Some positive and negative reinforcing properties of selected analgesics, indicating a scale of strong (+ + + +) to weak [(+)], and no effect (∅); no data, −.

abuse potential of these drugs in man. Since the overall effects of analgesics in humans, their benefits and risks, cannot be judged solely by the nature and strength of their reinforcing properties, an appraisal of the individual analgesics is possible only when all their pharmacological properties are considered. Thus the evaluation of a drug's direct effects on behavior supplements, in many respects, the evaluation of its reinforcing properties by providing the rationale for certain types of behavior during self-administration and by giving basic data on the anticipated therapeutic value of the drug.

For example, the agonists heroin, morphine, codeine, and dextropropoxyphene clearly belong to one group or type of drugs when their antinociceptive and morphine-substituting properties are compared. Among the agonist-antagonists, however, pentazocine and cyclazocine seem to be qualitatively related to each other and clearly different from nalorphine when only antinocicpetive properties are considered. On the other hand, a comparison of their influence on the withdrawal syndrome of the morphine-dependent rat reveals no major qualitative differences between all three compounds. Assessment of reinforcement capability clearly differentiates dextropropoxyphene from the other agonists described. Pentazocine can be differentiated from the agonists on one hand and cyclazocine and nalorphine on the other by a variety of self-administration procedures. Furthermore, it is interesting to note that the pattern of antinociceptive effects of the antipyretic analgesic phenacetin appears to be comparable to that of the agonists and that of nalorphine but it is clearly different from that of paracetamol as well as that of aminophenazone. As for its reinforcing properties, phenacetin seems to be more related to agonists than to the antipyretic analgesics aminophenazone and paracetamol.

Thus an assessment of both direct and functional effects on behavior describes the properties of analgesics more accurately than a consideration of either effect alone and optimizes the predictive value of such experiments for drug action in man.

Despite the wealth of recent methodological progress, there still remains the risk of observing false positives and false negatives. This risk, however, might be minimized by further improvements in methodology but, as in all animal experiment procedures, including toxicology, it cannot be completely eliminated.

Although there are a number of drawbacks, self-administration procedures have attained a significant importance, and an effective research strategy for the development of a new and better pharmacotherapy of pain must include the assessment of reinforcing properties.

REFERENCES

1. Deneau, G., Yanagita, T., and Seevers, M. H. (1969): Self-administration of psychoactive substances by the monkey—A measure of psychological dependence. *Psychopharmacologia,* 16:30–48.
2. Goldberg, S. R., Hoffmeister, F., Schlichting U., and Wuttke, W. (1971): Aversive properties of nalorphine and naloxone in morphine-dependent monkeys. *J. Pharmacol. Exp. Ther.,* 179:268–276.

3. Griffith, R. R., Brady, J. V., and Snell, J. O. (1978): Progressive-ratio performance maintained by drug infusions. *Psychopharmacology,* 56:5–13.
4. Hoffmeister, F. (1968): Untersuchungen über die analgetischen morphinantagonistischen und morphinartigen Wirkungen von Morphinantagonisten an normalen und morphinabhängigen Tieren. *Pharmakopsychiatr. Neuropsychopharmakolog.,* 1:239–260.
5. Hoffmeister, F. (1968): Tierexperimentelle Untersuchungen über den Schmerz und seine pharmakologische Beeinflussung. *Arzneim. Forsch.,* 16 (Suppl.): 57.
6. Hoffmeister, F. (1977): Self-administration of codeine plus acetylsalicylic acid in rhesus monkeys with unlimited access to the drug. *Pharmacol. Biochem. Behav.,* 6:179–182.
7. Hoffmeister, F. (1979): Progressive ratio performance in the rhesus monkey maintained by opiate infusions. *Psychopharmacology (in press).*
8. Hoffmeister, F., Kroneberg, G., Schlichting, U., and Wuttke, W. (1974): Zur Pharmakologie des Analgetikums Propiramfumarat [*N*-(1-Methyl-2-piperidino-äthyl)-*N*-(2-pyridyl)-propionamid-fumarat]. *Arzneim. Forsch.,* 24:600–624.
9. Hoffmeister, F., and Schlichting, U. (1972): Reinforcing properties of some opiates and opioids in rhesus monkeys with histories of cocaine and codeine self-administration. *Psychopharmacologia,* 23:55–74.
10. Hoffmeister, F., and Wuttke, W. (1973): Negative reinforcing properties of morphine antagonists in naive rhesus monkeys. *Psychopharmacologia,* 33:247–258.
11. Hoffmeister, F., and Wuttke, W. (1973): Self-administration of acetylsalicylic acid and combinations with codeine and caffeine in rhesus monkeys. *J. Pharmacol. Exp. Ther.,* 186:267–275.
12. Hoffmeister, F., and Wuttke, W. (1974): Self-administration: Positive and negative reinforcing properties of morphine-antagonists in the rhesus monkey. In: *Advances in Biochemical Psychopharmacology, Vol. 8, Narcotic Antagonists,* edited by M. C. Braude et al., pp. 361–369. Raven Press, New York.
13. Hoffmeister, F., and Wuttke, W. (1975): Further studies on self-administration of antipyretic analgesics and combinations of antipyretic analgesics with codeine in rhesus monkeys. *J. Pharmacol. Exp. Ther.,* 193:870–875.
14. Hoffmeister, F., and Wuttke, W. (1975): Psychotropic drugs as negative reinforcers. *Pharmacol. Rev.,* 27:419–428.
15. Johanson, C. E., and Schuster, C. R. (1975): A choice procedure for drug reinforcers: Cocaine and methylphenidate in the rhesus monkey. *J. Pharmacol. Exp. Ther.,* 193:676–688.
16. Keats, A. S., and Telford, J. (1956): Nalorphine, a potent analgesic in man. *J. Pharmacol. Exp. Ther.,* 117:190–196.
17. Pickens, R., Meisch, R. A., and Thompson, T. (1978): Drug self-administration: An analysis of the reinforcing effects of drugs. In: *Drugs of Abuse,* edited by L. L. Iversen, S. D. Iversen, and S. H. Snyder, Plenum, New York.
18. Woods, J. H. (1977): Narcotic-reinforced responding: A rapid screening procedure. *Report to the Committee on Problems of Drug Dependence,* pp. 420–437. National Academy of Sciences, Washington, D.C.
19. Yanagita, T. (1973): An experimental framework for evaluation of dependence liability of various types of drugs in monkeys. *Bull. Narc.,* 25:57–64.
20. Yanagita, T., and Takahashi, S. (1973): Dependence liability of several sedative-hypnotic agents: Response-drug contingencies. *J. Pharmacol. Exp. Ther.,* 185:307–316.

Mechanisms of Pain and Analgesic Compounds,
edited by R. F. Beers, Jr., and E. G. Bassett.
Raven Press, New York © 1979.

40. Cannabinoids as Analgesics

Louis S. Harris

Department of Pharmacology, Medical College of Virginia, Richmond, Virginia 23298

INTRODUCTION

For millennia man has used the leaves and flowering tops of the hemp plant, *Cannabis sativa,* for medicinal purposes. Indeed, until 1942 cannabis was listed in the U.S. Pharmacopeia. Owing to legal control problems and the development of a wide variety of new therapeutic agents, the medical use of cannabis fell into disrepute and was discontinued. One of the problems associated with the use of the plant material involved quality control. There was no good way of ensuring the purity and potency of the material. With the recent final, complete identification of the active principle of cannabis, Δ^9-tetrahydrocannabinol (Δ^9-THC) (7,8), and its subsequent total synthesis (8,25,27), a readily prepared, pure compound became available for pharmacological and clinical evaluation. This, coupled with the increased illicit use of marihuana, has led to dramatic increase of interest in the drug. A large number of recent books and reviews sum up the current state of the art in this regard (2,11,18,19,30). As for the therapeutic potential of cannabis, the report (3) of a recent symposium summarizes our broad current knowledge in this area.

Among the many therapeutic properties ascribed to cannabis was its use for the relief of pain, particularly pain associated with migraine headache, menstrual cramps, and toothache. Until recently, there were no adequate laboratory or clinical studies that would allow one to ascertain the analgesic efficacy of the drug. Early publications reported analgesic activity for Δ^9-THC approximating morphine in potency (1,9). Using the analgesic test procedures employed in our laboratory, we have not had the same results (6). In our hands, Δ^9-THC showed minimal activity in the hot plate and tail flick tests at doses below those that produced severe behavioral and psychomotor impairment. This may be caused by the fact that we run a more stringent test procedure. For instance, in the tail flick test we use a normal reaction time of 2 to 4 sec with a cutoff time of 10 sec in mice and 20 sec in rats (10,12). Using these criteria, until recently only the narcotic analgesics were active in the tail flick test. Indeed, there was such a good correlation between antinociceptive activity in these tests and analgesics in man that we could accurately predict the dose necessary to relieve pain in man. The development of the narcotic antagonist analgesics, which are inactive in the hot plate and tail flick tests as we run them, caused rethinking of our test procedures and led to the extensive use of the "writhing" or "abdominal stretching" test (13,23,24). This test revealed activity for the narcotic antagonists. However, Δ^9-THC is again essentially inactive in this test unless doses that produce behavioral and motor impairment are used. Despite this controversy, Δ^9-THC was still of great interest because we believed that, unlike the narcotic analgesics, it did not produce physical dependence. On the other hand, we found that a profound tolerance to most of the central nervous system effects of Δ^9-THC developed, although there was no cross-tolerance to morphine (4,16,17).

In the last five years there have been four relatively well-controlled studies of the analgesic activity of Δ^9-THC in man. One study by Noyes and his colleagues (20), using patients with chronic pain of metastatic carcinoma, reported good analgesic activity. Figure 1 illustrates the data they obtained. However, a relatively high incidence of side effects was reported, including sedation, drowsiness, fall in blood pressure, and, surprisingly, bradycardia. Two other controlled studies reported no analgesic activity. One, by Regelson et al. (28), reported cancer patients to have an increased sense of well-being, increased appetite, and less nausea and vomiting after chemotherapeutic agents and radiation. The second study, by Raft and his colleagues (26), utilized both surgical and experimental pain paradigms and compared intravenous Δ^9-THC to diazepam and a placebo. They measured the effects of the drugs on extraction pain and on experimental pain produced by pressure and shock. For the experimental pain study, they measured the detection of pain and the amount of pain tolerated. In the case of surgical pain, all subjects preferred diazepam (0.157 mg/kg) to the high dose of Δ^9-THC (0.44 mg/kg). Three of 10 subjects receiving the

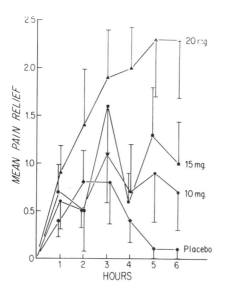

FIG. 1. Mean (± SEM) hourly pain relief in 10 patients following administration of THC. (From Noyes et al., ref. 20.)

TABLE 1. *Change in pain responses[a] after drug administration: Comparisons of THC and diazepam with placebo*

	Detection		Tolerance	
All subjects	Cutaneous stimulus	Pressure stimulus	Cutaneous stimulus	Pressure stimulus
Placebo (N = 10)	−1.1%	−5.4%	+2.8%	+0.2%
Diazepam (N = 10)	+6.3%	+6.2%	+1.4%	−6.6%
THC, 0.022 mg/kg (N = 10)	+11.2%[b]	+7.7%[b]	+1.5%	−0.1%
THC, 0.044 mg/kg (N = 9)[c]	+11.3%[b]	+20.2%[d]	+1.6%	+7.6%

[a] Percent change from base-line predrug measures.
[b] Change differing from placebo; t-test, $p < 2.5$.
[c] One patient excluded.
[d] Change differing from placebo; t-test, $p < 0.5$.
Data from Raft et al., ref. 26.

low dose of Δ^9-THC (0.22 mg/kg) reported good to excellent pain relief. In general, however, it was felt that Δ^9-THC was, at best, a poor analgesic under these circumstances. In the case of the experimental pain (Table 1) there was a clear indication of an increased detection threshold for both diazepam and Δ^9-THC but no evidence of an analgesic effect on pain tolerance threshold for any of the medications. Even when they separated the positive and negative responders to THC in surgical pain, the responses of these individuals to experimental pain were not different. Finally, Hill and her colleagues (14), using electric shocks applied to the fingers, reported an increased sensitivity to pain after smoking marihuana. Whether this effect was caused by constituents in the smoke other than Δ^9-THC remains to be determined. In summary, as far as the natural products are concerned, I believe it is fair to state that these cannabinoids are not useful analgesics.

OBSERVATIONS AND DISCUSSION

Some 10 years ago my colleagues and I began a systematic chemical manipulation of the cannabinoid structure in an attempt to enhance therapeutic utility and decrease side effect liability (5,21,22). One therapeutic area that interested us, of course, was analgesia. Figure 2 shows a variety of heterocyclic analogs of tetrahydrocannabinol with relatively good antinociceptive activity in laboratory animals. It should be noted that, as we indicated earlier, this antinociceptive data was generated using less stringent methodology in terms of control reaction time and cutoff times. There is, however, no question that these six compounds show more analgesic activity than Δ^9-THC. A more complete explication of the structure-activity relationships of these series of compounds can be found in the review by Pars et al. (22). One of these compounds, SP-106, was worked up for clinical trial and has now been evaluated in three laboratories for analgesic activity in man. The first study, carried out by Staquet and his colleagues (29),

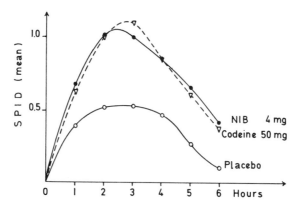

ANALGESIC ACTIVITY OF SELECTED NITROGEN AND SULFUR ANALOGS

STRUCTURE	ED_{50} - MG/KG, PO		
	HOT PLATE (MOUSE)	ANTI WRITHING (MOUSE)	TAIL FLICK (RAT)
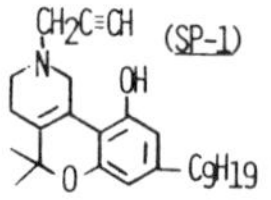 (SP-1)	7.7	4.3	13.8
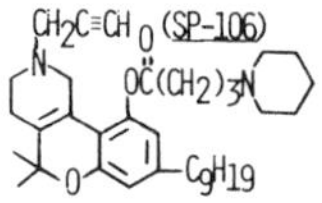 (SP-106)	4.2	12.0	12.5
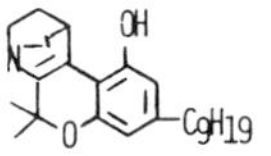	4.3	10.3	27.7
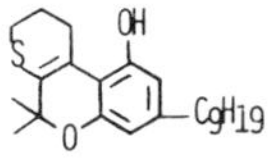	5.7	8.6	2.7
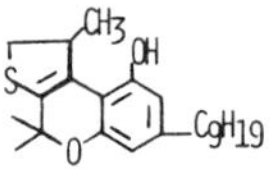	1.4	4.7	1.4

FIG. 2. Antinociceptive activities of selected heterocyclic cannabinoids.

utilized patients with pain from advanced metastatic carcinoma, and used a double-blind crossover design. Two separate experiments were performed, the first comparing oral SP-106 (4 mg), codeine (50 mg), and a placebo. The results of this study are shown in Fig. 3. From the pain intensity differences obtained

FIG. 3. Mean total pain intensity differences (SPID) following administration of NIB (a nitrogen-containing benzopyran derivative), codeine, or placebo on three different days. (From Staquet et al., ref. 29.)

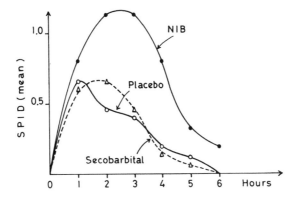

FIG. 4. Time effect curves for oral SP-106 and codeine expressed in terms of mean hourly pain relief scores. (From Staquet et al., ref. 29.)

in this experiment, one can conclude that SP-106 and codeine are indistinguishable from each other and both are more effective than a placebo in relieving pain. The second experiment compares SP-106 with secobarbital and a placebo (Fig. 4); it was observed that secobarbital did not differ from the placebo whereas SP-106 produced a clearly significant reduction in pain intensity.

A second study, in postoperative and cancer pain, was carried out by Houde and his colleagues (15). They compared oral SP-106 with codeine using a double-blind crossover design and reported good analgesic activity (Fig. 5) at much lower doses than those used by Staquet et al. (29). It should be noted, however, that the number of patients studied was not sufficient to obtain a meaningful

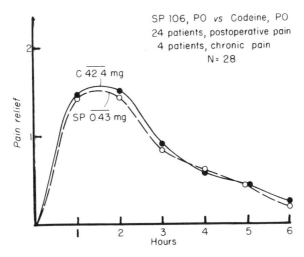

FIG. 5. Time effect curves for oral SP-106 and codeine expressed in time of mean hourly pain relief scores. (R. W. Houde, *personal communication.*)

estimate of the relative potency of the two drugs. Neither study noted any side effects of SP-106 administration that differed in frequency or severity from those of the other active medications employed. Of particular interest is the fact that dysphoria, injected conjunctiva, and tachycardia were not observed. Although these results look promising, it should be pointed out that Houde *(personal communication),* on increasing the dosage of SP-106, was unable to generate a dose-response relationship. This is consistent with the observations of Beaver *(personal communication),* who could find only variable degrees of analgesia with a variety of doses of the drug. Again, at doses up to 4 mg, no real side effects were noted. Doses greater than 4 mg were not attempted since phase I clinical studies of higher dose levels had not been conducted. These studies have recently been completed and indicate that oral doses up to 15 mg are well tolerated. We will have to wait until clinical analgesic evaluations have been carried out at elevated doses before conclusions can be reached concerning the clinical efficacy of SP-106 as an analgesic.

SUMMARY

It is obvious that a wide variety of cannabinoid structures are now available, many of which have antinociceptive activity in laboratory animals. A number of these are currently being evaluated in the clinic for a variety of therapeutic indications. There is reason to hope that one of these compounds will prove to be an effective analgesic in man and demonstrate a lower dependence liability than the narcotic analgesics.

ACKNOWLEDGMENTS

Work from the author on this manuscript was supported, in part, from a National Institute on Drug Abuse grant (DA-00490) and a grant from SISA, Inc.

REFERENCES

1. Bauxbaum, D., Sanders-Bush, E., and Efron, D. (1969): Analgesic activity of tetrahydrocannabinol (THC) in the rat and mouse. *Fed. Proc.,* 28:735.
2. Braude, M. C., and Szara, S. (editors) (1977): *Pharmacology of Marihuana, Vols. 1 and 2.* Raven Press, New York.
3. Cohen, S. and Stillman, R. C. (editors) (1976): *The Therapeutic Potential of Marihuana.* Plenum, New York.
4. Dewey, W. L., Harris, L. S., Howes, J. F., and Kennedy, J. S. (1969): Pharmacological effects of some constituents of marihuana. *Pharmacologist,* 11:278.
5. Dewey, W. L., Harris, L. S., Howes, J. F., Kennedy, J. S., Granchelli, F. E., Pars, H. G., and Razdan, R. F. (1970): Pharmacology of some marihuana constituents and two heterocyclic analogues. *Nature,* 226:1265–1267.
6. Dewey, W. L., Harris, L. S., and Kennedy, J. S. (1972): Some pharmacological and toxicological effects of *l-trans-Δ8-* and *l-trans-Δ9-*tetrahydrocannabinol in laboratory rodents. *Arch. Int. Pharmacodyn. Ther.,* 196:133–145.

7. Gaoni, Y., and Mechoulam, R. (1964): Isolation, structure and partial synthesis of an active constituent of hashish. *J. Am. Chem. Soc.,* 86:1646–1647.
8. Gaoni, Y., and Mechoulam, R. (1971): The isolation and structure of Δ^1-tetrahydrocannabinol and other neutral cannabinoids from hashish. *J. Am. Chem. Soc.,* 93:217–224.
9. Grunfield, Y., and Edery, H. (1968): Psychopharmacological activity of the active constituents of hashish and some related cannabinoids. *Psychopharmacologia,* 14:200–210.
10. Harris, L. S., Dewey, W. L., Howes, J. F., Kennedy, J. S., and Pars, H. (1969): Narcotic-antagonist analgesics: Interactions with cholinergic systems. *J. Pharmacol. Exp. Ther.,* 169:17–22.
11. Harris, L. S., Dewey, W. L., and Razdan, R. K. (1977): Cannabis: Its chemistry, pharmacology, and toxicology. In: *Drug Addiction II,* edited by W. R. Martin, pp. 371–429. Springer-Verlag, New York.
12. Harris, L. S., and Pierson, A. K. (1964): Narcotic antagonists in the benzomorphan series. *J. Pharmacol. Exp. Ther.,* 143:141–148.
13. Hendershot, L. C., and Forsacht, J. (1959): Antagonism of the frequency of phenylquinone-induced writhing in the mouse by weak analgesics and non-analgesics. *J. Pharmacol. Exp. Ther.,* 125:237–240.
14. Hill, S. Y., Schwin, R., Goodwin, D. W., and Powell, B. J. (1974): Marihuana and pain. *J. Pharmacol. Exp. Ther.,* 188:415–418.
15. Houde, R. W., Wallenstein, S. L., Rogers, A., and Kaiko, R. F. (1976): Annual report of the analgesic studies section of the Sloan-Kettering Cancer Center. *Report to the Committee on Problems of Drug Dependence,* pp. 149–168. National Academy of Sciences, Washington, D.C.
16. McMillan, D. E., Dewey, W. L., and Harris, L. S. (1972): Characteristics of tetrahydrocannabinol tolerance. *Ann. NY Acad. Sci.,* 191:83–99.
17. McMillan, D. E., Harris, L. S., Frankenheim, J. M., and Kennedy, J. S. (1970): 1-trans-Δ^9-Tetrahydrocannabinol in pigeons: Tolerance to the behavioral effects. *Science,* 169:501–503.
18. Mechoulam, R. (editor) (1973): *Marihuana: Chemistry, Pharmacology, Metabolism and Clinical Effects.* Academic Press, New York.
19. Nahas, G. G. (1976): *Marihuana: Chemistry, Biochemistry and Cellular Effects.* Springer-Verlag, New York.
20. Noyes, R., Jr., Brunk, S. F., Baram, D. A., and Canter, A. (1975): Analgesic effects of delta-9-tetrahydrocannabinol. *J. Clin. Pharmacol.,* 15:139–143.
21. Pars, H. G., Granchelli, F. E., Keller, J. K., and Razdan, R. K. (1966): Physiologically active nitrogen analogs of tetrahydrocannabinols. Tetrahydrobenzopyrano [3,4-*d*] pyridines. *J. Am. Chem. Soc.,* 88:3664–3665.
22. Pars, H. G., Razdan, R. K., and Howes, J. F. (1977): Potential therapeutic agents derived from the cannabinoid nucleus. *Adv. Drug Res.,* 11:97–189.
23. Pearl, J., Aceto, M. D., and Harris, L. S. (1968): Prevention of writhing and other effects of narcotics and narcotic antagonists in mice. *J. Pharmacol. Exp. Ther.,* 160:217–230.
24. Pearl, J., and Harris, L. S. (1966): Inhibition of writhing by narcotic antagonists. *J. Pharmacol. Exp. Ther.,* 154:319–323.
25. Petrazilka, T., Haefliger, W., and Sikemeier, C. (1969): Synthese von Haschisch: Inhaltsstoffen. *Helv. Chim. Acta,* 52:1102–1134.
26. Raft, D., Gregg, J., Ghia, J., and Harris, L. S. (1977): Effects of intravenous tetrahydrocannabinol on experimental and surgical pain. *Clin. Pharmacol. Ther.,* 121:26–33.
27. Razdan, R. K., and Handrick, G. R. (1970): A stereospecific synthesis of (−)-Δ^1- and (−)-$\Delta^{1,6}$-tetrahydrocannabinols. *J. Am. Chem. Soc.,* 92:6061–6062.
28. Regelson, W., Butler, J. R., Schulz, J., Kink, T., Peek, L., Green, M. L., and Zalis, M. O. (1976): Delta-9-THC as an effective anti-depressant and appetite stimulating agent in advanced cancer patients. In: *Pharmacology of Marihuana, Vol. 2,* edited by M. C. Braude and S. Szara, pp. 763–776. Raven Press, New York.
29. Staquet, M., Gantt, C., and Machin, D. (1978): Effect of a nitrogen analog of tetrahydrocannabinol on cancer pain. *Clin. Pharmacol. Ther.,* 23:397–401.
30. Waller, C. W., Johnson, J. J., Buelke, J., and Turner, C. E. (1976): *Marihuana: An Annotated Bibliography.* Macmillan, New York.

Mechanisms of Pain and Analgesic Compounds,
edited by R. F. Beers, Jr., and E. G. Bassett.
Raven Press, New York © 1979.

41. Morphine and Nonaddicting Analgesics: A Current Perspective

D. R. Jasinski

National Institute on Drug Abuse, Division of Research, Addiction Research Center, Lexington, Kentucky 40583

From 1929 through 1976, a collection of academic, governmental, and industrial scientists of diverse disciplines worked on a common goal of finding new analgesics, antitussives, and antidiarrheals (1,5,15). Their purpose was twofold: to reduce reliance on the opium poppy for drugs to relieve pain and suffering, and to eliminate the problem of addiction through medically supplied or diverted opiates. In 1976 and 1977 this program was disrupted, if not terminated, because of two critical events. The National Academy of Sciences/National Research Council terminated their support of the Committee on Problems of Drug Dependence, and the prisoner research program at the Addiction Research Center was eliminated. As a consequence, this volume offers a propitious opportunity to reflect on the achievements of the search for morphine substitutes, and more important, to convey the perspectives gained from this scientific activity.

The pharmacological strategy of developing morphine substitutes includes:

(a) Identification of the salient pharmacological features of morphine leading to abuse;
(b) Development of bioassay systems to measure these effects;
(c) Assay of new therapeutic compounds for these effects.

The two pharmacological properties of morphine that lead to abuse are physical dependence and euphoria. Physical dependence is evidenced by a characteristic stereotyped withdrawal syndrome with symptoms that are discomforting to the addict subject. The addict learns to relieve these symptoms with further morphine administration, and in turn, a drive state is established. The administration of opiates to nontolerant, nondependent postaddicts results in "euphoria" or a characteristic state of well-being, contentment, enhanced self-image, and, at times, elation. In experimental studies, this euphoria following morphine administration is not reported by nonaddict normal volunteers (19).

In essence, the abuse potential of a drug is determined by measuring its ability to produce morphine-like euphoria and physical dependence. Within this concept lies the concept of relative abuse potential—certain substances that are pharmacologically equivalent to morphine may have a lower liability to be abused.

When opium and its derivatives were placed under legal control, neither pharmacological equivalence among the agents nor potency differences was recognized (5). Codeine was widely used as an antitussive and analgesic but its incidence of abuse, compared with that of morphine or heroin, was nil or nonexistent (5). Over the years, it has been recognized that codeine can produce euphoria and physical dependence and is pharmacologically equivalent to morphine and, further, is abused (5). The lower abuse liability of codeine is not related to a lack of ability to produce morphine-like effects. It is felt to be related to a lower potency than morphine, a lower solubility, a greater tissue irritant property, side effects that limit ability to obtain strong morphine-like effects, and availability predominantly as an oral preparation in low dosage units. More important, codeine historically served as a criterion drug for control purposes (5). Agents having a greater ability to produce morphine-like euphoria and physical dependence were controlled. Those with a lower ability to produce euphoria and physical dependence than codeine were exempted from control. Subsequently, the synthetic substances meperidine, methadone, and levorphanol were shown to have the abuse potential of morphine (5). Derivatives of these compounds (diphenoxylate from meperidine and propoxyphene from methadone) were found to be morphine-like drugs of low abuse potential. Diphenoxylate is insoluble in water, has a slow onset of action, and is available only as an oral preparation in low dosage units (2). Propoxyphene is less potent than codeine, has greater tissue irritant properties, produces convulsant and psychotic effects in addiction studies, and is marketed as an oral preparation in low dosage units (9). Dextromethorphan (the dextrorotatory codeine analog of levorphanol) was found to have antitussive activity but to lack the analgesic, euphoriant, and physical dependence–producing properties of morphine (4,8,12).

For the last 25 years, the search for new morphine substitutes has centered on the narcotic antagonists (5). Some of these compounds can produce analgesia and other effects that resemble those produced by morphine (14). The two prototypic compounds nalorphine and cyclazocine produced dysphoric, rather than euphoric, effects in postaddicts (17). Further, they produced a type of physical dependence that is distinct from that of morphine, is not discomforting, and does not lead to drug seeking (17,18). Pentazocine was marketed as an analgesic of low abuse potential since it did not produce strong morphine-like properties, but, in large doses, produced effects similar to those of nalorphine (3). It was later demonstrated that pentazocine in low doses did have the ability to produce a degree of morphine-like euphoria even though larger doses produced the characteristic dysphoric effects of nalorphine (6). In addition, pentazocine experimentally produced physical dependence that resembled both that of morphine and of nalorphine (6). The withdrawal syndrome was only mildly discomforting, but led to some drug-seeking behavior. Pentazocine, however, was judged to have the lowest abuse potential of any available morphine-like analgesic (6).

The judgment that codeine had less abuse potential than morphine, and, that relative to this paradigm, dextromethorphan, propoxyphene, diphenoxylate, and pentazocine were compounds of equal or lower abuse potential than codeine has been challenged by the reported incidence of abuse of some of these drugs over the past five years. A few years ago, I surveyed (5) the available epidemiological data on the incidence of abuse of morphine substitutes and found that in all studies, codeine, propoxyphene, and pentazocine were compounds of reported high incidence of abuse. The interpretation of these data, however, required recognition that these particular compounds are prescribed to a much greater extent and are under less control than morphine. To interpret these data, the availability of the various drugs relative to morphine was estimated by determining the amount of drugs produced, adjusting this amount for the euphorigenic potency of the drugs relative to morphine, and calculating the ratio of these morphine-equivalent amounts to the amount of morphine (5). A portion of these data is shown in Table 1. Codeine has a lower incidence of abuse than morphine. Propoxyphene has an incidence of abuse probably equal to that of codeine. Pentazocine, on the other hand, has a significantly lower incidence of abuse than either codeine or propoxyphene. For all practical purposes, diphenoxylate and dextromethorphan have almost no incidence of abuse. From an analysis of these data, as well as data from other surveys, two conclusions were drawn (5): (a) Agents that are pharmacologically equivalent to morphine in ability to produce euphoria and physical dependence will also be abused, and (b) valid judgments of relative abuse potential of morphine-like substances can be based on the relative ability to produce morphine-like euphoria and physical dependence.

In the mid 1960s, Martin (13,14) speculated that morphine-like drugs could differ in intrinsic activity. Subsequently, such partial agonists of morphine were found.

One of these, propiram, produced morphine-like subjective effects, euphoria, and physical dependence. The intensity of the abstinence syndrome was mild (7). Propiram acted as an antagonist and precipitated abstinence in subjects

TABLE 1. *Abuse incidence and availability of various morphine substitutes indicating their lower abuse potential[a]*

Drug	Relative availability (1973)	Relative abuse incidence (1973–1975)
Morphine	1.0	1.0
Codeine	5.0	1.0
d-Propoxyphene	9.5	2.3
Diphenoxylate	0.5	0
Dextromethorphan	?	0
Pentazocine	4.6	0.4

[a]From Jasinski, ref. 5.

dependent on large doses of morphine but substituted for morphine and suppressed abstinence in subjects dependent on low levels of morphine. Propiram was concluded to be a partial agonist of morphine (7). On the basis of its relative ability to produce euphoria and physical dependence, the abuse potential of propiram was judged to be less than that of codeine and *d*-propoxyphene (7). Since neither propiram nor any other partial agonist of morphine has been marketed, it is impossible to validate this judgment from abuse incidence studies.

A more interesting partial agonist of the morphine type is the oripavine derivative, buprenorphine (11,16). In volunteer prisoner postaddicts (10), single doses of buprenorphine constricted pupils, produced morphine-like subjective effects and euphoria, was 25 to 50 times more potent than morphine, and may have been relatively less effective than morphine in producing subjective effects when doses of both were increased. Further, buprenorphine was longer acting than morphine, with a duration of action equal to or greater than that of methadone. Chronic administration of buprenorphine produced morphine-like subjective, behavioral, and physiological changes. It was less toxic than morphine, methadone, codeine, and propoxyphene. Subcutaneous administration of naloxone in doses up to 4 mg did not precipitate abstinence during chronic administration of buprenorphine. Abrupt withdrawal in a dose of 8 mg/day s.c. (equivalent to 200 to 400 mg morphine sulfate daily) indicated little, if any, withdrawal of clinical significance. Significant abstinence signs and symptoms were seen only in the 15th through the 21st day of withdrawal, with an intensity less than that reported for withdrawal from maximal subtoxic doses of codeine and propoxyphene. During chronic administration of buprenorphine, single doses of morphine (up to 120 mg s.c.) were without effect, indicating that chronic buprenorphine is capable of blocking the effects of morphine and other narcotics through the two mechanisms of cross-tolerance and competitive antagonism. Because buprenorphine produces minimal, if any, clinically significant physical dependence, the relative abuse potential of buprenorphine is significantly lower than that of codeine and propoxyphene (10). The production of morphine-like subjective effects acceptable to addicts, a long duration of action, the production of low levels of physical dependence such that patients may be easily detoxified, a lower toxicity than other drugs used for maintenance therapy, and the ability to block the effects of other narcotics led to the proposal that buprenorphine has potential for treating narcotic addiction (10).

In this overview of the scientific activity conducted to find morphine substitutes, clear accomplishments can be delineated. The reliance on the opium poppy for drugs to relieve pain and suffering has been reduced, if not eliminated, by the development of synthetic substitutes. Valid pharmacological methods exist for judging the abuse potential of morphine substitutes. Only compounds of little or no abuse potential have been introduced, uncontrolled, into therapeutics. The resulting widespread predominant use of these drugs (20), in all likelihood, has reduced the incidence and consequences of drug abuse that occur through the diversion of medically prescribed drugs for pain and suffering.

REFERENCES

1. Eddy, N. B. (1973): *The National Research Council Involvement in the Opiate Problem, 1928–1971.* National Academy of Sciences, Washington, D.C.
2. Fraser, H. F., and Isbell, H. (1961): Human pharmacology and addictiveness of ethyl 1-(3-cyano-3,3-phenylpropyl)-4-phenyl-4-piperidine carboxylate hydrochloride (R-1132, diphenoxylate). *Bull. Narc.* 13:29–43.
3. Fraser, H. F., and Rosenberg, D. E. (1964): Studies on the human addiction liability of 2'-hydroxy-5,9-dimethyl-2-(3,3-dimethylallyl)-6,7-benzomorphan (Win 20,228), a weak narcotic antagonist (II-C-2). *J. Pharmacol. Exp. Ther.,* 143:149–156.
4. Isbell, H., and Fraser, H. F. (1953): Action and addiction liabilities of dromoran derivatives in man. *J. Pharmacol. Exp. Ther.,* 107:524–530.
5. Jasinski, D. R. (1977): Assessment of the abuse potentiality of morphine-like drugs (methods used in man). In: *Drug Addiction. I. Handbook of Experimental Pharmacology, Vol. 45,* edited by W. R. Martin, pp. 197–258. Springer-Verlag, Berlin.
6. Jasinski, D. R., Martin, W. R., and Hoeldtke, R. D. (1970): Effects of short- and long-term administration of pentazocine in man. *Clin. Pharmacol. Ther.,* 11:385–403.
7. Jasinski, D. R., Martin, W. R., and Hoeldtke, R. (1971): Studies of the dependence-producing properties of GPA-1657, profadol and propiram in man. *Clin. Pharmacol. Ther.,* 12:613–649.
8. Jasinski, D. R., Martin, W. R., and Mansky, P. A. (1971): Progress report on the assessment of the antagonists nalbuphine and GPA-2087 for abuse potential and studies of the effects of dextromethorphan in man. *Report to the Committee on Problems of Drug Dependence, Vol. 1,* pp. 143–178. National Research Council, Washington, D.C.
9. Jasinski, D. R., Pevnick, J. S., Clark, S. C., and Griffith, J. D. (1977): Therapeutic usefulness of propoxyphene napsylate in narcotic addiction. *Arch. Gen. Psychiatry,* 34:227–233.
10. Jasinski, D. R., Pevnick, J. S., and Griffith, J. D. (1978): Human pharmacology and abuse potential of the analgesic buprenorphine: A potential agent for treating narcotic addiction. *Arch. Gen. Psychiatry,* 35:501–516.
11. Lewis, J. W. (1974): Ring C-bridged derivatives of thebaine and oripavine. In: *Advances in Biochemical Psychopharmacology, Vol. 8, Narcotic Antagonists,* edited by M. C. Braude, L. S. Harris, E. L. May, J. P. Smith, and J. E. Villarreal, pp. 123–136. Raven Press, New York.
12. Mansky, P. A., and Jasinski, D. R. (1970): Effects of dextromethorphan in man. *Pharmacologist,* 12:231.
13. Martin, W. R. (1963): Strong analgesics. In: *Physiological Pharmacology, Vol. 1,* edited by W. S. Root and E. G. Hofman, pp. 275–312. Academic Press, New York.
14. Martin, W. R. (1967): Opioid antagonists. *Pharmacol. Rev.,* 19:463–521.
15. Martin, W. R. (1977): General problems of drug abuse and drug dependence. In: *Drug Addiction. I. Handbook of Experimental Pharmacology, Vol. 45,* edited by W. R. Martin, pp. 3–40. Springer-Verlag, Berlin.
16. Martin, W. R., Eades, C. G., Thompson, J. A., Huppler, R. E., and Gilbert, P. E. (1976): The effects of morphine- and nalorphine-like drugs in the nondependent and morphine-dependent chronic spinal dog. *J. Pharmacol. Exp. Ther.,* 197:517–532.
17. Martin, W. R., Fraser, H. F., Gorodetzky, C. W., and Rosenberg, D. E. (1965): Studies of the dependence-producing potential of the narcotic antagonist 2-cyclopropylmethyl-2'-hydroxy-5,9-dimethyl-6,7-benzomorphan (cyclazocine, Win 20,740; ARC II-C-3). *J. Pharmacol. Exp. Ther.,* 150:426–436.
18. Martin, W. R., and Gorodetzky, C. W. (1965): Demonstration of tolerance to and physical dependence on *N*-allylnormorphine (nalorphine). *J. Pharmacol. Exp. Ther.,* 150:437–442.
19. Martin, W. R., and Sloan, J. W. (1977): Neuropharmacology and neurochemistry of subjective effects, analgesia, tolerance, and dependence produced by narcotic analgesics. In: *Drug Addiction. I. Handbook of Experimental Pharmacology, Vol. 45,* edited by W. R. Martin, pp. 43–158. Springer-Verlag, Berlin.
20. Seitner, P. G., Martin, B. C., Cochin, J., and Harris, L. (1975): *Survey of Analgesic Drug Prescribing Patterns.* Drug Abuse Council, Inc., Washington, D.C.

Mechanisms of Pain and Analgesic Compounds,
edited by R. F. Beers, Jr., and E. G. Bassett.·
Raven Press, New York © 1979.

42. Discussion

Moderator: Julián E. Villarreal

M. C. Braude: Dr. Harris, when you were talking about the SP compounds, I understand there were two major structural modifications. The first one is an introduction of nitrogen into the molecule, and the second a change in the side chain to increase solubility. What is the effect of lengthening of the side chain on the analgesic or pharmacological activity?

L. S. Harris: As you might have guessed, we did a great deal of work in modifying that side chain. By and large, the work parallels the classical studies done many years ago by Roger Adams and Lord Todd when they were synthesizing their 3-substituted compounds. Our derivative has a dimethylheptyl side chain, but other compounds with more complex side chains have more potency. However, you reach a point of no return—the activity either levels off or decreases. There is currently an extremely large variety of compounds that have been prepared for such studies.

N. Khazan: To expand on Dr. Braude's question, have we achieved partial or complete differentiation between CNS, cardiovascular, and analgesic effects of any of these cannabinoids?

L. S. Harris: Well, we have succeeded in dissociating, in experimental animals, the cardiovascular responses from the analgesic responses. However, we have no adequate tests—if you will—in animals to assess the so-called cannabinoid-like psychoactive effects.

We don't know the entire story. We have had only two compounds of this series in human clinical trials. Both produce, in adequate doses, some degree of cannabinoid-like activity. In trials of the compound that has had the most extensive testing, however, this activity was not reached until the doses administered were much higher than one would have expected to use.

K. L. Casey: It was my impression that most or all of the drugs of abuse are, by nature euphorogenic. I think Dr. Jasinski made the statement—and I think it is a common experience related by people who begin taking heroin or morphine—that they do have dysphoria or experience nausea, and these effects are overridden by the subsequent strong euphorogenic action of the drug and thus they become addicts.

Are there any compounds that are drugs of abuse yet not basically euphorogenic?

D. R. Jasinski: I don't think we have data to adequately answer your question. I think sometimes it depends on what population is under study.

The subjective changes—that is, alteration in mood and feeling states—of narcotics have been studied in the addict population. We know that there is a similar set of feeling states that occurs with amphetamine and probably with the barbituates. We do not have data, what I would call hard data, with either tetrahydrocannabinol or with the hallucinogens. It would be very difficult to go back and undertake additional hallucinogenic studies. However, anecdotal evidence suggests that there is a particular type of euphoria.

One interesting drug is cyclazocine, a relatively effective analgesic. This compound, when studied in experimental circumstances, was not morphine-like. There was a huge amount of money spent trying to use this as a treatment for addicts. You couldn't give it away. You couldn't keep them on it because they just didn't like it.

There is another phenomenon, not well documented but which has influenced the perspective in this field. I am referring to studies that were conducted not in addicts but in "normals." When they are under experimental circumstances, the people to whom morphine is given commonly respond with feelings of detachment and lethargy which are relatively unpleasant or at least something not desirable.

Now, if you take people in pain or in a stress situation and give them a shot of morphine, this is something else. They now find it somewhat pleasurable. This has led to a lot of speculation about what the pathophysiology and specific effects of addiction are.

L. S. Harris: I would like to comment on another important issue. Recently, with the help of many people like Drs. Hoffmeister, Woods, and Yanagita, we have developed animal tests for demonstrating the reinforcing properties of drugs, that is, drug self-administration. The data looks very good for most classes of drugs except for the hallucinogens or the cannabinoid-type of drug where the major portion of the users find these effects "pleasurable," yet the animals don't self-administer them.

J. E. Villarreal: Don Jasinski and I have argued before about the question of a necessary relationship between subjective pleasurable effects and compulsive drug use. Cigarette smoking is very compulsive and yet smoking does not produce anything resembling the effects of narcotics or amphetamines in addicts.

D. R. Jasinski: You are talking, I think, about two different sets of things; this is not going to be a philosophical debate but I would argue that the concept of euphoria is not elation. I think this is a mistake. I think that these feeling states are not those of elation. I would suggest that, if you were to not smoke a cigarette, became nervous and then smoked a cigarette, the feelings of contentment following the cigarette and relaxation would be called euphoric.

J. E. Villarreal: Wouldn't such feelings simply be the result of satisfying an impulse, and not the origin of the impulse?

D. R. Jasinski: I think that what I was alluding to is that those of us who feel those euphoric responses which are only seen in the addict population (or whatever we mean by addict population), probably indicates that there is an underlying pathology within the addict which is not seen in the "normal." I don't think the fact that one can achieve the dry state to cigarettes in "normals" is part of these mechanisms which are particularly there.

I don't have a clear answer for this, Julián. I know we talk about a phenomenon which we see. I don't know of anyone who has looked for euphoria with cigarette smoking and I hope to do studies in this area.

W. A. Check: Dr. Jasinski, I have recently seen some letters about what is called the opium stockpile, which is apparently some reserve of opium-derived drugs supposedly needed for medical treatment.

Are you planning to become independent of poppy derivatives so that such a stockpile is no longer critical or was that an overextension of what you were saying?

D. R. Jasinski: No, I was concluding that until the 1950s, we were very dependent on opium for medical needs. I don't think any morphinologist or pharmacologist could really argue that, excepting the economic, political, and social aspects, we could not adequately relieve pain and suffering with synthetic drugs if we had to.

Even though we still rely on the opium poppy—and there may be political, economic, and social reasons to continue—it is not really necessary. If all the opium poppies in the world were destroyed tomorrow, and all the stockpiles of opium were to disappear, we still would be able to relieve pain and suffering as effectively as we could do with morphine.

L. S. Harris: The one exception may be codeine, which has a rather unique part in our medical practice, both in this country and around the world.

R. W. Houde: Dr. Villarreal, I hesitate to use cigarette smoking as an example. Why don't you consider the use of other analgesics that are not classified as addictive, such as APC or aspirin? Do you believe that abuse liability is present in these compounds? Certainly, abuse of analgesics has been reported. Perhaps it is applicable to what Dr. Hoffmeister was discussing earlier.

I am always worried about the problem of evaluating the potential of physical dependence and of reinforcing agents in light of the variety of contingencies existing in the real world.

Do the members of the panel feel that their tests for a drug's reinforcing abilities or its ability as a substitute for preventing or suppressing physical dependence are applicable in the real world, when we speak of abuse liability rather than satisfying certain physical dependency?

D. R. Jasinski: The issue here is more one of a sociological or a cultural necessity to do this or that. This is the point I was making: that to a great extent, much of the original motivation for the search for new drugs was due to the fact that drugs which were very effective in relieving suffering and pain were diverted from medicinal use. In addition, there was a serious cultural problem.

It was not so much the drug's reinforcing properties or a societal segment that was indifferent to those abusing drugs, but mostly the so-called sociopathic behavior and the consequences to our society resulting from actions of people who seek and shoot dope, thereby diverting large quantities of medical supplies.

It is said that the history of this situation was that doctors and pharmaceutical industries introduced heroin. I think many people have been concerned over the years about the introduction of another heroin onto the scene. We should all realize that we have the technical and scientific know-how to accomplish this. This is old history.

The context of the argument with Julian about cigarettes does not have the same connotation or the same sociological implications as the seeking and using of heroin.

A person smoking cigarettes continues to function in our particular society and is able to function normally. This normal functioning would be more difficult under heroin self-administration, although I think all of us know physicians who have been morphine addicts and continue to practice medicine.

There have been some relatively prominent people who were victims of this practice. So, judgments are made within a social contact and a social behavior. We know that certain drugs are associated with these generally undesirable behaviors and the classic example is the narcotics; I would contrast narcotics with, for example, the benzodiazopines. We have a different attitude now when one observes people abusing these drugs. Does that answer your question?

R. W. Houde: What I was really asking was about the appropriateness of our testing. Do you consider APC abuse to represent drug abuse? Does it show up as a reinforcing drug in our test procedures?

D. R. Jasinski: Dr. Houde, I was trying to answer your specific question. Considering people who chronically ingest aspirin, it is not the particular phenomenon of repetitively ingesting a substance or a drug. It is like eating popcorn or peanuts. The problem that you are concerned about is predicting use by a certain segment of the population. Our society has decided the use of certain drugs by this population is undesirable. This occurs particularly with heroin and drugs which have the same properties.

We do not make the same social judgment about someone who may be taking aspirin repetitively and chronically, or consider this to be detrimental to our society. I think this is the distinction that I was making.

The drive state may be just as strong or perhaps even stronger. My own suspicion is that the drive state for nicotine is as strong as that for heroin.

We do not condemn people for using nicotine, as we do for heroin. I think our attitude in society is changing. We are beginning to realize that tobacco consumption represents economic and social costs to our society. We have begun to take certain social measures that restrict the use of tobacco as we develop a different attitude towards tobacco consumption.

L. S. Harris: I think there is, in addition to that issue, a methodological problem that Ray Houde has been stressing and that you have been trying to avoid although you are the one who brought it up. One might get an entirely different profile of any class of drug, depending on the state of the subjects using the drug. For instance, you state that morphine in a person without pain is generally dysphoric; yet to a person in pain and suffering it may be euphoric. This might be true for aspirin, too. We have never tested it under those circumstances.

Some of the reinforcing properties that Dr. Hoffmeister observes by various manipulations of drug combinations suggests that compounds like phenacetin may have some reinforcing properties. I agree with you that we have been negligent because, as Don stated, we were concerned about social or sociopathic behavior. I think we will have to reexamine many compounds in different models; we may find many of them to be more reinforcing or euphorogenic than we thought before, depending on the particular model used.

D. R. Jasinski: I agree with this. For someone in chronic pain, does aspirin become a reinforcing agent? I would argue, yes.

J. H. Woods: I will refer to the reason why we ignore the questions just discussed. Most of the psychologists who became interested in drug self-administration techniques some time ago thought that there would be all kinds of variables that would influence self-administration and change its patterns. In fact, we have been consumed by the importance of differences in pharmacological properties and the work, naturally, has been aimed primarily at clarifying the effects of pharmacological variables.

J. E. Villarreal: I believe Dr. Hoffmeister in his presentation mentioned the criteria we might use for identifying dangerous drugs; that is, those drugs that are self-administered in a wide variety of circumstances and that do not require special behavioral situations to be self-administered.

F. Hoffmeister: I think the shortcomings of all these procedures have been expressed already. In my mind, reinforcing properties *per se* are neither positive nor negative events. They might be necessary in a given situation while unnecessary—or even to be avoided—in other situations. Until now what has emerged from many laboratories is nothing more than statements about whether, under given conditions, a compound will have negative or positive reinforcing properties.

The mere fact that a drug has a positive reinforcing property is, primarily, nothing negative. I see the problem to be our current inability to utilize, in animal experiments, all the different environmental contingencies that influence the drug-taking behavior of humans. If this could be done, I think we could accurately estimate under which contingency and/or conditions a compound might be a hazard to public health.

The trouble is that we have to be confined to preset contingencies and that we can describe a pattern. The relevance of this pattern for a potential abuse is still an open question and has to be proved in man.

Subject Index